GLOBAL VIEW OF THE FIGHT AGAINST INFLUENZA

GLOBAL VIEW OF THE FIGHT AGAINST INFLUENZA

PETAR M. MITRASINOVIC
EDITOR

Nova Science Publishers, Inc.
New York

NOTICE TO THE READER

The Publisher has taken reasonable care in the preparation of this book, but makes no expressed or implied warranty of any kind and assumes no responsibility for any errors or omissions. No liability is assumed for incidental or consequential damages in connection with or arising out of information contained in this book. The Publisher shall not be liable for any special, consequential, or exemplary damages resulting, in whole or in part, from the readers' use of, or reliance upon, this material. Any parts of this book based on government reports are so indicated and copyright is claimed for those parts to the extent applicable to compilations of such works.

Independent verification should be sought for any data, advice or recommendations contained in this book. In addition, no responsibility is assumed by the publisher for any injury and/or damage to persons or property arising from any methods, products, instructions, ideas or otherwise contained in this publication.

This publication is designed to provide accurate and authoritative information with regard to the subject matter covered herein. It is sold with the clear understanding that the Publisher is not engaged in rendering legal or any other professional services. If legal or any other expert assistance is required, the services of a competent person should be sought. FROM A DECLARATION OF PARTICIPANTS JOINTLY ADOPTED BY A COMMITTEE OF THE AMERICAN BAR ASSOCIATION AND A COMMITTEE OF PUBLISHERS.

LIBRARY OF CONGRESS CATALOGING-IN-PUBLICATION DATA

ISBN: 978-1-60741-952-5
Available upon request

Published by Nova Science Publishers, Inc. ✦ *New York*

To my dear mother, Milena, and the memory of my wonderful father, Milorad, who sincerely believed in the strength of knowledge.

Mojoj dragoj majci Mileni i uspomeni na mog izvanrednog oca Milorada koji je iskreno verovao u moć znanja.

This book is especially dedicated to the memory of my renowned colleague, outstanding scientist and great man, Dr. Graeme Laver. Graeme worked on his contribution to my book until September 26, 2008 when he passed away in London at the age of 79 while en route to an influenza virus conference in Portugal.

Ova knjiga je posebno posvećena mom slavnom kolegi, izvanrednom naučniku i sjajnom čoveku Prof. Dr. Gramiju Lejveru. Grami je radio na svom rukopisu za moju knjigu neposredno pre 26.09.2008 kada je preminuo u Londonu u 79-oj godini za vreme putovanja na konferenciju u Portugal.

Prof. Dr. Petar M. Mitrasinovic

CONTENTS

FOREWORD

Dr. Graeme Laver, former professor of biochemistry and molecular biology at the Australian National University in Canberra and Fellow of the Royal Society of London, passed away in Britain on September 26, 2008 while en route to an influenza virus conference in Portugal. In the memory of Prof. Laver, one of the leading avian influenza experts, this foreword is an extract from a recent e-mail communication describing the essence of this book in the best possible sense.

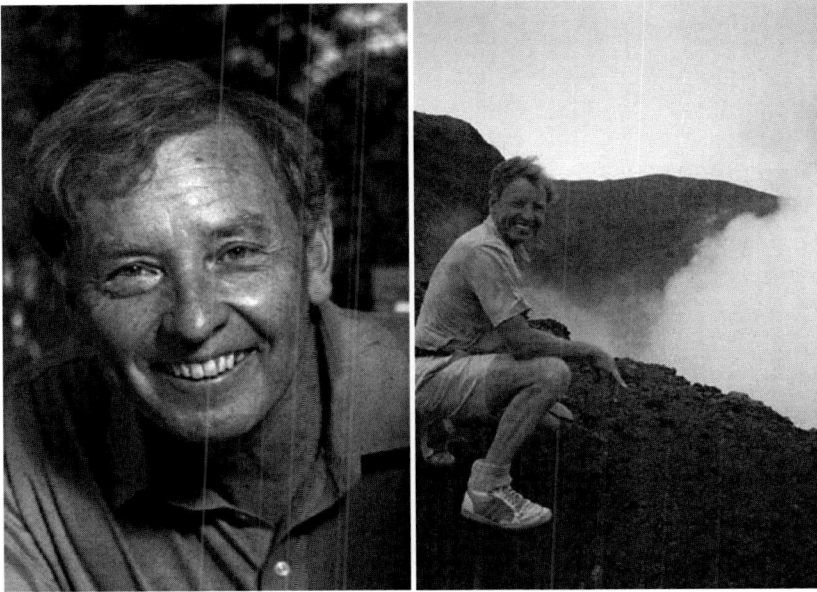

William Graeme Laver (left); visiting the Yasur volcano, one of the world's most active volcanoes, in southern Vanuatu (right). Graeme Laver was fascinated by volcanoes, and also enjoyed organizing influenza conferences, so many of his conferences were held near volcanoes. Adrian J. Gibbs, an eminent virology professor who worked with Graeme at the John Curtin School of Medical Research and knew him for more than 40 years, recalled that "It was pretty exciting!" "Every few seconds there would be a considerable BOOM. As it got dark, you could see each boom was accompanied by a lot of red hot rocks flying through the air. We were essentially dangling our legs into the crater as we waited for darkness. Graeme, as you can see, just loved it."!!

From: Graeme Laver <graeme.laver@bigpond.com>
To: Petar M. Mitrasinovic <petar.mitrasinovic@gmail.com>
Sent: Aug 11, 2008 2:37 AM
Subject: Re: Invitation for Chapter/Article Contribution to Global View of the Fight
    against Influenza
Mailed-by: bigpond.com

Dear Petar,

Thank you for your invitation to me to contribute an article to your publication *Global View of the Fight against Influenza.*

I would be happy to write an essay-style review, if that would be acceptable to you, rather than a comprehensive review of the subject. The title of my article could be "The Origin and Control of Pandemic Influenza". This would cover what we know (not much!) about how human pandemic flu viruses arise, and then a bit of history about the way in which the new flu drugs, the neuraminidase-inhibitors, were developed and how these should be used, both in a pandemic and in seasonal flu outbreaks. There is a lot of misinformation out there that needs correcting.

I have a question for you with regard to the use of oseltamivir (Tamiflu) and zanamivir (Relenza) to treat seasonal flu infections in your country, and in other European countries you might be familiar with. The question is, do people know about these drugs and are there ways they can get them 6 to 12 hours after they experience symptom onset? That is when they are most effective. In Australia, the Government insists that Tamiflu can only be obtained after the patient first obtains a doctor's prescription, a procedure that takes so long the drug is rendered ineffective. There is no need for a doctor's prescription and we are trying very hard to have this requirement changed.

Is it likely that you will be attending the Third European Influenza Conference, to be held this year in Portugal on September 14–17?

Best wishes,

Graeme Laver,
61 2 6227 0061
graeme.laver@bigpond.com

PREFACE

Flu, caused by the influenza virus, has worried mankind for centuries. The virus, dubbed "Spanish influenza" (H1N1), caused the 1918 influenza pandemic in which more than 40 million people died worldwide. Since then there have been two other major pandemics—in 1957 "Asian flu" (H2N2) caused the death of about two million people and in 1968 "Hong Kong flu" (H3N2) killed about one million people. In 1976, "swine flu" (H1N1) did not cause a pandemic. Of particular concern currently is a lethal avian influenza virus known as "bird flu". Avian influenza is an infectious disease of birds caused by particular strains of the influenza virus. There are 15 different types of avian influenza virus. The types causing the most deaths are known as highly pathogenic avian influenza (HPAI). The disease occurs worldwide, and is most commonly found in migratory water birds. Water birds are generally resistant to infection caused by avian influenza, but the virus can cause severe disease when it spreads to poultry and other birds. In rare cases, avian influenza can infect humans. The first cases of humans being infected by H5N1 were detected in Hong Kong in 1997. Eighteen people were infected, six of whom died. In that instance the virus did not spread from person to person. There have since been more outbreaks of human infection according to World Health Organization sources. One was in Hong Kong (H9N2) in 1999 and two cases of infection without deaths occurred. There were three outbreaks of human infection in 2003, in Hong Kong (H5N1, two cases, one death), in the Netherlands (H7N7, 84 cases, one death) and in Hong Kong (H9N2, one case). Several outbreaks took place in 2004, one in Vietnam and others in Thailand and Indonesia (H5N1, 34 cases, 23 deaths). To date there have been no confirmed cases of human-to-human transmission into the general community, although there have been "family" clusters of avian influenza in Vietnam, Thailand and Indonesia. These cases involved very close contact with an infected person and, as the family members were all exposed to the same potential animal and environmental sources of infection as well as to each other, it is impossible to know whether transmission was human-to-human. So far, avian flu has occurred mostly among Asian poultry workers who had direct contact with infected birds. However, in one possible case in Thailand, researchers suspected human-to-human transmission of the virus. If this virus does manage to adapt genetically initiating person-to-person transmission it will spread like wildfire throughout the world. Such a pandemic might well arise in the future by a still-undiscovered mechanism, which makes flu research so fascinating. Herein we discover a global view of the fight against influenza by featuring key aspects and contemporary methods of flu research that can aid us to prepare for a potential pandemic more effectively. In this light, the multidisciplinary character of this book is reflected by the chapters written by eminent experts from medicine, public health business, pharmacy, chemistry, molecular and structural biology, mathematics, and statistics.

As infected birds continue to migrate, public health officials worry that an avian strain could become better at spreading between humans, making it uncontrollable. In a rapidly spreading pandemic caused by an unknown strain, vaccination is not a realistic plan. Vaccines require months to create because it is necessary to identify a virus and grow antibodies against it. Besides, vaccine needs to be distributed, which takes time. A vaccine for the avian virus is being developed, but none is yet available. Thus, the question of vital importance is: in the absence of a specific avian flu vaccine, could antiviral drugs obstruct a pandemic should the virus spread from birds to humans? The two classes of anti-viral drugs to treat influenza are adamantanes and neuraminidase inhibitors. Adamantanes, including amantadine and rimantadine, are less expensive and more readily available, but they would likely not be useful in an avian pandemic. Adamantanes are established as not being effective against most of the isolated avian flu viruses, and their use can cause serious side effects such as seizures. More importantly, adamantanes are capable of encouraging drug-resistant strains to emerge, and these strains can transmit from person to person. The class of neuraminidase inhibitors consists of the drugs zanamivir and oseltamivir, having the commercial names Relenza and Tamiflu, respectively. If administered early before the virus infects too many cells, these drugs prevent the release of influenza virus from infected cells to healthy ones, and their action is associated with very little toxicity. By being far less likely to promote the development of drug-resistant variants than adamantanes, the key virtue of neuraminidase inhibitors is their substantial effectiveness at treating and protecting against all strains of influenza, including avian influenza. For example, neuraminidase inhibitors would have been effective against the virus that caused the devastating 1918 influenza pandemic, and have been effective against the avian viruses of 1997 to 1999 and the avian viruses of 2004. In a possible pandemic caused by avian influenza, neuraminidase inhibitors would probably be the only useful drug. However, the problem is that the anti-viral drugs are not available in sufficient amounts to stop a pandemic, and there is little capacity to increase their production in a time of need. Hence, leading adepts urgently call on agencies, governments and nations to create stockpiles of neuraminidase inhibitors that can be quickly delivered to an outbreak. One idea is to develop international stockpiles managed by the World Health Organization. Prof. Graeme Laver, a renowned world expert on origin and control of pandemic influenza and a key contributor to the development of the anti-flu drug Relenza, had accepted our invitation on August 11, 2008 to elucidate what we know (essentially, not much) about how human pandemic flu viruses arise. "Since there is a lot of misinformation out there that needs correcting", as Graeme stated in one of our personal communications (see the Foreword), his idea was to recall herein a bit of history on the way in which the neuraminidase inhibitors were developed and how these should be used, both in pandemic and in seasonal flu outbreaks. Unfortunately, the death of Prof. Laver, one of the giants of Canberra's John Curtin School of Medical Research, on his way to an international influenza conference in Portugal on September 26, 2008, precluded the delivery of his contribution to us. Thus, in the first chapter, Graeme's long-time friend and collaborator Prof. Robert G. Webster, another leading avian influenza expert, gives interesting insights into the importance of Graeme Laver's research, life and mission. Prof. Adrian J. Gibbs, an eminent virology professor who worked with Prof. Laver at the John Curtin School of Medical Research and knew him for more than 40 years, was recently informed by Graeme's daughter, Penny, that about 50% of

Graeme's manuscript had actually been completed before traveling to Portugal. Exclusively for our book, Penny and Adrian brought the unfinished manuscript to completion by describing vital discoveries by which Graeme worked out the major foundation of influenza biology (chapter 2). We would like to thank Penny and Adrian for the exceptional effort. To illustrate the unique, essay-like writing style of Prof. Laver, chapter 3 features his short paper "Flu Drugs: Pathway to Discovery" that is reproduced from the 2007 March issue of the journal *Education in Chemistry* by permission of The Royal Society of Chemistry.

To successfully attack influenza A viruses—which are known for their rapid mutations, frequent reassortments and some RNA recombination cases—understanding the molecular evolution of the viruses appears to be a necessary condition, as is generally agreed among various scientific communities that have been thus far represented at a number of trans-disciplinary conferences and congresses. Since the present availability of the genomic sequences provides a great chance for us to understand these evolutionary processes much better than ever before, chapter 4 reviews recent advances and challenges in the molecular evolution of both seasonal influenza and avian influenza viruses. Since 2003, highly pathogenic H5N1 influenza viruses have been the cause of large-scale death in poultry and the subsequent infection and death of more than 140 humans. Chapter 5 summarizes the latest reports and represents current opinion on the pathology and pathogenesis of avian influenza H5N1 infection in humans for the past few years, and reports on autopsies on H5N1 infected victims. A substantial amount of original data elucidates the identification of multiple organ infections, vertical (mother-to-fetus) transmission of the virus, viral receptor distributions, and immune response by the infected subjects, thus shedding new light on the nature of this disease. Chapter 6 clarifies the role of an important receptor, such as dendritic cell-specific ICAM-3 grabbing non-integrin, in mediating avian H5N1 virus transmission.

At present, there are only three licensed anti-influenza drugs, namely zanamivir (Relenza), oseltamivir (Tamiflu), and amantadine/rimantadine. The latter targets the M2 ion channel, whereas the other compounds target neuraminidase and were designed through structure-based enzyme inhibitor programmes. The seventh chapter elaborates the activity of neuraminidase inhibitor oseltamivir against all subtypes of influenza viruses using experimental animal and avian models with a special emphasis on the effectiveness of oseltamivir treatment against infection caused by highly pathogenic H5N1 and H7N7 influenza viruses. The fact that several tens of different crystal structures of both sole neuraminidases and neuraminidases complexed with various inhibitors are currently available in the Protein Data Bank has enabled the binding mode predictions of known anti-viral molecules, as well as extensive investigations of the effect of small changes in protein structure on the predicted binding modes using computational methods. Chapter 8 demonstrates the way in which new valuable insights into the molecular mechanism of the resistance of H5N1 influenza A virus neuraminidase to oseltamivir can be obtained by applying the state-of-the-art modeling strategies, and elucidates how these novel insights can be correlated with the available experimental data. Chapter 9 focuses on the role that structural biology and crystallography have played in the development of the antiviral drugs, the emergence of resistance to them and recent research toward the development of new inhibitors of influenza viruses that target other proteins, haemagglutinin and polymerase. Chapter 10 considers the structure-based design of novel, more potent H5N1 neuraminidase inhibitors and establishes the future directions for the successful development of such inhibitors.

Universal flu vaccines have been proposed, but none currently exists on the market. There is a fundamental problem in the development of a vaccine that has not been solved so far. The more the pandemic virus differs antigenically from the vaccine virus, the less effective the vaccine will be. If the pandemic is caused by a virus of a different subtype, the vaccine will be no good at all. The fact that many manufacturers are making a split H5N1 influenza virus or "subunit" vaccine when they should be making a whole, inactivated virus vaccine is closely related to its dose-dependent effectiveness. At low doses, the whole virus vaccine is very much better at inducing an antibody response than the split virus vaccine, while at high doses there is little difference between the two. The whole virus vaccine can cause some unwanted side reactions, worse in some people than in others, but it is unlikely that any H5N1 vaccine would be used for mass immunization before a pandemic. The advantage of making a whole virus vaccine is that in an emergency the lower dose required means there would be much more vaccine to go around for everyone. Chapters 11, 12 and 13 deal with all of the vital aspects by reviewing current and featuring novel approaches to vaccine development and quantitative analysis. We are aware that global effort and support are currently indispensable in order to get closer to the successful development of new influenza therapeutics. The National Institute of Allergy and Infectious Diseases (NIAID) of the National Institute of Health (NIH) in Bethesda, MD, U.S.A. has conducted and supported basic and applied influenza research for more than 50 years. The NIAID research has led to new therapies, vaccines, diagnostic tests, and other technologies that have improved the health of millions of people in the United States and around the world. Chapter 14 features the NIAID resources that are available to the global research community to support development of novel influenza therapeutics.

Since the current drugs have limited curative potential, improved therapies are needed for attacking influenza. Besides infecting pulmonary areas, influenza virus affects extrapulmonary areas in association with basement membrane disruption by matrix metalloproteinases capable of degrading collagen type IV. Hence, an effective strategy for fighting influenza must be targeted not only to blocking virus replication, but also to protecting connective tissue and inhibiting virus spread without inflicting toxicity to host cells. Chapter 15 examines the effectiveness of micronutrients, a unique mixture containing ascorbic acid, green tea extract, lysine, proline, N-acetyl cysteine, and selenium, and their synergy in controlling actions of influenza A virus, viral multiplication and cellular invasive parameters of infected and non-infected cells. Consequently, the non-toxic micronutrient mixture is shown to have the potential for treating influenza, not only by decreasing viral multiplication in infected cells but also by blocking the enzymatic degradation of the extracellular matrix in order to limit virus spread. In other words, it reveals a possible strategy for eradicating endemic public health problems through effective, cause-oriented natural therapies.

Influenza, as an important infectious disease, is known for its enormous economic impact on population health. The major public health concern is the next influenza pandemic and the way in which such a crisis should be controlled. Chapter 16 considers the efficiency of intervention policies against influenza pandemic. In the context of our recent communication with Prof. Lorenzen (the author of chapter 16), it is important to note a detail regarding the geographical spread of the avian influenza virus H5N1 type Asia. Even though several highly pathogenic strains of the specific virus have evolved in China since 1996, only one of them was able to spread to the West. The first isolated strain was obtained in May of 2005 from bar-headed geese breeding at the huge mountain saltwater Qinghai Lake in central China, and reached Europe and Africa in the first half of 2006. With regard to its evolution, the main scientific arguments rejecting the migratory bird hypothesis (a widely-accepted point of view) and supporting the transnational poultry industry hypothesis are currently being considered by all ministers of the European Union who are involved in agrarian topics associated with the problem of biosecurity. Anyway, there is no doubt that effective measures against the emergence of some influenza pandemic must be based on correct scientific evidence. Chapters 17 and 18 show that mathematical models can be a valuable means of both warning about and estimating potential risk of the disease spread. Furthermore, possible strategies for mitigating damage of the pandemic are proposed. Chapter 19 describes preventive measures and discusses their applicability in healthcare facilities with resource-limited settings. Chapter 20 introduces a system view on economy, politics and influenza by exploring the current situation in South Africa.

This book represents a comprehensive account of the up-to-date research achievements in the fight against flu. Its contents cover several critical issues, including (1) the molecular evolution of influenza viruses; (2) the origin and control of pandemic influenza; (3) the pathology and pathogenesis of avian influenza H5N1 infection in humans; (4) the high resistance of H5N1 influenza A virus to the currently approved anti-viral drugs; (5) the structure-based design of novel, more potent, H5N1 neuraminidase inhibitors; (6) the current progress and pitfalls in the development and quantitative analysis of adequate vaccines; (7) the US National Institute of Allergy and Infectious Diseases (NIAID) resources for the global research community to support development of novel influenza therapeutics; (8) the improved strategies of eradicating endemic public health problems through effective, cause-oriented natural therapies; and (9) the prevention policies against influenza pandemic with their applications. Written by 50 eminent scientists from well-known research institutions from around the world (14 different countries—U.S.A., China, Russia, Japan, Australia, Canada, England, Ireland, Germany, Serbia, Taiwan, Korea, Thailand, and South Africa), this book indicates the future directions in which the war against influenza is to be developed, thus ensuring its scientific priority. This book is intended to serve as a valuable professional reference for healthcare professionals, health science administrators, scientific industry leaders, lab directors, and researchers of various backgrounds, including medicine, pharmacy, chemistry, biology, biotechnology, and molecular modeling.

Prof. Dr. Petar M. Mitrasinovic

ACKNOWLEDGMENTS

It is a pleasure to thank a number of people who helped us in this endeavor. First of all, we gratefully acknowledge our dear colleagues, eminent scientists Graeme Laver (1929–2008), Robert G. Webster, Adrian J. Gibbs, Xiu-Feng (Henry) Wan, Sievert Lorenzen, Yasuhiro Takeuchi, Anucha Apisarnthanarak, Thomas Gstraunthaler, Jiang Gu, Elena A. Govorkova, Noel A. Roberts, Rupert Russell, Yi-Ming Arthur Chen, Andrei Korobeinikov, Alexei V. Pokrovskii, Slobodan Paessler, Runtao He, Terry D. Cyr, Sean (Xuguang) Li, Amy Krafft, Aleksandra Niedzwiecki, Matthias Rath, and their collaborators for accepting our invitation and investing valuable time in writing excellent contributions. They deserve most of the credit for making this book possible. However, the sad news that Graeme Laver is no longer with us arrived on September 26, 2008. We, all of his friends and colleagues, will miss him very much with a strong belief that Graeme has become one of the legends. We especially thank Linda C. Lambert, Chief of Respiratory Diseases Branch, Division of Microbiology and Infectious Diseases, National Institute of Allergy and Infectious Diseases, U.S.A. and Marie-Paule Kieny, Director of Initiative for Vaccine Research, World Health Organization, Switzerland for their kind advice and suggestions pertaining to the identification of prospective contributors. We are considerably indebted to many colleagues worldwide whose constructive ideas, opinions and criticisms, exchanged in fruitful mutual communications and discussions in the last eight months, have turned out to be of vital importance for assembling the edited collection on such a fascinating field of research on time. We sincerely apologize for not being able to mention a huge number of names specifically. Many thanks are offered to Nova Science Publishers, Inc. for recognizing the need for this book based on its scientific priority. We owe very much to all of the members of our family for their unforgettable understanding, support and love throughout all of the stages of preparing the book for publication.

Prof. Dr. Petar M. Mitrasinovic
Belgrade, Serbia, March 31, 2009

PART I:
DEDICATED TO WILLIAM GRAEME LAVER
(1929-2008)

Chapter 1

WILLIAM GRAEME LAVER (GRAEME), PhD, FRS, 1929–2008[*]

Robert G. Webster[†]

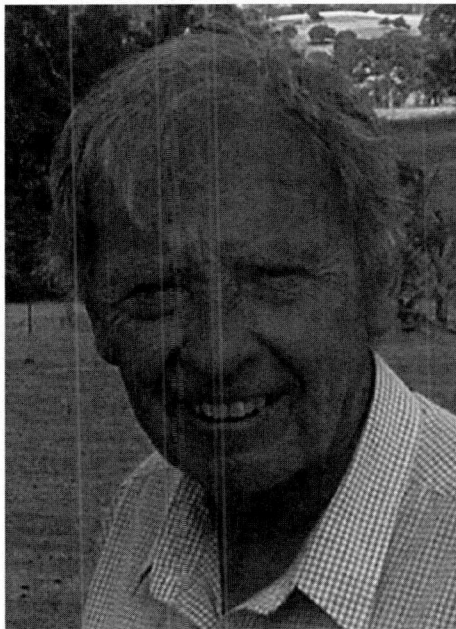

While Graeme Laver claims to have been motivated by scientific curiosity rather than by humanitarian endeavors, his fundamental understanding of the influenza virus led to the current options used to control both seasonal and pandemic influenza globally. These include the development of one of the first subunit influenza vaccines still being produced in

---

[*] Reprinted from *Virology*, Vol. 385, Robert G. Webster, Obituary: William Graeme Laver (Graeme) PhD, FRS, 1929-2008, vii-viii. Copyright (2009), with permission (2152010265812) from Elsevier.
[†] E-mail: robert.webster@stjude.org

Australia and to the development of the first of a family of drugs against the influenza viral neuraminidase.

Graeme was a superb bench scientist who grew up through the ranks at the Walter and Eliza Hall Institute (Hall Institute) in Melbourne, Australia. His parents, Laurence and Madge Laver, owned a potato farm at Kinglake, Victoria and in his early years Graeme was schooled by correspondence. The family lost the farm during the depression and they moved to Melbourne where Graeme attended Ivanhoe Grammar School. At the age of 16, Graeme began work as a "bottle washer" and general laboratory helper at the Hall Institute and matriculated (graduated) by attending night school. He continued working at the Hall Institute and supported himself through Melbourne University graduating with a BSc. Subsequently he completed an MSc in biochemistry at Melbourne University and was supported in his PhD at London University by a Commonwealth Scientific and Industrial Research Organization (CSIRO) scholarship.

Throughout his entire life, Graeme was an adventurer; during his student years as a mountaineer he met his wife, Judy. After completing his PhD in London he and Judy in 1955 drove a small "Standard 10" (English Standard Motor Company) across country back to Australia through Europe, Turkey, Iran, Afghanistan, Pakistan and India to Mumbai (Bombay), and then traveled by ship to Australia. They camped en route and were occasionally advised to move on due to bandits and "enjoyed" whole legs of camel, and as guests of honor the eyeballs at impromptu feasts. Upon arrival in Mumbai, Graeme found a letter at the post office from Frank Fenner offering him a job at the John Curtin School of Medical Research at the Australia National University (ANU) in Canberra, Australia.

He accepted the position in the Department of Microbiology at ANU and teamed up with Stephen Fazekas de St. Groth and myself (Rob Webster) to work on the influenza virus. Graeme used his extensive background in chemistry to study the structure of the virus. Being a lipid-containing virus, he used lipid solvents to take the virus apart. At that time ether was being used to disrupt the virus to make vaccines. Graeme found that ether was a very poor disrupting agent and turned to the mild detergent sodium deoxycholate and the "particles were completely disrupted". This important contribution appeared in the Discussion and Preliminary report section of *Virology* (*Virology* 1961, 14, 499-502) and formed the basis for the subunit vaccine currently used in Australia. This vaccine was non-reactogenic in children as compared with the earlier whole virus inactivated vaccine. The ANU paid 10 shillings each to Laver and Webster and patented the process. Studies with Robin Valentine of the National Institute of Medical Research in London determined the morphology of hemagglutinin (HA) and neuraminidase (NA) and their clusters in rosettes (*Virology* 1969, 38, 105).

Studies on the natural history of influenza viruses and the establishment of the role of migratory waterfowl as reservoirs of influenza viruses was begun using Ochterloney plates on The Great Barrier Reef islands off the Queensland coast of Australia. Faint precipitin bands in the agar gel between disrupted influenza virus and the sera from mutton birds (*Puffinus pacificus*) appeared right there on the reef. An earlier die off of mutton birds on the coast near Bateman's Bay, New South Wales may have served as the initial pointer for an influenza virus had been isolated from dead terns in South Africa (A/Tern/South Africa/61 [H5N3]). Multiple trips to the Great Barrier Reef resulted in, first, the confirmation of antibodies to the NA of human H2N2 influenza in the mutton bird sera, and later in the isolation of multiple influenza A viruses. These findings provided the original evidence for the role of migratory waterfowl as the reservoirs of all influenza A viruses.

Influenza viruses are notoriously variable. Our current knowledge of the mechanism of both antigenic drift and shift of influenza virus came from Graeme's peptide mapping and antigenic studies. In the early 1960s antigenic shift and drift were not distinguished; antigenic shift was considered to be a more pronounced antigenic change-presumably by mutation in the circulating virus. After the emergence of the Hong Kong H3N2 pandemic in 1968 comparison of the isolated HA with that of the preceding H2N2 virus showed vast differences in peptide maps indicating that there was no way that H3 could have arisen from H2 by mutation (*Virology* 1972, 48, 445). Further analysis of influenza viruses from horses (A/Equine/Miami/1/63 [H3N8]) and ducks (A/Duck/Ukraine/1/63 [H3N8]) antigenically related to the newly emerged human H3 viruses showed that while the HA1 portions of the HA had differences by peptide mapping the HA2, portions of the molecule were essentially identical (*Virology* 1973, 51, 383), providing the initial evidence that the HA came from an animal source by reassortment.

To mimic antigenic drift swine influenza virus was grown in the presence of antisera made essentially monoclonal by partial adsorption with homologous antigen. Virus grown in the presence of this serum was antigenically distinct and peptide mapping showed that the HAs were almost identical except for one or two peptides that had shifted position (*Virology* 1968, 34, 193). This provided the first biochemical evidence that antigenic drift occurred by mutation in the HA. Subsequent studies with monoclonal antibodies to the HA showed that escape mutants had single amino acid changes in defined regions (epitopes) on the HA permitting antigenic mapping of the HA molecule. Electron microscopy studies of these antibodies with isolated HA in conjunction with Nick Wrigley established that the antibody binding sites were on the outer tip of the HA molecule.

Continuation of Graeme's initial structural studies of influenza viruses led to the crystallization of the "heads" of the NA and this keynote paper appeared in *Virology* in 1978 (*Virology* 1978, 96, 78). These studies led to the resolution of the three dimensional structure of the NA with Peter Colman and Jose Varghese (*Nature* 1983, 303, 35) enabling Mark von Itzstein to design the first anti-influenza drug zanamivir (Relenza) based on NA structure. Although Relenza is efficacious against all influenza A and B viruses, its route of administration as an aerosol powder was not well accepted and development of an orally available anti-neuraminidase drug oseltamivir (Tamiflu) by Gilead Sciences was based in part on crystals derived from a novel influenza virus isolated from a noddy tern on The Great Barrier Reef. Photographs of these NA crystals appeared on the cover of many journals and Graeme and the photographer Julie Macklin were awarded the Nikon "Small World" prize in 1987. In 1996 in recognition of the contribution to the development of anti-neuraminidase drugs Graeme together with Peter Colman, Mark von Itzstein and Paul Janssen were awarded the Australia Prize.

In addition to his studies on influenza viruses Graeme also made contributions to our knowledge of adenoviruses and parainfluenza viruses. One of his passions later in life was the growth of perfect crystals of sialidases-including the NA's of influenza. He worked with Russian scientists to grow NA crystals on the MIR space station at zero gravity. The resulting crystals were little better than those grown on earth but Graeme's sense of adventure in cutting through Australian, United States and Soviet red tape was his personal achievement. Graeme's outdoor activities in addition to mountaineering and birding on Barrier Reef Islands included the raising of beef cattle on their family farm at Murrumbateman-near Canberra,

Australia. Graeme loved to collect and chop his own firewood, he grew grapes for wine and had a large vegetable garden fertilized by rich compost.

In recognition of his many contributions to our knowledge of influenza viruses, Graeme Laver was elected to the Royal Society of London in 1987. His final goal was to have anti-influenza drugs made available over-the-counter (OTC) in Australia. He argued that when the next human influenza pandemic spreads that the drugs must be immediately available in patient's own medicine cabinets and that distribution from stockpiles would be too slow. Authorities argued against his proposal saying that this would lead to antiviral resistance. The current emergence of resistance to Tamiflu in seasonal H1N1 influenza from Northern Europe where little Tamiflu was used argues against selection by the drug. Graeme died as he lived challenging the foundations of knowledge and the search for novel approaches. At the age of 79 he was on his way to the Third European Influenza Conference in Vilamoura, Portugal (September 14–17, 2008) when he collapsed en route. The airport authorities at Heathrow Airport, London cleared the airspace to get him to medical attention rapidly. He lived long enough to realize the mayhem he had caused but was unaware that he had terminal abdominal cancer. He had hoped to meet with colleagues to promote the distribution of anti-influenza drugs OTC.

One of Graeme's great successes was the organization of small scientific meetings at key times in superb venues. He organized 10 such meetings at places like Rougement, Baden, Thredbo (Australia), Cold Sydney Harbor, Beijing, Hawaii and London. Probably the most memorable was the Thredbo meeting in the Snowy Mountains of New South Wales, Australia when various HA sequences were being worked on in several laboratories. As participants arrived they were given a box of amino acid cards and told to post their sequence around the room. The participants were first in shock but soon "got with it" and had a lot of fun comparing their sequences and working out possible consequences of the differences. Graeme was rarely a diplomat and often upset people with his quest for understanding questions at the fundamental level. There was one certainty to working with Graeme: your ideas were sometimes ridiculed before being accepted and you could never get away with merely accepting conventional thinking. He had an extraordinary ability to get to the heart of a scientific question and to design the direct experiment.

Graeme had many international collaborators; in the early years he was given use of a NASA communications satellite and later global telephone coverage. He contributed enormously to the "animal influenza" aspects of the World Health Organization program on influenza with Martin Kaplan and Bernard Easterday. His contributions to our knowledge of the structure, origin and methods of control of both seasonal and pandemic influenza are continuing through his multiple collaborators.

— Robert G. Webster, Ph.D., FRS
Rose Marie Thomas Endowed Chair
Division of Virology
Department of Infectious Diseases
St. Jude Children's Research Hospital

In: Global View of Fight against Influenza
Editor: Petar M. Mitrasinovic

Chapter 2

THE ORIGIN AND CONTROL OF PANDEMIC INFLUENZA[*]

Graeme Laver (1929–2008)

ABSTRACT

During the past 100 years there have been three major pandemics of influenza. These occurred in 1918, 1957 and 1968. The viruses that caused the 1957 and 1968 pandemics were found to be hybrids. Their major virion proteins were closely related to those previously found in human and avian influenza viruses. It is assumed these viruses arose by gene re-assortment, but where, how and when this happened is not known. Until we know the gene sequences of pre-1918 human influenzas we will not know whether the 1918 flu was or was not a hybrid too.

It seems that the world is now overdue for the next influenza pandemic. When this might happen and the nature of the virus that will be responsible for it are completely unknown. It is clear, however, that the world's human population will have no immunity against a "new" virus if one should suddenly arise, and effective vaccines might take months to make. In the meantime, anti-influenza drugs exist that should provide an effective defence against the new virus until vaccines become available. These drugs are the neuraminidase-inhibitors, Tamiflu (oseltamivir) and Relenza (zanamivir) and this review will describe how these were deliberately created, how they work and how they should be used, both in a pandemic and for the seasonal flu outbreaks that occur around the world every winter.

---

[*] The abstract and first section of this chapter were drafted by Graeme Laver before his death on September 26, 2008 (Webster, 2009). The second section is reprinted with the permission of The Johns Hopkins University Press. The chapter concludes with a synopsis of Graeme Laver's views on preparations for countering an influenza pandemic, and were collated and edited by Penny Laver and Adrian Gibbs.

SECTION 1. INTRODUCTION

You suddenly start to shiver with a high fever, a throbbing headache, your limbs and joints are aching and you have a dry cough. You also have a sore throat and maybe some sneezing. You feel absolutely terrible. Yes, you have caught the flu! But as you lie there in utter misery, you are comforted by the thought that sooner or later you will start to get better. But what if you don't? What if you get worse and go on to die? Thousands do, every year, and until recently, if you caught the flu there was very little you could do about it.

The Spanish Influenza pandemic of 1918–19, killed about 40 million people worldwide. Many died in the most horrific manner, in many cases only a few hours after first experiencing symptoms similar to those listed above. Victims struggled to clear their airways of the bloody froth that poured from their lungs, to no avail. Blood spurted from the nose, purple blisters appeared on the skin, and death came in a matter of hours. The lungs of these unfortunate people – and remember, there were 40 million or so victims – were up to six times their normal weight and looked like "melted red-currant jelly". It was truly a most horrible death.

At the time the agent responsible was not known—the first human influenza virus was not isolated until 1933—there was no good means of preventing infection, and there was no cure once flu symptoms appeared. People were obviously desperate for a "cure" for this deadly infection and the newspapers of the time carried advertisements for treatments that had no effect whatsoever. Nowadays the situation is greatly improved. Safe and effective anti-influenza drugs are available that, if taken early after symptom onset, will specifically bind to and disable the virus, so aborting the infection and allowing the patient to recover.

Two of these drugs, Relenza (zanamivir) and Tamiflu (oseltamivir) that are effective against all influenza viruses, were deliberately created by a process of rational, structure-based, drug design and here I will describe some of the scientific events that lead to their creation, what the drugs are, how they work and how they should be used.

The Origin of Influenza Pandemics

Early accounts of influenza pandemics are few and far between (Potter, 2001) (F.B. Smith personal communication). In Europe the first influenza epidemic with a reasonably clear description occurred in 1173 in Italy and France. Further epidemics in Europe are said to have occurred in 1414, 1557 and 1675–1676. France experienced further epidemics in 1788–1790 and in 1830–1832.

The first great flu pandemic to be widely recorded was the Russian flu pandemic of 1889–1893. In Great Britain, the winters of 1891 and 1892 were the worst. Symptoms varied, but victims commonly experienced sudden fever which lasted 3–5 days, and sometimes for a fortnight, chills, thumping muscular pains, especially in the back, runny nose and eyes, sneezing or dry coughing, prostration for up to a fortnight, loss of appetite and photophobia. "Headache" and "melancholia" were also reported.

The epidemic was characterised by huge morbidity. London, one of the worst affected cities had, at one stage, one-third of its population incapacitated by influenza. There were also deaths. In 1891, 125,000 people died from influenza and in 1892, 250,000 flu deaths were recorded in Great Britain.

This epidemic, and the ones preceding it, were probably caused by "new" flu viruses that spread into, and then through, the human population, as it had no immunity to the new virus. The virus spread like wild-fire until, presumably, the immunity of the population developed and the virus died out.

The greatest recorded influenza pandemic occurred in 1918–1919. "Spanish flu" killed 40 million people world-wide, many under the most horrible circumstances. Where did this virus come from, and what made it so virulent?

In an extraordinary piece of scientific detective work, Taubenberger and his colleagues determined the sequence of all of the genes of the 1918 virus. Fragments of these genes were isolated from specimens of the virus that had remained in the lungs of people who died from influenza in 1918 and had been preserved buried in the permafrost in arctic Alaska, or in tissue samples stored in jars held in pathology museums in the USA. Using this gene sequence information the entire 1918 virus (or at least a virus containing the protein coding regions of the 1918 virus's genes) has been re-created in the laboratory and some of its characteristics have been determined. The team also suggested that the Spanish Influenza virus had an avian precursor virus that was able to infect humans, in other words the 1918 virus was a lethal avian virus that had jumped from birds to man in a very short time. This was used as an argument for the idea that the H5N1 avian virus currently causing millions of deaths among poultry and which kills a large proportion of the small number of humans it has infected, was also likely to jump from birds to man like the 1918 virus was postulated to have done (Taubenberger et al., 2005). However, no direct evidence, sequencing or other, has yet proved that such a mechanism occurred when the 1918 virus emerged (Antonovics et al., 2006; Gibbs and Gibbs, 2006), or that any avian influenza virus, such as the highly pathogenic H5N1 virus, has the potential to do so.

Thus, we do not know how the 1918 Spanish Influenza virus arose.

Nor is it known why the virus was so virulent. One suggestion is that it replicated in the body to much higher titres than "normal" human flu viruses. Experiments in animals with the re-constructed 1918 virus suggest that this was the case. It is well known that Type A influenza viruses can vary widely in their growth rates and a fast growing virus, producing huge numbers of virus particles in infected individuals might trigger a rapid and deadly cytokine storm in a very short time (Kobasa et al., 2004; Tuvim et al., 2009).

What about the other two most recent pandemics? What was their origin?

The virus that caused the pandemic of Hong Kong influenza in 1968 was a subtype H3N2 virus. This virus possessed the same neuraminidase as the previously circulating Asian H2N2 viruses, but careful analysis showed that the hemagglutinin was antigenically completely different from that of the H2N2 viruses.

Where did the "new" H3 antigen come from? Some suggested that there were "bridging strains" that resulted in H2 giving rise to H3, but no evidence for such viruses was ever found.

Crude sequencing experiments using peptide mapping, the only technique available at the time, showed that the sequences of the H2 and H3 antigens were so different that it was very unlikely that H3 arose from H2 by mutation. It was then discovered that the human H3 antigen was similar in its amino acid sequence to the hemagglutinin of a duck influenza virus. In other words the 1968 Hong Kong virus was a hybrid, having genes from both human and bird influenza viruses. Later, the Asian H2N2 virus was also found to be such a hybrid virus.

But that is all we know. It is assumed that these hybrid viruses were formed by re-assortment between human and animal viruses, but when this happened, in what host the double infection occurred and exactly where in the world the re-assortment event took place, we have no idea.

Something other than simple re-asssortment between animal and human influenza viruses might be required for a "new" pandemic virus to emerge.

In Southern China all the Type A viruses exist, mainly as seemingly harmless infections of water birds. Influenza epidemics among humans also frequently occur in Southern China. So, there must be many opportunities for infections by mixtures of avian and human viruses to occur. And yet, for 40 years, no new pandemic virus has arisen.

Therefore, the way in which past influenza pandemic viruses have arisen and how future "new" viruses might get into the human population is not at all clear.

SECTION 2. FROM THE GREAT BARRIER REEF TO A "CURE" FOR THE FLU: TALL TALES BUT TRUE[1]

Abstract

How we discovered that sea birds on the Great Barrier Reef are riddled with influenza viruses, and how one of these led to a new drug now being used in the battle against the flu are recounted.

I was in Sydney, attending a cocktail party thrown by the pharmaceutical company Hoffmann-La Roche to launch its new anti-influenza drug Tamiflu. As one does on these occasions, I got talking to a young lady from the marketing division of Roche, who asked,"Why are you here? What is your involvement with Tamiflu?"

I said, "If I told you, you wouldn't believe me.''

"Try me," she replied, so this is what I said:

One summer I went to a deserted coral island on Australia's Great Barrier Reef with friends and colleagues. One of these was Adrian Gibbs, a veritable giant of a man, skilled in catching airborne objects. He caught a white-capped noddy tern, stuck a cotton wool swab up its backside, from which we isolated an influenza virus. The neuraminidase from this virus was sent into space to crystallize on the Soviet space station *Mir*, and from the crystals the structure of the virus's neuraminidase was discovered. This information was then used by Gilead Sciences in California to create the anti-influenza drug now called Tamiflu which was taken over by Roche and is what you are now toasting at this party.

"Oh," she exclaimed, and went off to talk to someone else. Clearly she did not believe a word I said.

The story started in the late 1960s, when RobWebster and I were walking along a sandy beach on the south coast of New South Wales in Australia. We noticed that every 10 to 15 meters or so there was a dead mutton bird (shearwater) washed up on the beach. Knowing

---

[1] (Laver, 2004) Reprinted with permission of The Johns Hopkins University Press.

that terns in South Africa had been killed by an influenza virus in 1961, we wondered if these birds, too, had died from a flu infection.

Avian influenza, or fowl plague, was the first influenza virus to be isolated, in 1900, but fowl plague was not recognized as being caused by a type A influenza virus until 1955, years after the first human influenza virus was isolated in 1933. Then, in 1956, two other avian influenza A viruses were isolated from domestic ducks, following which an increasing number of influenza viruses were isolated from domestic chickens, turkeys, ducks, quail, pheasants, and pigeons. It was believed, however, that these bird viruses all originated from human strains of influenza and had got into the domesticated birds because of their close proximity to people.

Apart from the one incident in South Africa in 1961, where terns were found dying from influenza, there were no reports of influenza viruses being isolated from wild birds, and no accounts of attempts to do this. Two people, however, pushed this idea: Martin Kaplan of the World Health Organization, and Helio Pereira, who headed the Department of Virology at the National Institute for Medical Research, Mill Hill, London.

I was skiing with Pereira one winter in Argentiere, France, and we talked about trying to isolate flu from wild birds. We toyed with the idea of doing this on the coral islands of the Great Barrier Reef. Why there? Can you think of a more unlikely place to look for flu? Beautiful islands in an azure sea, hot sand, a baking sun, and a warm coral lagoon. What better place to do flu research! After skiing, we visited Martin Kaplan at the WHO in Geneva, and after a good deal of smooth talking managed to wheedle $500 out of him to help pay for an expedition to the Reef.

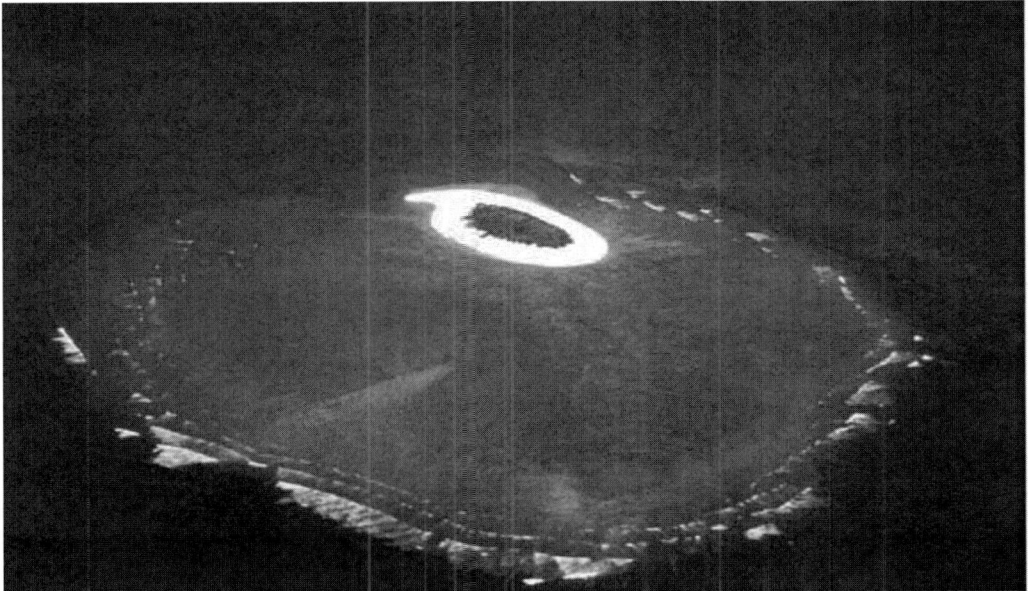

Figure 1. An aerial view of Tryon Island, an uninhabited coral cay in the Capricorn group at the southern end of the Great Barrier Reef, about 45 miles (72 km) off the Queensland coast (lat 23°15′ S, long 151°47′ E). Many thousands of birds nest on these islands during the breeding season, including shearwaters, which nest in burrows in the ground.

This was just as well, as my Head of Department at the Australian National University, when asked for funds for an expedition to look for flu on the Great Barrier Reef, said, "Laver is hallucinating." He also said that in any case I wouldn't be able to catch the birds. But I knew that thousands upon thousands of mutton birds or shearwaters nested on the coral cays of the Reef in burrows in the sand, and that all you had to do to catch these wild, free-flying sea birds was to bend over and pick them up.

As it turned out, Pereira wasn't able to come to Australia at the time the mutton birds were nesting so I went with an assistant, Alice Murdoch, for three weeks in December 1969. We set up camp on the uninhabited coral cay Tryon Island, 50 miles off the coast of Queensland (Figure 1). We collected sera from 201 shearwaters and tested these on the spot in double immuno-diffusion tests with a preparation of influenza type A ribonucleoprotein (RNP), which had been made in the lab before coming to the island. All type A influenza viruses have the same RNP antigen, and following infection, antibodies to RNP can be found in the sera of infected individuals. To our great surprise, we saw faint precipitin lines in some of the gel diffusion plates. These were too weak and fuzzy to form the basis of a publication,but they were strong enough to encourage further testing of the sera for flu antibodies. Back in the lab the question was which viral antigen to test the sera against. We ruled out hemagglutination inhibition tests, the ones most people would have used, because sera often contain high levels of non-specific inhibitors of flu hemagglutinin, and these might have muddied the waters. Instead, we chose to look for the ability of the shearwater sera to inhibit influenza virus neuraminidase. But which neuraminidase?

Several antigenically distinct influenza type A neuraminidase subtypes were already known, and we had to guess which was the right one to use. A previous experiment by Webster pointed the way. In 1967, with Pereira and Bela Tumova, Webster had found that some avian influenza viruses possessed neuraminidase antigens that were immunologically similar to that of the "Asian" (1957) H2N2 strain of human influenza. We mixed samples of influenza virus neuraminidase of the human 1957 N2 subtype with sera from the shearwaters on Tryon Island and looked for inhibition of neuraminidase activity. We tested about 30 sera, and in each case the test gave the familiar bright red color produced by active neuraminidase. And then, suddenly, we got one test that was completely colorless. Something in that bird's serum had completely eliminated the activity of the neuraminidase. It was one of those rare "Eureka" moments that make scientific research so exciting.

It didn't take long to prove that this inhibition of the neuraminidase was due to specific antibody to human influenza virus neuraminidase of the N2 subtype. This led to the inescapable conclusion that this shearwater bird had been infected sometime in the past with a virus possessing N2/1957 neuraminidase. Out of the 201 shearwater sera collected on Tryon Island in December 1969, and 119 sera from neighboring Heron Island, collected by my research assistant Catherine Dasen, a total of 18 had antibody that inhibited N2/1957 neuraminidase. It then became imperative that we should try to isolate live virus from the birds, and a number of expeditions were organized to do just that. At the end of 1970, Webster and I collected 172 sera and tracheal swabs from shearwaters on Phillip Island near Melbourne, Australia, and a total of 321 sera and 148 tracheal swabs from a variety of pelagic birds on the Great Barrier Reef. We found a number of sera with antibody to "Asian" (N2/1957) neuraminidase, confirming the previous findings, but no virus was isolated from any of the tracheal swabs. Then, in 1971, another expedition was undertaken to Tryon Island, to collect 201 tracheal swabs from shearwaters nesting on the island. During the day, the shearwaters spent their time out at sea fishing, returning to their nesting burrows when the sun went down. The daily routine for us, therefore, was to swim and sunbathe during the day and then, following the traditional sherry party on the beach at dusk, to spend two hours or so catching and swabbing the birds before returning to camp for dinner prepared by our excellent cooking team. The swabs were then stored in liquid nitrogen before being transported back to the lab.

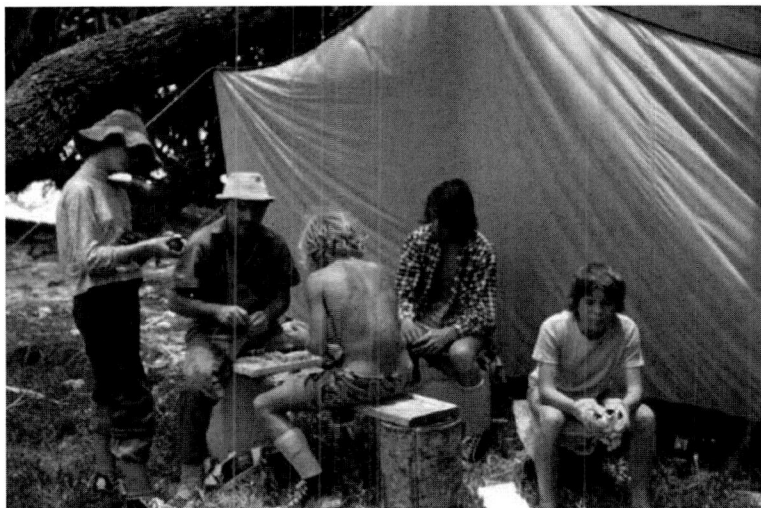

Figure 2. Dr. Walter Dowdle, CDC Atlanta, collecting serum samples and swabs from White Capped Noddy Terns on Lady Musgrave Island on the Great Barrier Reef. The children who caught the terns are (left to right) Judith Skeat, Rowan Laver, Matthew Barnard and Penny Laver.

Finding volunteers to undertake the arduous work involved was not difficult. Small children who came along were particularly helpful, as their light weight enabled them to walk among the burrows and capture the birds without breaking through and damaging the nests (Figure 2).

Material from the swabs was inoculated into 10-day-old embryonated chicken eggs, and after two days' incubation at 37 degrees, the allantoic fluid around the embryo was harvested and tested for influenza virus. Most of the eggs were negative, but you can imagine our excitement when we eventually found one egg full of an influenza type A virus, which had come from the trachea of a completely healthy shearwater bird nesting on Tryon Island, remote from human habitation. This finding suggested that the natural hosts of influenza A might be wild aquatic birds, and that many more type A viruses might exist in these pelagic bird populations.

Human influenza is, of course, a respiratory virus, and it is therefore understandable that we looked for viruses in the bird's respiratory secretions. However, Webster then found that in domestic ducks, avian influenza viruses replicated in cells lining the bird's gut, rather than in the lungs or trachea, and he suggested that it might be a better idea to swab the other end of the bird, and to collect material from the cloaca rather then from the trachea. So in later expeditions to the Reef we did just that, and this eventually led to the isolation of a number of influenza A viruses from the Reef birds, some of which had not been characterized previously.

One virus was of particular interest and importance. The 70th cloacal swab collected by Gibbs from a white capped noddy tern on North West Island in December 1975 yielded a type A influenza virus of subtype H11N9. Type A influenza viruses exist in a number of subtypes with serologically quite different surface antigens, hemagglutinin (H) and neuraminidase (N). So far, 15 H and nine N subtypes have been discovered, and viruses can be classified into H1N2, H3N2, H3N6, and so on. Viruses of the H1N1, H2N2, and H3N2 subtypes are known to have caused human flu pandemics. Because N9 neuraminidase had not previously been described, we were curious to examine this in more detail. But first pure N9 neuraminidase had to be isolated from the virus. To do this, the N9 neuraminidase of the H11N9 noddy tern virus was first segregated into a re-assortant virus, H1N9, using Webster's famous recipe: "Antigenic hybrids of influenza A viruses with surface antigens to order." It was much easier to purify the neuraminidase from the re-assortant virus than from the parent. N9 neuraminidase "heads" were then isolated from the H1N9 virus, purified, and crystallized using a high-salt phosphate buffer recipe suggested by Peter Colman. How these neuraminidase crystals were used in the creation of the anti-viral drug, Tamiflu, will now be described.

In 1978, I had crystallized N2 neuraminidase from the human H2N2 influenza virus, and Peter Colman and his colleagues had determined its three-dimensional structure by X-ray crystallography. This showed the enzyme to have a conserved catalytic site, which meant that if a neuraminidase inhibitor, a "plug drug," could be developed as an anti-viral drug for viruses with N2 neuraminidase, this drug should be effective against all influenza viruses - even those that had not yet appeared in man. From knowledge of the three-dimensional structure of the catalytic site of N2 neuraminidase, Mark von Itzstein and his colleagues designed and synthesized a potent and specific inhibitor of the enzyme. This inhibitor, known as Relenza, is now being used worldwide to treat influenza infections. However, Relenza is not orally bioavailable; it is a powder that has to be puffed into the lungs, a procedure that does not appeal to many people. Gilead Sciences in California and BioCryst pharmaceuticals in Alabama therefore set out to create an influenza virus neuraminidase inhibitor that could be administered as a pill, or a suspension or solution that could be swallowed.

The story now shifts back to the Great Barrier Reef birds. The virus from Gibbs' noddy tern on North West Island, possessed neuraminidase of the N9 subtype, which formed the most beautiful large crystals that diffracted X-rays to 1.9 Å resolution. N9 crystals were, in fact, the best influenza neuraminidase crystals ever obtained. In an attempt to get N9 crystals of even bigger size and of higher quality, we grew them in space in conditions of microgravity. The first crystals were grown on the American space shuttle, but these experiments came to an end following the *Challenger* accident. I then travelled to Moscow and arranged to have N9 neuraminidase crystals grown on the Soviet space station, *Mir*. Growing crystals in space for X-ray diffraction analysis was a new experience for the Russians, and the appropriate apparatus for this had to be designed and built. This was accomplished in a remarkably short time, and on June 8, 1988, N9 neuraminidase was put on a rocket and sent into space to crystallize on *Mir* in microgravity. Three months later the N9 crystals were returned to earth and a sample sent to BioCryst and the University of Alabama for X-ray analysis. The results showed that the crystals grown in space were no bigger, and of only slightly higher quality, than N9 crystals grown on earth. We therefore abandoned further attempts to grow crystals in space, and although the data set from the *Mir* N9 crystal was used by BioCryst in their initial drug design experiments, further work used N9 crystals grown in

Australia, which is a long way away from the United States, but not yet in space. The influenza virus neuraminidase inhibitor developed by BioCryst has not so far been approved for clinical use. Gilead Sciences in California also used N9 neuraminidase crystals grown in Canberra in the design and synthesis of a carbocyclic, orally bioavailable neuraminidase inhibitor, now marketed under the name Tamiflu. Tamiflu is administered as a pill for adults or a suspension for children, and is being used worldwide for the treatment of influenza infections. It is, in fact, the best defence we will have if the H5N1 bird flu virus, currently causing havoc in Southeast Asia, ever acquires the ability to spread in the human population and kill people as efficiently as it kills chickens. Tamiflu might, of course, have been developed using N2 neuraminidase crystals, but when Adrian Gibbs caught the noddy tern that yielded the N9 crystals, it made the job a whole lot easier.

So the story I told the young lady at the Tamiflu launch celebration was indeed more or less true. But the isolation of influenza viruses from birds on the Great Barrier Reef was of as much importance in understanding the ecology of influenza as it was in the design of anti-viral drugs. It led to Rob Webster's demonstration that healthy wild ducks on lakes in Northern Canada are infected with every known subtype of influenza type A virus, and that these viruses can be isolated, not only from the birds themselves, but also from the lake water on which they swim. Further work by Webster and others has now established that wild aquatic birds are indeed the natural hosts of type A influenza, and probably have been for many millions of years. They act as a reservoir of antigens for the formation of "new" human pandemic influenza viruses. Knowing this now gives us a better understanding of how to control pandemic influenza.

Additional reading: (Laver and Garman, 2002; Laver, 2004; Laver et al., 1999)

SECTION 3. CONTROL OF INFLUENZA

Penny Laver[2] and Adrian J. Gibbs[3]

Graeme Laver's views on the control of influenza were summarized in his submissions to the 2006 enquiry, "Pandemic influenza: science to policy", held jointly by The Royal Society of London and the British Academy of Medical Sciences (http://royals (http://royalsociety.org/downloaddoc.asp?id=3544), and also in his submissions to the National Drugs and Poisons Schedule Committee (NDPSC) of the Australian Government's Department of Health and Ageing (Therapeutic Goods Administration) (http://www.tga.gov.au/ndpsc/record/rr200806.htm)

He commented to the UK enquiry that "many of the measures Governments are proposing to control a pandemic, if one should suddenly erupt, are unlikely to succeed. Closing schools might create more problems than it solves, fever clinics seem to be a waste of time and thermal imaging devices at airports would not detect recently infected people who show no symptoms and have no fever but are shedding virus in large amounts. It is true that there is no evidence that such people are also good transmitters, but it would be safe to

---

[2] Correspondence: pennylaver@bigpond.com
[3] Correspondence: adrian_j_gibbs@hotmail.com

assume this is the case." He concluded that the use of anti-viral drugs followed as soon as possible by vaccination was the best strategy.

Two types of anti-influenza drugs are in use or being tested at present (http://en.wikipedia.org/wiki/Influenza_treatment). They are the M2 inhibitors (adamantane derivatives) and the neuraminidase inhibitors. Of the latter only Relenza (zanamivir) and Tamiflu (oseltamivir) have so far been approved for use. Oseltamivir phosphate, is swallowed, absorbed from the gut and metabolised in the liver to the active oseltamivir carboxylate, whereas zanamivir is used as a fine powder that is inhaled, and is therefore restricted to the respiratory tract.

Laver saw several issues that restricted the value of these drugs. Firstly "Although only a few human H5N1 infections have been treated with Tamiflu, some mutant viruses resistant to the drug have been found. These mutants were still sensitive to Relenza. So Tamiflu might not be the drug of choice in a "bird flu" pandemic. On the other hand, there is some evidence that the H5N1 virus might replicate in organs other than in the respiratory system. In this case, Relenza might be less effective than Tamiflu."

Since his submission to the UK enquiry, strains of influenza virus with resistance to both classes of anti-viral drugs have been found, and it is clear that these are potentially a significant problem (de Jong et al., 2005; Hayden, 2008; Moscona, 2005; Sheu et al., 2008), and the reasons why mutants of the N1 neuraminidase are resistant to oseltamivir, but not zanamivir, has been confirmed by studies of its structure (Collins et al., 2008). However "The current emergence of resistance to Tamiflu in seasonal H1N1 influenza from Northern Europe where little Tamiflu was used argues against selection by the drug" (Webster, 2009).

Laver was also particularly concerned with the decision of the Australian health authorities to require that a doctor must prescribe the anti-influenza drugs before a person can obtain them from a pharmacist; 'over-the-counter' (OTC) sales are banned. This requirement inevitably adds to the time required to obtain and administer the drug despite clear evidence that the sooner after infection that a person takes the drug, the better the outcome (Aoki et al., 2003). Thus the health authority's OTC ban inevitably diminishes the efficacy of the drugs. Furthermore Laver commented to the UK enquiry that "Governments around the world are stockpiling Tamiflu in huge amounts. The Australian Government has 3.9 million treatment courses. But the strategy to use this stockpile is wrong. If used correctly, there would already be enough Tamiflu in the stockpile for everyone in Australia who might need it in a pandemic situation. The plan was to use the stockpile to give Tamiflu to "essential workers" to be used prophylactically for a period of 6 weeks. This is, of course, a complete waste of a valuable drug. What happens, after 6 weeks when the stockpile is used up and the pandemic is still raging? What about people in the community, not on the essential worker's list who fall ill or whose children fall ill?"

Laver's preferred solution was "to have Tamiflu available in every pharmacy in the country where people who needed it, essential workers and others not on the list, could get the drug quickly". He suggested that "a rapid, sensitive and accurate point-of-care diagnostic test for influenza should be available in the pharmacy. So people who think they might have caught the flu, can go immediately to the pharmacy, be rapidly tested, and if positive be given Tamiflu, if negative be denied the drug. As a bonus, people who do have flu, take Tamiflu quickly and recover, should then be immune to re-infection with the same virus for the rest of the epidemic or pandemic" (Treanor et al., 2000).

The Australian Government's NDPS Committee banned OTC sale of oseltamivir on the grounds that it would select resistant mutants of the virus, and diminish the value of the drug for use during a pandemic. On this issue, and over many years, Laver sought to have the OTC ban lifted. As recently as August 2008, in response to the latest refusal to lift the OTC ban, he asked the committee and its staff simple direct questions such as:

"Please explain why the committee believes that if oseltamivir is supplied OTC by a pharmacist to treat genuine influenza, then there will be a greater chance of the virus developing resistance than if oseltamivir is prescribed by a GP?"

"In Australia, how long would "appropriate physical diagnosis" by a GP take? Could this be achieved 6 to 12 hours after symptom onset? Does the committee realise that every hour the virus is replicating, the greater the damage done to the body and the greater the risk of a deadly "cytokine storm". Surely it would be in everybody's interest to stop virus replication as soon as possible".

"What procedure does the committee have in mind to make sure flu victims are able to get really early treatment, if OTC in pharmacies is not allowed?"

"If oseltamivir is taken inappropriately, to treat a common cold for example, then how can this cause the influenza virus to become resistant?"

He seems never to have had satisfactory replies.

It is clear that many of the problems with anti-viral drugs foreseen by Laver are becoming reality. In Australia the drugs are still not sold "over the counter", although in New Zealand they are. Drug resistant strains in influenza virus have come to dominate the H1N1 population of the U.S.A.; in winter 2007/8 only 11% of influenza virus isolates were oseltamivir-resistant, whereas 99% are in 2008/9, although none of the few H3N2 isolates also tested have shown resistance. As a result, the latest (early 2009) advice from the Centers for Disease Control and Prevention, Atlanta, U.S.A. for clinicians (http://www.cdc.gov/flu/professionals/antivirals/) is to use zanamivir or a combination of oseltamivir and rimantadine, as these would provide effective treatment against all known circulating influenza viruses.

The practical difficulties of making vaccines to protect against novel pandemic strains of influenza virus also concerned Laver because a significant time is inevitably required to isolate a virus and then produce adequate quantities of a suitable immunogen for mass vaccination. He suggested that an inactivated virion vaccine should be used, despite problems of toxicity, because it might be produced more quickly and be more effective than a subunit vaccine, and he noted that although a "universal" flu vaccine has been proposed on several occasions, none existed. His views are shared by other virologists and immunologists and many novel vaccines and vaccination strategies are now being discussed and tested (Carter and Plosker, 2008; Doherty and Kelso, 2008; Huber and McCullers, 2008; Nichol and Treanor, 2006; Sui et al., 2009; Zheng et al., 2009).

REFERENCES

Antonovics, J., Hood, M.E. and Baker, C.H. (2006) Was the 1918 flu avian in origin? *Nature* 440, e9.

Aoki, F.Y., Macleod, M.D., Paggiaro, P., Carewicz, O., El Sawy, A., Wat, C., Griffiths, M., Waalberg, E. and Ward, P. (2003) Early administration of oral oseltamivir increases the benefits of influenza treatment. *Journal of Antimicrobial Chemotherapy* 51, 123-129.

Carter, N.J. and Plosker, G.L. (2008) Prepandemic influenza vaccine H5N1 (split virion, inactivated, adjuvanted) [Prepandrix]: a review of its use as an active immunization against influenza A subtype H5N1 virus. *BioDrugs* 22, 279-292.

Collins, P.J., Haire, L.F., Lin, Y.P., Liu, J., Russell, R.J., Walker, P.A., Skehel, J.J., Martin, S.R., Hay, A.J. and Gamblin, S.J. (2008) Crystal structures of oseltamivir-resistant influenza virus neuraminidase mutants. *Nature* 453, 1258-1261.

de Jong, M.D., Thanh, T.T., Khanh, T.H., Hien, V.M., Smith, G.J.D., Chau, N.V., Cam, B.V., Qui, P.T., Ha, D.Q., Guan, Y., Malik Peiris, J.D., Hien, T.T. and Farrar, J. (2005) Oseltamivir resistance during treatment of influenza A (H5N1) infection. *New England Journal of Medicine* 353, 2667-2672.

Doherty, P.C. and Kelso, A. (2008) Toward a broadly protective influenza vaccine. *Journal of Clinical Investigation* 118, 3273-3275.

Gibbs, M.J. and Gibbs, A.J. (2006) Was the 1918 pandemic caused by a bird flu? *Nature* 440, E8.

Hayden, F. (2008) Developing new antiviral agents for influenza treatment: what does the future hold? *Clinical Infectious Diseases* 48, S3–13.

Huber, V.C. and McCullers, J.A. (2008) Vaccines against pandemic influenza: what can be done before the next pandemic? *Pediatric Infectious Disease Journal* 27, Suppl: S113-117.

Kobasa, D., Takada, A., Shinya, K., Hatta, M., Halfmann, P., Theriault, S., Suzuki, H., Nishimura, H., Mitamura, K., Sugaya, N., Usui, T., Murata, T., Maeda, Y., Watanabe, S., Suresh, M., Suzuki, T., Suzuki, Y., Feldmann, H. and Kawaoka, Y. (2004) Enhanced virulence of influenza A viruses with the haemagglutinin of the 1918 pandemic virus. *Nature* 431, 703-707.

Laver, G. and Garman, E. (2002) Pandemic influenza: Its origin and control. *Microbes and Infection* 4, 309-316.

Laver, W.G. (2004) From the Great Barrier Reef to a "cure" for the flu: tall tales but true. *Perspectives in Biology and Medicine* 47, 590-596.

Laver, W.G., Bischofberger, N. and Webster, R.G. (1999) Disarming flu viruses. *Scientific American* 280, 78-87.

Moscona, A. (2005) Oseltamivir resistance — disabling our influenza defenses. *New England Journal of Medicine* 353, 2633-2636.

Nichol, K.L. and Treanor, J.J. (2006) Vaccines for seasonal and pandemic influenza. *Journal of Infectious Diseases* 194, S111–S118.

Potter, C.W. (2001) A history of influenza. *Journal of Applied Microbiology* 91, 572-579.

Sheu, T.G., Deyde, V.M., Okomo-Adhiambo, M., Garten, R.J., Xu, X., Bright, R.A., Butler, E.N., Wallis, T.R., Klimov, A.I. and Gubareva, L.V. (2008) Surveillance for neuraminidase inhibitor resistance among human influenza A and B viruses circulating worldwide from 2004 to 2008. *Antimicrobial Agents and Chemotherapy* 52, 3284–3292.

Sui, J., Hwang, W.C., Perez, S., Wei, G., Aird, D., Chen, L.-M., Santelli, E., Stec, B., Cadwell, G., Ali, M., Wan, H., Murakami, A., Yammanuru, A., Han, T., Cox, N.J., Bankston, L.A., Donis, R.O., Liddington, R.C. and Marasco, W.A. (2009) Structural and functional bases for broad-spectrum neutralization of avian and human influenza A viruses. *Nature Structural and Molecular Biology* doi:10.1038/nsmb.1566.

Taubenberger, J.K., Reid, A.H., Lourens, R.M., Wang, R., Jin, G. and Fanning, T.G. (2005) Characterization of the 1918 influenza virus polymerase genes. *Nature* 437, 889-893.

Treanor, J.J., Hayden, F.G., Vrooman, P.S., Barbarash. R., Bettis, R., Riff, D., Singh, S., Kinnersley, N., Ward, P. and Mills, R.G. (2000) Efficacy and safety of the oral neuraminidase inhibitor oseltamivir in treating acute influenza: a randomized controlled trial. *JAMA* 283, 1016-1024.

Tuvim, M.J., Evans, S.E., Clement, C.G., Dickey, B.F. and Gilbert, B.E. (2009) Augmented lung inflammation protects against influenza A pneumonia. *PLoS ONE* 4, e4176.

Webster, R.G. (2009) Obituary: William Graeme Laver (Graeme) Ph.D. FRS 1929–2008. *Virology* 385, vii-viii.

Zheng, L., Wang, F., Yang, Z., Chen, J., Chang, H. and Chen, Z. (2009) A single immunization with HA DNA vaccine by electroporation induces early protection against H5N1 avian influenza virus challenge in mice. *BMC Infectious Diseases* 9(e17).

In: Global View of Fight against Influenza
Editor: Petar M. Mitrasinovic

ISBN: 978-1-60741-952-5
© 2009 Nova Science Publishers, Inc.

Chapter 3

FLU DRUGS: PATHWAY TO DISCOVERY[*]

Graeme Laver (1929–2008)

IN SHORT

- Isolation and crystallisation of neuraminidase on the surface of influenza virus leads to the first effective drugs for controlling flu
- Chemists identified an active site in the enzyme which when 'plugged' by a drug stopped the enzyme working and the virus multiplying

"Whether or not bird flu will be transmitted from human to human is still not known. If it does, with no effective vaccine available our only defence will be the antiviral drugs Relenza and Tamiflu."

—*Graeme Laver*

Flu, caused by the influenza virus, has plagued mankind for centuries. In 1918–19 the virus, dubbed Spanish flu, killed about 40 million people worldwide. Since then there have been two other major pandemics—in 1957 "Asian flu" killed about two million people and in 1968 "Hong Kong flu" killed about one million people. Of great concern at the moment is a lethal avian influenza virus, or "bird flu", which has killed millions of domestic poultry, some wild birds and some mammals, including humans. To date, however, people infected with this virus have not been able to infect other people. If this virus does manage to adapt genetically to do this, it will spread like wildfire throughout the world and the antivirals Relenza and Tamiflu appear to be our best lines of attack. Here we discover how these drugs were developed and how they can be used effectively.

---

[*] *Education in Chemistry,* Issue 2007 March - Reproduced by permission of The Royal Society of Chemistry

VIRUSES TAKE OVER HOST CELLS

Virus particles are essentially nucleic acid (as RNA/DNA) packed into a protein matrix. All viruses have surface antigens (proteins) that can interact with moieties on the surface of their target cells, and are the means by which the virus gets into the cell. The pandemics of 1957 and 1968 were caused by viruses that had surface antigens to which no one had any immunity, allowing the viruses to spread unhindered throughout the world. The destruction of the host cells and the immune response to the virus give rise to the symptoms of the viral infection. In the case of the influenza virus these are high fever, shivering attacks, muscle pains, headache and a dry cough.

In the 1940s George Hirst, working at the Rockefeller Institute, New York, discovered that the influenza virus could attach to receptors on red blood cells in the cold, causing the cells to clump together. When the virus-red cell complexes were warmed to 37°C the cells dispersed and the virus separated. This happened because of a receptor-destroying enzyme on the surface of the virus. This enzyme was eventually identified as a sialidase or neuraminidase by Alfred Gottschalk at the Walter and Eliza Hall Institute, Melbourne, Australia. Specifically, the enzyme cleaved sialic acid from the receptors, destroying their capacity to bind virus particles. Scientists quickly realised that if a 'poison' could be developed that stopped this enzyme working, it might provide a cure for the flu. It took more than 50 years for this idea to be realised.

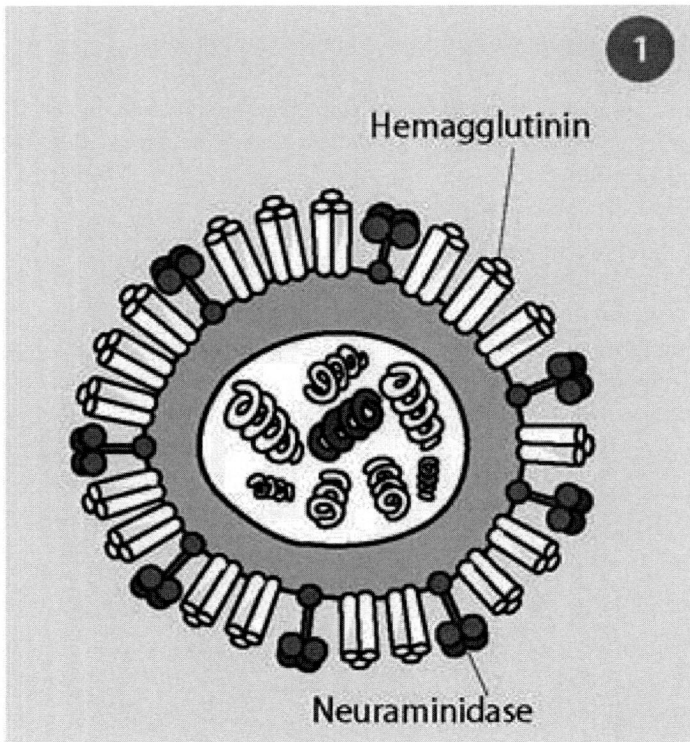

Figure 1. Diagram of the influenza virus, showing surface antigens.

PROGRESS: HAEMAGGLUTININ ANTIGEN IDENTIFIED

Initially scientists thought that the virus bound to cells via an enzyme-substrate interaction. Slowly, this explanation was shown to be incorrect and it was finally proved by Robin Valentine and myself, working at the National Institute for Medical Research, Mill Hill, London, by using electron microscopy, that there were two distinct antigens with different functions on the surface on the influenza virus. One was the glycoprotein, haemagglutinin, which attaches the virus to receptors on the cells, and the other, the enzyme neuraminidase, destroys these receptors and allows the new virus particles to be released from the cells (see Figure 1).

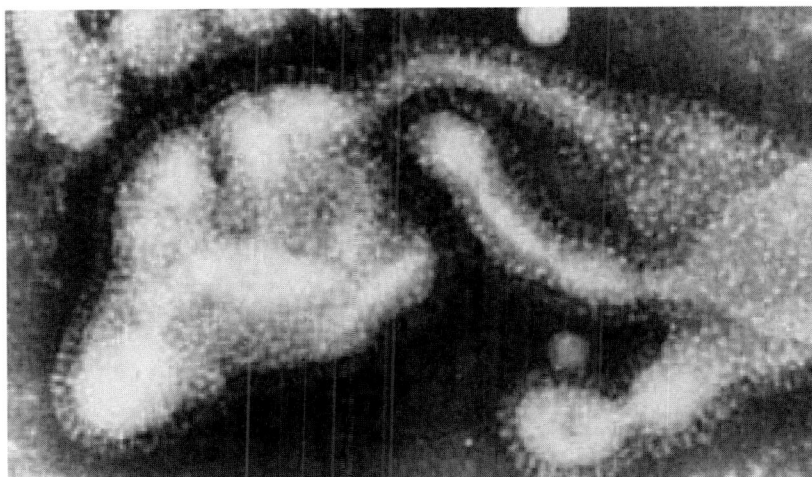

Figure 2. Electron micrograph of influenza virus.

The electron micrographs showed that the influenza virus particles are covered by a layer of surface projections or "spikes" (see Figure 2). These are of two kinds. One of the spikes, a triangular rod-shaped molecule, has haemagglutinin activity, while the other spike, a mushroom-shaped molecule, with a square box-like head sitting on top of long thin stalk, is the enzyme, neuraminidase. The end of the stalk is hydrophobic which allows the neuraminidase to be attached to the lipid membrane of the virus. Each influenza virus particle is covered by about 2000 haemagglutinin and 500 neuraminidase spikes.

The head of the neuraminidase spike, which contains all the enzymic activity of the molecule, can be released from some influenza virus strains by digesting the virus particles with a protease. The released heads can then be purified and in some cases crystallised. In 1978 I grew the first neuraminidase crystals of influenza virus and, five years later, Peter Colman and his colleagues at the CSIRO Division of Protein Chemistry, Melbourne, solved the three dimensional structure by using x-ray diffraction (Figure 3). This structure revealed that the neuraminidase was a tetramer composed of four identical monomers, each containing a single polypeptide chain. In the centre of each monomer was a deep cleft, or canyon able to bind sialic acid. This was the active, catalytic site of the enzyme.

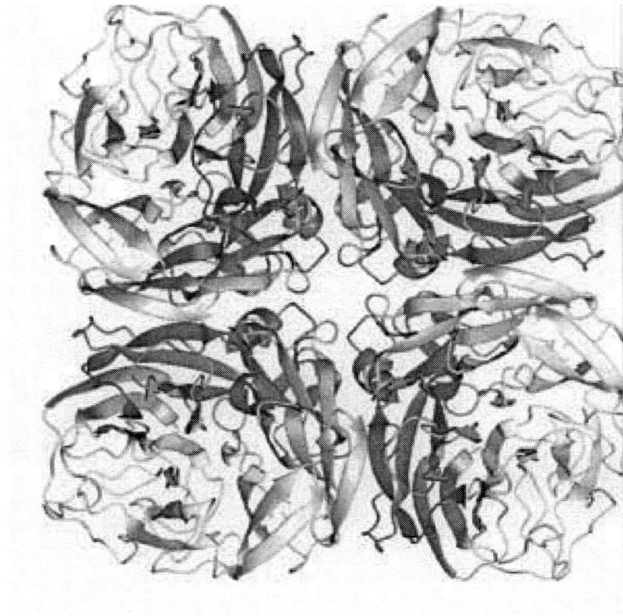

Figure 3. X-ray crystal structure of neuraminidase tetramer.

A CRUCIAL DISCOVERY

It turns out that influenza viruses undergo enormous variation, mainly in the two surface antigens. Because of this influenza vaccines need to be updated every year. To date 16 flu A haemagglutinin subtypes (H1-H16) and nine neuraminidase subtypes (N1-N9) have been found in Nature, some in people, but most in viruses infecting wild water birds. (Note Spanish flu was designated H1N1, Asian flu, H2N2, Hong Kong flu H3N2, and the lethal avian or "bird flu", H5N1).

Within each subtype there are many different strains. The amino acid sequences of the neuraminidase from a variety of different influenza viruses show enormous variation, some sequences being as much as 75 per cent different. Nevertheless, scattered along the neuraminidase polypeptide at various positions were amino acids that were the same for all strains. When the neuraminidase polypeptide folded into its three dimensional structure, these 'conserved' amino acids were seen to be lining the walls of the catalytic site canyon (Figure 4). This meant that if an inhibitor of the enzyme, a "plug drug", could be created for one neuraminidase, it would be effective against the neuraminidase of all influenza viruses, even those which had not yet appeared in humans. This was a crucial discovery.

However, there was little point in trying to develop such a 'plug drug' to treat flu infections unless the neuraminidase played an important role in the replication of the virus. Several experiments by Rob Webster and myself (John Curtin School of Medical Research, Canberra), Rudi Rott (Institut für Virologie, Giessen), and Peter Palese and Dick Compass (Mount Sinai School of Medicine, New York), confirmed that it did. Although inhibiting the neuraminidase did not stop the virus from infecting cells, the activity of the enzyme was essential for newly formed virus particles to be released from infected cells and spread in the body to infect other cells. This is because flu viruses infect cells by first binding to receptors on cells via haemagglutinin. The virus then gains entry to the cell by fusing its membrane with the cell membrane, a process also mediated by the haemagglutinin.

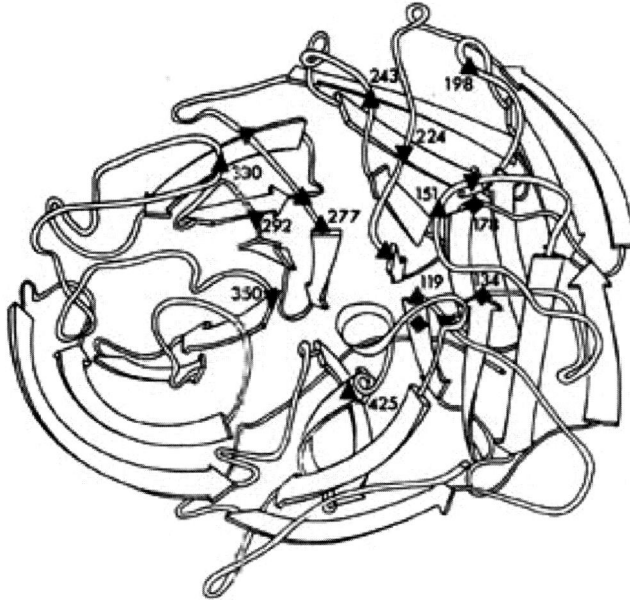

Figure 4. Ribbon diagram of neuraminidase, showing conserved active sites.

The receptors to which the haemagglutinin binds are composed of chains of sugar molecules with terminal sialic acid residues (Figure 5). The neuraminidase removes the sialic acid from the receptors on cells where the virus is replicating, allowing the newly formed virus particles to escape. But these virus particles also have carbohydrate side chains with terminal sialic acid residues, and these also need to be removed to stop the virus particles sticking together. So the function of the neuraminidase is not only to release the virus from infected cells but also to allow it to spread in the body.

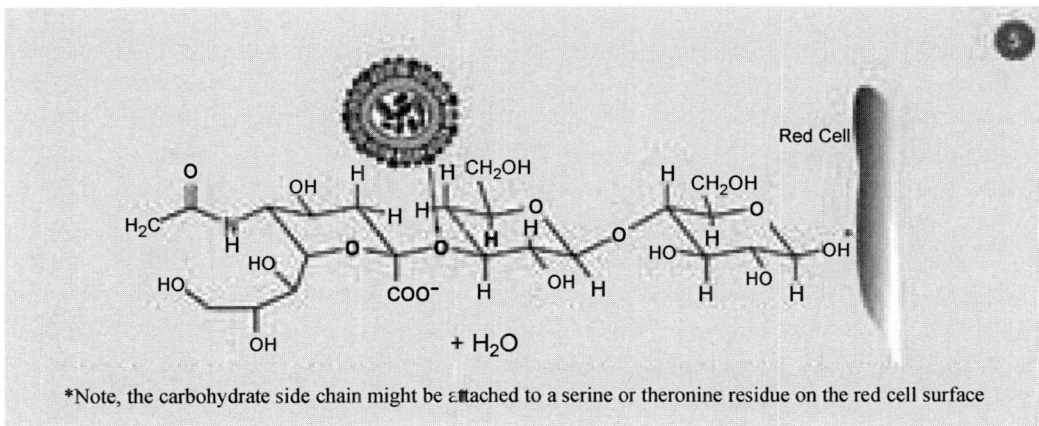

*Note, the carbohydrate side chain might be attached to a serine or theronine residue on the red cell surface

Figure 5. The influenza virus binds via haemagglutinin to terminal sialic acid residues on cell receptors.

RELENZA: THE FIRST "PLUG DRUG"

The first neuraminidase inhibitor, or "plug drug", was created from a knowledge of the crystal structure of a human flu virus neuraminidase, subtype N2. Sialic acid (*N*-acetyl neuraminic acid, NANA) [1], the substrate of neuraminidase, is itself a mild inhibitor of the enzyme but the dehydrated derivative, deoxy-dehydro-*N*-acetyl neuraminic acid, DANA [2], the transition state analogue, is a better inhibitor.

Mark von Itzstein and his colleagues at the Victorian College of Pharmacy in Melbourne used computational chemistry techniques to probe the active site of the enzyme in an attempt to design structurally modified derivatives of DANA that would bind tightly to the amino acids in the catalytic site and so prove to be potent and specific inhibitors of the enzyme. They used the software program GRID to determine energetically favourable interactions between various functional groups and residues in the catalytic site canyon. This showed that there was a negatively charged zone in the neuraminidase active site that aligned with the C4 hydroxyl group of DANA. We therefore replaced this hydroxyl with a positively charged amino group; the 4-amino DANA [3] was 100 times better an inhibitor than DANA, owing to the formation of a salt bridge with a conserved glutamic acid (119) in the active site. They then noticed that Glu 119 was at the bottom of a conserved pocket in the active site, which was just big enough to accommodate a more basic functional positively charged group, such as a guanidino group, that was also larger than the amino group.

Von Itzstein's colleague, Wen Yang Wu, synthesised 4-guanidino DANA [4], and found it to be 1000 times better an inhibitor of flu neuraminidase than DANA, and was specific for the flu enzyme, i.e., it did not inhibit other sialidases found in mammalian cells, some other viruses, bacteria or parasites. 4-Guanidino DANA was named Zanamivir and, after passing clinical trials, is now marketed under the name Relenza.

However, while the presence of the guanidino group made Relenza such a good inhibitor, it also meant it was not orally bioavailable and, if swallowed, was unable to be absorbed from the gut. Relenza therefore had to be administered as a powder that was puffed into the lungs.

TAMIFLU TABLETS

Choung Kim and his colleagues at Gilead Sciences in California then set out to develop a neuraminidase inhibitor that could be swallowed as a pill. Meanwhile, I had organised series of expeditions to Australia's Great Barrier Reef and had isolated, for the first time, a number of avian influenza viruses from wild sea birds, remote from human habitation. One of these viruses had a previously undiscovered neuraminidase, subtype N9, which formed the best crystals of any flu neuraminidase so far examined (Figure 6).

X-ray crystallography of sialic acid bound in this flu neuraminidase showed that the glycerol side chain of the substrate occupied a large pocket in the catalytic site of the neuraminidase protein, made up of a number of hydrophobic amino acids. It also revealed that the C7 position of the sialic acid molecule had no interaction with any of the amino acids in this site. Gilead scientists therefore made carbocyclic sialic acid analogues in which the CHOH group at the C7 position of the glycerol side chain was replaced by an oxygen atom. Then, to create a molecule with hydrophobic groups that would interact well with amino acids in the large hydrophobic pocket, they attached various lipophilic side chains to the oxygen linker that had been introduced at the 7 position.

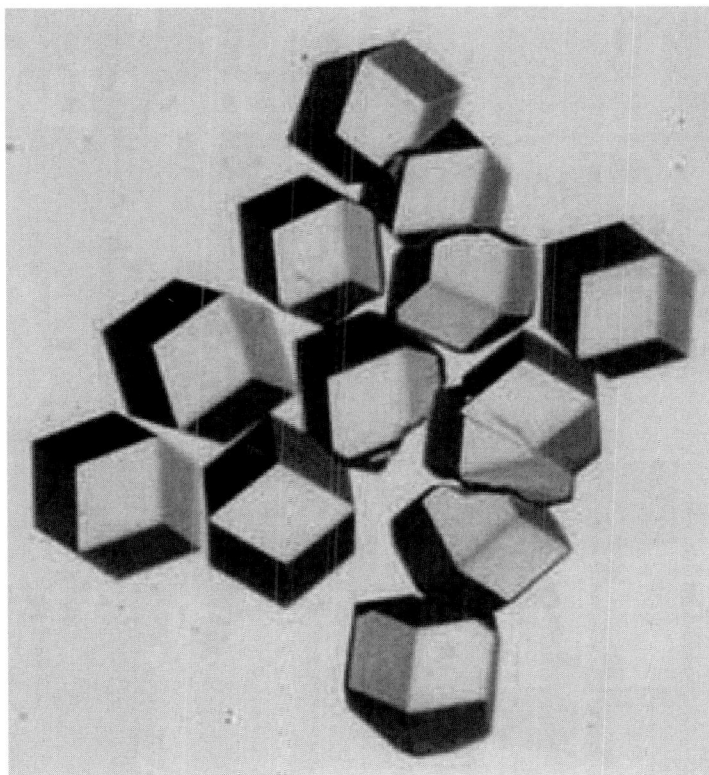

Figure 6. Crystals of neuraminidase 'heads' from bird flu virus.

The carboxylate and acetamido groups corresponding to the same groups on DANA were retained on the new carbocyclic compound and an amino group was introduced at position C4. The final compound chosen, GS4071, had a 3-pentyl side chain and was a potent and specific inhibitor of flu neuraminidase. This compound differed from Relenza in that it was not a sugar, but still suffered from the disadvantage that, because the presence of the amino and carboxyl groups gave it the properties of a zwitterion, it was not orally bioavailable and was unable to be absorbed from the gut.

Gilead scientists solved this problem by converting the carboxyl group to the ethyl ester. The resulting pro-drug, oseltamivir (Tamiflu) can be swallowed as a pill, it is absorbed from the gut and the ester is hydrolysed in the liver to give the active inhibitor that finds its way into the respiratory secretions.

AND FINALLY

Relenza and Tamiflu are safe and effective treatments for influenza, but they need to be given early after the first symptoms appear. Six to 12 hours is ideal. In most countries the drugs can only be obtained with a doctor's prescription, and usually the time taken to get a prescription renders them ineffective. Ideally, they should be available "over-the-counter" in pharmacies without a prescription but only to those people who have genuine influenza. This could be achieved if rapid, sensitive, accurate and inexpensive point-of-care diagnostic tests were also available in pharmacies. Effort is now being put into making this "test and treat" routine procedure for influenza infections throughout the world.

There is the fear that the influenza virus will develop resistance to the drugs. Inappropriate use will not lead to resistance, but widespread appropriate use might. So far, viruses resistant to Tamiflu have arisen in the human population, but these have not yet spread in the community and the hope is that they never will. Time will tell.

Professor Graeme Laver can be contacted at 3047 Barton Highway, Murrumbateman, NSW 2582, Australia (e-mail: graeme.laver@bigpond.com.

REFERENCES

[1]   G. Laver, *Future Virology*, 2006, **1** (5), 577.
[2]   E. Garman and G. Laver, *Current Drug Targets*, 2004, **5**, 119.
[3]   Moscona, *New England J. Med.*, 2005, **353**, 1363.
[4]   M. A. Williams *et al*, *Bioorganic and Med. Chem. Lett.*, 1997, **7**, 1837.

PART II:
VIRUS EVOLUTION AND PATHOGENESIS OF H5N1 INFECTION IN HUMANS

In: Global View of Fight against Influenza
Editor: Petar M. Mitrasinovic

ISBN: 978-1-60741-952-5
© 2009 Nova Science Publishers, Inc.

Chapter 4

ADVANCES IN MOLECULAR EVOLUTION OF INFLUENZA A VIRUS

Xiu-Feng Wan[1,2], Michael Emch[3] and Zi-Ming Zhao[1]*

[1]School of Biology, Georgia Institute of Technology, Atlanta, GA, USA
[2]Department of Basic Sciences, College of Veterinary Medicine,
Mississippi State University, MS, USA
[3]Department of Geography, University of North Carolina, Chapel Hill, NC, USA

ABSTRACT

Influenza A viruses are known for their rapid mutations, frequent reassortments, and RNA recombinations. The availability of the genomic sequences provides an opportunity for us to understand evolutionary process better than in the past. In this chapter, we will review recent research progresses and challenges in molecular evolution for both seasonal influenza and avian influenza viruses. The topics discussed include positive selection, reassortant identification, genotyping, RNA recombination, and the molecular clock in influenza A virus. Both common and uncommon features of previous pandemic strains, seasonal influenza viruses, swine influenza viruses, avian influenza viruses (especially H5N1), and other influenza A viruses are reviewed. The challenges for influenza molecular evolution studies will also be discussed.

1. INTRODUCTION

Influenza A virus is a negative-stranded RNA virus that belongs to the *Orthomyxoviridae* family [1]. Influenza A virus has eight genomic segments with varying lengths from about 890 to 2,341 nucleotides which encode at least 11 proteins. Influenza A virus has three major evolutionary events: mutation, reassortment, and recombination. The mutations in the influenza surface proteins HA and NA are also referred to as antigenic drift, since the mutations can cause a change of antigenicity, thus making vaccines ineffective. The muta-

---

* Correspondence to: wanhenry@yahoo.com or wan@cvm.msstate.edu.

tions in internal segments may increase their compatibility, thus, viral fitness. The mutations in NA or M genes may also lead to the resistance of influenza to drugs, such as Amantadine/rimantadine and Oseltamivir (Tamiflu). Genetic reassortment refers to the exchange of one or more discrete RNA segments into multipartite viruses, and it occurs frequently between influenza A viruses and between influenza B viruses [2-6]. Reassortments between two co-infecting influenza A viruses can possibly generate 2^8 genotypes in their offspring (Figure 1). Recombination will be referred to insertion or exchange of RNA fragment between influenza segments or between influenza segment and other RNA sources, e.g., host 28s ribosomal RNA [7]. It has been accepted that mutations and recombinations in influenza viruses facilitate the emergence of highly pathogenic strains, while genetic reassortment speeds generation of pandemic influenza strains. The alternation or combination of these evolutionary events lead to a rapid emergence of novel flu genotypes [8-11].

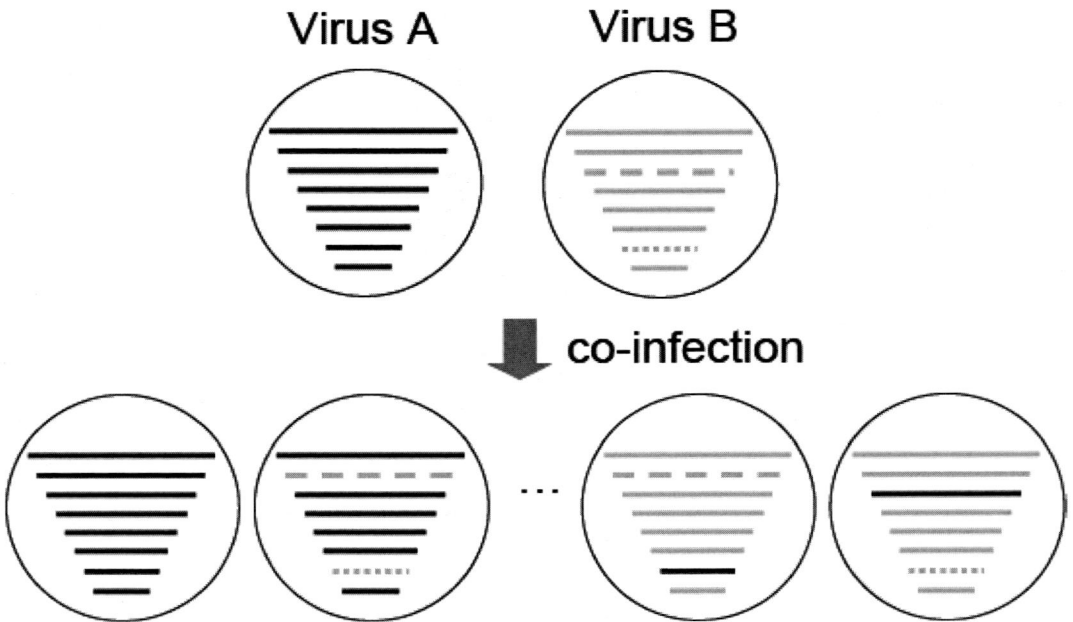

Figure 1. The reassortment occurs between two co-infected influenza viruses.

Evolutionary analyses of the influenza A virus have focused on unveiling these three types of evolutionary events and their association with either an epidemiological or ecological question. Availability of the genomic sequences provides a great opportunity for us to understand these evolutionary processes much better than in the past. These studies have broadened our knowledge of influenza biology and retrospectively have helped us design better influenza surveillance programs, select vaccine strains more effectively, and make a better plan for influenza prevention and control.

In this chapter, we review the advances in technologies and tools used to investigate influenza molecular evolution as well as major findings using these methods. The topics discussed include positive selection, reassortant identification, genotyping, RNA recombination, and the molecular clock in influenza A virus. Both common and uncommon features of previous pandemic strains, seasonal influenza viruses, avian influenza viruses (especially H5N1), and other types of influenza A viruses, such as swine influenza viruses, equine and canine influenza viruses are reviewed. Challenges in influenza molecular evolution studies will also be discussed.

2. ADVANCES IN COMPUTATIONAL TECHNOLOGIES FOR INFLUENZA EVOLUTIONARY ANALYSES

2.1. Phylogenetic Reference

Numerous computational tools have been developed for molecular evolution. Based on the distance and tree construction methods, these tools can be categorized into neighbor-joining, parsimony, minimum evolution, maximum likelihood, and Bayesian methods. The comparisons of these tools are reviewed in Holder and Lewis [12]. More than 400 phylogeny packages and Web servers are listed in Dr. Joseph Felsenstein's collection: http://evolution. genetics.washington.edu/phylip/software.html. During the past decade, these tools have been explored and applied widely in influenza evolutionary analyses. Before phylogenetic tree construction, users generally had to generate a multiple sequence alignment using software such as Clustal W [13], T-coffee [14], MUSCLE [15] or other multiple sequence alignment programs. It is well known that multiple sequence alignment is not trivial task, and the accuracy of multiple sequence alignments is less than 70% in simulation analysis [16, 17]. However, the divergence in influenza A virus sequences is relatively low and these generally do not have a problem in obtaining a reliable alignment, although inaccurate alignments among regions with deletions, such as cleavage sites in HA, are not uncommon. In practice, we need to manually examine alignments to ensure the accuracy of these regions. We may even align protein sequences first and revert back to nucleotide sequence alignments.

During the past five years, the number of influenza sequences has been increasing at an exponential rate. Until February 18 of 2009, the influenza virus resource (http://www. ncbi.nlm.nih.gov/genomes/FLU/FLU.html) included 18,137 HA sequences of the influenza A virus. None of the available sequence alignment and phylogenetic programs is suitable for analyses of such a large number of sequences. Thus, it is common to select prototype sequences for evolutionary analyses, and this selection, without proper computational assistance, may lead to a biased phylogeny inference and incorrect biological conclusion. *Basic Local Alignment Search Tool* (BLAST) [18] is a common tool used to identify sequences with high similarity. However, BLAST is not a phylogenetic program but a basic local alignment search tool and therefore should not be used for influenza genotyping (section 2.2).

Recently, we presented a new distance measurement based on complete composition vector (CCV) and applied it to influenza studies [19-22] as well as bacteria [23], HIV [24], and foot-and-mouth disease virus [25]. Our study showed that CCV accurately assessed the genetic distances between influenza viruses and that the phylogenetic tree from CCV reflected a similar topology as the tree from a multiple sequence alignment [22]. Since CCV computes the distance based on the distance between string probability and expected probability from nucleotide frequency, CCV distance measurements are more robust and the genetic distance between viruses will not vary even if the number of taxa increases. Thus, CCV is very suitable for prototype sequence selection as well influenza phylogeny analyses.

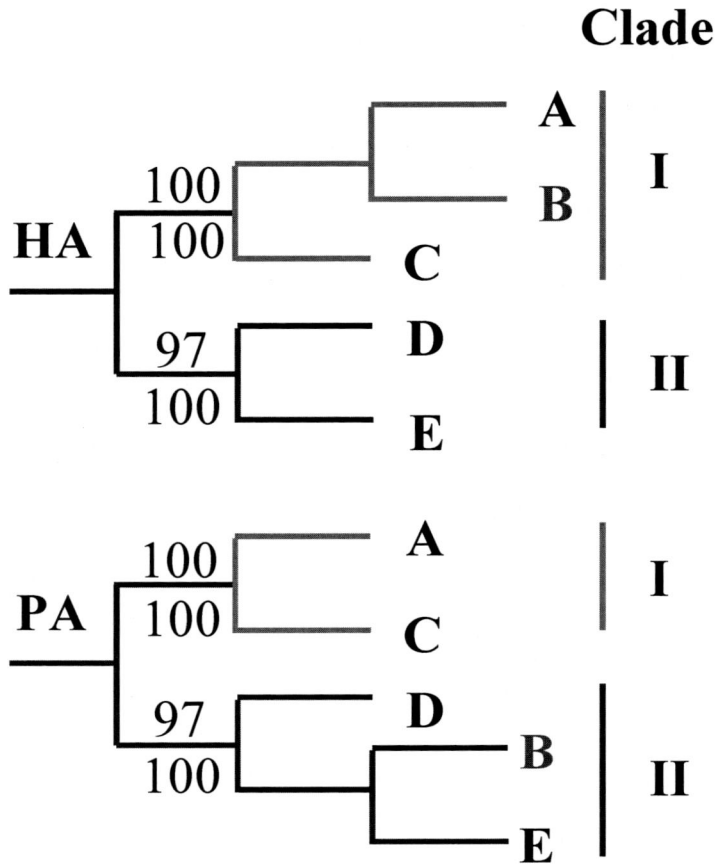

Figure 2. Reassortment identification based on conflicts of phylogenetic tree topologies.

2.2. Reassortant Detection and Influenza Genotyping

The traditional approach to reassortment identification generally involves two steps: (1) phylogenetic inference as described in the previous section; and (2) tree topology analyses. The conflicting tree topologies between gene segments will be identified as potential reassortments. In Figure 2, HA genes of virus A, B, and C form lineage I while HA genes of virus D and E form lineage II. However, PB2 gene of virus B, D, and E are grouped into the same lineage. Thus, there is a reassortment event in either the HA or PB2 gene of virus B. The bootstrap value and/or the Bayesian posterior probability are usually used in statistical assessment. Generally, the bootstrap value has a less risk in supporting a false phylogenetic hypothesis than Bayesian posterior probability [26]. The determination of donor and receptor genes during reassortment analyses will depend on not only phylogenetic tree topology but also the spatio-temporal information of associated virus strains. At some cases, influenza subtypes are used as simple criteria for evaluation of reassortment events. For instance, if an internal gene in H5N1 avian influenza virus is located with a clade of H9N2 avian influenza virus, a potential reassortment will be proposed.

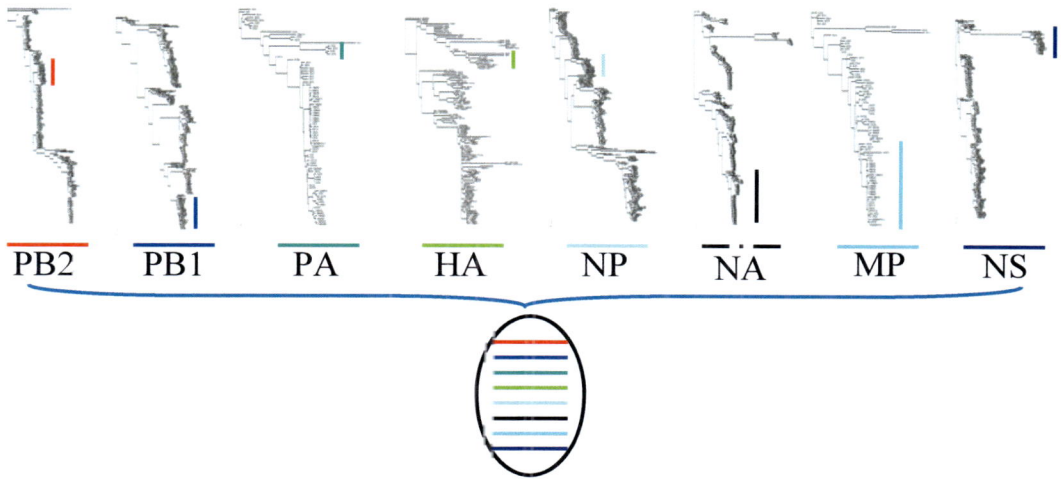

Figure 3. Influenza genotyping involves analyses of phylogenetic trees for all eight segments.

Generally speaking, the influenza genotyping process involves phylogenetic analyses (reassortment, mutation, and recombination) of all eight individual influenza segments. The distinct combination of individual genetic information will be assigned a genotype (Figure 3). For instance, if there is a reassortment event within two viruses that are compared, these two viruses will be assigned into two distinct genotypes. Such a genotyping procedure is time consuming and depends heavily on the prototype sequences selected from the database. Thus, it is not unusual that the analyses from different laboratories, or even the analyses from the same laboratory but with different datasets, have conflicting results.

In order to overcome the limitations in the traditional genotyping method, we proposed a new quantitative genotyping system based on CCV and module identification [22]. This method is based on a hypothesis that influenza viruses form normal distributions in a hierarchical order (Figure 4). Figure 4A shows the Bayesian analyses of HA genes of H5N1 highly pathogenic avian influenza viruses, which form five peaks indicating five levels of overlapping normal distributions [22]. As shown in Figure 4B, the genetic distance between influenza viruses within the pink squares may form a normal distribution. The viral populations in different peak squares form normal distributions with similar means and standard deviations. Similarly, the viruses in yellow squares form normal distributions but with a larger mean value. If the normal distributions for the viruses in pink squares correspond to pink peak in Figure 4A, the normal distributions for the viruses in yellow squares may correspond to yellow peak in Figure 4A. This hierarchical genotyping schema may reflect Darwinian natural selection and adaptation responding to different ecological niches [22]. This quantitative genotyping strategy automates the genotyping process for the first time. The disadvantage of this method is that the module identification is computationally intensive.

A.

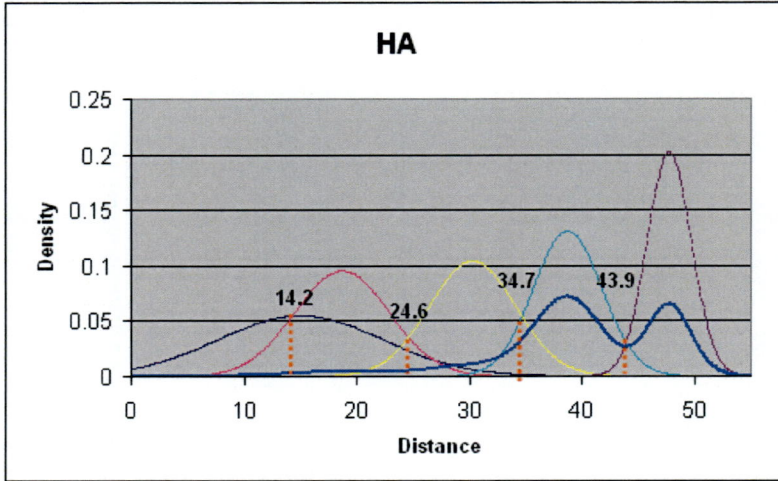

B.

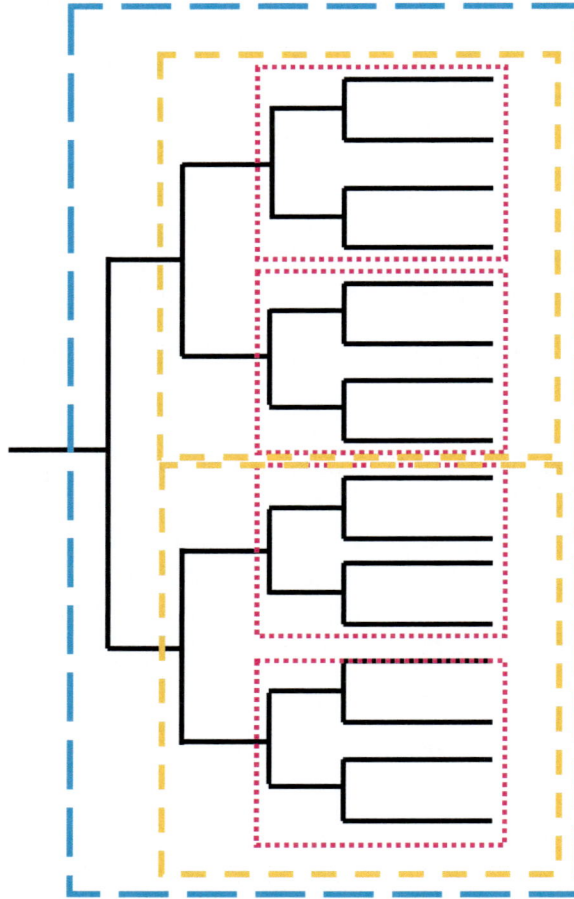

Figure 4. Influenza A virus forming hierarchical normal distributions during molecular evolution (A). The taxa with the same color (B) have a similar normal distribution.

Recently, we have developed another new reassortment identification algorithm using a clustering algorithm based on minimum spanning tree (MST) methods [21]. MST algorithms have a unique advantage over most of the other clustering algorithms in which we do not need to define the number of clusters before the clustering process. In addition to being a very efficient method for clustering, MST algorithms can handle any shapes of clusters even with the background noise created by the outlier points. Thus, it is fit for influenza reassortment identification and genotype analysis since we are not sure how many genotypes are present in nature. Interestingly, we found that the results from MST were similar to those in module identification when analyzing HA of H5N1 highly pathogenic avian influenza viruses. Using this newly constructed method, we identified 34 potential reassortment clusters among 2,641 PB2 segments of influenza A viruses [21]. Among the 83 serotypes tested, at least 56 serotypes (67.46%) exchanged their fragments with another serotype of avian influenza viruses. More frequent reassortments were found to occur in wild birds, especially migrating birds.

2.3. Recombination Detection

Influenza recombination includes both homologous recombination and non-homologous recombination. Non-homologous recombination has been shown to connect the peptide region between HA1 and HA2, which can affect the cleavability of HA and thus the infectivity and pathogenesis of the virus [7, 27, 28]. For instance, an H7N3 avian influenza outbreak in Chile was caused by recombination between HA and NP genes of the H7N3 avian influenza virus [29], and another outbreak in British Columbia was caused by recombination between HA and M genes in H7N3 avian influenza virus [30]. There are a few reported homologous recombination cases for avian influenza viruses H5N1 and H9N2 [31], swine influenza H1N2 and H2N2 [32], and seasonal influenza virus H1N1 and H3N2 [32, 33]. The 1918 Spanish flu H1N1 virus was shown to be a recombinant from swine and avian influenza viruses [34, 35]. However, this still remains unclear since others argue this might not be from recombination but unequal evolutionary rates [36]. Thus, the recombination in influenza A viruses seems to be much less clear than two other evolutionary events, mutation and reassortment.

As a single negative-strand RNA virus, influenza A virus was reported to have a low homologous recombination rate [33]. It was proposed that the association of ribonucleoprotein complex with viral RNA might prevent polymerase from switching templates during replication [37]. Two other hypotheses have also been proposed for the rare homologous recombination cases in influenza viruses: (1) homologous recombination needs at least two co-infected viruses; (2) most recombinants may be more deleterious or less fit than the clonal replicates [38]. However, frequent reassortments in influenza viruses show that it is not uncommon for two influenza viruses to co-infect the same cell. Thus, it is still not clear why the recombination rate is low or rare in influenza. On the other hand, we may not eliminate the biases from the limitations of current detection methods, which may show inconsistent results for the same dataset.

The challenges for recombination detection include at least two factors: recombination of short sequences and homologous genetic background in parental strains. Although many different recombination programs are available, recombination of short fragments, e.g. less than 100 nucleotides, are still not trivial since less information can be used in such short sequences to differentiate divergence of genetic origin. Influenza viruses are generally short, and the longest segment is up to 2,342 nucleotides. Thus, it is especially challenging to detect recombination in influenza viruses. When the parental strains are genetically homologous, it will be difficult to identify the recombination in their recombinant. During influenza outbreaks, many co-infected viruses could have originated from the same introduction. Thus, recombination events could be missed during the analysis.

During the past two decades, various methods have been proposed to detect genome recombination, including viral RNA recombination. Based on Posada et al. [39], these recombination detection methods may be classified into five categories, namely *similarity*, *distance*, *phylogenetic*, *compatibility*, and *nucleotide substitution distribution* methods. *Similarity* methods detect recombination by calculating synonymous substitutions. If the synonymous substitutions within a region are more frequent than the average, this region would be the recombination region. These methods are only appropriate for coding region analysis. *Distance* methods, such as PhylPro [40] and DIVERT [41], predict recombination by using a sliding window to estimate genetic distances. These categories of methods are computationally efficient since they do not need to construct phylogeny trees. The *phylogenetic* methods, such as SplitsTree [42], TOPAL [43], SIMPLOT [44], RDP [45], PLATO [46], RECPARS [47], and TRIPLE [48], predict recombination by detecting conflicting phylogeny tree topologies. The detailed strategies are quite similar to those in reassortment detection using a phylogenetic tree, but recombination detection uses adjacent sequences to construct phylogenetic trees whereas reassortment employs entire gene segments. The *compatibility* methods, such as Reticulate [49] and Partition matrix (PM) [50], detect recombination on a site-by-site basis. PM generates a partition matrix by determining the consistency of parsimoniously informative sites in a set of aligned sequences with binary partitions inferred from the sequences. *Substitution distribution* methods either check a cluster of substitutions with or without an expected statistical distribution. These methods include GENECONV [51], HOMOPLASY TEST [52], PIST [53], RUNS TEST [54], LARD [55], and DualBrothers [56]. Recently, Boni et al.[57] developed a non-parametric method, called 3SEQ, which groups the sequences into triplets and assesses a null hypothesis that the evolutionary history of this triplet is clonal. 3SEQ [57] is suitable for detecting recombinations in a large number of sequences, which is usually the case for influenza viruses.

2.4. Mutation and Positive Selection Detection

The lack of fidelity in RNA polymerases generates a high number of variants during RNA replication. These random mutations form quasispecies. However, many of these mutations are lethal and would not survive the influenza life cycle. If it does not lead to an amino acid change, this mutation is synonymous. Otherwise, the mutation is non-synonymous. Non-synonymous mutations can result from either random mutations or natural selection by environmental stimuli faced by viruses. For each codon, if the rate of synonymous substitutions (dS) is larger than that of non-synonymous substitutions (dN), the selection will be negative; if dS is smaller than dN, the selection will be positive; otherwise, the selection will be neutral.

The strain with positive selection may have fitness advantages over other viruses under negative or neutral selection. The surface proteins HA and NA of human influenza virus were likely positively selected by human immune system [58]. These positively selected sites will help influenza virus escape the immunological protection. The immunological selection can be validated *in vitro* by presenting monoclonal antibody in viral cultures, and the resulting mutants *in vitro* are also called escape mutants [59]. Positive selections have been widely present in seasonal influenza viruses H3N2 [60-64], avian influenza viruses H5N1 [20, 65-67] and H9N2 [68]. However, rare positive selections have been reported in seasonal influenza H1N1 [62, 63, 69]. Most of the positively selected sites detected in HA are located in antigenic sites. The positive selections are also found in internal genes, and these are believed to increase viral fitness and compatibility between influenza segments [64].

Many methods have been developed for positive selection analysis and applied in influenza viruses. The basic idea is to estimate the dS/dN ratio, which is commonly denoted as ω. However, the variations from these predictions may result from the difference between statistical methods. Most of these methods were proposed to target individual amino acid sites. These methods can be categorized into parsimony [58, 70], likelihood [71-74], and Bayesian [75, 76] methods. Comparison between these methods showed that parsimony methods were more reliable [77, 78]. The assumption for positive selection is for a single codon change at the third position of the codon, which may result in an amino acid change or no amino acid change. The aforementioned methods do not consider the gene splicing cases in influenza viruses, in which two proteins may be encoded by overlapping but frame shifted segments. The known pairs include NS1 and NS2, M1 and M2, and PB1 and PB1-F. A method has been developed for detecting positive selection among these overlapping genes [79]. Their studies suggest this method may reduce the false positive rate of positive selection prediction for these overlapping genes. Since the positive selection in proteins may not be independent, methods have been developed to target positive selection within certain regions in linear sequence [80] or 3D structure [81]. The 3D window analysis was shown to be more sensitive than single-site analysis and 1D window analysis when analyzing the positive selections in influenza H3N2 HA and NA genes [81]. The details of the statistical methods are beyond the scope of this chapter.

PAML (http://abacus.gene.ucl.ac.uk/software/paml.html) is one of the most commonly used software package for estimating dS/dN. PAML allows incorporation of nucleotide-based models and amino acid-based likelihood analysis with rate variation among sites.

2.5. Evolutionary Rate Estimation and Molecular Clock

Evolutionary rate estimation is based on two assumptions that the viruses in the analyses should be from a single introduction and that these viruses have been present in the same host population for a long enough period. The second assumption is critical since influenza viruses may not always have a consistent evolutionary speed in different host species. For instance, influenza A virus may have a relatively slower evolutionary rate in avian hosts than mammal hosts. Within the natural reservoirs, feral waterfowl and shorebirds, influenza A virus was shown to reach evolutionary stasis [82]. There were a few cases of "frozen evolution" [83] [19], which indicates that the viral genomes remain highly similar or even identical over a long time period, probably due to frozen replication. For instance, we recently determined that the NP gene in H5N1 avian influenza virus was identical to NP gene segments from the H6N2 ad H2N2 avian influenza virus isolated in Hong Kong about 30 years ago[19]. During the disease outbreak period, influenza virus is more likely to have a faster evolutionary rate since the viruses have a higher replication rate by spreading to more hosts. The H3 of human seasonal influenza A virus has an evolutionary rate over 5.7×10^{-3} substitutions/nucleotide per year [84]. The H5 and N1 of H5N1 highly pathogenic avian influenza virus have a evolutionary rate of 4.77×10^{-3} and 5.19×10^{-3} substitutions/nucleotide per year, respectively [85].

To estimate the molecular clock, we typically hypothesize that influenza viruses have a constant evolutionary rate over all branches of the phylogenetic tree. Recently, the software package BEAST implements two other options, the uncorrelated lognormal relaxed clock and the uncorrelated exponential relaxed clock. These two new hypotheses allow evolutionary rates to vary along branches within lognormal and exponential distributions [86]. Many other models have also been proposed for molecular clock estimates [87]. In general, to obtain a reliable result, we will need to compare the results from different models.

Our recent study showed that Gs/Gd/96-like viruses and other H5N1 highly pathogenic avian influenza viruses are related to the viruses detected earlier [88]. A/swan/ Hokkaido/51/96(H5N3) and A/duck/Hokkaido/55/96(H1N1) were detected in Japan in 1996 while A/goose/Guangdong/1/1996 (Gs/Gd/96-1) and A/goose/Guangdong/2/1996 (Gs/Gd/96-2) were identified in southern China during the same year. The phylogenetic analyses showed these viruses shared the same progenitor genes (e.g., HA or NA) from A/turkey/England/50-92/91 (H5N1)-like virus. The nucleotide substitution models for ML and NJ were selected using MODELTEST 3.7 [89]. Time divergence estimation using PAML[72] and Multidivtime [90] showed that H5 of A/swan/Hokkaido/51/96 (H5N3) and Gs/Gd/96-1 diverged about 4 years ago (Figure 5A), and that N1 of A/duck/Hokkaido/55/96(H1N1) and Gs/Gd/96-1 diverged about 2.3 years ago (Figure 5B).

A.

HA

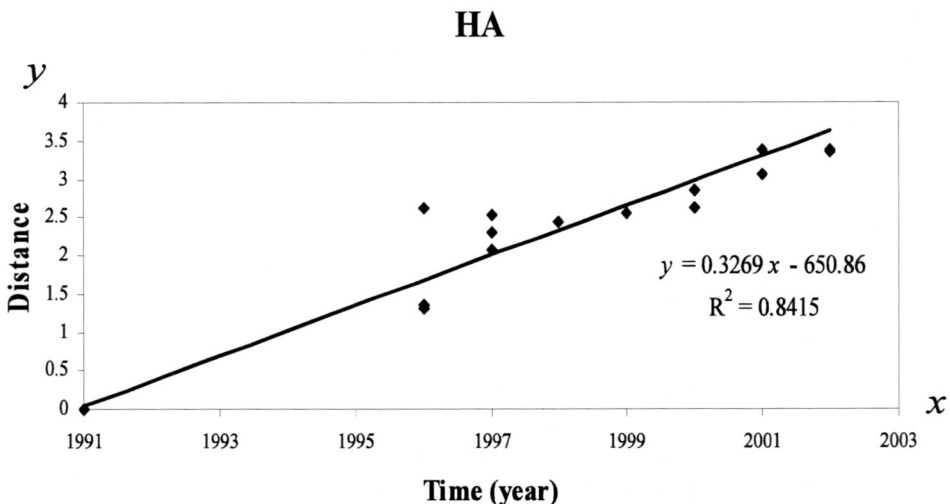

$$y = 0.3269 x - 650.86$$
$$R^2 = 0.8415$$

Time (year)

B.

NA

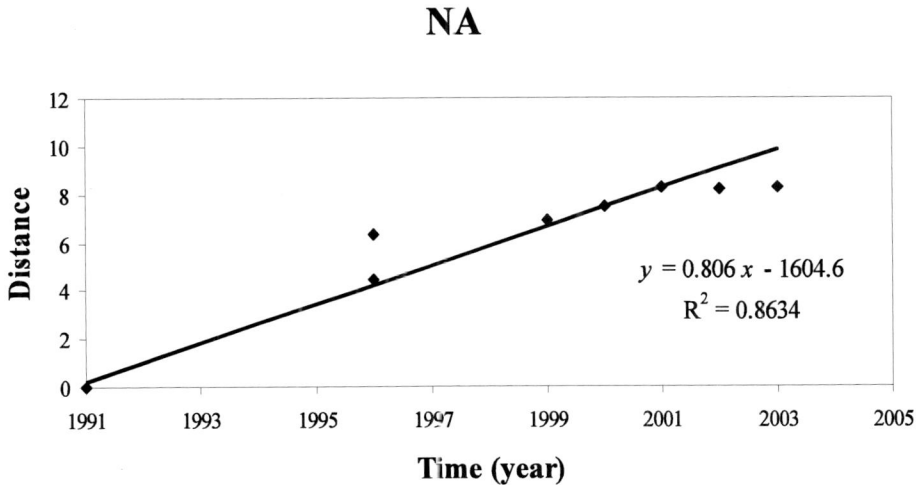

$$y = 0.806\,x - 1604.6$$
$$R^2 = 0.8634$$

Figure 5. Divergent time of HA (A) and NA (B) genes of H5N1 avian influenza virus from their putative precursor virus A/turkey/England/52-92/1991 (H5N1).

2.6. Predictive Influenza Evolution

One of the most important goals for molecular evolutionary studies is to predict future evolution based on current sequence data. This type of prediction may be useful in vaccine strain selection. However, this task is non-trivial due to two factors: (1) unknown selective pressure in nature and (2) sequence sampling biases (section 4). Though, Bush et al. (1999) [61] showed that, using a retrospective test, they can predict whether a HA lineage would more likely be circulating in the future. Their predictions were based on the number of positively selected codons at antigenic site A/B or a receptor binding site. Their results also showed that the strain with a fast mutation rate does not necessarily have better fitness and that the positive selections on the sites other than antigenic binding will have less impact on the viral fitness. The results were exciting but the test was not designed to predict an epidemic strain causing influenza outbreak.

3. PROGRESS IN EVOLUTIONARY STUDIES OF INFLUENZA A VIRUS

3.1. Pandemic Influenza

In the last century, three influenza pandemics occurred in 1918, 1957, and 1968, respectively. These diseases have caused millions of deaths and dramatic economic losses. Although the origin of the 1918 H1N1 influenza virus is still debated (as shown in section 2.3), it is generally accepted that the H1N1 influenza virus is related to avian influenza viruses. Both the 1957 H2N2 and 1968 H3N2 influenza pandemic strains were reassortants from the circulating H1N1 strains before 1957 [91]. H2N2 pandemic strains probably emerged from H2N2 avian influenza virus (PB1, HA, NA) and H1N1 human influenza virus (PB2, PA, NP, MP, and NS); H3N2 pandemic influenza virus might be a reassortment from H3 avian influenza virus (HA, PB1) and circulating H2N2 human influenza virus (PB2, PA, NA, NP, MP, and NS).

What will cause next pandemic influenza virus is a critical question not only for influenza scientists but also for the general public. It is unclear whether future pandemic influenza viruses will be an avian influenza virus, for instance, H5N1 and H9N2 avian influenza virus, a reassortant between avian influenza virus and a contemporary human influenza virus, or other subtypes of the influenza A virus. The reassortants between A/Hong Kong/486/97 (H5N1) (HA and NA) and A/Victoria/3/75 (H3N2) (6 internal genes) were not able to cause transmission between ferrets [92]. The 63 laboratory reassortants between A/Thailand/ 16/2004 (H5N1) and A/Wyoming/3/2003 (H3N2) showed that these two viruses are compatible in vitro but only 13 of them are virulent to mice [93].

3.2. Seasonal Influenza

During the past three decades, seasonal influenza epidemics were mainly caused by H3N2 and H1N1 influenza A virus, and influenza B virus. H3N2 influenza virus is related to the 1968 pandemic influenza virus and H1N1 virus to the 1977 influenza epidemics. During the past 10 seasons in US, three were H1N1. In the 2008–2009 season, H1N1 virus is more prevalent than H3N2. Many papers have been published regarding to the evolution of seasonal influenza viruses. Here we only discuss some recent discoveries in H3N2 and H1N1 evolution.

3.2.1. Antigenic Drift and Shift

Since 1968, H3N2 viruses were shown to have similar evolutionary trends: the phylogeny of HA of these viruses has a major trunk, and emerging genotypes always replaced the previously circulating one although multiple clusters may be present in the same season [61, 63]. Although the genetic evolution of HA is gradual, the antigenic evolution is punctuated [94, 95]. Such an evolutionary character is related to human host immunity. The positive selections are discussed in the previous section. The antigenic drift in H1N1 is less than H3N2, and there were rare positive selections identified in the H1N1 virus.

The availability of complete genomes of influenza viruses gave us a better opportunity to study the correlation between influenza evolution and epidemic outbreaks. There have been reassortments between co-circulating genotypes of H3N2 or H1N1 viruses [96-98]. The H3N2 and H1N1 outbreaks were complicated with these reassortment events and periodic selective sweep [97, 99].

3.2.2. Emergence of H3N2 Virus Not Grown in Chicken Embryonic Eggs

Because A/Fujian/411/2002 (H3N2)-like viruses were not able to grow in chicken embryonic eggs, the 2003/2004 vaccine did not include A/Fujian/411/2002 (H3N2)-like viruses and this results in ineffectiveness of prevention of H3N2 outbreaks. Although the structural changes from the mutations in these viruses have not been determined, mutagenesis studies show that the mutations in HA or HA and NA positions (e.g., G186V/V226I, H183L/V226A [100] or G186V, S219F, V226I, V309I in HA and E119Q, Q136K in NA

[101]) may reduce the growth ability in chicken embryonic eggs. Two residue HA (H155T, Q156H) were reported to be responsible for the antigenic drift from A/Panama/2007/99 to A/Fujian/411/02-like influenza viruses, and these two mutations also affect the growth ability of A/Fujian/411/02-like in chicken embryonic eggs [102].

3.2.3. Emergence of Drug Resistance Strains

Adamantane/rimantadine resistance in influenza A viruses is not new. The adamantine resistance in influenza A gene is related to a single residue S31N in M2 gene. The global surveillance showed that adamantine resistance strains were less than 1% before 1995 [103]. However, in 2004, the H3N2 adamantine strains rose up to 12.3% worldwide and in 2005 to 92% in US [104]. These H3N2 resistance strains belong to a single lineage. Since adamantine is not used frequently in many countries, it is more likely this emergence comes not from selective pressure but fitness mutations, which was probably related to 4 + 4 reassortment events in these viruses [105]. Additional 17 mutations across viral genomes were also identified along with S31N.

Oseltamivir (Tamiflu) resistance is another emerging problem for influenza prevention and treatment. Oseltamivir resistance is related to residue H274Y (H275Y in N1) in NA. From November 2007 to January 2008, oseltamivir resistant H1N1 strains were approximately 14% in Europe [106]. These resistant strains have spread globally since then. During the 2008–2009 influenza season, more than 98.5% of H1N1 isolates were oseltamivir resistant in the US [107]. Due to lack of wide usage of oseltamivir, current oseltamivir resistance might have resulted from fitness mutations.

3.3. Avian Influenza Viruses

3.3.1. H5N1 Highly Pathogenic Avian Influenza Virus

3.3.1.1. Emergence of H5N1 Highly Pathogenic Avian Influenza Virus from Low Pathogenic Avian Influenza Virus

In May 1996, the first two H5N1 highly pathogenic avian influenza viruses causing current pandemic threats, A/goose/Guangdong/1/96(H5N1) (Gs/Gd/96-1) and A/goose/Guangdong/2/96(H5N1) (Gs/Gd/96-2) (so called Gs/Gd/96-like viruses), were identified from farmed geese at Guangdong, China [108]. One year later, in late April and May of 1997, two outbreaks with high mortality were reported in chicken farms located in northwestern area of Hong Kong [109]. The first human case of H5N1 avian influenza was confirmed in May of 1997 and 17 more in November and December of 1997. This led to the depopulation of about 1.5 million birds in Hong Kong. In 1999, H5N1 highly pathogenic avian influenza viruses reemerged in waterfowl in Hong Kong [110]. In February 2003, two human cases were confirmed caused by an H5N1 genetic variant in Hong Kong. Since the end of 2003, the disease has spread all over eastern and southeastern Asia [111]. In May of 2005, another H5N1 genetic variant was identified in Qinghai Lake [112] and has since spread to the Mideast, Europe, and Africa. These viruses have also caused enormous outbreaks in birds, million of which, including both wild and domestic birds, have been culled or died of the disease. By March 8 of 2009, H5N1 highly pathogenic avian influenza viruses have also caused 409 laboratory confirmed human cases, 256 of which were fatal [113]. The fear of influenza pandemic has been increasing along with the increasing number of human cases caused by these H5N1 avian influenza viruses.

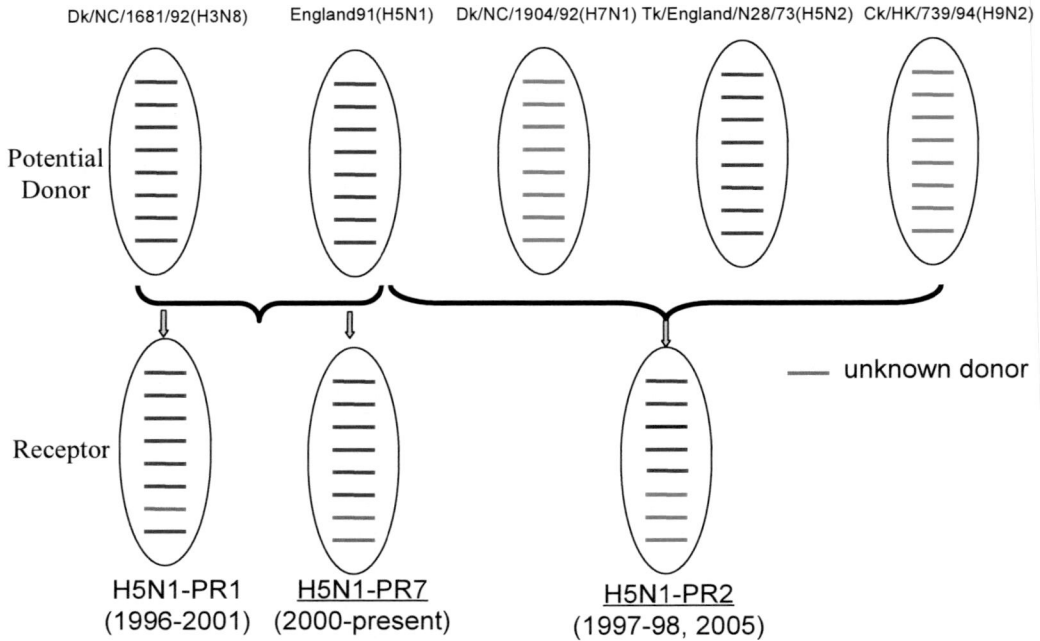

Figure 6. Simplified diagram showing reassortments involved in generation of three genotypes (H5N1-PR1, H5N1-PR2, and H5N1-PR7) of H5N1 highly pathogenic avian influenza viruses.

Recently, we have attempted to track down the progenitor genes for Gs/Gd/96-like viruses [88]. Our results showed that both HA and NA genes of current H5N1 highly pathogenic avian influenza viruses were likely derived from A/turkey/England/50-92/91(H5N1) (E91-like viruses). However, the possible progenitor genes for five other genes, including PB2, PB1, PA, NP and NS, were from A/duck/Nanchang/1681/92(H3N8) (NC92-like viruses), which were isolated in southern China about 3 years earlier than Gs/Gd/96-like viruses. The MP genes of Gs/Gd/96-like viruses were from an unknown lineage (Figure 6). This reassortant, Gs/Gd/96-like virus (also named H5N1-PR1) [88], was last detected in the waterfowl in 2001 in Hong Kong [110].

In contrast to Gs/Gd/96-like viruses, the potential progenitor genes for HK97 viruses (H5N1-PR2) are very diverse: HA from E91-like viruses; PB1 and NP from NC92-like viruses; NA from unknown lineage; PB2 from A/chicken/Korea/38349.p96323/96 (H9N2)-like viruses; NA from an unknown lineage; PA, MP, and NS genes from A/chicken/Hong Kong/739/1994 (H9N2) viruses. HK97 H5N1 avian influenza viruses only share lineages with Gs/Gd/96-like viruses over HA, PB1, and NP [88] (Figure 6). Thus, the 1997 Hong Kong outbreaks more likely originated from a different reassortment event than the Gs/Gd/96 isolates.

HK97 H5N1 avian influenza viruses were named H5N1 PR-2. This reassortant disappeared after slaughtering 1.5 million chickens in Hong Kong and by stopping live poultry trade for 7 weeks [109]. The reappearance of H5N1-PR2 in Vietnamese eggs in 2005 possibly came from HK97-like virus inactivated vaccine usage or laboratory contamination [88, 114].

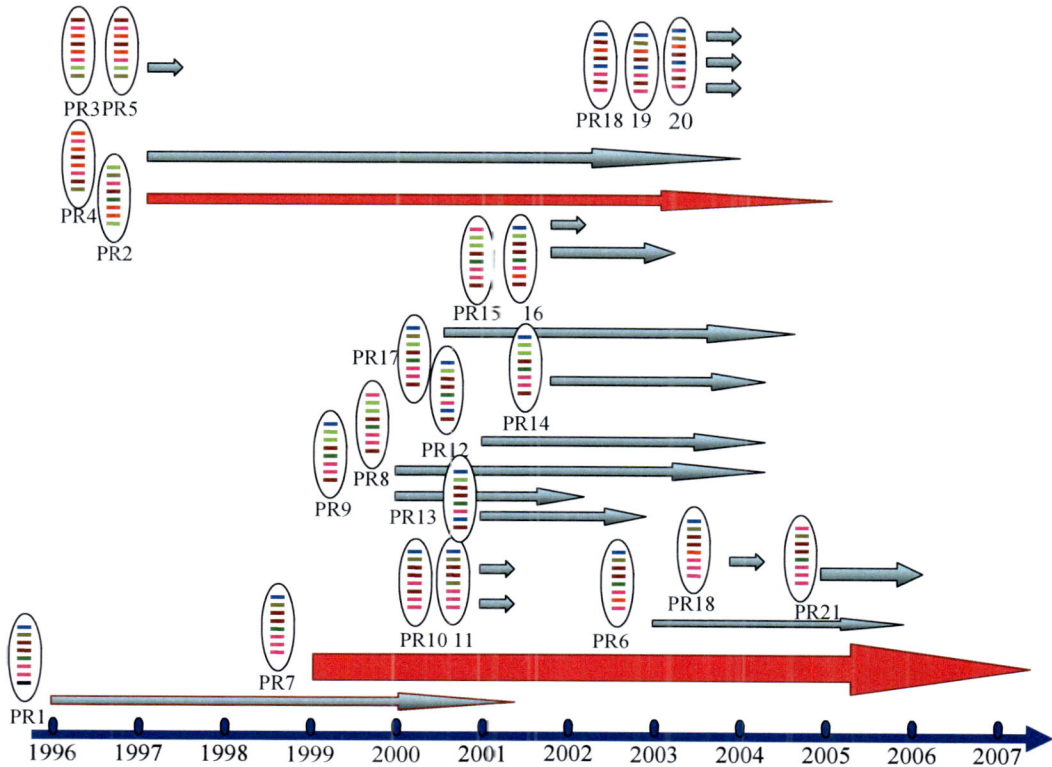

Figure 7. Emergence pathway of H5N1 highly pathogenic avian influenza viruses.

Through tracking down the progenitor genes, the H5N1 highly pathogenic avian influenza viruses can be sorted into at least 21 reassortants [88]. New reassortants still keep emerging. The emergence of new H5N1 genotypes is illustrated in Figure 7. Among these 21 reassortants, H5N1-PR7 has been dominant since 1999. The viruses in H5N1-PR7 caused most of the reported outbreaks in both domestic and wild birds. They were also identified from all confirmed human cases since 2002. The genetic characterization showed the only lineage difference between H5N1-PR7 and H5N1-PR1 (Gs/Gd/96-like) viruses is located in NS gene, and this single lineage difference possibly limited the transmission of Gs/Gd/96-like viruses among chickens.

These progenitor genes are also involved in generating reassortants in the low pathogenic avian influenza viruses, such as A/swan/Hokkaido/51/96 (H5N3), A/duck/Hokkaido/55/96 (H1N1), A/duck/Mongolia/54/01(H5N2), and A/chicken/Hebei /1/02 (H7N2). The details for the H5N1 genotypic diversity are described in our recent report [88].

It is interesting that Gs/Gd/96-like viruses were only identified in goose, waterfowl, and environmental samples (such as fecal samples collected from the poultry cage floors). As described previously, Gs/Gd/96-2 was not able to be transmitted between chickens in a pen mate experiment [108]. The failure to identify these avian influenza virus genotypes in the Guangdong province from 1996 to 1998 indicated that Gs/Gd/96-like viruses might not be able to be spread to chickens easily. However, due to lack of continuing surveillance of avian influenza viruses in birds, especially waterfowls, in southern China, it is unknown how these viruses were or are present in bird populations.

3.3.1.2. Molecular Evolution of H5N1 Highly Pathogenic Avian Influenza Virus

Since the first detection of H5N1 highly pathogenic avian influenza virus, this virus has undergone dramatic changes. At least 10 clades (Clade 0 to 9) and more subclades have been identified [115]. The distributions of H5 HA clades/sub-clades have shown a strong spatio-temporal trend [19, 116]. For instance, Clade 1 and 2.3 H5N1 viruses were predominant in Southeast Asia, including Vietnam, Laos, Cambodia, Thailand, and China, until 2005; Clade 2.1 in Indonesia since 2005; Clade 2.2 in China, Europe, Middle East, and Africa since 2005. Statistical analyses also suggests that the phylogenetic clusters of H5N1 viruses were associated with local evolutionary radia [117].

Frequent reassortments were not only identified between H5N1 avian influenza viruses and other subtypes of low pathogenic avian influenza viruses but also within H5N1 avian influenza viruses [20, 85, 118, 119]. Phylogeographic studies have revealed potential evolutionary and migration histories of H5N1 highly pathogenic avian influenza viruses. Vietnamese and Indonesian H5N1 viruses have been shown to have originated from two different southern Chinese provinces, Yunnan and Hunan [119]; in addition to southern China as the primary epicenter, Qinghai and Nigeria were shown to be the secondary epicenters of these H5N1 viruses [117, 120]. The two dimensional transmission of H5N1 viruses has also been shown to have occurred across the Eurasian landmass [119].

We studied genesis and geography of H5N1 avian influenza viruses in Vietnam from 2001 to 2007 [20]. Vietnam is one of the countries which has suffered the most from H5N1 highly pathogenic avian influenza viruses, which were first identified in the country in 2001 [20]. During the 2003/2004 H5N1 avian influenza outbreaks, almost the entire poultry population of Vietnam was destroyed; 109 H5N1 human cases have been confirmed in the country, 54 of which were fatal. Our study showed at least six clades/subclades of H5 highly pathogenic avian influenza viruses HA (Clade 0, 1, 2.3.2, 2.3.4, 3, and 5) and 9 reassortants of H5N1 highly pathogenic avian influenza viruses emerged in Vietnam from 2001 to 2007 [19, 20, 121]. HA genes introduced later are likely to reassort with the NA and/or internal segments from those pre-existing H5N1 avian influenza viruses. One of these emerging genotypes was always predominant and caused the outbreaks before the next introductions. However, it is very common that multiple genotypes co-exist during the same period. These H5N1 viruses formed two phylogenetic clusters across both northern and southern Vietnam after they were introduced into northern Vietnam and spread to southern Vietnam [20, 65]. In Vietnam, it is interesting that these genotypes usually emerged in northern Vietnam and then spread into southern Vietnam. On the other hand, some genotypes are predominant longer than others in the bird population. For instance, genotype VN3, which was introduced into Vietnam at the end of 2003, has never disappeared in the bird population in Vietnam. This suggests certain genotypes of H5N1 may have a better fitness in the bird population than other genotypes. On the other hand, H5N1 has undergone positive selections not only in HA but only other gene segments, which may suggest an adaptive trend of these viruses in the ecological niche, e.g., bird population.

3.3.2. Other Subtypes of Avian Influenza Viruses

The transmission of low pathogenic avian influenza viruses in wild birds, especially ducks, has been documented since the early 1960s. Almost all subtypes of HA and NA have been documented in ducks. Recent rapid increases of influenza surveillance in wild birds have given us more information about the distributions of influenza A viruses, especially low pathogenic avian influenza viruses. Frequent reassortments occurred in these low pathogenic avian influenza viruses [21], especially those isolates in the birds across flyways in North America. It would be interesting to understand how the viruses are transmitted between the Americas and other continents, especially Asia since this would reveal how and when H5N1 highly pathogenic avian influenza viruses will spread to the American continents. However, earlier studies have shown that the chance for transcontinental transmission is rare (less than 0.01%) [122, 123]. Nevertheless, a recent study found that there in 38 viruses isolated in northern pintails, 44.7% have one or more segments closely related to Asian lineages identified before [124]. The reason for different detection rates might be related to the sampling targets, e.g. species and sensitivity of RT-PCR.

3.3. Evolution of Influenza A Virus in Other Hosts

Before the direct evidence of human infection of H5N1 highly pathogenic avian influenza viruses, swine have been considered to be a necessary intermediate vessel for avian influenza viruses to infect and adapt to human populations. It is not uncommon to identify (1) a human influenza virus (fully human-like origins) [125]; (2) reassortant with swine influenza virus and human influenza virus [126] (e.g., reassortments between human H3N2 and swine H1N1 virus); (3) reassortment between human H3N2 and swine H1N2 [125, 127]; and (4) triple reassortants between human, swine and avian influenza viruses (e.g., a H3N2 triple reassortant was identified in an American H3N2 swine population containing avian-like (PA and PB2), swine-like (M, NP, and NS), and human-like (HA, NA, and PB1) gene segments [128]).

The H3N8 influenza virus has been identified in greyhounds and foxhound dogs [129, 130], and these viruses were genetically related to the equine H3N8 viruses. There were only a few residue changes in these canine H3N8 isolates when comparing to the contemporary equine H3N8 virus. Continuing surveillance needs to be conducted to determine whether these viruses have adapted and spread to dogs.

4. IMPACTS OF SAMPLING BIAS ON INFLUENZA EVOLUTIONARY ANALYSIS

An unbiased influenza sequence dataset is the baseline for influenza evolutionary analyses. However, it is almost impossible to generate unbiased data from our current surveillance strategy under financial restrictions. These errors or biases put us at risk for drawing flawed conclusions. Commonly, these errors or biases may be introduced into the sequence datasets in four categories: (1) virus sampling, (2) viral isolation method, (3) virus selection for sequencing, and (4) sequencing errors.

Influenza viruses are commonly isolated from outbreaks or epidemics. Especially for avian influenza viruses in waterfowls (i.e., the natural reservoir), limited surveillance has been done until recently. In human seasonal influenza, some countries have a very small surveillance program or none at all. In current influenza databases, most influenza A viruses are isolated via chicken embryonic eggs. The MDCK cell line is also utilized to isolate influenza viruses, especially those that do not grow well in chicken embryonic eggs, such as Fujian-like H3N2 human isolates and canine H3N8 influenza A viruses. The incubation of these samples in chicken embryonic eggs was shown to have introduced host-mediated mutations which were not present in the viruses from the original hosts. These host-mediated mutations will increase the false positive rate of positive selection analyses [131]. Through comparisons of 152 HA1 sequence isolates from eggs and those from MDCK cell line, Bush et al. [131] found that there were at least 22 codons that may be introduced into sequences through egg passage. These changes were identified in the tips of influenza trees.

Advances in sequencing technologies and the promotion of influenza genomic sequencing from National Institute of Allergy and Infectious Diseases (NIAID), the sequence data in public influenza database have grown exponentially. However, due to the limitations of resources (human and financial), not all viral isolates are sequenced. For instance, less than 20% of human isolates sampled by the Centers for Disease Control and Prevention of the United States are sequenced each week. Even for these sequenced isolates, only HA, NA and M are sequenced for most of them. The additional errors may be introduced by sequencing errors and human proof-reading of these sequences. It is not uncommon to find a "mistaking" gap or insertion or unrecognized nucleotides (N) in the public influenza sequences, especially for those earlier submissions.

5. IMPACTS OF INFLUENZA EVOLUTION ON EMERGENCE OF INFLUENZA PANDEMIC STRAINS

It has been hypothesized that certain genomic signatures may be shared across influenza viruses. For instance, due to a fast evolution rate in influenza A virus and relatively slow evolutionary rate in the host, influenza A virus from the same host may show a similar receptor binding feature. Human influenza virus has a different carbohydrate binding profile from avian influenza virus [132]. In order to adapt to different hosts, these viruses have to mutate their receptor binding sites to bind to the receptor binding sites in the new hosts. Typical examples are H9N2 and H5N1 avian influenza virus, which are acquiring the binding ability of human receptors [133, 134]. Some genetic markers were identified to be conserved in H5N1 highly pathogenic avian influenza viruses when compared with the 1918, 1957, and 1968 pandemic influenza viruses [135]. These markers were present across different segments in those pandemic strains and H5N1 highly pathogenic avian influenza viruses, which might suggest that these avian influenza viruses have obtained "modest adaptations" to humans since their first identification in humans in 1997. However, it is still not certain whether these adaptations may lead to another pandemic strain in the near future.

6. CONCLUSION

During the past several decades, many advances have been made in molecular evolution of influenza viruses. We thus now have a much better understanding of influenza molecular evolution. However, three critical evolutionary questions or challenges directly related to public health still need to be answered. The vaccine strain selection might be the first and most important challenge for seasonal influenza. With advances in biological technologies, we have improved our ability to generate more sequences as well as other phenotypic analyses, especially hemagglutinin inhibition (HI) assays. However, we need to know which strain will cause the next influenza epidemics, but this is a great challenge because of limited knowledge about influenza selective pressures. We still do not understand why and when certain influenza lineages die out. The second challenge is that we do not understand how different subtypes of influenza viruses—such as H1N1, H3N2, and influenza B viruses—co-circulate in the human populations and what drives or maintains these co-circulations. The third question concerns which influenza viruses may cause the next pandemic, especially regarding the specific reassortment from current influenza genetic pools in nature that may be able to cause human-to-human transmission; the human population lacks immunity against these reassortants.

REFERENCES

[1]   Flint SJ, L.W. Enquist, V.R. Racaniello & A.M. Skalka. *Principles of virology: molecular biology, pathogenesis, and control of animal viruses*. 2nd ed: ASM press 2004.

[2]   McCullers JA, Saito T, Iverson AR. Multiple genotypes of influenza B virus circulated between 1979 and 2003. *Journal of virology*. 2004 Dec;78(23):12817-28.

[3]   Li C, Yu K, Tian G, Yu D, Liu L, Jing B, et al. Evolution of H9N2 influenza viruses from domestic poultry in Mainland China. *Virology*. 2005 Sep 15;340(1):70-83.

[4]   Brown IH, Harris PA, McCauley JW, Alexander DJ. Multiple genetic reassortment of avian and human influenza A viruses in European pigs, resulting in the emergence of an H1N2 virus of novel genotype. *The Journal of general virology*. 1998 Dec;79 (Pt 12):2947-55.

[5]   Matsuzaki Y, Mizuta K, Sugawara K, Tsuchiya E, Muraki Y, Hongo S, et al. Frequent reassortment among influenza C viruses. *Journal of virology*. 2003 Jan;77(2):871-81.

[6]   Widjaja L, Krauss SL, Webby RJ, Xie T, Webster RG. Matrix gene of influenza a viruses isolated from wild aquatic birds: ecology and emergence of influenza a viruses. *Journal of virology*. 2004 Aug;78(16):8771-9.

[7]   Khatchikian D, Orlich M, Rott R. Increased viral pathogenicity after insertion of a 28S ribosomal RNA sequence into the haemagglutinin gene of an influenza virus. *Nature*. 1989 Jul 13;340(6229):156-7.

[8]   Guan Y, Poon LL, Cheung CY, Ellis TM, Lim W, Lipatov AS, et al. H5N1 influenza: a protean pandemic threat. *Proceedings of the National Academy of Sciences of the United States of America*. 2004 May 25;101(21):8156-61.

[9]   Wan XF, Ren T, Luo KJ, Liao M, Zhang GH, Chen JD, et al. Genetic characterization of H5N1 avian influenza viruses isolated in southern China during the 2003-04 avian influenza outbreaks. *Archives of virology*. 2005 Jun;150(6):1257-66.

[10] Webster RG, Bean WJ, Gorman OT, Chambers TM, Kawaoka Y. Evolution and ecology of influenza A viruses. *Microbiol Rev*. 1992 Mar;56(1):152-79.

[11] Guan Y, Peiris JS, Lipatov AS, Ellis TM, Dyrting KC, Krauss S, et al. Emergence of multiple genotypes of H5N1 avian influenza viruses in Hong Kong SAR. *Proceedings of the National Academy of Sciences of the United States of America*. 2002 Jun 25;99(13):8950-5.

[12] Holder M, Lewis PO. Phylogeny estimation: traditional and Bayesian approaches. *Nature reviews*. 2003 Apr;4(4):275-84.

[13] Thompson JD, Higgins DG, Gibson TJ. CLUSTAL W: improving the sensitivity of progressive multiple sequence alignment through sequence weighting, position-specific gap penalties and weight matrix choice. *Nucleic acids research*. 1994 Nov 11;22(22): 4673-80.

[14] Notredame C, Higgins DG, Heringa J. T-Coffee: A novel method for fast and accurate multiple sequence alignment. *Journal of molecular biology*. 2000 Sep 8;302(1):205-17.

[15] Edgar RC. MUSCLE: multiple sequence alignment with high accuracy and high throughput. *Nucleic acids research*. 2004;32(5):1792-7.

[16] Lassmann T, Sonnhammer EL. Quality assessment of multiple alignment programs. *FEBS Lett*. 2002 Oct 2;529(1):126-30.

[17] Nuin P, Wang Z, Tillier E. The accuracy of several multiple sequence alignment programs for proteins. *BMC Bioinformatics*. 2006;7:471.

[18] Altschul SF, Gish W, Miller W, Myers EW, Lipman DJ. Basic local alignment search tool. *Journal of molecular biology*. 1990 Oct 5;215(3):403-10.

[19] Wan XF, Chen G, Luo F, Emch M, Donis R. A quantitative genotype algorithm reflecting H5N1 Avian influenza niches. *Bioinformatics*. 2007 Sep 15;23(18):2368-75.

[20] Wan XF, Nguyen T, Davis CT, Smith CB, Zhao ZM, Carrel M, et al. Evolution of highly pathogenic H5N1 avian influenza viruses in Vietnam between 2001 and 2007. *PLoS ONE*. 2008;3(10):e3462.

[21] Wan XF, Ozden M, Lin G. Ubiquitous reassortments in influenza a viruses. *Journal of bioinformatics and computational biology*. 2008 Oct;6(5):981-99.

[22] Wan X-F, Wu X, Lin G, Holton SB, Desmone RA, Shyu CR, et al. Computational Identification of Reassortments in Avian Influenza Viruses. *Avian diseases*. 2007;51:434-9.

[23] Wu X, Goebel R, Wan X-F, G. L. Whole Genome Composition Distance for HIV-1 Genotyping. In: Xu, editor. *Proceedings of the IEEE Computational Systems Bioinformatics*; 2006; Stanford, California; 2006. p. 179-90.

[24] Wu X, Wan X-F, Wu G, Xu D, Lin G. Phylogenetic analysis using complete signature information of whole genomes and clustered Neighbour-Joining method. *International Journal of Bioinformatics Research and Application*. 2006;2:219-48.

[25] Lin G, Cai Z, Wu J, Wan XF, Xu L, Goebel R. Identifying a few foot-and-mouth disease virus signature nucleotide strings for computational genotyping. *BMC Bioinformatics*. 2008;9:279.

[26] Douady CJ, Delsuc F, Boucher Y, Doolittle WF, Douzery EJ. Comparison of Bayesian and maximum likelihood bootstrap measures of phylogenetic reliability. *Molecular biology and evolution*. 2003 Feb;20(2):248-54.

[27] Orlich M, Gottwald H, Rott R. Nonhomologous recombination between the hemagglutinin gene and the nucleoprotein gene of an influenza virus. *Virology*. 1994 Oct;204(1):462-5.

[28] Mitnaul LJ, Matrosovich MN, Castrucci MR, Tuzikov AB, Bovin NV, Kobasa D, et al. Balanced hemagglutinin and neuraminidase activities are critical for efficient replication of influenza A virus. *Journal of virology*. 2000 Jul;74(13):6015-20.

[29] Suarez DL, Senne DA, Banks J, Brown IH, Essen SC, Lee CW, et al. Recombination resulting in virulence shift in avian influenza outbreak, Chile. *Emerging infectious diseases*. 2004 Apr;10(4):693-9.

[30] Pasick J, Handel K, Robinson J, Copps J, Ridd D, Hills K, et al. Intersegmental recombination between the haemagglutinin and matrix genes was responsible for the emergence of a highly pathogenic H7N3 avian influenza virus in British Columbia. The *Journal of general virology*. 2005 Mar;86(Pt 3):727-31.

[31] He CQ, Xie ZX, Han GZ, Dong JB, Wang D, Liu JB, et al. Homologous recombination as an evolutionary force in the avian influenza A virus. *Molecular biology and evolution*. 2009 Jan;26(1):177-87.

[32] He CQ, Han GZ, Wang D, Liu W, Li GR, Liu XP, et al. Homologous recombination evidence in human and swine influenza A viruses. Virology. 2008 Oct 10;380(1):12-20.

[33] Boni MF, Zhou Y, Taubenberger JK, Holmes EC. Homologous recombination is very rare or absent in human influenza A virus. *Journal of virology*. 2008 May;82(10):4807-11.

[34] Gibbs MJ, Armstrong JS, Gibbs AJ. The haemagglutinin gene, but not the neuraminidase gene, of 'Spanish flu' was a recombinant. *Philosophical transactions of the Royal Society of London*. 2001 Dec 29;356(1416):1845-55.

[35] Gibbs MJ, Armstrong JS, Gibbs AJ. Recombination in the hemagglutinin gene of the 1918 "Spanish flu". *Science* (New York, NY. 2001 Sep 7;293(5536):1842-5.

[36] Worobey M, Rambaut A, Pybus OG, Robertson DL. Questioning the evidence for genetic recombination in the 1918 "Spanish flu" virus. *Science* (New York, NY. 2002 Apr 12;296(5566):211 discussion

[37] Pons MW. Isolation of influenza virus ribonucleoprotein from infected cells. Demonstration of the presence of negative-stranded RNA in viral RNP. *Virology*. 1971 Oct;46(1):149-60.

[38] Chare ER, Gould EA, Holmes EC. Phylogenetic analysis reveals a low rate of homologous recombination in negative-sense RNA viruses. *The Journal of general virology*. 2003 Oct;84(Pt 10):2691-703.

[39] Posada D, Crandall KA, Holmes EC. Recombination in evolutionary genomics. *Annual review of genetics*. 2002;36:75-97.

[40] Weiller GF. Phylogenetic profiles: a graphical method for detecting genetic recombinations in homologous sequences. *Molecular biology and evolution*. 1998 Mar;15(3):326-35.

[41] Worobey M, Holmes EC. Evolutionary aspects of recombination in RNA viruses. The *Journal of general virology*. 1999 Oct;80 (Pt 10):2535-43.

[42] Huson DH. SplitsTree: analyzing and visualizing evolutionary data. *Bioinformatics*. 1998;14(1):68-73.

[43] Milne I, Wright F, Rowe G, Marshall DF, Husmeier D, McGuire G. TOPALi: software for automatic identification of recombinant sequences within DNA multiple alignments. *Bioinformatics*. 2004 Jul 22;20(11):1806-7.

[44] Lole KS, Bollinger RC, Paranjape RS, Gadkari D, Kulkarni SS, Novak NG, et al. Full-length human immunodeficiency virus type 1 genomes from subtype C-infected seroconverters in India, with evidence of intersubtype recombination. *Journal of virology*. 1999 Jan;73(1):152-60.

[45] Martin DP, Williamson C, Posada D. RDP2: recombination detection and analysis from sequence alignments. *Bioinformatics*. 2005 Jan 15;21(2):260-2.

[46] Grassly NC, Holmes EC. A likelihood method for the detection of selection and recombination using nucleotide sequences. *Molecular biology and evolution*. 1997 Mar;14(3):239-47.

[47] Hein J. Reconstructing evolution of sequences subject to recombination using parsimony. *Math Biosci*. 1990 Mar;98(2):185-200.

[48] Kuhner MK, Lawlor DA, Ennis PD, Parham P. Gene conversion in the evolution of the human and chimpanzee MHC class I loci. *Tissue Antigens*. 1991 Oct;38(4):152-64.

[49] Jakobsen IB, Easteal S. A program for calculating and displaying compatibility matrices as an aid in determining reticulate evolution in molecular sequences. *Comput Appl Biosci*. 1996 Aug;12(4):291-5.

[50] Jakobsen IB, Wilson SR, Easteal S. The partition matrix: exploring variable phylogenetic signals along nucleotide sequence alignments. *Molecular biology and evolution*. 1997 May;14(5):474-84.

[51] Sawyer S. Statistical tests for detecting gene conversion. *Molecular biology and evolution*. 1989 Sep;6(5):526-38.

[52] Maynard Smith J, Smith NH. Detecting recombination from gene trees. *Molecular biology and evolution*. 1998 May;15(5):590-9.

[53] Worobey M. A novel approach to detecting and measuring recombination: new insights into evolution in viruses, bacteria, and mitochondria. *Molecular biology and evolution*. 2001 Aug;18(8):1425-34.

[54] Takahata N. Comments on the detection of reciprocal recombination or gene conversion. *Immunogenetics*. 1994;39(2):146-9.

[55] Holmes EC, Worobey M, Rambaut A. Phylogenetic evidence for recombination in dengue virus. *Molecular biology and evolution*. 1999 Mar;16(3):405-9.

[56] Minin VN, Dorman KS, Fang F, Suchard MA. Dual multiple change-point model leads to more accurate recombination detection. *Bioinformatics*. 2005 Jul 1;21(13):3034-42.

[57] Boni MF, Posada D, Feldman MW. An exact nonparametric method for inferring mosaic structure in sequence triplets. *Genetics*. 2007 Jun;176(2):1035-47.

[58] Fitch WM, Leiter JM, Li XQ, Palese P. Positive Darwinian evolution in human influenza A viruses. *Proceedings of the National Academy of Sciences of the United States of America*. 1991 May 15;88(10):4270-4.

[59] Lentz MR, Air GM, Laver WG, Webster RG. Sequence of the neuraminidase gene of influenza virus A/Tokyo/3/67 and previously uncharacterized monoclonal variants. *Virology*. 1984 May;135(1):257-65.

[60] Bush RM, Fitch WM, Bender CA, Cox NJ. Positive selection on the H3 hemagglutinin gene of human influenza virus A. *Molecular biology and evolution*. 1999 Nov;16 (11):1457-65.

[61] Bush RM, Bender CA, Subbarao K. Cox NJ, Fitch WM. Predicting the evolution of human influenza A. *Science* (New York, NY. 1999 Dec 3;286(5446):1921-5.

[62] Wolf YI, Viboud C, Holmes EC, Koonin EV, Lipman DJ. Long intervals of stasis punctuated by bursts of positive selection in the seasonal evolution of influenza A virus. *Biology direct*. 2006;1:34.

[63] Bragstad K, Nielsen LP, Fomsgaard A. The evolution of human influenza A viruses from 1999 to 2006: a complete genome study. *Virology journal*. 2008;5:40.

[64] Suzuki Y. Natural selection on the influenza virus genome. *Molecular biology and evolution*. 2006 Oct;23(10):1902-11.

[65] Smith GJ, Naipospos TS, Nguyen TD, de Jong MD, Vijaykrishna D, Usman TB, et al. Evolution and adaptation of H5N1 influenza virus in avian and human hosts in Indonesia and Vietnam. *Virology*. 2006 Jul 5;350(2):258-68.

[66] Ciccozzi M, Montieri S, Facchini M, Rezza G, Donatelli I, Campitelli L. Evolutionary analysis of HA and NS1 genes of H5N1 influenza viruses in 2004-2005 epidemics. *Avian diseases*. 2007 Mar;51(1 Suppl):455-60.

[67] Campitelli L, Ciccozzi M, Salemi M, Taglia F, Boros S, Donatelli I, et al. H5N1 influenza virus evolution: a comparison of different epidemics in birds and humans (1997-2004). *The Journal of general virology*. 2006 Apr;87(Pt 4):955-60.

[68] Jackwood MW, Stallknecht DE. Molecular epidemiologic studies on North American H9 avian influenza virus isolates from waterfowl and shorebirds. *Avian diseases*. 2007 Mar;51(1 Suppl):448-50.

[69] Sugita S, Yoshioka Y, Itamura S, Kanegae Y, Oguchi K, Gojobori T, et al. Molecular evolution of hemagglutinin genes of H1N1 swine and human influenza A viruses. *Journal of molecular evolution*. 1991 Jan;32(1):16-23.

[70] Suzuki Y, Gojobori T. A method for detecting positive selection at single amino acid sites. *Molecular biology and evolution*. 1999 Oct;16(10):1315-28.

[71] Suzuki Y. New methods for detecting positive selection at single amino acid sites. *Journal of molecular evolution*. 2004 Jul;59(1):11-9.

[72] Yang Z. PAML: a program package for phylogenetic analysis by maximum likelihood. *Comput Appl Biosci*. 1997 Oct;13(5):555-6.

[73] Yang Z. Maximum likelihood estimation on large phylogenies and analysis of adaptive evolution in human influenza virus A. *Journal of molecular evolution*. 2000 Nov;51(5):423-32.

[74] Zhang J, Nielsen R, Yang Z. Evaluation of an improved branch-site likelihood method for detecting positive selection at the molecular level. *Molecular biology and evolution*. 2005 Dec;22(12):2472-9.

[75] Yang Z, Nielsen R, Goldman N, Pedersen AM. Codon-substitution models for heterogeneous selection pressure at amino acid sites. *Genetics*. 2000 May;155(1):431-49.

[76] Yang Z, Wong WS, Nielsen R. Bayes empirical bayes inference of amino acid sites under positive selection. *Molecular biology and evolution*. 2005 Apr;22(4):1107-18.

[77] Suzuki Y, Nei M. Simulation study of the reliability and robustness of the statistical methods for detecting positive selection at single amino acid sites. *Molecular biology and evolution.* 2002 Nov;19(11):1865-9.

[78] Zhang J. Frequent false detection of positive selection by the likelihood method with branch-site models. *Molecular biology and evolution.* 2004 Jul;21(7):1332-9.

[79] Sabath N, Landan G, Graur D. A method for the simultaneous estimation of selection intensities in overlapping genes. *PLoS ONE.* 2008;3(12):e3996.

[80] Clark AG, Kao TH. Excess nonsynonymous substitution of shared polymorphic sites among self-incompatibility alleles of Solanaceae. *Proceedings of the National Academy of Sciences of the United States of America.* 1991 Nov 1;88(21):9823-7.

[81] Suzuki Y. Three-dimensional window analysis for detecting positive selection at structural regions of proteins. *Molecular biology and evolution.* 2004 Dec;21(12):2352-9.

[82] Hatchette TF, Walker D, Johnson C, Baker A, Pryor SP, Webster RG. Influenza A viruses in feral Canadian ducks: extensive reassortment in nature. *The Journal of general virology.* 2004 Aug;85(Pt 8):2327-37.

[83] Endo A, Pecoraro R, Sugita S, Nerome K. Evolutionary pattern of the H 3 haemagglutinin of equine influenza viruses: multiple evolutionary lineages and frozen replication. *Archives of virology.* 1992;123(1-2):73-87.

[84] Fitch WM, Bush RM, Bender CA, Cox NJ. Long term trends in the evolution of H(3) HA1 human influenza type A. *Proceedings of the National Academy of Sciences of the United States of America.* 1997 Jul 22;94(15):7712-8.

[85] Vijaykrishna D, Bahl J, Riley S, Duan L, Zhang JX, Chen H, et al. Evolutionary dynamics and emergence of panzootic H5N1 influenza viruses. *PLoS pathogens.* 2008;4(9):e1000161.

[86] Drummond AJ, Ho SY, Phillips MJ, Rambaut A. Relaxed phylogenetics and dating with confidence. *PLoS biology.* 2006 May;4(5):e88.

[87] Lepage T, Bryant D, Philippe H, Lartillot N. A general comparison of relaxed molecular clock models. Molecular biology and evolution. 2007 Dec;24(12):2669-80.

[88] Zhao Z, Garcia M, Guan Y, Shortridge KF, Wan XF. Genetic preparedness for current pandemic threats. Submitted.

[89] Posada D, Crandall KA. MODELTEST: testing the model of DNA substitution. *Bioinformatics.* 1998;14(9):817-8.

[90] Thorne JL, Kishino H. Divergence time and evolutionary rate estimation with multilocus data. *Syst Biol.* 2002 Oct;51(5):689-702.

[91] Webster RG, Shortridge KF, Kawaoka Y. Influenza: interspecies transmission and emergence of new pandemics. *FEMS Immunol Med Microbiol.* 1997 Aug;18(4):275-9.

[92] Maines TR, Chen LM, Matsuoka Y, Chen H, Rowe T, Ortin J, et al. Lack of transmission of H5N1 avian-human reassortant influenza viruses in a ferret model. *Proceedings of the National Academy of Sciences of the United States of America.* 2006 Aug 8;103(32):12121-6.

[93] Chen LM, Davis CT, Zhou H, Cox NJ, Donis RO. Genetic compatibility and virulence of reassortants derived from contemporary avian H5N1 and human H3N2 influenza A viruses. *PLoS pathogens.* 2008 May;4(5):e1000072.

[94] Smith DJ, Lapedes AS, de Jong JC, Bestebroer TM, Rimmelzwaan GF, Osterhaus AD, et al. Mapping the antigenic and genetic evolution of influenza virus. *Science* (New York, NY. 2004 Jul 16;305(5682):371-6.

[95] Koelle K, Cobey S, Grenfell B, Pascual M. Epochal evolution shapes the phylodynamics of interpancemic influenza A (H3N2) in humans. *Science* (New York, NY. 2006 Dec 22;314(5807):1898-903.

[96] Nelson MI, Simonsen L, Viboud C, Miller MA, Taylor J, George KS, et al. Stochastic processes are key determinants of short-term evolution in influenza a virus. *PLoS pathogens*. 2006 Dec;2(12) e125.

[97] Nelson MI, Viboud C, Simonsen L, Bennett RT, Griesemer SB, St George K, et al. Multiple reassortment events in the evolutionary history of H1N1 influenza A virus since 1918. *PLoS pathogens*. 2008 Feb 15;4(2):e1000012.

[98] Holmes EC, Ghedin E, Miller N, Taylor J, Bao Y, St George K, et al. Whole-genome analysis of human influenza A virus reveals multiple persistent lineages and reassortment among recent H3N2 viruses. *PLoS biology*. 2005 Sep;3(9):e300.

[99] Rambaut A, Pybus OG, Nelson MI, Viboud C, Taubenberger JK, Holmes EC. The genomic and epidemiological dynamics of human influenza A virus. *Nature*. 2008 May 29;453(7195):615-9.

[100] Lu B, Zhou H, Chan W, Kemble G, Jin H. Single amino acid substitutions in the hemagglutinin of influenza A/Singapore/21/04 (H3N2) increase virus growth in embryonated chicken eggs. *Vaccine*. 2006 Nov 10;24(44-46):6691-3.

[101] Widjaja L, Ilyushina N, Webster RG, Webby RJ. Molecular changes associated with adaptation of human influenza A virus in embryonated chicken eggs. *Virology*. 2006 Jun 20;350(1):137-45.

[102] Jin H, Zhou H, Liu H, Chan W, Adhikary L, Mahmood K, et al. Two residues in the hemagglutinin of A/Fujian/411/02-like influenza viruses are responsible for antigenic drift from A/Panama/2007/99. *Virology*. 2005 May 25;336(1):113-9.

[103] Ziegler T, Hemphill ML, Ziegler ML, Perez-Oronoz G, Klimov AI, Hampson AW, et al. Low incidence of rimantadine resistance in field isolates of influenza A viruses. *The Journal of infectious diseases*. 1999 Oct;180(4):935-9.

[104] Deyde VM, Xu X, Bright RA, Shaw M, Smith CB, Zhang Y, et al. Surveillance of resistance to adamantanes among influenza A(H3N2) and A(H1N1) viruses isolated worldwide. *The Journal of infectious diseases*. 2007 Jul 15;196(2):249-57.

[105] Simonsen L, Viboud C, Grenfell BT, Dushoff J, Jennings L, Smit M, et al. The genesis and spread of reassortment human influenza A/H3N2 viruses conferring adamantane resistance. *Molecular biology and evolution*. 2007 Aug;24(8):1811-20.

[106] Lackenby A, Hungnes O, Dudman SG, Meijer A, Paget WJ, Hay AJ, et al. Emergence of resistance to oseltamivir among influenza A(H1N1) viruses in Europe. *Euro Surveill*. 2008 Jan 31;13(5).

[107] Dharan NJ, Gubareva LV, Meyer JJ, Okomo-Adhiambo M, McClinton RC, Marshall SA, et al. Infections With Oseltamivir-Resistant Influenza A(H1N1) Virus in the United States. *JAMA*. 2009 Mar 2.

[108] Wan X-F. Isolation and characterization of avian influenza viruses in China. [Master thesis]. Guangzhou: South China Agricultural University; 1998.

[109] Sims LD, Ellis TM, Liu KK, Dyrting K, Wong H, Peiris M, et al. Avian influenza in Hong Kong 1997-2002. *Avian diseases*. 2003;47(3 Suppl):832-8.

[110] Webster RG, Guan Y, Peiris M, Walker D, Krauss S, Zhou NN, et al. Characterization of H5N1 influenza viruses that continue to circulate in geese in southeastern China. *Journal of virology*. 2002 Jan;76(1):118-26.

[111] Li KS, Guan Y, Wang J, Smith GJ, Xu KM, Duan L, et al. Genesis of a highly pathogenic and potentially pandemic H5N1 influenza virus in eastern Asia. *Nature*. 2004 Jul 8;430(6996):209-13.

[112] Chen H, Smith GJ, Zhang SY, Qin K, Wang J, Li KS, et al. Avian flu: H5N1 virus outbreak in migratory waterfowl. *Nature*. 2005 Jul 14;436(7048):191-2.

[113] [WHO] WHO. Cumulative number of confirmed human cases of avian influenza A/(H5N1) reported to WHO. 2008 [cited 2008 July 22]; Available from: http://www.who.int/csr/disease/avian_influenza/country/cases_table_2008_06_19/en/in dex.html

[114] Li Y, Lin Z, Shi J, Qi Q, Deng G, Li Z, et al. Detection of Hong Kong 97-like H5N1 influenza viruses from eggs of Vietnamese waterfowl. *Archives of virology*. 2006 Aug;151(8):1615-24.

[115] WHO/OIE/FAO. Toward a unified nomenclature system for highly pathogenic avian influenza virus (H5N1). *Emerging infectious diseases*. 2008 Jul;14(7):e1.

[116] WHO/OIE/FAO_H5N1_Evolution_Working_Group. Toward a unified nomenclature system for highly pathogenic avian influenza virus (H5N1). *Emerging infectious diseases*. 2008 Jul;14(7):e1.

[117] Wallace RG, Fitch WM. Influenza A H5N1 immigration is filtered out at some international borders. *PLoS ONE*. 2008;3(2):e1697.

[118] Zhao ZM, Shortridge KF, Garcia M, Guan Y, Wan XF. Genotypic diversity of H5N1 highly pathogenic avian influenza viruses. *The Journal of general virology*. 2008 Sep;89(Pt 9):2182-93.

[119] Wang J, Vijaykrishna D, Duan L, Bahl J, Zhang JX, Webster RG, et al. Identification of the progenitors of Indonesian and Vietnamese avian influenza A (H5N1) viruses from southern China. *J Virol*. 2008 Apr;82(7):3405-14.

[120] Wallace RG, Hodac H, Lathrop RH, Fitch WM. A statistical phylogeography of influenza A H5N1. *Proc Natl Acad Sci U S A*. 2007 Mar 13;104(11):4473-8.

[121] Le MT, Wertheim HF, Nguyen HD, Taylor W, Hoang PV, Vuong CD, et al. Influenza A H5N1 clade 2.3.4 virus with a different antiviral susceptibility profile replaced clade 1 virus in humans in northern Vietnam. *PLoS ONE*. 2008;3(10):e3339.

[122] Krauss S, Obert CA, Franks J, Walker D, Jones K, Seiler P, et al. Influenza in migratory birds and evidence of limited intercontinental virus exchange. *PLoS pathogens*. 2007 Nov;3(11):e167.

[123] Winker K, McCracken KG, Gibson DD, Pruett CL, Meier R, Huettmann F, et al. Movements of birds and avian influenza from Asia into Alaska. *Emerging infectious diseases*. 2007 Apr;13(4):547-52.

[124] Koehler AV, Pearce JM, Flint PL, Franson JC, Ip HS. Genetic evidence of intercontinental movement of avian influenza in a migratory bird: the northern pintail (Anas acuta). *Molecular ecology*. 2008 Nov;17(21):4754-62.

[125] Yu H, Hua RH, Zhang Q, Liu TQ, Liu HL, Li GX, et al. Genetic evolution of swine influenza A (H3N2) viruses in China from 1970 to 2006. *Journal of clinical microbiology*. 2008 Mar;46(3):1067-75.

[126] Sun L, Zhang G, Shu Y, Chen X, Zhu Y, Yang L, et al. Genetic correlation between H3N2 human and swine influenza viruses. *J Clin Virol.* 2009 Feb;44(2):141-4.

[127] Zell R, Bergmann S, Krumbholz A, Wutzler P, Durrwald R. Ongoing evolution of swine influenza viruses: a novel reassortant. *Archives of virology.* 2008;153(11):2085-92.

[128] Richt JA, Lager KM, Janke BH, Woods RD, Webster RG, Webby RJ. Pathogenic and antigenic properties of phylogenetically distinct reassortant H3N2 swine influenza viruses cocirculating in the United States. *Journal of clinical microbiology.* 2003 Jul;41(7):3198-205.

[129] Crawford PC, Dubovi EJ, Castleman WL, Stephenson I, Gibbs EP, Chen L, et al. Transmission of equine influenza virus to dogs. *Science* (New York, NY. 2005 Oct 21;310(5747):482-5.

[130] Daly JM, Blunden AS, Macrae S, Miller J, Bowman SJ, Kolodziejek J, et al. Transmission of equine influenza virus to English foxhounds. Emerging infectious diseases. 2008 Mar;14(3):461-4.

[131] Bush RM, Smith CB, Cox NJ, Fitch WM. Effects of passage history and sampling bias on phylogenetic reconstruction of human influenza A evolution. Proceedings of the National Academy of Sciences of the United States of America. 2000 Jun 20;97(13):6974-80.

[132] Stevens J, Blixt O, Glaser L, Taubenberger JK, Palese P, Paulson JC, et al. Glycan microarray analysis of the hemagglutinins *from modern and pandemic influenza viruses reveals different receptor specificities. Journal of molecular biology.* 2006 Feb 3;355(5):1143-55.

[133] Stevens J, Blixt O, Chen LM, Donis RO, Paulson JC, Wilson IA. Recent avian H5N1 viruses exhibit increased propensity for acquiring human receptor specificity. J*ournal of molecular biology.* 2008 Sep 19;381(5):1382-94.

[134] Wan H, Sorrell EM, Song H, Hossain MJ, Ramirez-Nieto G, Monne I, et al. Replication and transmission of H9N2 influenza viruses in ferrets: evaluation of pandemic potential. PLoS ONE. 2008;3(8):e2923.

[135] Finkelstein DB, Mukatira S, Mehta PK, Obenauer JC, Su X, Webster RG, et al. Persistent host markers in pandemic and H5N1 influenza viruses. *Journal of virology.* 2007 Oct;81(19):10292-9.

In: Global View of Fight against Influenza
Editor: Petar M. Mitrasinovic

ISBN: 978-1-60741-952-5
© 2009 Nova Science Publishers, Inc.

Chapter 5

PATHOGENESIS OF AVIAN INFLUENZA (H5N1) INFECTION IN HUMANS

Ruishu Deng[1] and Jiang Gu[1, 2,]*

[1]Department of Pathology, School of Basic Medical Sciences,
Peking University, Beijing, China
[2]Shantou University Medical College, Shantou, China

ABSTRACT

H5N1 influenza virus is highly pathogenic to humans and has posed an increasing pandemic threat to mankind. However, the pathogenesis of this newly emerging infectious disease remains unclear. This chapter describes major pathological findings, receptor distributions, viral tropism and transmission, and the body's response to the infection. Key pathogenetic mechanisms are reviewed and discussed.

INTRODUCTION

H5N1 avian influenza A virus has crossed the species barrier to cause high human fatalities and posed an increasing pandemic threat since it first occurred in Hong Kong in 1997. During the first outbreak in Hong Kong, 18 individuals were infected and six died [1]. The avian influenza re-emerged among humans in Hong Kong in January 2003, causing two cases of infection and one death [2]. Thus far, the World Health Organization has reported 412 confirmed cases, with a fatality rate of above 60%. H5N1 influenza is still a relatively novel disease with poorly understood pathology and pathogenesis. In this chapter, major pathological findings reported in published postmortem studies of human H5N1 cases are summarized. In addition, virus distribution and receptor specificity are also discussed. The

---

* Corresponding author: Jiang Gu, MD, PhD, Dean, Shantou University Medical College, Shantou, China; Professor of Pathology, School of Basic Medical Sciences, Peking University Health Science Center, Beijing, China; President, Chinese Pathologist Association (CPA). Tel: (86)10-8280-2998; E-mail: jianggu@bjmu.edu.cn

major pathogenetic mechanisms that may play key roles in the pathogenesis of this disease are postulated. Viral transmission and prevention of this disease are also discussed.

TRANSMISSION

Direct avian-to-human viral transmission is the predominant means of human infection. Limited, nonsustained human-to-human transmissions have probably occurred when close contact with a severely ill patient takes place without any protection. In addition, environment-to-human transmission remains possible [3, 4].

Avian to Human Transmission

During the 1997 Hong Kong outbreak, exposure to live poultry within a week before the onset of illness was recognized as the risk factor [5]. Recently, a history of direct contact with poultry was commonly found for most patients. Slaughtering, defeathering, or preparing sick poultry for cooking; playing with or holding diseased or dead poultry; handling asymptomatic infected fighting cocks or ducks; and consuming raw or undercooked poultry or poultry products have all been shown to be potential risk factors [4, 6-9].

Limited Human-to-Human Transmission

It has been reported that clusters of human influenza A (H5N1) illness with at least two epidemiologically linked cases occurred in 10 countries [4, 6, 9-12]. In these clusters, raging from two to eight individuals, most persons probably acquired infection from common-source exposures to poultry. However, limited, nonsustained human-to-human transmission has been reported. When this happened, there was always a close contact with a severely ill index patient without any protection [10, 11].

Environment-to-Human Transmission

For a certain number of H5N1 cases, the source of exposure was unclear. Though not firmly identified, several other modes of environment-to-human transmission are theoretically possible [3]—for example, oral ingestion, direct intranasal or conjunctival contact of virus-contaminated water during swimming, or use of untreated poultry feces as fertilizer [3].

HISTOPATHOLOGY

Postmortem analyses are sparse worldwide. Only nine full autopsies, including one autopsy of a fetus [2, 11, 13-17], six limited autopsies [17, 18] and two cases of postmortem organ biopsies [19-21] have been reported. The main histopathological findings of these reports are summarized in Table 1.

Table 1. Summary of main histopathical findings

Region or country	Year	Case	Sex/age	Disease duration	Major histopathological findings	Ref.
Hong Kong	1997	1(BA)	M/3y	11d	Liver: microvesicular fatty changes, multiple Councilman bodies with some inflammatory cells. Kidneys: vacuolation and vesicular change of proximal tubules (consistent with Reye's syndrome). Bone marrow: active granulopoiesis with left shift, active erythropoiesis, increase in reactive histiocytes with occasional haemophagocytic activity	
Hong Kong	1997	2(BA)	M/54y	11d	Lungs: areas of hemorrhage, fibrinous exudates in air spaces, reactive pneumocytes, sparse interstitial lymphocytic infiltration. Kidneys: extensive acute tubular necrosis	C,C-11
Hong Kong	1997	3(FA)	F/13y	29d	Lungs: firm, consolidated, extensive hemorrhage, focal cystic changes, organizing DAD, interstitial fibrosis, cystically dilated air spaces, reactive pneumocytes, interstitial lymphoplasmacytic infiltration, few histiocytes with reactive hemophagocytic activity. Liver: extensive central lobular necrosis, activated Kupffer's cells with occasional hemophagocytic activity. Kidney: extensive acute tubular necrosis. Brain: edema, hemophagocytic histiocytes over the meninges, demyelinated areas. Bone marrow: hypoplastic, histiocytic hyperplasia with diffuse reactive histiocytes with reactive hemophagocytic activity. Lymph nodes: hemophagocytosis, focal necrosis	Chr,chri-6
Hong Kong	1997	4(FA)	F/25y	28d	Lungs, liver, kidneys: similar to those of case 31. Brain: mildly swollen. Bone marrow: hypercellular, active hematopoiesis, reactive hemophagocytic histiocytes. Lymph nodes: reactive hemophagocytic, extra-medullary hematopoiesis, focal necrosis	C,C-6
Hong Kong	2003	5(FA)	M/33y	6d	Lungs: oedema, haemorrhage, fibrin exudation, focal type-2 pneumocyte hyperplasia, intra-alveolar macrophages, interstitial CD3 +T lymphocytes. bronchial and hilar lymph nodes: parafollicular reactive histiocytes with haemophagocytosis Bone marrow: hypercellular, reactive haemophagocytosis	C,C-3,14
Thailand	2004	6(FA)	M/6y	17d	Lungs: proliferative phase of diffuse alveolar damage, interstitial pneumonia, focal hemorrhage, bronchiolitis, reactive hyperplasia pneumocytes. lymph nodes, spleen, and bone marrow: slight histiocytic hyperplasia without hemophagocytic activity. Liver: mild fatty changes, activated Kupffer cells, lymphoid infiltration. Brain: edema, small foci of necrosis. Other organs: no remarkable changes.	C,C-8

Table 1. Summary of main histopathological findings (continued)

Region or country	Year	Case	Sex/age	Disease duration	Major histopathological findings	Ref.
Thailand	?	7(FA)	M/48y	6d	Lungs: exudative phase of diffuse alveolar damage, atypical pneumocytes with large bizarre and clumping Nuclei, Bronchiolitis and pleuritis, Hemophagocytic activity. Hemophagic activity in lungs, liver, and bone marrow	C,C-9
Thailand	2004	8(FA)	F/26y	9d	Lungs: diffuse alveolar damage, interstitial pneumonia. Liver: cholestasis, congestion, and hemophagocytic activity. Spleen: congestion and depletion of lymphoid cells.	C,C-4
Thailand	2004	9,10,11 (LA)	NS	NS	Lungs: DAD, reactive fibroblasts, hemorrhage. Spleen: atypical lymphocytes	C-C-10
China	2005	12 (FA)	F/24	9d	Lungs: diffuse alveolar damage, focal desquamation of epithelial cells without evidence of type II pneumocyte hyperplasia, variable numbers of macrophages in the alveoli, moderate numbers of scattered neutrophils, rare lymphocytes in the interstitial spaces. Spleen, lymph nodes, and mucosal lymphoid tissue in the gastrointestinal tract: substantially depleted lymphoid tissue. Liver: spotty necrosis. Kidneys: extensive tubular necrosis. Placenta: scattered foci of syncytiotrophoblast necrosis, sometimes with associated dystrophic calcification, focal acute necrotizing deciduitis. Other organs: no remarkable findings. Fetus: most tissues showed no specific histopathological findings except edema and very small numbers of scattered interstitial neutrophils in the lungs.	
China	2005	13(FA)	M/35y	27d	Lungs: similar to case 12 except for patchy foci of consolidated bronchopneumonia and areas of fibrosis. Spleen, lymph node, kidneys: similar to those of case 12. No pronounced histological changes, apart from hypertrophy in the thymus.	C,C-7
Vietnam	2003–2004	14(LA)	F/12	6d	Lungs: exudative phase diffuse alveolar damage, hyaline membrane formation, hemmorhagic necrosis.	Vie
Vietnam	2003–2004	15(LA)	M/5	17d	Lungs: proliferative phase diffuse alveolar damage, hyaline membrane formation.	
Vietnam	?	16(LA)	M/4	16d	Lungs: similar to that of case 15 except for microabscess.	

The Respiratory Tract

The lungs are the major and primary organ of injury. Prominent change in lungs is diffuse alveolar damage in different phases, i.e., the acute exudative phase for patients dying in the first two weeks, organizing phase and the final fibrotic stage for patients dying in the third week or later [2, 11, 13-17, 22]. In the exudative phase of diffuse alveolar damage, edema, fibrous exudates, and hyaline membranes formation are predominant, whereas the reactive hyperplasia of type II and interstitial fibrosis are remarkable features of the organizing phase and later fibrotic stage [2, 11, 13-17, 22]. Viral inclusions or other cytopathic changes have not been observed in cases of proliferative pneumocytes [13, 15, 19, 22]. However, infection of type II pneumocytes occurred in other cases [13, 15]. Apoptoses in alveolar cells and infiltrating leukocytes have been reported to be prominent findings in a small number of cases [16]. The major exudating cell types in the alveoli were macrophages [2, 14] and infiltration of lymphocytes into the interstitial areas, with or without neutrophils are present [2, 13, 14, 19]. Scattered histiocytes with hemophagocytic activity have been observed in the lungs of some cases [13]. In addition, the above features, bronchiolitis with squamous metaplasia, pulmonary congestion with varying degrees of hemorrhage have also been present in some patients [14, 16, 22].

Hemato-Lymphoid System

Reactive hemophagocytic syndrome have been noted prominent in the spleen, lymph node and bone marrow [2, 11, 13, 16, 19, 21], whereas in recent autopsies this phenomenon has been less prominent or even absent [14, 15]. Lymphoid depletion and atypical lymphocytes occur in spleen, lymph nodes, and lymphoid tissues at autopsy [1, 2, 13, 17]. The bone marrow varied from hypocellular [2, 21] to hypercellular [13]. The spleen typically presents congestion and white pulp atrophy with depletion of lymphocytes [11, 13, 14, 22]. Apoptotic lymphocytes have been commonly observed in this organ [16]. In some cases lymph nodes show focal necrosis [13] and loss of germinal centers [14].

Other Organs

Kidneys present acute tubular necrosis in several cases [13, 14, 19, 22]. In liver, activated Kupffer cells, cholestasis, necrosis and fatty changes have been found [13-16]. Usually, the brain is edematous without any significant histopathological change [13, 14] except demyelinated areas and reactive histiocytes and foci of necrosis in two cases [13, 15]. No significant pathology was noted in other organs [2, 4, 14, 15].

Among reported H5N1 human subjects, there was a unique case of a 24-year-old pregnant female who died nine days after onset of symptoms; the fetus died in utero. Both the mother and the fetus were fully autopsied [14]. The placenta did not display specific histopathological features except for foci of syncytiocytotrophoblast necrosis, necrotizing deciduitis, and diffuse villitis. Most fetal tissues presented a normal appearance except for some edema and a few scattered interstitial neutrophils in the lungs [14].

Taken together, the above histopathological changes are not unique to H5N1 influenza and they may be caused by infection of other organisms such as severe acute respiratory syndrome (SARS) coronavirus (SARS-CoV) or by other factors such as aspiration or oxygen toxicity. Therefore, pathologic findings alone cannot be used as the sole criterion for diagnosis of H5N1 infection. More specific tests to ascertain pathogens such as RT-PCR, virus isolation and in situ hybridization to detect the virus or ELISA and western blot to detect the antibodies are absolutely necessary. On the other hand, pathologic findings described above reflected only changes at the end stage of this disease when the autopsy analysis was performed. These histopathological characteristics do not reflect the dynamic changes in all phases of the disease.

VIRUS TROPISM

Morphological methods combined with molecular biological techniques are commonly used to investigate virus tropism. Immunohistochemistry (IHC) and in situ hybridization are methods for in situ detection of viral antigens and genomic sequences in various organs [2, 11, 13-16]. Hemagglutinin (HA) and nucleocapsid protein (NP) and their corresponding viral geneomic segments are usually chosen as the targets in these methods [2, 11, 13-16]. In addition, RT-PCR, strand-specific RT-PCR, and nucleic acid sequence-based amplification H5 detection assays (NASBA) are commonly used molecular biological methods [2, 13-16]. In contrast to previous reports that H5N1 infection was confined to the lungs [2, 13], recent studies indicated that the virus disseminated beyond the respiratory tract [14-16].

The Respiratory Tract

A number of studies have detected both viral antigens and genomic sequences in epithelial cells of the trachea [15] and alveoli [2, 11, 14-16]. Both ciliated and nonciliated cells of tracheal epithelium have been identified as the targets of infection [14]. Similarly, type II pneumocytes have also been identified as target cells by double labeling with antibodies to surfactant protein [14, 15]. Both RT-PCR and NASBA have confirmed viral RNA in the trachea and the lungs [14-16]. The detection of positive-stranded RNA and the presence of the positive signals in the nuclei of the infected cells indicates active viral replication in the epithelial cells of the lungs [14-16].

Peripheral Lymphoid Organs

In the lymph nodes, T lymphocytes have been confirmed to be infected by H5N1 virus using in situ hybridization. [14] Morphologically, the virus was not detected in the spleen [14]. However, RT-PCR and NASBA were positive for both lymph node and spleen [14]. This discrepancy may be attributed to different detecting sensitivity of the methods.

Blood

The possible occurrence of viremia in the course of human H5N1 infection has been supported by several studies [23-26]. Virus has been isolated successfully from sera of four human H5N1 cases [23, 24, 26]. A recent study suggested neutrophils as a vehicle for viral replication and dissemination [27]. In this report, viral antigens and RNA were observed in neutrophils in the placental blood of a pregnant woman. Morphologic methods and molecular biological ones have been used in this particular study. The infected neutrophils were verified by virtue of morphologic features and double labeling of a neutrophil marker (CD15) with in situ hybridization [27]. This finding provided a reasonable explanation for the possible mechanism of viral spread beyond the respiratory system. As this was a study based on a unique case of pregnancy, the universality of this phenomenon warrants further investigation.

Brain

Neurons of the brain have also been reported to be infected by H5N1 virus based on detection of viral RNA and antigen in them [14]. RT-PCR detected both negative- and positive-stranded RNA in the brain [14], and H5N1 virus has been isolated from cerebrospinal fluid [24]. These are evidence for the transmission of the H5N1 virus to the central nervous system. However, the specific pathway of this transmission remains unclear. The viruses might be carried to the brain via circulation, or alternatively via the afferent fibers of the olfactory, vagal, trigeminal, and sympathetic nerves after replication in the lungs, as has been observed in a mouse model [28].

Intestines

Intestinal epithelial cell was found to be infected by H5N1 virus using morphological and molecular biological methods [14]. Digestive tract symptoms were frequently observed in these patients and viral shedding was reported in stool samples [1, 24, 29, 30]. Two Vietnamese patients presented with severe digestive tract symptoms and diarrhea rather than respiratory symptoms at onset of the disease [24]. Infection of the intestine was thought to be the result of ingesting infected secretions from the respiratory tract. Avian influenza viruses maintain sialidase activities at the low pH conditions of the stomach [31], and passing through the upper digestive tract, the survival viruses might infect the gut. On the other hand, blood transmission of the virus could not be excluded.

Other Organs

Viral RNA and antigens have not been detected in heart, kidneys, and liver by morphological means. However, viral RNA was detected in those organs using molecular biological techniques [14]. This discrepancy might be attributed to different detecting sensitivity of the techniques used [32, 33].

Placenta and Fetus

Thorough investigation of the autopsy tissue samples of the pregnant female and her fetus yielded significant discoveries [14]. In the placenta, viral antigens and sequences were detected in Hofbauer cells and cytotrophoblasts, but not in syncytiotrophoblasts [14]. In addition, vertical transmission (from mother to fetus) was confirmed with abundant and extensive presence of the virus in the lungs of the fatus [14]. The mechanisms for this transplacental transmission might be similar to that for the cytomegalovirus which is also known to infect mainly cytotrophoblasts and Hofbauer cells [34]. Two possible routs were suggested for the transmission of cytomegalovirus: (1) transcytosis across syncytio trophoblasts to cytotrophoblasts in chorionic villi and (2) via invasive cytotrophoblasts within the uterine wall [34]. The reported infection of neutrophils by H5N1 in the placental blood of this case suggests anther possible route for transplacental transmission [27].

RECEPTOR

Sialic acid linked galactose is the most commonly accepted receptor for influenza virus. Avian influenza viruses preferentially bind to cell-surface glycoproteins containing terminal sialyl-galactosyl residues linked by 2–3-linkage, whereas human viruses bind to those containing terminal 2–6-linked sialyl-galactosyl moieties [33, 35-39]. It was initially thought that avian influenza viruses were incapable of causing human infection. In 1997, the H5N1 virus crossed the species barrier for the first time and caused 18 human infections and 6 deaths [1].

Initially, receptor distribution patterns of avian and human influenza viruses were thought to be different in the respiratory tract with vian influenza virus receptors primarily distribute in the lower respiratory tract, whereas the human influenza virus receptors are mainly expressed in the upper respiratory tract [33, 40-42]. This difference may decreases the susceptibility of humans to avian influenza virus infection [42]. More recently, avian influenza virus receptors were detected on epithelial cells of trachea and bronchi [33, 36, 37, 43-46], and epithelial cells of the upper respiratory tract were found to be infected by the virus in abundancy (14).

In line with multiple organ infections [14], virual receptors were found to be expressed in extra-pulmonary tissues [47-50]. Neurons, pancreatic epithelial cells and bile duct epithelial cells were found to express avian influenza receptors [48, 49]. Endothelial cells in many organs throughout the body were also found to express such receptors [47]. In particular, epithelial cells of the intestinal mucosa were reported to express the avian influenza virual receptor [50, 51]. T cells [52] and Kuffer cells were also found to express these receptors [47].

It is speculated that in additional to the typical avian influenza virus receptor, other receptors or co-receptors may play a role in the interaction between the virus and the target cells. Though the receptor distribution pattern broadly resembled that of infected cells, there are some discrepancies between the two. Classical avian influenza virus receptors were present abundantly on the endothelial cells of various organs whereas the viruses were absent from those cells [47]. In addition, the limited number of infected pneumocytes was sharply different from the widespread and abundant expression of avian influenza virus receptors detected in the lungs [14, 47]. Furthermore, H5N1 viruses were detected in placental macrophages, alveolar macrophages, and cytotrophoblasts whereas receptors were absent from those cells [14, 47]. These discrepancies support the assumption of possible existence of other receptor or co-receptors on the infected cells.

PATHOGENESIS

Virus-Induced Tissue Injury

Avian influenza virus replication may induce tissue damage through cytolytic or apoptotic mechanisms. These might be similar to common H3N2 or H1N1 influenza virus. Active viral replication in respiratory tract was reported in laboratory tests on hospitalized patients and postmortem studies. H5N1 virus was isolated from the tracheal, nasopharyngeal aspirate and postmortem lungs of H5N1 influenza patients [6, 10, 25, 29]. Positive strand virus RNA was detected in the postmortem tracheal epithelial cells and alveolar epithelial cells of human H5N1 cases [14]. Furthermore, H5N1 viruses were found to infect ex vivo nasopharynx and lungs efficiently [41]. In contrast to the respiratory tract, little was known of H5N1 viral replication in extra-pulmonary organs. The infection of neutrophils suggests that white blood cells might be a vehicle for ex-pulmonary dissemination [27].

The replication process of H5N1 virus was incompletely understood [25]. The highest viral loads were detected in the fatal cases, suggesting a correlation between viral replication and negative disease outcome [25, 33]. Studies of hospitalized patients suggested that viral RNA can be detected from 1 day up to 15 days after disease onset [3, 10]. Limited data showed that H5N1 infected patients had detectable viral RNA in the respiratory tract for up to 3 weeks, presumably because of negligible pre-existing immunity and possibly viral evasion of immune responses [4, 14, 25]. Prolonged viral replication was also indicated by viral RNA detection, particularly the presence of positive strand viral sequence in postmortem samples of one fatal patient who died on the 27th day after the onset of illness [14].

Host Cytokines and Chemokines Response

Host innate immune responses may contribute to the pathogenesis of human H5N1 influenza. In vivo and in vitro studies indicated that increased production of proinflammatory cytokines and chemokines may play an important role. Such responses may contribute in part to the acute respiratory distress syndrome (ARDS), and multiple organ failure [3] and were consistent with hemophagocytotic activity observed in autopsized cases [2, 11, 13, 16, 19, 21]. Elevated seral levels of proinflammatory cytokines and chemokines were detected in some H5N1 patients [2, 13, 15, 25,]. In the 2003 Hong Kong outbreak, elevated seral levels of interferon-inducible protein 10, monocyte chemoattractant protein 1, and monokine induced by interferon-γ were found three to eight days after the onset of illness [2]. In a large group of Vietnamese patients, seral levels of macrophage- and neutrophil-attractant chemokines, proinflammatory and anti-inflammatory cytokines were found higher than those of patients infected with common influenza virus [25]. Furthermore, they were correlated positively with pharyngeal viral loads, suggesting that high levels of cytokines and chemokine response may be induced by high viral loads [25]. Up-regulation of multiple cytokines were found to be induced by H5N1 influenza virus as compared to common influenza viruses, supporting the role of an exaggerated immune response in the pathogenesis of H5N1 influenza [9, 17, 41, 42]. Animal experiments also provided support for critical contribution of cytokines and chemokines in the pathogenesis of this disease [53-55]. Nevertheless, the role of cytokines and chemokines in the pathogenesis of H5N1 influenza was debated by a couple of animal and postmortem human studies [56, 57]. Mice with deficient induction of interleukin-6, macrophage inflammatory protein 1α, tumor necrosis factor α or its receptors, and mice treated with glucocorticoids had similar mortality as compared to wild-type animals. What's more, those without interleukin-1 receptors had increased mortality. These data indicated that inhibition of cytokine response did not protect against lethal H5N1 influenza infection [56]. A recent postmortem study showed distinctly different patterns of infection in the lungs of a pregnant woman (died 9 days after onset of symptom) and a male case (died 27 days after onset of symptom) [57]. The male case had increased cytokine/chemokine expression but much reduced viral load in the lungs, while the pregnant female had diminished cytokine/chemokine expression but a significantly increased viral load in the lungs. It was speculated that "cytokine storm" alone could not be a sufficient explanation for the severe lung injury seen in this disease [57]. Overall, the contribution of host cytokine and chemokine response to the pathogenesis remains incompletely understood.

Oxidative Stress and Toll-like Receptor 4 for Acute Lung Injury

As a part of normal physiology and a defense mechanism to external thread of microorganisms and chemicals, biological systems continuously generate reactive oxygen to ward off these agents and in turn are exposed to the deleterious effects of these oxidants. On the other hand, the subtle systems are endowed with a battery of endogenous agents, the antioxidants, to counterbalance those oxidants [58]. The disequilibrium between oxidants and antioxidants in favor of the oxidants, "oxidative stress", may lead to tissue injury with oxidation of protein, DNA and lipids [59]. In the entire human body, the lung is the only organ which has the highest exposure to atmospheric oxygen. Owing to its large surface area and blood supply, the lung is susceptible to oxidative injury [58]. What's more, surfactants, the abundant material in the lung for maintaining normal lung function, are prone to be oxidized by virtue of the predominance of phospholipids in them [60]. It was reported that surfactant oxidation and dysfunction likely contributed to the development of ARDS [61, 62]. Most patients who died of H5N1 infection developed ARDS, the most severe form of acute lung injury [3]. Therefore, oxidative stress and subsequent oxidation of surfactant may play an important role in the pathogenesis of ARDS in H5N1 patients. A recent study suggested a common signal pathoway for ARDS caused by multiple lung pathogens such as chemical agents, H5N1 avian influenza, or SARS. It was reported that acute lung injury was triggered by signaling of oxidized phospholipids through TLR4-TRIF-TRAF6 in several strains of acid induced acute lung injury mouse models [63]. In the same study, inactivated H5N1 avian influenza virus is found to be able to induce oxidation of phospholipids and acute lung injury [63]. In addition, in situ oxidized phospholipids have been detected in lungs of several patients infected with H5N1 avian influenza virus and SARS-coronavirus [63]. These provide evidences for the contributions of oxidative stress in the course of H5N1 infection for ARDS.

Apoptosis

Induction of apoptosis was an effective way of host response against invading viruses. With the death of host cells, virus replication was inhibited, thus the limitation of virus dissemination [16]. As for common influenza virus, apoptosis was observed for epithelial cells and lymphocytes in several in vitro studies [64-68]. However, whether and to what extent apoptosis contributes to the highly virulence property of influenza (H5N1) viruses are not clear [16]. In vitro and autopsy studies indicated the possible involvement of this mechanism in severe tissue injury [16, 66, 69, 70]. An increase in apoptotic cells in the spleen of mice infected with virulent H5N1 was observed and deduced as a possible cause of lymphocyte death and subsequent lymphopenia in mammals [71]. In another in vitro experiment, tumor necrosis factor–related apoptosis-inducing ligand (TRAIL), a functional death receptor, was shown to be up-regulated in human monocyte-derived macrophages infected by H5N1 virus comparing to those infected with H1N1 virus [69]. These H5N1 virus-infected macrophages showed increased capability of inducing apoptosis on co-cultured T lymphocytes. Virus involvement in enhanced sensitization of T lymphocytes to death receptor ligand-induced apoptosis has also been demonstrated [69]. Both sensitization and up-regulation of TRAIL were thought to contribute to lymphopenia frequently observed in H5N1 patients [69]. In addition, a delayed onset of apoptosis was shown in H5N1 infected macrophages comparing to H1N1 counterparts. This might be a mean for the pathogens to have longer survival in the infected cells and may contribute to the pathogenesis of H5N1 infection in humans [70]. Furthermore, apoptosis was observed in human autopsy alveolar epithelial cells and leukocytes in the lungs, and in the spleen and the intestinal tissues [16]. This phenomenon may occur as a result of direct viral replication or up-regulation of cytokines and chemokines [16]. The specific rationale for the occurrence of apoptosis remains unclear and further studies are warrant.

Reduced Cytotoxicity of CD8[+] Lymphocytes

Hyperproduction of proinflammatory cytokines (including IFN-γ and macrophage-derived cytokines) and hemophagocytic syndrome were reported in human H5N1 fatal cases. These presentations were also commonly found in virus infections of perforin-deficient mice or persons with perforin gene defect, such as familial hemophagocytic lymphohistiocytosis [72-75]. Perforin is a key component of the lytic granules in cytotoxic CD8[+] T lymphocytes and plays a critical role in cell-mediated cytotoxicity against viral infection. Thus, insufficient expression of perforin and consequently reduced cytotoxicity of CD8[+] T Lymphocytes was hypothesized to be associated with severe manifestations of human H5N1 influenza [76]. According to in vitro experiments, in contrast to H3N2 and H1N1 viruses, a recombinant hemagglutinin (H5) from a H5N1 virus suppressed perforin expression, which resulted in impaired cytotoxic activity causing failure of clearance of H5N1 virus or HA (H5) protein-bearing cells [76]. The persistence of H5-presenting cells provided sustained stimulation leading to excessive production of IFN-γ, which may contribute to macrophage over-activation and subsequent hypocytokinemia and hemophagocytosis observed in some H5N1 patients [76]. However, host cellular immune response, including activation of all kinds of immune cells such as antigen presenting cells and cytotoxic CD8+ T Lymphocytes, is a very complicated process. The data obtained from limited in vitro experiments is far from sufficient to draw any conclusion. A large number of animal experiments and more autopsy studies are necessary to elucidate the mechanism.

CONCLUSION

From the occurrence of the first case of H5N1 human infection until now, only a limited number of studies reporting pathological findings in human H5N1 have been published. Recent reports together with early findings lead to improved understanding of pathology and pathogenesis of this disease. Histopathological features observed are unspecific for H5N1 infection and are common for severe inflammation of the lungs caused by other pathogens. Multiple organ infection was an important feature of this disease. Dissemination of this virus to the brain and vertical transmission to the fetus have important clinical implications. Recently-proposed oxidative stress and subsequent tissue injury add to the knowledge of pathogenesis. However, many aspects of the pathogenesis remain unknown. In light of the sustained threat of a potentially devastating influenza pandemic, further investigations into the pathology and pathogenesis are still urgently needed.

ACKNOWLEDGEMENTS

We thank Juxiang Ye, Lu Yao, and Yingying Zhao for their help in the preparation of this chapter.

REFERENCES

[1] Yuen, K.Y., et al., Clinical features and rapid viral diagnosis of human disease associated with avian influenza A H5N1 virus. *Lancet*, 1998. 351(9101): p. 467-71.

[2] Peiris, J.S., et al., Re-emergence of fatal human influenza A subtype H5N1 disease. *Lancet*, 2004. 363(9409): p. 617-9.

[3] Beigel, J.H., et al., Avian influenza A (H5N1) infection in humans. *N Engl J Med*, 2005. 353(13): p. 1374-85.

[4] Abdel-Ghafar, A.N., et al., Update on avian influenza A (H5N1) virus infection in humans. *N Engl J Med*, 2008. 358(3): p. 261-73.

[5] Bridges, C.B., W. Lim, and e.a. Hu-Primmer J, Risk of influenza A (H5N1) infection among poultry workers, Hong Kong, 1997-1998. *J Infect Dis* 2002. 185: p. 1005-10.

[6] Oner, A.F., et al., Avian influenza A (H5N1) infection in eastern Turkey in 2006. *N Engl J Med*, 2006. 355(21): p. 2179-85.

[7] Dinh, P.N., H.T. Long, and e.a. Tien NTK, Risk factors for human infection with avian influenza A H5N1, Vietnam, 2004. *Emerg Infect Dis*, 2006. 12: p. 1841-7.

[8] Areechokchai, D., et al., Investigation of avian influenza (H5N1) outbreak in humans — Thailand, 2004. *MMWR Morb Mortal Wkly Rep*, 2006. 55(Suppl 1:3-6).

[9] edyaningsih, E.R., et al., Epidemiology of cases of H5N1 virus infection in Indonesia, July 2005-June 2006. *J Infect Dis*, 2007. 196(4): p. 522-7.

[10] Kandun, I.N., et al., Three Indonesian clusters of H5N1 virus infection in 2005. *N Engl J Med*, 2006. 355(21): p. 2186-94.

[11] Ungchusak, K., et al., Probable person-to-person transmission of avian influenza A (H5N1). *N Engl J Med*, 2005. 352(4): p. 333-40.

[12] Olsen, S.J., K. Ungchusak, and e.a. Sovann L, Family clustering of avian influenza A (H5N1). *Emerg Infect Dis*, 2005. 11: p. 1799-801.

[13] To, K.F., et al., Pathology of fatal human infection associated with avian influenza A H5N1 virus. *J Med Virol*, 2001. 63(3): p. 242-6.

[14] Gu, J., et al., H5N1 infection of the respiratory tract and beyond: a molecular pathology study. *Lancet*, 2007. 370(9593): p. 1137-45.

[15] Uiprasertkul, M., et al., Influenza A H5N1 replication sites in humans. *Emerg Infect Dis*, 2005. 11(7): p. 1036-41.

[16] Uiprasertkul, M., et al., Apoptosis and pathogenesis of avian influenza A (H5N1) virus in humans. *Emerg Infect Dis*, 2007. 13(5): p. 708-12.

[17] Chotpitayasunondh, T., et al., Human disease from influenza A (H5N1), Thailand, 2004. *Emerg Infect Dis*, 2005. 11(2): p. 201-9.

[18] Liem, N.T., et al., H5N1-infected cells in lung with diffuse alveolar damage in exudative phase from a fatal case in Vietnam. *Jpn J Infect Dis*, 2008. 61(2): p. 157-60.

[19] Chan, P.K., Outbreak of avian influenza A(H5N1) virus infection in Hong Kong in 1997. *Clin Infect Dis*, 2002. 34 Suppl 2: p. S58-64.

[20] Subbarao, K., et al., Characterization of an avian influenza A (H5N1) virus isolated from a child with a fatal respiratory illness. *Science*, 1998. 279(5349): p. 393-6.

[21] Ku, A.S. and L.T. Chan, The first case of H5N1 avian influenza infection in a human with complications of adult respiratory distress syndrome and Reye's syndrome. *J Paediatr Child Health*, 1999. 35(2): p. 207-9.

[22] Ng, W.F., et al., The comparative pathology of severe acute respiratory syndrome and avian influenza A subtype H5N1—a review. *Hum Pathol*, 2006. 37(4): p. 381-90.

[23] Buchy, P., et al., Influenza A/H5N1 virus infection in humans in Cambodia. *J Clin Virol*, 2007. 39(3): p. 164-8.

[24] de Jong, M.D., et al., Fatal avian influenza A (H5N1) in a child presenting with diarrhea followed by coma. *N Engl J Med*, 2005. 352(7): p. 686-91.

[25] de Jong, M.D., et al., Fatal outcome of human influenza A (H5N1) is associated with high viral load and hypercytokinemia. *Nat Med*, 2006. 12(10): p. 1203-7.

[26] Chutinimitkul, S., et al., H5N1 influenza A virus and infected human plasma. Emerg Infect Dis, 2006. 12(6): p. 1041-3.

[27] Zhao, Y., et al., Neutrophils May Be a Vehicle for Viral Replication and Dissemination in Human H5N1 Avian Influenza. *Clin Infect Dis*, 2008.

[28] Park, C.H., et al., The invasion routes of neurovirulent A/Hong Kong/483/97 (H5N1) influenza virus into the central nervous system after respiratory infection in mice. *Arch Virol.*, 2002. 147(7): p. 1425-36.

[29] Tran, T.H., et al., Avian influenza A (H5N1) in 10 patients in Vietnam. *N Engl J Med*, 2004. 350(12): p. 1179-88.

[30] Apisarnthanarak, A., et al., Atypical avian influenza (H5N1). Emerg Infect Dis, 2004. 10(7): p. 1321-4.

[31] Takahashi, T., et al., Duck and human pandemic influenza A viruses retain sialidase activity under low pH conditions. *J Biochem*, 2001. 130(2): p. 279-83.

[32] Nicholls, J.M., et al., Time course and cellular localization *of SARS-CoV nucleoprotein and RNA in lungs from fatal cases of SARS*. PLoS Med, 2006. 3(2): p. e27.

[33] Korteweg, C. and J. Gu, Pathology, molecular biology, and pathogenesis of avian influenza A (H5N1) infection in humans. *Am J Pathol*, 2008. 172(5): p. 1155-70.

[34] Fisher, S., et al., Human cytomegalovirus infection of placental cytotrophoblasts in vitro and in utero: implications for transmission and pathogenesis. *J Virol*, 2000. 74(15): p. 6808-20.

[35] Rogers, G.N. and J.C. Paulson, Receptor determinants of human and animal influenza virus isolates: differences in receptor specificity of the H3 hemagglutinin based on species of origin. *Virology*, 1983. 127: p. 361-373.

[36] Baum, L.G., J.C. Paulson et al., Sialyloligosaccharides of the respiratory epithelium in the selection of human influenza virus receptor specificity. *Acta Histochem* 1990. Suppl, 40: p. S35-S38.

[37] Couceiro, J.N., J.C. Paulson, and L.G. Baum, Influenza virus strains selectively recognize sialyloligosaccharides on human respiratory epithelium, the role of the host cell in selection of hemagglutinin receptor specificity. *Virus Res,*, 1993. 29: p. 155-165.

[38] Matrosovich, M., et al., Early alterations of the receptor-binding properties of H1, H2, and H3 avian influenza virus hemagglutinins after their introduction into mammals. *J Virol*, 2000. 74: p. 8502-8512.

[39] Connor, R., et al., Receptor specificity in human, avian, and equine H2 and H3 influenza virus isolates. *Virology* 1994. 205: p. 17-23.

[40] Van Riel, D., et al., H5N1 virus attachment to lower respiratory tract. *Science* 2006: p. 312:399.

[41] Nicholls, J.M., et al., Tropism of avian influenza A (H5N1) in the upper and lower respiratory tract. *Nat Med*, 2007. 13(2): p. 147-9.

[42] Shinya, K., et al., Avian flu: influenza virus receptors in the human airway. *Nature*, 2006. 440(7083): p. 435-6.

[43] Matrosovich, M.N., et al., Human and avian influenza viruses target different cell types in cultures of human airway epithelium. *Proc Natl Acad Sci USA*, 2004. 101: p. 4620-4624.

[44] Thompson, C., et al., Infection of human airway epithelium by human and avian strains of influenza a virus. *J Virol* 2006. 80: p. 8060-8068.

[45] Ibricevic, A., et al., Influenza virus receptor specificity and cell tropism in mouse and human airway epithelial cells. *J Virol* 2006. 80: p. 7469-7480.

[46] Zhang, L., et al., Infection of ciliated cells by human parainfluenza virus type 3 in an in vitro model of human airway epithelium. *J Virol*, 2005. 79: p. 1113-1124.

[47] Yao, L., et al., Avian influenza receptor expression in H5N1-infected and non-infected human tissues. *FASEB J* 2008. 22: p. 733-740.

[48] Eash, S., et al., Differential distribution of the JC virus receptor-type sialic acid in normal human tissues. *Am J Pathol* 2004. 164: p. 419-428.

[49] Ulloa, F. and F. Real, Differential distribution of sialic acid in alpha2,3 and alpha2,6 linkages in the apical membrane of cultured epithelial cells and tissues. *J Histochem Cytochem* 2001. 49: p. 501-510.

[50] Roth, J., Cellular sialoglycoconjugates: a histochemical perspective. *Histochem J* 1993. 25: p. 687-710.

[51] Sata, T., et al., Expression of alpha 2,6-linked sialic acid residues in neoplastic but not in normal human colonic mucosa. A lectin-gold cytochemical study with Sambucus nigra and Maackia amurensis lectins. *Am J Pathol*, 1991. 139: p. 1435-1448.

[52] Garcı́a-Sastre, A., et al., Influenza A virus lacking the NS1 gene replicates in interferon-deficient systems. *Virology*, 1998. 252: p. 324-330.

[53] Conenello, G.M., et al., A single mutation in the PB1-F2 of H5N1 (HK/97) and 1918 influenza A viruses contributes to increased virulence. *PLoS Pathog*, 2007. 3(10): p. 1414-21.

[54] Lipatov, A.S., et al., Pathogenesis of Hong Kong H5N1 influenza virus NS gene reassortants in mice: the role of cytokines and B- and T-cell responses. *J Gen Virol*, 2005. 86(Pt 4): p. 1121-30.

[55] Szretter, K.J., et al., Role of host cytokine responses in the pathogenesis of avian H5N1 influenza viruses in mice. *J Virol*, 2007. 81(6): p. 2736-44.

[56] Salomon, R., E. Hoffmann, and R.G. Webster, Inhibition of the cytokine response does not protect against lethal H5N1 influenza infection. *Proc Natl Acad Sci U S A*, 2007. 104(30): p. 12479-81.

[57] Deng, R., et al., Distinctly different expression of cytokines and chemokines in the lungs of two H5N1 avian influenza patients. *J Pathol*, 2008. 216(3): p. 328-36.

[58] Rahman, I., S.K. Biswas, and A. Kode, Oxidant and antioxidant balance in the airways and airway diseases. *Eur J Pharmacol*, 2006. 533(1-3): p. 222-39.

[59] Sies, H., Oxidative stress: oxidants and antioxidants. *Exp Physiol*, 1997. 82(2): p. 291-5.

[60] Rodriguez Capote, K., F.X. McCormack, and F. Possmayer, Pulmonary surfactant protein-A (SP-A) restores the surface properties of surfactant after oxidation by a mechanism that requires the Cys6 interchain disulfide bond and the phospholipid binding domain. *J Biol Chem*, 2003. 278(23): p. 20461-74.

[61] Gunther, A., et al., Surfactant alterations in severe pneumonia, acute respiratory distress syndrome, and cardiogenic lung edema. *Am J Respir Crit Care Med*, 1996. 153(1): p. 176-84.

[62] Lewis, J.F. and R. Veldhuizen, The role of exogenous surfactant in the treatment of acute lung injury. *Annu Rev Physiol*, 2003. 65: p. 613-42.

[63] Imai, Y., et al., Identification of oxidative stress and Toll-like receptor 4 signaling as a key pathway of acute lung injury. *Cell*, 2008. 133(2): p. 235-49.

[64] Takizawa, T., et al., Induction of programmed cell death (apoptosis) by influenza virus infection in tissue culture cells. *J Gen Virol*, 1993. 74 (Pt 11): p. 2347-55.

[65] Fesq, H., et al., Programmed cell death (apoptosis) in human monocytes infected by influenza A virus. *Immunobiology*, 1994. 190(1-2): p. 175-82.

[66] Hinshaw, V.S., et al., Apoptosis: a mechanism of cell killing by influenza A and B viruses. *J Virol*, 1994. 68(6): p. 3667-73.

[67] Nichols, J.E., J.A. Niles, and N.J. Roberts, Jr., Human lymphocyte apoptosis after exposure to influenza A virus. *J Virol*, 2001. 75(13): p. 5921-9.

[68] Lowy, R.J., Influenza virus induction of apoptosis by intrinsic and extrinsic mechanisms. *Int Rev Immunol*, 2003. 22(5-6): p. 425-49.

[69] Zhou, J., et al., Functional tumor necrosis factor-related apoptosis-inducing ligand production by avian influenza virus-infected macrophages. *J Infect Dis*, 2006. 193(7): p. 945-53.

[70] Mok, C.K., et al., Differential onset of apoptosis in influenza A virus H5N1- and H1N1-infected human blood macrophages. *J Gen Virol*, 2007. 88(Pt 4): p. 1275-80.

[71] Tumpey, T.M., et al., Depletion of lymphocytes and diminished cytokine production in mice infected with a highly virulent influenza A (H5N1) virus isolated from humans. *J Virol*, 2000. 74(13): p. 6105-16.

[72] Katano, H. and J.I. Cohen, Perforin and lymphohistiocytic proliferative disorders. *Br J Haematol*, 2005. 128(6): p. 739-50.

[73] Osugi, Y., et al., Cytokine production regulating Th1 and Th2 cytokines in hemophagocytic lymphohistiocytosis. *Blood*, 1997. 89(11): p. 4100-3.

[74] Jordan, M.B., et al., An animal model of hemophagocytic lymphohistiocytosis (HLH): CD8+ T cells and interferon gamma are essential for the disorder. *Blood*, 2004. 104(3): p. 735-43.

[75] Henter, J.I., et al., Hypercytokinemia in familial hemophagocytic lymphohistiocytosis. *Blood*, 1991. 78(11): p. 2918-22.

[76] Hsieh, S.M. and S.C. Chang, Insufficient perforin expression in CD8+ T cells in response to hemagglutinin from avian influenza (H5N1) virus. *J Immunol*, 2006. 176(8): p. 4530-3.

ISBN: 978-1-60741-952-5

© 2009 Nova Science Publishers, Inc.

Chapter 6

THE INTERACTIONS BETWEEN AVIAN H5N1 INFLUENZA VIRUS AND DENDRITIC CELL-SPECIFIC ICAM-3 GRABBING NON-INTEGRIN (DC-SIGN)

Sheng-Fan Wang[1] and Yi-Ming Arthur Chen[2]

[1]Department of Biotechnology and Laboratory Science in Medicine,
[2]Institute of Microbiology and Immunology,
National Yang-Ming University, Taipei, Taiwan

ABSTRACT

Dendritic cell-specific ICAM-3 grabbing non-integrin (DC-SIGN) has been identified as a receptor for human immunodeficiency virus type 1, hepatitis C virus, Ebola virus, cytomegalovirus, dengue virus, and the SARS coronavirus. In this chapter, we discuss experiments on the interactions between DC-SIGN and H5N1 viruses using pseudotyped and reverse-genetics (RG) technologies. In addition, electronic microscopy and functional assay were employed to elucidate the morphology and function of pseudotyped viruses containing hemagglutinin (HA) and neuraminidase (NA) proteins from H5N1 strains. Results from a capture assay showed that DC-SIGN-expressing cells as well as dendritic cells from human peripheral blood are capable of transferring H5N1 pseudotyped and RG virus particles to target cells; this action can be blocked by anti-DC-SIGN monoclonal antibodies. In summary, DC-SIGN mediates infections both in cis and in trans for avian H5N1 virus transmission.

INTRODUCTION

The global spread of highly pathogenic avian influenza A H5N1 viruses in poultry and sporadic human infections are viewed as parts of a pandemic threat [1, 2]. Currently, H5N1 viruses are viewed as animal pathogens concentrated in poultry and wild birds; most H5N1 human cases have been the result of direct contact with diseased poultry [3, 4]. Between 2003 and April 2008, there were 381 human cases and 240 deaths reported [5, 6]. General influenza virus binding to cellular receptors is mediated by viral hemagglutinin and sialic acid (SA) receptors on cell surfaces. Avian flu viruses generally show a preference for binding to α-2,3-linked SA, whereas human influenza viruses prefer α-2,6-linked SA as a receptor [7].

The H5N1 virus triggers severe systemic infections resulting in a high mortality rate in humans, and its clinical manifestations differ from those associated with influenza A virus infection [5, 8]. Human influenza A viruses usually cause upper respiratory illness and seldom induce systemic infections. In contrast, H5N1-infected patients usually have high fever, few respiratory symptoms, pulmonary infiltrates, and lymphopenia; a small number have shown acute respiratory distress syndrome and sepsis [5, 8]. Results from clinical laboratory diagnoses indicate the presence of H5N1 viral RNA in patient plasma, and the virus has been isolated from plasma specimens [9, 10]. This suggests H5N1 dissemination from a primary infection site (the lungs) to other organs, where they cause systemic diseases [11-15]. The spreading mechanism and cells responsible for the systemic dissemination of the H5N1 influenza virus are still unclear.

Table 1. DC-SIGN binding pathogens

Pathogen	Antigen
Viruses	
HIV-1	Envelope gp120
HIV-2	Envelope gp120
SIV-1	Envelope gp120
Ebola virus	Glycoprotein (GP)
Dengue virus	gE Envelope protein
Hepatitis C virus (HCV)	E1/E2
Cytomegalovirus (CMV)	gB Envelope protein
SARS-CoV	Spike(S) glycoprotein
Influenza A virus	Hemagglutinin protein
Bacteria	
Helicobacter pylori	*Lipopolysaccharides* (LPS)
Klebsiella pneumoniae	*Lipopolysaccharides* (LPS)
Mycobacterium tuberculosis	M. tuberculosis mannose-capped lipoarabinomannan (ManLAM)
Parasites	
Leishmania pifenoi	LPG
Schistosoma mansoni	SEA
Yeast	
Candida albicans	N/A

N/A: None available

Dendritic cells (DCs), a type of professional antigen presenting cell, play an important role in immune system homeostasis [16-18]. When pathogens invade a host, DCs sense and capture them via two pattern recognition receptors: toll-like receptors and C-type lectins [17-19]. A C-type lectin known as dendritic cell-specific ICAM-3 grabbing non-integrin (DC-SIGN) (CD209) is an important factor in DC immune regulation [16]. Researchers have recently described a crosstalk system between DC-SIGN and toll-like receptors leading to T-cell activation or repression [19, 20]. DC-SIGN may be capable of capturing or internalizing pathogens as a means of mediating antigen presentation for T-cell activation and proliferation. During interactions between DC-SIGN and pathogens, the latter would take advantage of this mechanism for immune escape [21]. DC-SIGN was initially identified as an attachment molecule for the human immunodeficiency virus [22], but has since been identified as a receptor for several viruses, including Ebola, hepatitis C, dengue, cytomegalovirus, human herpes type 8, and the SARS coronavirus, among others (Table1) [17, 23-25]. In addition to enhancing viral infections in trans [26, 27], it also serves as a receptor for virus entry and replication in DCs [28, 29]. According to van Kooyk et al.'s [30] report, the carbohydrate-recognition domain (CRD) located in the DC-SIGN cytoplasmic region is responsible for its interaction with the glycoprotein envelope of the above-mentioned viruses. DC-SIGN binds distinct carbohydrate structure, such as mannose-containing glycoconjugates and fucose-containing Lewis blood group antigens, suggesting that it governs a broad pathogen-recognition pattern [30]. Since the HA protein of H5N1 is a glycoprotein, we hypothesized that DC-SIGN interacts with the HA protein, consequently facilitating viral infection or dissemination. In this chapter, we will discuss the possible interaction between DC-SIGN molecules and H5N1 HA proteins.

PREDICTION OF N-LINKED GLYCOSYLATION ON HEMAGGLUTININ OF H5N1 INFLUENZA STRAIN A/VIETNEM/1203/04

The binding of DC-SIGN to pathogens depends on the presence of either high-mannose N-linked carbohydrate chains or fucosylated oligosaccharides on the envelope glycoproteins of the pathogens. We hypothesized interaction between the glycosylated envelope of avian influenza H5N1 viruses and the CRD domain of DC-SIGN. Predictions of N-linked glycosylation on H5N1 hemagglutinin protein were performed using the NetNGlyc 1.0 Server. The hemagglutinin amino acid sequence from the avian influenza H5N1 A/Vietnam/1203/04 strain (accession no. ABW90135) was uploaded to the website, and total N-linked glycosylation sites were predicted following the Asn-X-Ser/Thr rule as previously described [31]. The 3D hemagglutinin structure file was downloaded from the Protein Data Bank (File name: 2FK0). N-linked glycosylation sites were labeled on the structure shown via the DS ViewerPro Trial program. As show in Figure 1, nine N-glycosylation sites on HA — seven in the HA1 domain (amino acid residues 26, 27, 39, 170, 181, 209 and 302) and two in the HA2 domain (residues 500 and 559)—were predicted using the NetNGlyc 1.0 program. The external globular structure is primarily composed of the HA1 domain; N-glycosylation sites 26, 27, 39, 170, 181, 209 and 302 are likely candidates for interaction with DC-SIGN (Figure 1B).

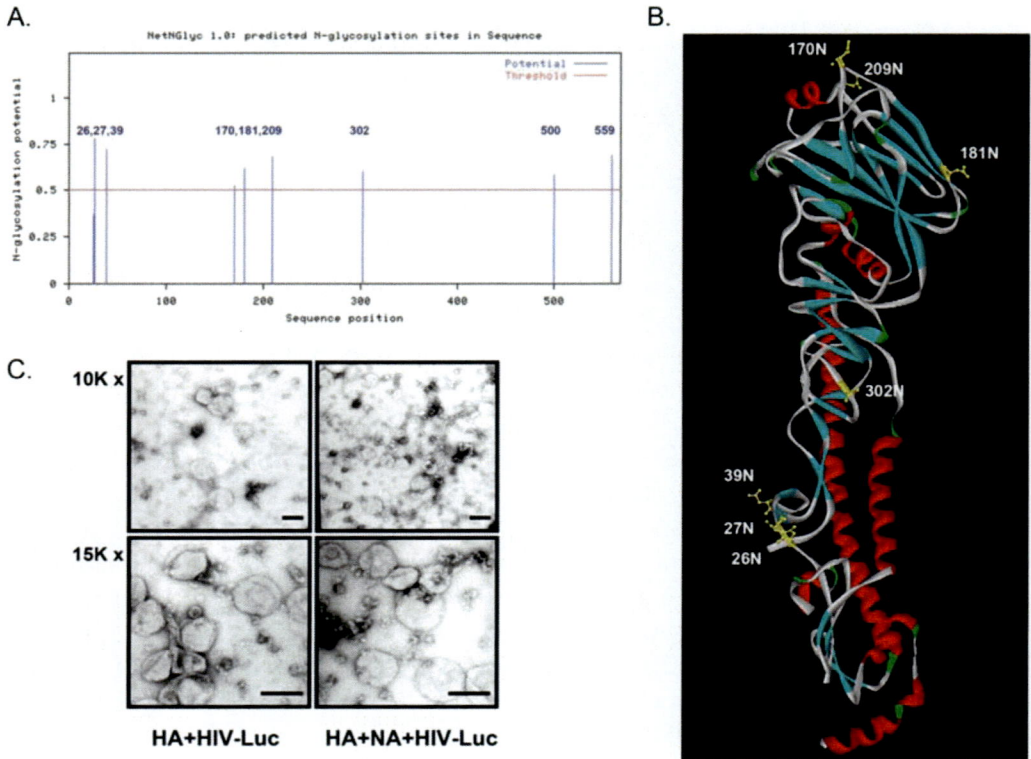

Figure 1. Prediction of N-linked glycosylation on hemagglutinin of H5N1 influenza strain A/Vietnem/1203/04 by NetNGlyc 1.0 Server, displayed on 3D structure with DS ViewerPro Trial program. (A) Of the nine N-glycosylation sites, seven were in the HA1 domain and two in the HA2 domain. Numbers represent a.a site in amino acid sequence (lower panel) and relative structure site (upper panel). (B) Each N-glycosylation site on the hemagglutinin structure was labeled; numbers indicate relative amino acid site. (C) Different combinations of HIV-Luc plasmid with HA (H5N1) or NA (H5N1) plasmid were used to transfect HEK293T cells for H5 pseudotyped virus particle production. Images were taken from grids under a transmission electron microscope after coating and uranyl acetate staining. Upper panel: 10,000X; lower panel: 15,000X; proportional scale: 100 nm.

ESTABLISHMENT OF H5N1 PESUDOTYPED VIRUSES

The pseudotyped virus system is useful for analyzing functional domains for the receptor-binding property of viral envelopes. Pseudotyped lentiviral particles expressing heterologous viral glycoproteins have been reported for SARS [25], HCV [32], Ebola [28], and dengue viruses [33], among others. It has also been reported that lentiviral particles pseudotyped with HA from H5N1 (H5) have entry characteristics (i.e., receptor usage, pH requirements, and neutralization) that are similar to those for the real H5N1 [34].

Plasmids with different genomic segments of H1N1 (A/PR8/34) and H5N1 (A/Vietnam/1203/04) influenza viruses (pHW191-PB2, pHW192-PB1, pHW193-PA, pHW194-HA, pHW195-NP, pHW196-NA, pHW197-M, pHW198-NS, pHW1203-HA and pHW1203-NA) were generously provided by Dr. Robert G. Webster at the St. Jude Children's Research Hospital in Memphis, USA. The plasmid pNL-Luc-E⁻R⁻ contains an env-defective HIV-1 genome with a firefly luciferase reporter gene. We therefore used a HIV-1-defective genome to generate two types of pseudotyped viruses: HA alone and HA/NA of the H5N1 virus.

Pseudotyped viral particle production and concentration were performed as described previously [25, 34]. Briefly, standard calcium phosphate precipitation was used to transfect HEK293T cells with pNL-Luc-E'R' vector and selectively with pHW1203-HA (H5N1) or pHW1203-NA (H5N1) vectors. Cell supernatant containing pseudotyped HIV-1 particles with H5 envelope glycoprotein HA or HA/NA proteins were collected 48 h posttransfection and purified through a 0.45 μm filter. Supernatant was concentrated by ultracentrifugation at 25,000 rpm for 2.5 h, after which concentrated pseudotyped H5 particles were studied with transmission electron microscopy or used for infectivity, hemagglutinin assay and capture assays.

Results from TEM examinations revealed that both H5 and H5N1 pseudotyped virus particles contained spike-like HA structures on their surfaces (Figure 1C). We also observed higher numbers of pseudotyped virus particles generated by HA/NA co-transfection compared to HA alone. Nefkens et al. [31] used a similar system to produce lentiviral pseudotyped viruses with HA from H5N1, adding neuraminidase to culture medium to harvest larger quantities. Their data is consistent with our observation that pseudotyped virus particles bearing both HA and NA proteins are much more easily released from cell surfaces compared to particles bearing the HA protein only.

Table 2. Hemagglutination and cell susceptibility of H5N1 pseudotyped virus

	Hemagglutinin assay [a]	Luminescence value [b]		
		HEK293T	MDCK	Vero
H5 pseudotyped virus				
TPCK(+)	Positive	26 ± 9.2	19.6 ± 4.4	2.3 ± 0.5
TPCK(-)	Negative	3 ± 1	1.6 ± 0.5	N/A
H5N1 pseudotyped virus				
TPCK(+)	Positive	129 ± 40.8 (**)	111 ± 30.5 (*)	4.3 ± 0.5
TPCK(-)	Negative	1.3 ± 0.5	1.3 ± 0.5	N/A

Footnotes:

[a] Hemagglutination activity of H5 or H5N1 pseudotyped viruses evaluated with hemagglutinin assay (0.5% turkey RBC), the HA titers of positive reaction was 1:2~1:8.

[b] In cell susceptibility, each cell was infected with 20 ng H5 or H5N1 pesudotyped viruses and infectivity was evaluated by luciferase acitivity. Comparison of infectivity between H5 and H5N1 pesudotyped virus in each cell lines (* indicates $p < 0.05$; ** indicates $p < 0.01$).

FUNCTIONAL CHARACTERIZATION OF H5N1 PSEUDOTYPED VIRUSES

We used a hemagglutinin test and cell susceptibility assay to compare the functional integrity of H5- and H5N1-pseudotyped viruses, and found that following TPCK treatment, both virus types expressed similar hemagglutinin activity, with titers ranging from 1:2 to 1:8. Both types displayed very low hemagglutinin activity without TPCK treatment (Table 2). It has been reported that HA precursors must be cleaved into HA1 and HA2 in order to become capable of binding to cellular receptors [35].

Regarding cell susceptibility, three cell lines (HEK293T, MDCK, and Vero) were tested with equal amounts of H5- and H5N1-pseudotyped viruses standardized by p24 antigen. Following p24 quantification with a Coulter HIV-1 p24 antigen assay, 100 ng of H5 pseudotyped virus particles were collected and incubated with HEK293T, MDCK, or Vero cells. Luciferase activity was measured in cell lysate after 48 h of incubation. Our results indicate that judging by luciferase enzyme activity, the H5N1-pseudotyped virus had significantly higher infectivity than the H5-pseudotyped virus ($p < 0.05$). In addition, both MDCK and HEK293T cells were more susceptible to pseudotyped virus infection than the Vero cells (Table 1). A possible explanation is that MDCK and HEK293T cells express more α-2,3-linked SA receptors than Vero cells (34). This explains our rationale to use the MDCK and HEK293T cells in our experiments.

DC-SIGN Molecule Mediates H5N1 Pseudotyped Viruses Infection In Cis

We used two cell lines—B-THP-1 and B-THP-1/DC-SIGN (a stable B-THP-1 clone expressing DC-SIGN molecules)—to investigate whether DC-SIGN is capable of mediating the binding and entry of H5N1 pseudotyped virus particles to target cells. Cells were incubated with H5N1 pseudotyped viruses; viral infectivity was determined with luciferase assays. Note that some of these cells or cell lines had been pretreated with DC-SIGN monoclonal antibody before we received them.

As shown in Figure 2A, B-THP-1/DC-SIGN cells expressed twice as much luciferase activity as the B-THP-1 cells, and the ability of the H5N1 pseudotyped virus to infect B-THP-1/DC-SIGN cells was reduced when the cells were pre-treated with an anti-DC-SIGN monoclonal antibody. Similar results were observed using the combination of THP-1 and THP-1/DC-SIGN cell lines (data not shown). To rule out the possibility that enhanced infectivity was due to differential expression levels of avian influenza viruses that bind only to the α2,3-linked SA receptor, both cell lines were stained with SNA (*Sambucus nigra* for α2,6-linked SA staining) and MAA (Maackia amurensis for α2,3-linked SA staining). As shown in Figure 2B, both cell lines had identical distributions of α-2,3- and α-2,6-linked SA receptors. To clarify whether DC-SIGN is a receptor that mediates the entry of H5N1 pseudotyped virus particles or if it simply enhances viral entry via SA receptors, we used vibrio cholerae sialidase to eliminate α-2,3-linked SA from the cells. Our results show that almost all of the α-2,3-linked SA was removed but DC-SIGN levels remained unchanged (Figure 2C). Following treatment with sialidase, B-THP-1 and B-THP-1/DC-SIGN cells were incubated with H5N1 pseudotyped virus particles; we detected very low luminescence levels in the resulting cell lysates (data not shown). This strongly suggests that H5N1 pseudotyped virus particles interact with DC-SIGN and facilitate viral entry into target cells in cis via SA receptors.

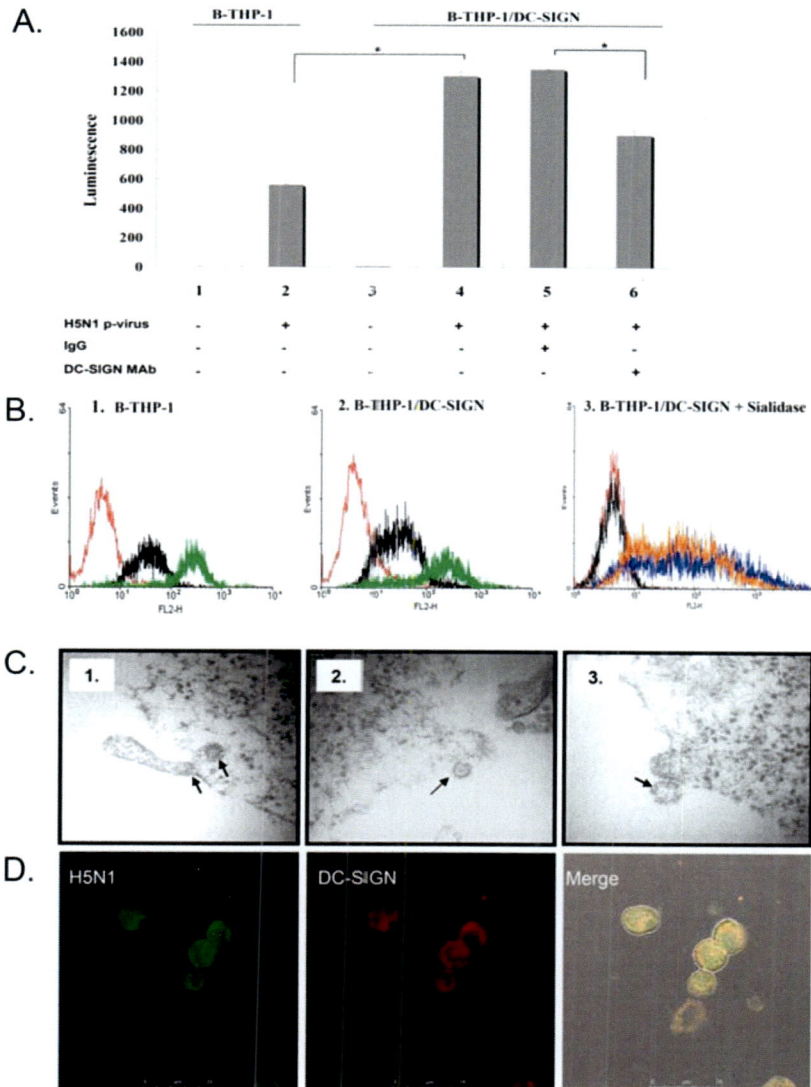

Figure 2. DC-SIGN as an attachment receptor for H5N1 pseudotyped virus and enhanced H5N1 pseudotyped virus infection in cis. (A) B-THP-1 cells and B-THP-1/DC-SIGN infected with the H5N1 pseudotyped virus (H5N1 p-virus), with or without anti-DC-SIGN MAb or IgG control preincubation, were used for infectivity assays. Bars represent B-THP-1/DC-SIGN pretreated with the following antibodies: 3, medium only; 5, IgG control; 6, anti-DC-SIGN MAb. (B) MAA and SNA were used to stain influenza virus receptor α-2,3- and α-2,6-linked SA on B-THP-1 and B-THP-1/DC-SIGN cells. Graphs 1 and 2: black and green lines represent MAA and SNA staining, respectively; red represents isotype control. Graph 3: black line represents MAA, orange and blue lines pre- and post-sialidase treatment, respectively. (C) H5N1 pseudotyped virus binding to DC-SIGN-expressing cells following the removal of the influenza receptor with sialidase. Images 1-3: arrows indicate H5N1 pseudotyped virus position in different sections of B-THP-1/DC-SIGN cells under TEM. (D) H5N1 pseudotyped virus and DC-SIGN colocalized staining under a confocal microscope. Green and red fluorescence represent H5N1 virus and DC-SIGN molecules on cell surfaces, respectively. Merged orange fluorescence on cell edges indicate their colocalization. Results shown are from one representative experiment out of three performed (*, $p<0.05$; **, $p<0.01$).

DC-SIGN SPECIFICALLY INTERACTS
WITH H5N1 HEMAGGLUTININ PROTEIN

Next we would like to prove that DC-SIGN molecule could specifically interact with the H5-HA protein. H5 pseudotyped viral binding to DC-SIGN- expressing cells was analyzed by transmission electron microscopy and immunofluorescence staining with laser-scanning confocal microscopy as described in (36). Briefly, following vibrio cholerae sialidase treatment, B-THP-1/DC-SIGN cells were incubated with pseudotyped H5N1 virus. After unbound particles were removed by washing with PBS. Some viral binding cells were observed under TEM. Alternatively, some were applied for IFA staining with FITC-conjugated anti-H5N1 polyclonal antibody and PE-conjugated anti-DC-SIGN monoclonal antibody. Then stained cells were observed using a confocal microscope.

Table 3. DC-SIGN could specifically capture H5N1 pseudotyped viruses

	B-THP-1/DC-SIGN		THP-1/DC-SIGN	
	P24 (pg/ml)	Inhibition (%)	P24 (pg/ml)	Inhibition (%)
IgG control	340	0	366	0
DC-SIGN MAb	260	23.55 ±2.3	262	28.65 ± 3.4

Footnotes: Inhibition rate was calculated by using the formula 100-[(P24 with anti-DC-SIGN/ P24 with isotyped control) x 100%] Each representative experiment of three independent experiments was shown. The percentages of viral binding were means of three independent experiments+ SD.

Transmission electron microscopy images demonstrate the attachment of many H5N1 pseudotyped virus particles to the surfaces of cells expressing DC-SIGN (Figure 2C); indirect immunofluorescent antibody assay (IFA) results further indicate a colocalization between H5N1 pseudotyped particles and DC-SIGN (Figure 2D). In addition to transmission electron microscopy and IFA colocalized staining, we also used HIV p24 quantification to study the binding of H5N1 pseudotyped virus particles to DC-SIGN, and found that p24 antigen levels in the cell lysates of DC-SIGN-expressing cells were significantly higher than those in the B-THP-1 and THP-1 control cells (Table 3). Furthermore, p24 levels were reduced in the presence of anti-DC-SIGN monoclonal antibodies, with inhibition percentages of 23% and 28% for B-THP-1/DC-SIGN and THP-1/DC-SIGN cells, respectively (Table 2). These results are similar to those found in a previous report on HCV pseudotyped virus binding to DC-SIGN [33]; those authors reported that the anti-DC-SIGN monoclonal antibody (MoAb 612X) had a 19-41% inhibitory effect on HCV pseudotyped virus binding to DC-SIGN.

DC-SIGN MOLECULE MEDIATES H5N1
PSEUDOTYPED VIRUSES INFECTION IN TRANS

We used a standard capture assay to determine whether DC-SIGN is capable of mediating H5N1 pseudotyped viral infection in trans, as described previously (25, 27). Briefly, donor cells were incubated with H5 pseudotyped viruses, then washed before being added to the target MDCK cells. Target cells were harvested and pseudotyped H5N1 virus quantification was performed using a luciferase reporter assay. As shown in Figure 3A (lanes 1, 2, 5 and 6), both B-THP-1/DC-SIGN and THP-1/DC-SIGN cells were capable of transferring H5N1 pseudotyped viruses to MDCK cells more efficiently than the B-THP-1 and THP-1 control cells. The differences in luciferase activity between cells with or without DC-SIGN expression were statistically significant ($p < 0.05$ and $p < 0.01$ for the B-THP-1 and THP-1 pairs, respectively). Furthermore, compared to cells treated with an IgG control antibody, luciferase activity decreased significantly when donor cells were pretreated with an anti-DC-SIGN monoclonal antibody (Figure 3A, lanes 3, 4, 7 and 8). Combined, the data indicate that DC-SIGN binds with H5N1 virus particles and facilitates the viral infection of their target cells in trans.

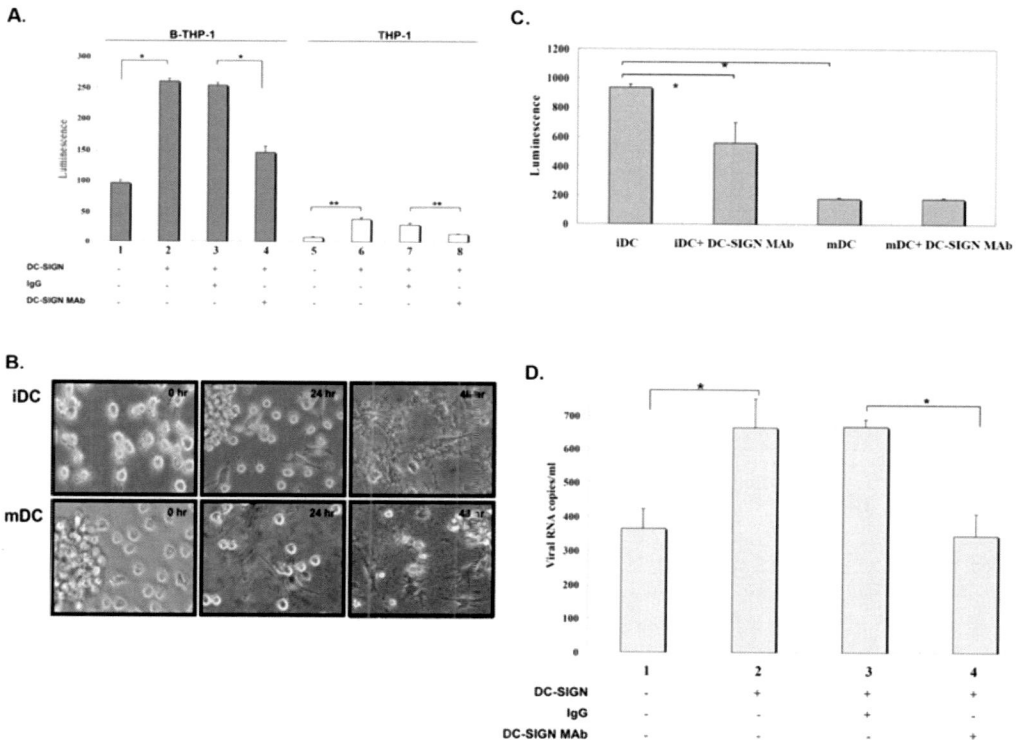

Figure 3. DC-SIGN mediates trans infection by H5N1 pseudotyped and reverse-genetics viruses. (A) The both sets of donor cells B-THP-1, B-THP-1/DC-SIGN and THP-1, THP-1/DC-SIGN were used in capture assay. The bars represent luciferase activity measured in MDCK cell lysates following co-culturing with donor cells in the presence or absence of MAb. (B) Immature and mature DCs were infected with H5N1 pseudotyped viruses for 0-48 h and cell morphology was observed under a light microscope. Upper and lower panels indicate iDCs and mDCs, respectively. (C) Immature and mature DCs with or without anti-DC-SIGN MAb treatment were used as donor cells to capture H5N1 pseudotyped virus particles and for co-culturing with MDCK cells. Luciferase activity was determined in MDCK lysates 48 h post-treatment. (D) The H5N1 reverse genetics strain A/Vietnam/1194/04 (10^5 copies/ml) was used for a capture assay. Virus-bound sialidase-treated B-THP-1/DC-SIGN and B-THP-1 donor cells were co-cultured with MDCK cells for 48 h; RT-PCR was used to quantify H5N1 viral RNA in MDCK cell lysates. Results shown are from one representative experiment out of three performed ($*$, $p < 0.05$).

DC-SIGN Expressed on Dendritic Cell (DC) Mediates H5N1 Pseudotyped and Reverse-Genetics (RG) Viruses Infection In Cis and In Trans

Interaction between DC-SIGN and H5N1 pseudotyped viruses was further confirmed using monocyte-derived DCs (MDCCs) purified from blood collected from healthy donors. Briefly, peripheral blood mononuclear cells (PBMCs) were isolated from blood donated by a healthy, anti-H5N1 negative donor. Monocytes were extracted from PBMCs with VARIOMACS anti-CD14 microbeads. Isolated human monocytes were cultivated in medium supplemented with human granulocyte-macrophage colony-stimulating factor (GM-CSF) and human interleukin-4(IL-4) for 6 days to trigger differentiation into immature DCs (iDCs). iDCs were confirmed with CD1a, CD40, CD54, HLA-DR, CD80, CD83, CD86 and DC-LAMP cell markers by flow cytometry and morphological characteristics. To induce the transformation of iDCs into mature DCs (mDCs), 0.1ug/ml lipopolysaccharide (LPS) was used to treat for further 1.5 days. mDCs were also confirmed using the above-mentioned cell markers and morphological characteristics [25].

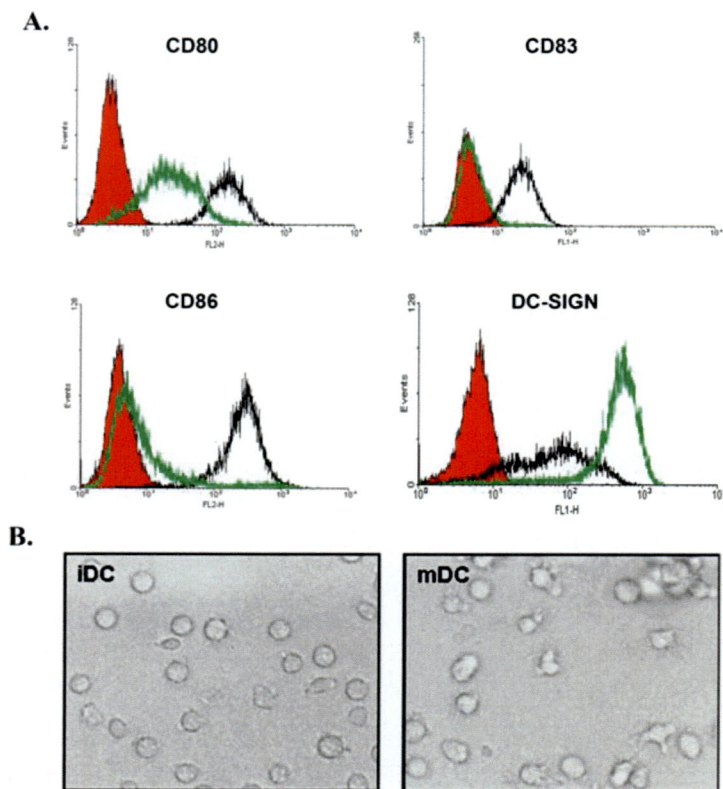

Figure 4. Differences in cell markers and morphologies between immature and mature DCs. (A) DCs were stained with anti-CD80, CD83, CD86, and anti-DC-SIGN monoclonal antibodies. Black and green lines represent mDCs and iDCs, respectively. (B) Morphologies were observed under a light microscope.

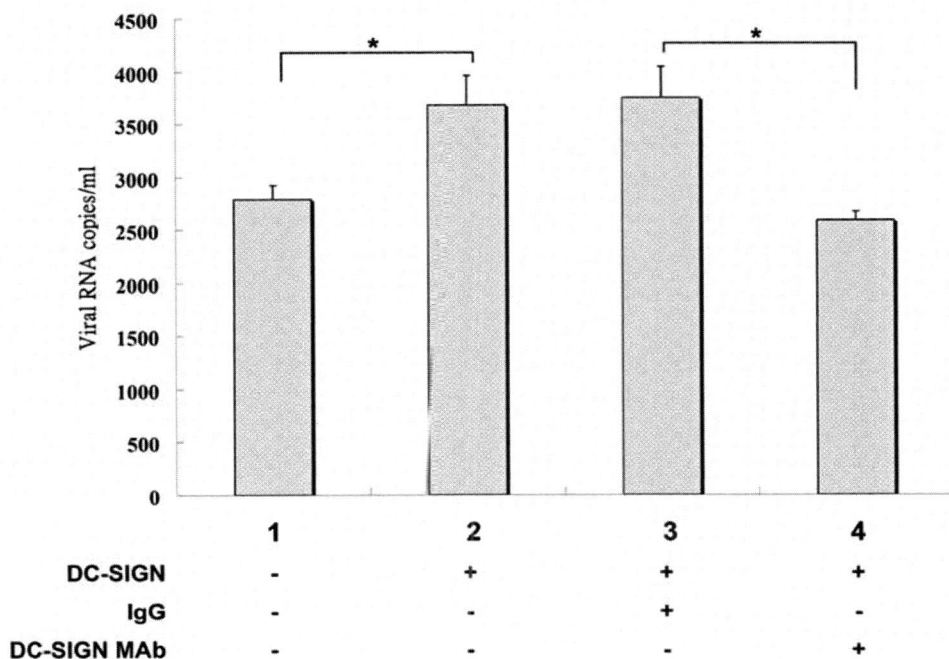

Figure 5. DC-SIGN mediates H5N1 reverse-genetics virus infection in cis. H5N1 reverse genetics strain A/Vietnam/1194/04 (10^5 copies/ml) was used for an infectivity assay. B-THP-1 cells and B-THP-1/DC-SIGN infected with the H5N1 reverse genetics virus, with or without anti-DC-SIGN MAb or IgG control preincubation, were used for infectivity assays. Viral RNA was quantified by real-time RT-PCR. Results shown are from one representative experiment out of three performed. (*, $p < 0.05$).

Compared to iDCs, mDCs expressed higher percentages of CD80, CD83, and CD86 cell markers (Figure 4A) and displayed both multiple pseudopods and irregular morphologies (Figure 4B); iDCs also expressed higher levels of DC-SIGN than mDCs (Figure 4A). Furthermore, the morphologies of both mDCs and iDCs changed dramatically 24 h post-infection with H5N1 pseudotyped viruses. At 48 h post-infection, both mDCs and iDCs adhered to the bottom of culture plates (Figure 3B). Following incubation with the H5N1 pseudotyped virus at 4°C for 1 hr, DCs were co-cultured with MDCK cells and the resulting luciferase activity of MDCK lysates was measured. The results show that iDCs had a significantly higher capture ability compared to mDCs (Figure 3C, lanes 1 and 3), and that this effect can be blocked by pre-treatment with anti-DC-SIGN monoclonal antibodies (Figure 3C, lane 2). Based on these findings, we conclude that iDCs play an important role in the dissemination of H5N1 pseudotyped virus infection due to its ability to capture and transfer viral infections to target cells. Finally, we used reverse-genetics (RG) to produce H5N1 A/Vietnam/1194/04 RG virus particles to confirm the phenomenon described in this chapter. As shown in Figure 5, B-THP-1/DC-SIGN cells had significantly higher copy numbers of H5N1 RG viruses than B-THP-1 cells 48 h post-infection (lanes 1 and 2, $p < 0.05$). Infection was significantly blocked when cells were pre-treated with anti-DC-SIGN monoclonal antibodies (lane 4). Results from a capture assay show that compared to the B-THP-1 control, the B-THP-1/DC-SIGN cells captured and transferred significantly higher numbers of H5N1 RG viruses to MDCK cells, and that the effect can be blocked by anti-DC-

SIGN monoclonal antibodies (Figure 3D). According to these results, DC-SIGN is capable of mediating H5N1 RG virus infection in cis and in trans. We found evidence indicating that DC-SIGN does not function as a main entry receptor in the same manner as α-2,3-linked SA for the avian H5N1 virus, but instead acts as a capture or attachment molecule for the virus and as an infection mediating factor both in cis and in trans.

Thitithanyanont et al. [37] previously showed that DCs express both α-2,3-linked and α-2,6-linked SA, and that H5N1 viruses are capable of escaping viral-specific immunity and dissemination to other organs through infection and replication in DCs. There are several existing reports indicating that iDCs and mDCs differ in viral infection susceptibility—for example, in HIV-1 [38, 39] and SARS CoV [38, 39]. Consistent with these studies, we found that iDCs had higher capture and transfer capabilities than mDCs. Thitithanyanont et al. also demonstrated that 24 h post-infection with the avian H5N1 virus, the majority of DCs died at a very low MOI [40]. Our results indicate that the H5N1 pseudotyped virus induced extensive activation of iDCs and mDCs after 48 h of incubation, but mDCs showed lower susceptibility to the H5N1 virus. The results also indicate that a reduction in DC-SIGN expression may lead to the phenomenon described in this report. Based on our findings, we suggest that iDCs residing in the lower respiratory tract or deep lung compartments are susceptible to H5N1 virus infection via the α-2,3-linked SA receptor and DC-SIGN. Infected iDCs then migrate to lymphoid tissues and other organs and transfer the H5N1 virus to other target cells expressing α-2,3-linked SA receptors, resulting in a systemic infection. Another recently published study suggests that $CD4^+$ T-cells may be an important target for H5N1 virus infection [40].

CONCLUSION

DC-SIGN may play an important role in enhancing H5N1 infection and be an attachment receptor for capturing H5N1 virus to other target cells during iDCs' activation and migration to other sites. In this chapter, we proved that pseudotyped viruses containing both H5N1 HA and NA proteins displayed hemagglutination and infection capability. In addition to enhancing H5N1 viral infectivity, we also observed that DC-SIGN expression facilitates virus transport to recipient cells via B-THP-1/DC-SIGN and human dendritic cells. These results suggest that DC-SIGN is an important attachment molecule mediating H5N1 virus infection in cis and in trans. It is useful for the development of preventive and therapeutic strategies for avian influenza infection. Further studies are needed to map the domains on the HA of H5N1 virus for its interaction with DC-SIGN.

ACKNOWLEDGMENTS

Our gratitude goes to the Vaccine Research and Development Center, National Health Research Institute, Taiwan for providing H5N1 A/Vietnam1194/04 RG strain, and to members of Dr. Shie-Liang Hsieh's lab for their advice and support for human DC isolation. This work was supported by a grant from the National Science Council, Republic of China (NSC 97-2321-B-010-003) and a grant from the Ministry of Education, Aim for the Top University Plan.

REFERENCES

[1] Gambotto A, Barratt-Boyes SM, de Jong MD, Neumann G, Kawaoka Y. Human infection with highly pathogenic H5N1 influenza virus. *Lancet.* 2008 Apr 26;371 (9622):1464-75.

[2] Korteweg C, Gu J. Pathology, Molecular Biology, and Pathogenesis of Avian Influenza A (H5N1) Infection in Humans. *Am J Pathol.* 2008 May;172(5):1155-70.

[3] Pawitan JA. Human H5N1 influenza. *N Engl J Med.* 2007 Mar 29;356(13):1375; author reply 6-7.

[4] Peiris JS, de Jong MD, Guan Y. Avian influenza virus (H5N1): a threat to human health. *Clin Microbiol Rev.* 2007 Apr;20(2):243-67.

[5] Beigel JH, Farrar J, Han AM, Hayden FG, Hyer R, de Jong MD, et al. Avian influenza A (H5N1) infection in humans. *N Engl J Med.* 2005 Sep 29;353(13):1374-85.

[6] Proenca-Modena JL, Macedo IS, Arruda E. H5N1 avian influenza virus: an overview. *Braz J Infect Dis.* 2007 Feb;11(1):125-33.

[7] Yao L, Korteweg C, Hsueh W, Gu J. Avian influenza receptor expression in H5N1-infected and noninfected human tissues. *FASEB J.* 2008 Mar;22(3):733-40.

[8] Gilbert M, Xiao X, Pfeiffer DU, Epprecht M, Boles S, Czarnecki C, et al. Mapping H5N1 highly pathogenic avian influenza risk in Southeast Asia. *Proc Natl Acad Sci USA.* 2008 Mar 25;105(12):4769-74.

[9] Chutinimitkul S, Bhattarakosol P, Srisuratanon S, Eiamudomkan A, Kongsomboon K, Damrongwatanapokin S, et al. H5N1 influenza A virus and infected human plasma. *Emerg Infect Dis.* 2006 Jun;12(6):1041-3.

[10] de Jong MD, Simmons CP, Thanh TT, Hien VM, Smith GJ, Chau TN, et al. Fatal outcome of human influenza A (H5N1) is associated with high viral load and hypercytokinemia. *Nat Med.* 2006 Oct;12(10):1203-7.

[11] Yuen KY, Chan PK, Peiris M, Tsang DN, Que TL, Shortridge KF, et al. Clinical features and rapid viral diagnosis of human disease associated with avian influenza A H5N1 virus. *Lancet.* 1998 Feb 14;351(9101):467-71.

[12] Chotpitayasunondh T, Ungchusak K, Hanshaoworakul W, Chunsuthiwat S, Sawanpanyalert P, Kijphati R, et al. Human disease from influenza A (H5N1), Thailand, 2004. *Emerg Infect Dis.* 2005 Feb;11(2):201-9.

[13] To KF, Chan PK, Chan KF, Lee WK, Lam WY, Wong KF, et al. Pathology of fatal human infection associated with avian influenza A H5N1 virus. *J Med Virol.* 2001 Mar;63(3):242-6.

[14] Uiprasertkul M, Puthavathana P, Sangsiriwut K, Pooruk P, Srisook K, Peiris M, et al. Influenza A H5N1 replication sites in humans. *Emerg Infect Dis.* 2005 Jul;11(7):1036-41.

[15] de Jong MD, Bach VC, Phan TQ, Vo MH, Tran TT, Nguyen BH, et al. Fatal avian influenza A (H5N1) in a child presenting with diarrhea followed by coma. *N Engl J Med.* 2005 Feb 17;352(7):686-91.

[16] Geijtenbeek TB, Torensma R, van Vliet SJ, van Duijnhoven GC, Adema GJ, van Kooyk Y, et al. Identification of DC-SIGN, a novel dendritic cell-specific ICAM-3 receptor that supports primary immune responses. *Cell.* 2000 Mar 3;100(5):575-85.

[17] Zhou T, Chen Y, Hao L, Zhang Y. DC-SIGN and immunoregulation. *Cell Mol Immunol*. 2006 Aug;3(4):279-83.

[18] Vicari AP, Caux C, Trinchieri G. Tumour escape from immune surveillance through dendritic cell inactivation. *Semin Cancer Biol*. 2002 Feb;12(1):33-42.

[19] Gringhuis SI, den Dunnen J, Litjens M, van Het Hof B, van Kooyk Y, Geijtenbeek TB. C-type lectin DC-SIGN modulates Toll-like receptor signaling via Raf-1 kinase-dependent acetylation of transcription factor NF-kappaB. *Immunity*. 2007 May;26(5): 605-16.

[20] Geijtenbeek TB, van Vliet SJ, Engering A, t Hart BA, van Kooyk Y. Self- and nonself-recognition by C-type lectins on dendritic cells. *Annu Rev Immunol*. 2004;22:33-54.

[21] van Gisbergen KP, Aarnoudse CA, Meijer GA, Geijtenbeek TB, van Kooyk Y. Dendritic cells recognize tumor-specific glycosylation of carcinoembryonic antigen on colorectal cancer cells through dendritic cell-specific intercellular adhesion molecule-3-grabbing nonintegrin. *Cancer Res*. 2005 Jul 1;65(13):5935-44.

[22] Curtis BM, Scharnowske S, Watson AJ. Sequence and expression of a membrane-associated C-type lectin that exhibits CD4-independent binding of human immuno-deficiency virus envelope glycoprotein gp120. *Proc Natl Acad Sci USA*. 1992 Sep 1;89(17):8356-60.

[23] Han DP, Lohani M, Cho MW. Specific asparagine-linked glycosylation sites are critical for DC-SIGN- and L-SIGN-mediated severe acute respiratory syndrome coronavirus entry. *J Virol*. 2007 Nov;81(21):12029-39.

[24] Kretz-Rommel A, Qin F, Dakappagari N, Torensma R, Faas S, Wu D, et al. In vivo targeting of antigens to human dendritic cells through DC-SIGN elicits stimulatory immune responses and inhibits tumor growth in grafted mouse models. *J Immunother*. 2007 Oct;30(7):715-26.

[25] Shih YP, Chen CY, Liu SJ, Chen KH, Lee YM, Chao YC, et al. Identifying epitopes responsible for neutralizing antibody and DC-SIGN binding on the spike glycoprotein of the severe acute respiratory syndrome coronavirus. *J Virol*. 2006 Nov;80(21):10315-24.

[26] Engering A, Geijtenbeek TB, van Vliet SJ, Wijers M, van Liempt E, Demaurex N, et al. The dendritic cell-specific adhesion receptor DC-SIGN internalizes antigen for presentation to T cells. *J Immunol*. 2002 Mar 1;168(5):2118-26.

[27] Geijtenbeek TB, Kwon DS, Torensma R, van Vliet SJ, van Duijnhoven GC, Middel J, et al. DC-SIGN, a dendritic cell-specific HIV-1-binding protein that enhances trans-infection of T cells. *Cell*. 2000 Mar 3;100(5):587-97.

[28] Alvarez CP, Lasala F, Carrillo J, Muniz O, Corbi AL, Delgado R. C-type lectins DC-SIGN and L-SIGN mediate cellular entry by Ebola virus in cis and in trans. *J Virol*. 2002 Jul;76(13):6841-4.

[29] Tassaneetrithep B, Burgess TH, Granelli-Piperno A, Trumpfheller C, Finke J, Sun W, et al. DC-SIGN (CD209) mediates dengue virus infection of human dendritic cells. *J Exp Med*. 2003 Apr 7;197(7):823-9.

[30] van Kooyk Y, Geijtenbeek TB. DC-SIGN: escape mechanism for pathogens. *Nat Rev Immunol*. 2003 Sep;3(9):697-709.

[31] Tsuchiya E, Sugawara K, Hongo S, Matsuzaki Y, Muraki Y, Nakamura K. Role of overlapping glycosylation sequons in antigenic properties, intracellular transport and

biological activities of influenza A/H2N2 virus haemagglutinin. *J Gen Virol*. 2002 Dec;83(Pt 12):3067-74.

[32]   Bartosch B, Dubuisson J, Cosset FL. Infectious hepatitis C virus pseudo-particles containing functional E1-E2 envelope protein complexes. *J Exp Med*. 2003 Mar 3;197(5):633-42.

[33]   Hu HP, Hsieh SC, King CC, Wang WK. Characterization of retrovirus-based reporter viruses pseudotyped with the precursor membrane and envelope glycoproteins of four serotypes of dengue viruses. *Virology*. 2007 Nov 25;368(2):376-87.

[34]   Nefkens I, Garcia JM, Ling CS, Lagarde N, Nicholls J, Tang DJ, et al. Hemagglutinin pseudotyped lentiviral particles: characterization of a new method for avian H5N1 influenza sero-diagnosis. *J Clin Virol*. 2007 May;39(1):27-33.

[35]   Elliot AJ, Steinhauer DA, Daniels RS, Oxford JS. Functional and antigenic analyses of the 1918 influenza virus haemagglutinin using a recombinant vaccinia virus expression system. *Virus Res*. 2006 Dec;122(1-2):11-9.

[36]   Barth H, Ulsenheimer A, Pape GR, Diepolder HM, Hoffmann M, Neumann-Haefelin C, et al. Uptake and presentation of hepatitis C virus-like particles by human dendritic cells. *Blood*. 2005 May 1;105(9):3605-14.

[37]   Thitithanyanont A, Engering A, Ekchariyawat P, Wiboon-ut S, Limsalakpetch A, Yongvanitchit K, et al. High susceptibility of human dendritic cells to avian influenza H5N1 virus infection and protection by IFN-alpha and TLR ligands. *J Immunol*. 2007 Oct 15;179(8):5220-7.

[38]   Granelli-Piperno A, Delgado E, Finkel V, Paxton W, Steinman RM. Immature dendritic cells selectively replicate macrophagetropic (M-tropic) human immunodeficiency virus type 1, while mature cells efficiently transmit both M- and T-tropic virus to T cells. *J Virol*. 1998 Apr;72(4):2733-7.

[39]   Spiegel M, Schneider K, Weber F, Weidmann M, Hufert FT. Interaction of severe acute respiratory syndrome-associated coronavirus with dendritic cells. *J Gen Virol*. 2006 Jul;87(Pt 7):1953-60.

[40]   Li YG, Thawatsupha P, Chittaganpitch M, Rungrojcharoenkit K, Li GM, Nakaya T, et al. Higher in vitro susceptibility of human T cells to H5N1 than H1N1 influenza viruses. *Biochem Biophys Res Commun*. 2008 Apr 30.

PART III:
ACTION OF CURRENT AND DESIGN OF NOVEL ANTI-VIRAL DRUGS

In: Global View of Fight against Influenza
Editor: Petar M. Mitrasinovic

ISBN: 978-1-60741-952-5
© 2009 Nova Science Publishers, Inc.

Chapter 7

THE ACTIVITY OF NEURAMINIDASE INHIBITOR OSELTAMIVIR AGAINST ALL SUBTYPES OF INFLUENZA VIRUSES

Noel A. Roberts[1] and Elena A. Govorkova[2]

[1] School of Biosciences, Cardiff University, Cardiff, UK
[2] Dept. of Infectious Diseases, St. Jude Children's Research Hospital, Memphis, Tennessee, USA

ABSTRACT

Influenza A viruses can potentially carry any pairing of 16 haemagglutinin (HA) and nine neuraminidase (NA) subtypes. Recent human epidemics have been limited to influenza A viruses of H1N1, H2N2, and H3N2 subtypes and influenza B viruses. However, in birds, reservoirs of influenza A viruses carrying all the other HA and NA subtypes can be found. Thus, influenza A virus composed of any combination of H1-H16 and N1-N9 could potentially transmit from birds to humans, creating a new pandemic virus. Nineteen highly conserved amino acids are common to the active site of all influenza virus NAs and thus make NA an attractive target for development of antiviral drugs. The NA inhibitor oseltamivir carboxylate (the active metabolite of oseltamivir) was designed to bind to this conserved region. Oseltamivir carboxylate is active in vitro against representative N1–N9 influenza A virus and influenza B virus NAs. Oseltamivir has been shown to be active in vivo against different subtypes of influenza viruses. In particular, experimental animal and avian models demonstrate the effectiveness of oseltamivir treatment against infection caused by highly pathogenic H5N1 and H7N7 influenza viruses. These and other data support the potential inhibitory activity of oseltamivir against all subtypes of influenza viruses.

INTRODUCTION

Influenza virus infection is not trivial. Annual deaths worldwide resulting from seasonal influenza virus infection are estimated at 250,000–500,000, with 3–5 million cases of severe illness and substantial burdens on healthcare resources and the economy [1]. In 1918–1919, an influenza pandemic caused about 50 million deaths worldwide. Other serious pandemic influenza viruses emerged in 1957–1958 and 1968–1969. These three pandemics of the twentieth century were all caused by different influenza A virus subtypes, H1N1, H2N2, and H3N2, respectively [2]. The influenza virus subtype that will cause the next pandemic is unknown, although H5N1 is currently thought to be a candidate [3]. Seasonal influenza outbreaks tend to be the result of milder infections with influenza A virus subtypes, which have caused recent pandemics, or influenza B virus. The ideal anti-influenza virus treatment should therefore be effective against any potential influenza virus subtype.

Influenza virus carries eight single-stranded RNA gene segments [4], two of which encode the viral surface glycoproteins neuraminidase (NA) and haemagglutinin (HA). There are nine NA (N1-N9) and 16 HA subtypes (H1-H16) of influenza A viruses and one NA and HA subtype of influenza B virus. Although influenza is a serious human infection, it is also a zoonotic disease and intrinsically an infection of birds, particularly aquatic birds [5]. Over the last century, human influenza virus infections have essentially been limited to influenza A subtypes H1N1, H2N2, and H3N2 and influenza B viruses; however, in birds, reservoirs of influenza A viruses carrying all the other NA and HA subtypes have been isolated [5]. All of the eight segmented genes of influenza A virus can potentially be re-assorted by co-infection in vivo in birds, humans, pigs, or other susceptible species, creating new viruses. This may also be achieved in vitro by either co-culture or reverse genetics [6, 7]. Thus, new strains of influenza, potentially very virulent to humans, could be transmitted directly from birds or could be generated in the laboratory by chance or otherwise, creating the source of future influenza pandemics. Recently, fairly limited but worrying infections of humans with avian influenza A viruses of the H5N1, H9N2, H7N3, and H7N7 subtypes have been reported [8, 9, 10]. Fortunately, these viruses have had little ability to transmit between humans, but minor random genetic changes or re-assortment following co-infection could suddenly change that characteristic. Most of the immune response to influenza infection is attributed to the two major surface proteins, NA and HA. Long-term lack of exposure of most humans to any influenza A subtypes other than H1N1, H2N2, and H3N2 leaves the population vulnerable to infection with influenza A viruses carrying NA or HA glycoproteins of the other subtypes. Currently available seasonal vaccines would likely be of little or no protective value and, without inspired pre-emption, vaccines to a new emergent pandemic strain would take about six months to become available. Thus, for the first few months of a new influenza pandemic it is likely that, in the absence of an antigenically closely matched pre-pandemic vaccine, treatment and prophylaxis with antiviral drugs will be the only means of defense. It is therefore important that the drugs available to treat influenza have activity against as wide a spectrum of influenza subtypes as possible.

Here we will review data demonstrating that the NA inhibitor oseltamivir is active in vitro and in vivo against all NA subtypes of influenza A and B viruses. Some previously unpublished data will be presented. For any influenza virus subtype there is the potential for the virus to become resistant to oseltamivir by mutation, usually in response to treatment with the drug. This topic will not be addressed here but has been reviewed previously [11, 12].

THE ROLE OF NEURAMINIDASE IN INFLUENZA VIRUS REPLICATION

NA is second to HA as the most abundant protein on the viral surface, with 50–100 molecules per virion. The viral NA, like HA protein, is a sialic acid binding protein [4]. However, in contrast to HA, which binds to cellular receptors containing terminal sialic acid residues initiating the viral fusion and entry process, the NA cleaves terminal sialic acid residues from glycoconjugates. In vitro studies indicate that viral NA has three related functions (Figure 1). It facilitates the release of newly synthesized virus particles by removing sialic acid residues from the surface of the infected cells, allowing virus to spread; it enhances viral infectivity by removing terminal sialic acid residues from the mucus in the respiratory tract, thus facilitating virus trafficking and allowing access to the respiratory epithelium; and it facilitates productive viral binding and entry to target cells [13]. Thus, although genetically engineered influenza virus deficient in the NA gene is able to replicate in vitro at a low level [14, 15], it is clear that NA plays a critical role in the infection and spread of influenza, making the inhibition of its activity a valid drug target.

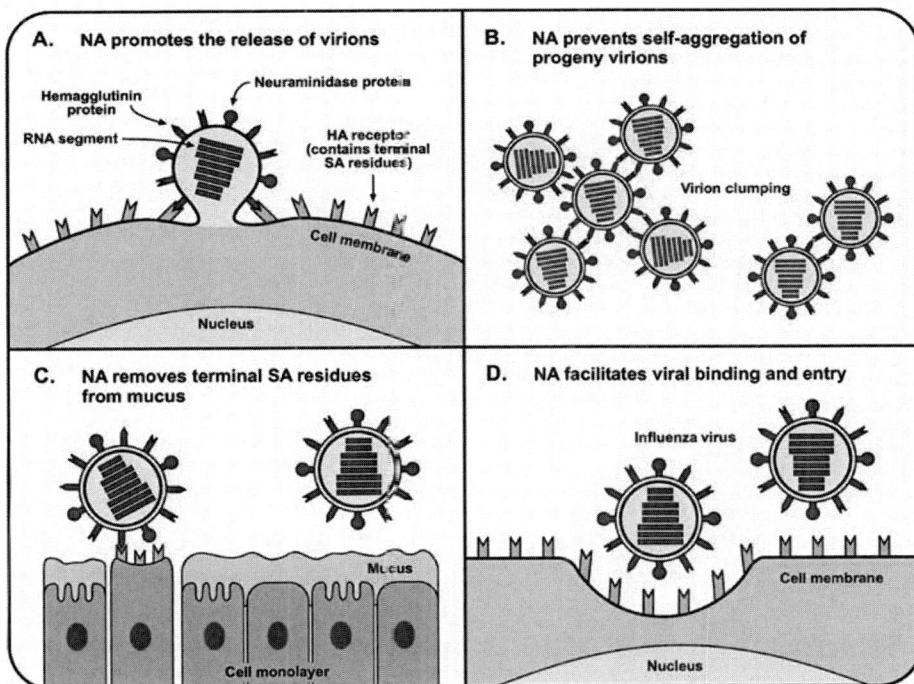

Figure 1. Schematic representation of influenza virus NA functions. Shown in panel (A) NA promotes the release of newly synthesized virus particles by removing sialic acid (SA) residues from the surface of the infected cells, allowing virus to spread; (B) NA prevents self-aggregation of progeny virions by removing the SA residues on oligosaccharide chains of the newly synthesised HA and NA; (C) NA removes terminal SA residues from the mucus in the respiratory tract; (D) it is postulated that NA facilitates productive viral binding and entry to target cells by removal of decoy receptors on mucins, cilia, and cellular glycocalix.

The NAs of influenza A and B viruses are structurally similar [16, 17]. They exist as tetramers consisting of four identical subunits. Each subunit is composed of a stalk region, containing the trans-membrane domain, which anchors the protein in the virus membrane, and a box-like globular head. The enzyme active site is present as a deep pocket on the distal surface of each monomer [18]. Although each monomer contains an active site, the NA functions only as a tetramer. The overall amino acid homology for the influenza virus NAs is low (~30%). However, the 19 amino acids that make up the catalytic site are highly conserved among all known influenza A and B NAs. These include catalytic residues (R118, D151, R152, R224, E276, R292, R371, and Y406; N2 numbering) that have a direct interaction with the substrate (sialic acid) and framework residues (E119, R156, W178, S179, D/N198, I222, E227, H274, E277, N294, and E425) that support the catalytic residues for functional binding and catalysis [18, 19]. The highly conserved nature of the influenza NA active site has led to the expectation that inhibitors of this enzyme would be active against a broad range of influenza A and B viruses.

RATIONAL DESIGN OF OSELTAMIVIR CARBOXYLATE

Influenza NA cleaves the α-2,3- or α-2,6-ketosidic linkage between a terminal sialic acid residue and an adjoining sugar residue (usually galactose). The catalytic mechanism has been studied at the molecular level [20, 21]. Based on these studies, it has been suggested that the catalytic mechanism proceeds through an oxonium cation transition-state intermediate (Figure 2). This intermediate binds in the enzyme active site in a distorted configuration due to interactions between the carboxylate of the substrate and a triad of conserved arginines (R118, R292, R371; N2 numbering) in the enzyme active site. A transition state analog, Neu5Ac2en (Figure 2), was chemically synthesized by incorporating a double bond into the ring structure of sialic acid. This compound inhibited NA activity in the low micromolar range and inhibited influenza virus replication in culture [22, 23], but was not active in animals infected with influenza virus [24].

The effort to identify a potent NA inhibitor was significantly aided by x-ray crystallographic studies of influenza A and B NAs and by the use of computational methods to facilitate the rational design of inhibitors. On the basis of x-ray crystallographic studies of influenza A and B virus NAs co-crystallized with sialic acid and Neu5Ac2en [23, 25], several sialic acid analogues were synthesized and tested as potential inhibitors of this enzyme. Zanamivir (GG167; 4-guanidino-Neu5Ac2en; Figure 2), the most potent of the earlier sialic acid-based inhibitors, effectively inhibits influenza A and B neuraminidase activity and virus replication in vitro at low nanomolar concentrations [26] and is active in animal models of influenza virus infection [27, 28]. The substantially greater potency of this compound than of Neu5Ac2en is due to strong interactions between the guanidino group of zanamivir and invariant charged residues (E119, E227, and D151) in the base of the active site [23]. However, the guanidino group also contributes substantially to the overall polarity of zanamivir, which is responsible for the poor oral bioavailability and rapid renal elimination of this compound [23]. Consequently zanamivir is applied topically to the respiratory tract by inhalation.

A.

B.

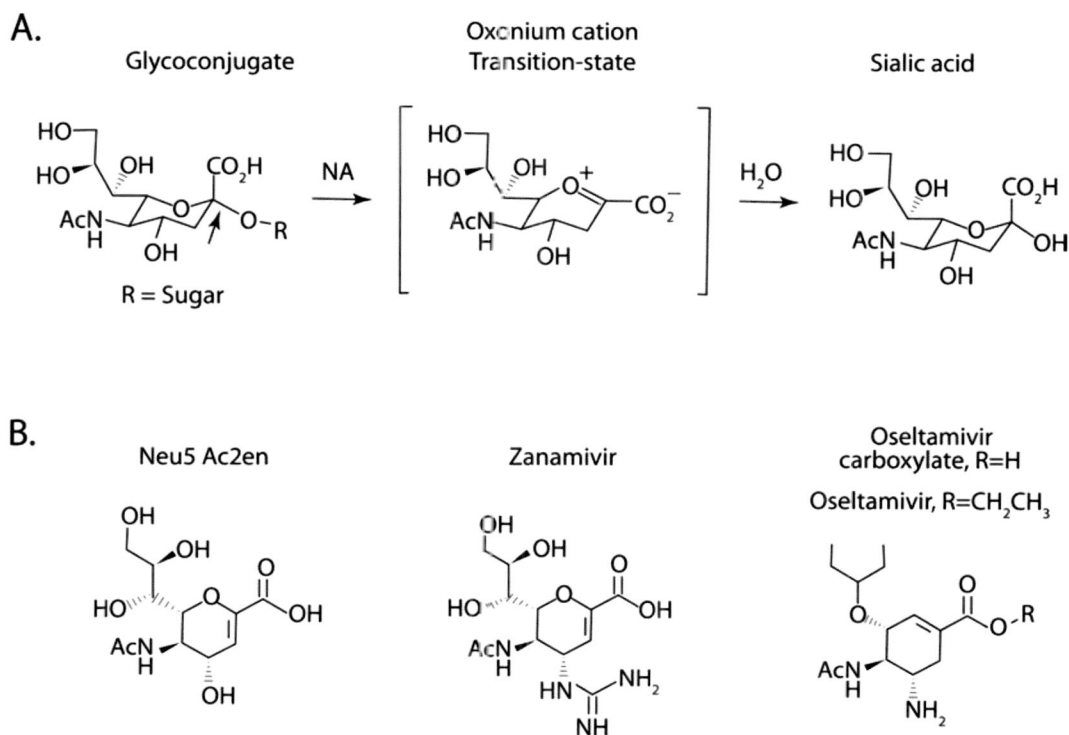

Figure 2. (A) Schematic representation of the proposed catalytic mechanism by which influenza NA cleave terminal sialic acid residues from glycoconjugates. (B) Structures of the transition state analog Neu5Ac2en, zanamivir, oseltamivir carboxylate, and its oral prodrug oseltamivir.

Because an oral compound would be more convenient and perhaps better able to uniformly deliver an inhibitor to all regions of the respiratory tract and other organs in which influenza viruses may potentially replicate [29], an effort was made to identify a potent, orally bio-available influenza NA inhibitor. The design strategy for oseltamivir carboxylate was to use knowledge of the enzyme active site and catalytic mechanism to generate a transition-state analogue using a more chemically stable carbocyclic ring structure, and to replace the polar glycerol moiety of the sialic acid-based inhibitors with a lipophilic side chain. The goal was to optimize hydrophobic interactions between the lipophilic side chain and conserved residues in the enzyme active site to maintain potency while increasing the overall lipophilic nature of the compound to enhance the potential for oral bioavailability. It was also recognized that highly polar substituents, such as a guanidino group, could not be incorporated into the inhibitor even though they would likely provide favorable interactions with conserved residues in the highly charged environment of the NA active site.

Oseltamivir carboxylate (Ro 64-0802, GS 4071; Figures 2 and 3) [30] is a potent and specific inhibitor of influenza virus NA and was derived from a rational synthetic chemistry program. It fulfilled all expected criteria except that tests in several species including humans showed low oral bioavailability. This problem was solved by preparing the ethyl ester of oseltamivir carboxylate (oseltamivir) which acts as a pro-drug for the active agent providing a drug giving good oral bioavailability of oseltamivir carboxylate and widespread tissue distribution [31, 32], particularly to both upper and lower respiratory tract, where it achieves high and sustained concentrations [33, 34].

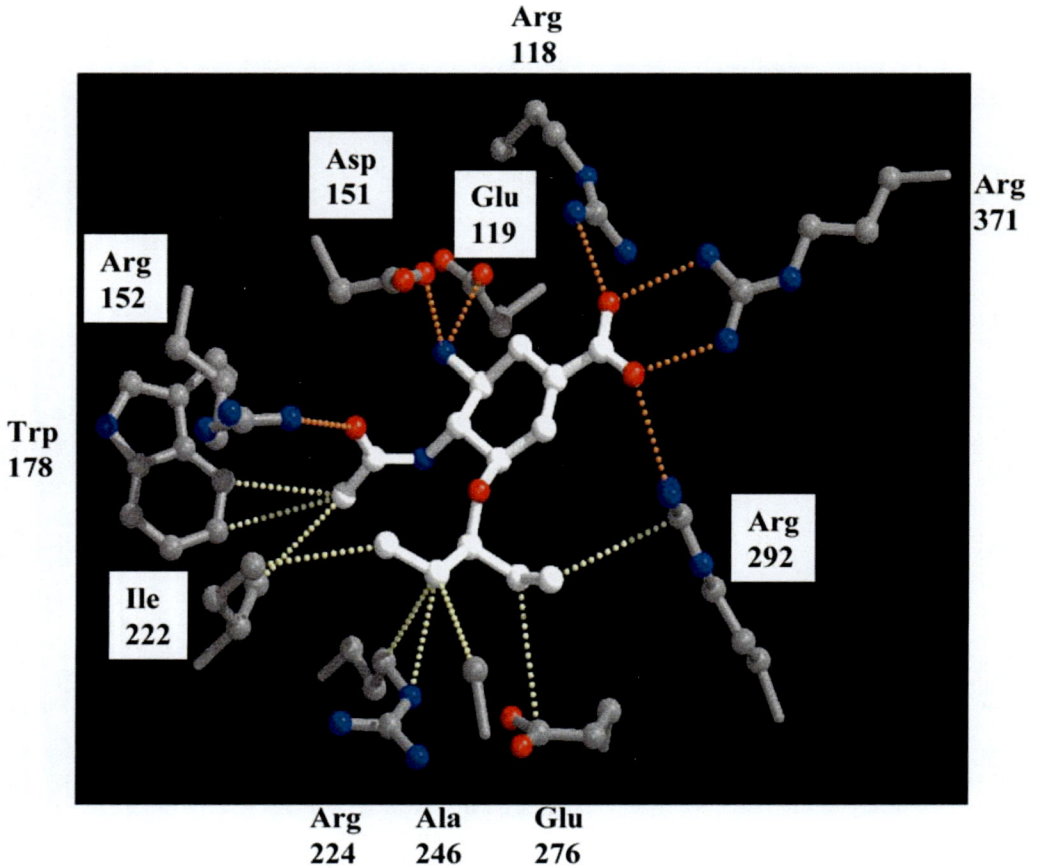

Figure 3. Binding interactions of oseltamivir carboxylate with amino acids in the active site of N9 neuraminidase of influenza virus. All amino acids with which oseltamivir carboxylate makes contact except Ala 246 are conserved in all neuraminidase subtypes. Figure taken from [35].

ACTIVITY OF OSELTAMIVIR CARBOXYLATE AGAINST ALL INFLUENZA NEURAMINIDASE SUBTYPES IN ENZYME INHIBITION ASSAYS

Following from the design of oseltamivir carboxylate to bind into the active site of NA, which is highly conserved among all subtypes, it would be expected that it would inhibit the NAs of all influenza virus subtypes. The activity of oseltamivir carboxylate against all nine influenza A virus NA subtypes, as well as influenza B virus NA, has been demonstrated [35]. As shown in Table 1, oseltamivir carboxylate is a potent inhibitor of all influenza NA subtypes, with IC_{50} values in the low nanomolar range when 50 μM MUNANA is used as a substrate in a fluorescence-based NA inhibition assay. In another study, the susceptibility to oseltamivir carboxylate of the NAs from influenza A viruses representing all NA subtypes was determined using a higher concentration of MUNANA (100 μM) as a substrate [36]. Although higher IC_{50} values were obtained with the higher substrate concentration, the results of both studies support the conclusion that the sensitivity of all influenza A and B NA subtypes are similar to those obtained for NAs currently represented on viruses that infect humans [37]. Importantly, none of the more than 4,500 naturally occurring influenza A or B viruses examined prior to the general availability of NA inhibitors have NA with low sensitivity to oseltamivir carboxylate [12, 37]. Again, this is consistent with the highly conserved nature of the NA active site.

Table 1. Susceptibility of different NA subtypes of influenza A and B viruses to oseltamivir carboxylate in vitro

Influenza virus	Subtype	Susceptibility to oseltamivir carboxylate (mean IC_{50}, nM) [a]
A/WS/33 [b]	H1N1	1.0
A/Japan/305/57 [b]	H2N2	0.3
A/Duck/Germany/1215/73 [c]	H2N3	0.3
A/Turkey/Ontario/6118/68 [c]	H8N4	0.4
A/Duck/Alberta/60/76 [c]	H12N5	1.5
A/Duck/Czechoslavakia/56 [c]	H4N6	0.4
A/Chick/Germany/N/49 [c]	H10N7	0.8
A/Duck/Ukraine/1/63 [c]	H3N8	0.8
A/NWS/G70C [d]	H1N9	0.3
B/Hong Kong/5/72 [b]	B	1.7

[a] Values represent average from two independent experiments using 2'-(4-methylumbelliferyl)-α-D-N acetylneuraminic acid (MUNANA) as substrate at a final concentration of 50 μM. Results were reported in [35].
[b] Human influenza virus.
[c] Avian influenza virus.
[d] Reassortant virus containing NA derived from an avian influenza virus.

Although oseltamivir carboxylate has been tested against only a representative number of N3 to N9 NAs, it has been tested against many thousands of isolates of N1 and N2 subtypes. One important observation from global surveillance data of influenza A virus NA susceptibility to oseltamivir carboxylate is that mean viral subtype susceptibility (e.g., mean IC_{50} values) changes little with the passage of time or between different continents of isolation. McKimm-Breshkin et al. [37] reported that the mean IC_{50} values for the inhibition of influenza N1 NAs for isolates from 1996, 1997, 1998, and 1999 were 1.59, 1.59, 1.43, and 1.32 nM, respectively. The corresponding values for N2 NAs were 0.46, 0.49, 0.36, and 0.36 nM, respectively. For the period 1996-1999, cumulative isolates from North America, Europe, Asia, Africa, South America, and Oceania gave N1 NA sensitivity values of 1.29, 1.42, 1.73, 1.30, 1.56, and 1.29 nM, respectively. The corresponding values for N2 NAs were 0.66, 0.69, 0.59, 0.53, 0.58, and 0.60 nM, respectively. Similarly, Hurt et al. [38] found little difference in mean IC_{50} values for the NA from influenza A viruses of N1 or N2 subtypes and influenza B isolates collected over the years from 1998 to 2002 in Australia and South East Asia and little difference in the susceptibility of influenza viruses to oseltamivir carboxylate between the two regions.

There is particular importance to confirming the activity of oseltamivir carboxylate against avian viruses that have infected humans and could potentially initiate a new influenza pandemic. In 1997, there was a first report of human infections with highly pathogenic avian H5N1 influenza viruses in Hong Kong, and 6 of 18 infected individuals died [8]; in 1999, two cases of avian H9N2 virus infection were reported in children in Hong Kong, and additional reports came from mainland China [9]. In 2003 in The Netherlands, H7N7 influenza viruses were transmitted from poultry to humans and caused mainly conjunctivitis, but there was one fatal case of acute respiratory distress syndrome [10]. Since 2003, human infection with avian H5N1 influenza viruses has been reported in 15 countries with overall >50% mortality rates [39]. Oseltamivir carboxylate has been tested against the NAs of representative viruses from these outbreaks/human cases and found to be active in the low nanomolar range in all cases (Table 2). Also, Tumpey et al. [40] were able to reconstruct the NA of the 1918 Spanish pandemic influenza A (H1N1) virus. This was tested for inhibition by oseltamivir carboxylate alongside the NAs of influenza A/WSN/33 (H1N1) and A/New Caledonia/20/99 (H1N1) viruses. All had a similar susceptibility to oseltamivir carboxylate with IC_{50} values in the range of 1-10 nM.

Table 2. Activity of oseltamivir carboxylate against the NA of human influenza viruses of H5N1, H9N2, and H7N7 subtypes

Influenza virus [a]	Subtype	Substrate for NA enzyme inhibition assay	Susceptibility to oseltamivir carboxylate (mean $IC_{50} \pm SD$, nM)	Reference
A/Hong Kong/156/97	H5N1	Fetuin	7.0 ± 0.9	69
A/Hong Kong /156/97	H5N1	MUNANA [b]	2.3 ± 0.3	43
A/Hong Kong /213/03	H5N1	MUNANA	2.3 ± 0.2	43
A/Hong Kong /1074/99	H9N2	Fetuin	15.0 ± 0.7	69
A/Netherlands/219/03	H7N7	Fetuin	1.3 ± 0.1	41
A/Hanoi/30408/05 [c]	H5N1	MUNANA	0.6	85
A/Vietnam/1203/04 [d]	H5N1	MUNANA	0.3 ± 0.1	86
A/Vietnam/1203/04	H5N1	MUNANA	0.1 ± 0.01	43
A/Vietnam/ JP14/05	H5N1	MUNANA	0.1 ± 0.06	43
A/Vietnam/JP4207/05	H5N1	MUNANA	0.1 ± 0.05	43
A/Vietnam/JP20-2/05	H5N1	MUNANA	0.1 ± 0.04	43
A/Vietnam/JPHN30321/05	H5N1	MUNANA	0.1 ± 0.07	43
A/Cambodia/408008/05	H5N1	MUNANA	0.1 ± 0.07	43

[a] Influenza viruses isolated from infected humans.
[b] 2'-(4-methylumbelliferyl)-α-D-N-acetylneuraminic acid (MUNANA).
[c] Data for oseltamivir carboxylate-sensitive clone.
[d] Recombinant influenza virus, generated by plasmid-based reverse genetics.

The NA of the highly pathogenic influenza H7N7 virus that caused the outbreak in poultry in The Netherlands in 2003 has also been tested against oseltamivir carboxylate [41]. Using fetuin as a substrate, an IC_{50} value of 1.29 nM was determined. This compared with a value of 0.33 nM for the NA of A/Chicken/Pennsylvania/21525/83 (H5N2) used as a positive control. Further assays by this group [42] using fetuin as a substrate showed that the IC_{50} value for A/Chicken/Pennsylvania/21525/83 (H5N2) virus varied from 0.55 to 0.95 nM in three further assays. The mean IC_{50} values for A/Chicken/Saudi Arabia/569017/00 (H9N2) and A/PR/8/34 (H1N1) were 1.13 nM and 2.33 nM, respectively.

When testing the sensitivities to oseltamivir carboxylate of a range of isolates of an individual subtype, although the mean IC_{50} values vary little, there are, as may be expected, variant outliers with sensitivities both slightly higher and lower then the means [37]. There may also be sensitivity differences with different clades of the same viral subtype, possibly due to minor, naturally occurring amino acid variants in the NA. In particular, the NAs of some 2003-2004 human H5N1 isolates from Vietnam and Cambodia, presumed clade 1 isolates, with variant amino acids E248G and Y252H were about 10-20 times more susceptible to oseltamivir carboxylate than those of other recent H5N1 isolates or currently circulating human H1N1 isolates [43].

We can find no published data on IC_{50} values for oseltamivir carboxylate against the NAs of those H5N1 viruses which have infected humans in Turkey and Egypt despite there being some clinical evidence of overall benefit of oseltamivir treatment against the latter infections [3]. However, some Egyptian H5N1 isolates from humans have carried a N294S variant/mutation in NA which confers a 12-15 fold increase in IC_{50} value in a NA inhibition assay (absolute IC_{50} values not reported) [44]. The N294S NA mutation has been observed only once in seasonal H3N2 influenza from an oseltamivir-treated subject [12, 45], not "frequently" as reported by Saad et al. [44].

Oseltamivir carboxylate was shown to be active in vitro not only against human H5N1 influenza virus isolates but also there are several reports of its activity against avian isolates. McKimm-Breschkin et al. [46] have reported a spread of activities for different clades of H5N1 viruses with the NA from clade 1 viruses from 2004 being approximately 5 times more sensitive to oseltamivir carboxylate than that from A/Mississippi/3/01 (H1N1) (which has typical sensitivity for a seasonal H1N1 virus [47]). The NA from H5N1 viruses of clade 1 from Cambodia 2005 have similar activity to A/Mississippi/3/01 (H1N1) virus, although NA from H5N1 viruses of clade 2 from Indonesia 2005 had an approximately 5 fold higher IC_{50} value than the NA from A/Mississippi/3/01. Oseltamivir carboxylate had a mean IC_{50} value of 11.5 nM using MUNANA as a substrate against the NA of these clade 2 viruses [46]. Independent data showed a significant clinical benefit in the use of oseltamivir to treat clade 2.1 influenza A (H5N1) infections in Indonesia over the period 2005-2007 [3, 48]. The particularly high sensitivity (low IC_{50} value) of NA from avian clade 1 2004 isolates confirmed the finding for the corresponding human isolates reported by Ramiex-Welti et al. [43].

In contrast, Hurt et al. [49] found little variation in the sensitivity of the NAs of 51 avian H5N1 isolates collected over a similar time in similar regions (mean IC_{50} value 0.33 nM using MUNANA as a substrate), with just two outliers, A/chicken/Vietnam/486A/04 (IC_{50} 3.59 nM) and A/chicken/Indonesia/Wates/77/05 (IC_{50} 5.38 nM). These viruses were shown to carry NA variants V116A and I117V, respectively. The IC_{50} for A/chicken/Indonesia/Wates/77/05 was reported as 25.6 nM by McKimm-Breschkin et al. [46].

In confirmation of the ability of oseltamivir carboxylate being able to inhibit all influenza virus NAs, x-ray crystallographic studies have directly demonstrated its binding into the active site of the group 1 NAs (N1, N4, and N8), the group 2 NAs (N2 and N9), and an NA from influenza B virus [17]. Given that oseltamivir carboxylate contains a bulky lipophilic side chain replacing the glycerol chain of the natural substrate, the influenza A virus NAs must undergo a conformational change to accommodate it [50]. To form a binding pocket for this side chain, the amino acid E276 must rotate and bond with the amino acid R224. However, no such significant reorientation is required for oseltamivir carboxylate to bind to influenza B virus NA. For the group 1 NAs, oseltamivir carboxylate can bind with the loop around residue 150 in either of two conformations (open or closed). The closed conformation is similar to the binding conformation in the group 2 NAs [17]. The binding of oseltamivir carboxylate to all types of influenza virus NA supports the NA inhibition data showing activity against all 9 influenza A plus influenza B NAs. The slightly different binding modes may be pertinent to the subtype-specific resistance mutations that can be selected by oseltamivir carboxylate, and in particular the lack of reorientation involved in binding to influenza B NAs may be reflected in the lack of resistance seen with influenza B viruses [12].

One important factor for any drug is its specificity of action, which at least in part contributes to the safety profile of the drug. Oseltamivir carboxylate is highly specific for the inhibition of NAs from influenza viruses. At about one million times the 1 nM IC_{50} value typical for inhibition of influenza virus NAs, oseltamivir carboxylate has little or no effect on the activity of NAs from the paramyxoviruses parainfluenza and Newcastle disease virus or against the NAs of bacteria *C. perfringens* and *V. cholerae* or, more importantly, against the mammalian NAs of human liver, rat liver, and uterus (previously unpublished data).

ANTIVIRAL ACTIVITY OF OSELTAMIVIR CARBOXYLATE IN CELL CULTURE

Many research groups have tried to assess the antiviral potency of oseltamivir carboxylate and other NA inhibitors against influenza viruses of different NA subtypes in Madin-Darby canine kidney (MDCK) epithelial cell-based assays. The antiviral activity of oseltamivir carboxylate is generally confirmed by cell culture experiments involving MDCK cells, but the assay system gives some anomalous results [51, 52, 53], particularly for low-passage clinical isolates. This is usually expressed as false insensitivity (resistance). It is likely that this results from the mismatch of the viral HA from clinical isolates preferring to bind to α-2,6-linked sialic acid receptors while those on MDCK and other common cell lines supporting influenza growth (e.g., Vero, MRC-5, and 293T cells) have predominantly α-2,3-linked sialic acid receptors (previously unpublished data). Poor binding to the cell receptors means progeny viruses can escape the cell without need of NA activity, and hence the viruses appear insensitive to NA inhibitors as a class. The newly developed cell lines with increased surface expression of human-like α-2,6-linked sialyl cell surface receptors [54, 55] may be better for cell culture assessment of the antiviral activity of NA inhibitors as a class. Oseltamivir carboxylate shows antiviral activity in the nanomolar range in these cells with a sensitivity that correlates well with the sensitivity of the viral NA. The compromised fitness of the influenza A/Wuhan/359/95 (H3N2) virus carrying an R292K NA mutation was detectable in MDCK-SIAT1 cells but not in MDCK cells [56]. The problem with mismatch between virus receptors in humans and in available cell-culture systems can also be overcome with the use of a novel cell culture-based system that morphologically and functionally recapitulates differentiated normal human bronchial epithelial (NHBE) cells ex vivo [57]. Ilyushina et al. [58] showed that NHBE cells could be used to evaluate the susceptibility of H5N1 viruses to NA inhibitors, avoiding false results.

Yamanaka et al. [59] showed that oseltamivir carboxylate is active against equine influenza viruses of the H7N7 and H3N8 subtypes. Activity was demonstrated by inhibition of the viral NA and antiviral activity in MDCK cells with IC_{50} and EC_{50} values in the low nanomolar range. In the case of one H3N8 virus, the NA was sensitive in the enzymatic assay, but the virus appeared insensitive to both oseltamivir carboxylate and zanamivir in the MDCK cell-based assay. The reason for this was not investigated but may be another case of the ambiguity of assay results in MDCK cells.

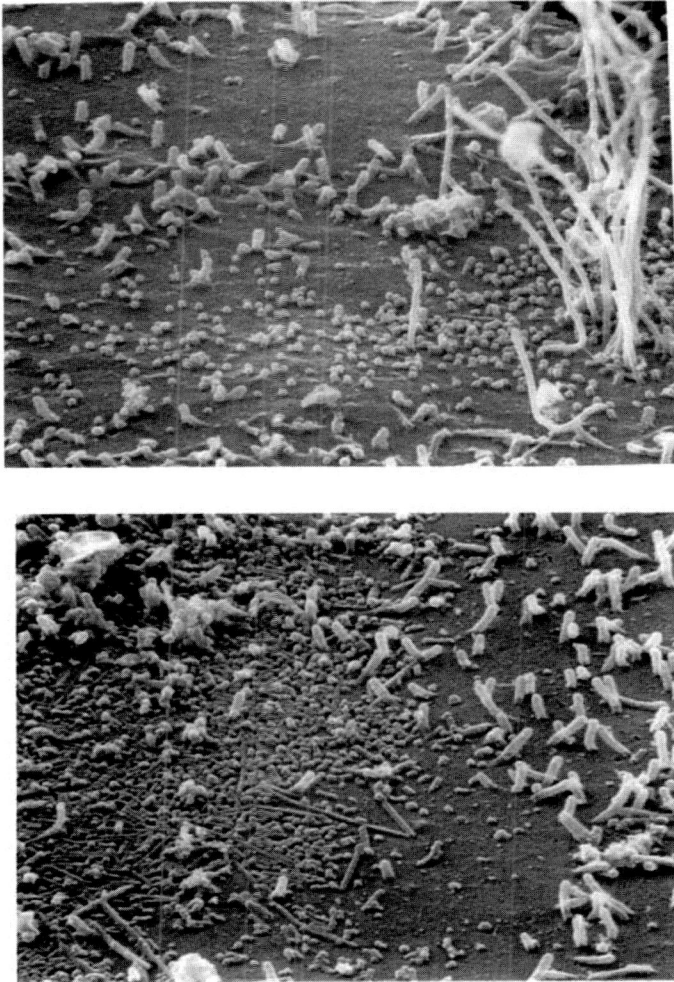

Figure 4. Action of oseltamivir carboxylate shown by electron microscopy. Electron micrograph of MDCK cells infected with influenza A/Sydney/97 (H3N2) virus in the absence (top) or presence (bottom) of oseltamivir carboxylate at 18 hours post infection. Rounded, isolated virus particles are present in the left of the top micrograph, and clumped virus attached flat to the cell surface is seen in the bottom micrograph. Original magnification x 13,000. Cell culture, infection and fixing performed by Prof. John Oxford, Retroscreen Virology, London, UK. Scanning electron microscopy by Dr. David John Hockley. Principal Scientist, Cell Biology and Imaging Section (CBI), National Institute for Biological Standards and Control (NIBSC), South Mimms, Herts, EN6 3QG, UK.

The pig is a potential host for influenza virus reassortment and interspecies transmission [60]. Bauer et al. [61] showed that the NAs of 7 porcine influenza A (H3N2) isolates collected between 1989 and 2001 were sensitive to oseltamivir carboxylate in a chemiluminescence enzyme inhibition assay. The corresponding viruses were also sensitive to oseltamivir carboxylate in cell culture assays in MDCK cells by both plaque reduction and virus yield end points. However, the rank order of sensitivity in the cell culture assays did not match that of the NA inhibition assays. The rank order also differed between the cell culture virology end points.

The antiviral activity of oseltamivir carboxylate in appropriate cell culture assays has been used to confirm the role of the viral NA in the life cycle of the influenza virus and the mode of action of oseltamivir carboxylate. In confirmation of the mode of action of oseltamivir carboxylate, evidence that its antiviral activity is due to inhibition of the viral NA was obtained from electron microscopy studies of the surface of influenza-infected cells in the absence or presence of inhibitor (Figure 4). In the absence of inhibitor, virus was observed as separate rounded virions on the surface of the cells. In the presence of oseltamivir carboxylate, virus was clumped together and attached flattened to the cell surface in the same way that others have reported for influenza viruses lacking NA function due to genetic deletion [62], growth of temperature-sensitive NA mutants at non-permissive temperatures [63], or the presence of other NA inhibitors [64]. In contrast to the early finding of Liu et al. [62], the NA inhibitory activity of oseltamivir carboxylate in single cycle cell culture assays has been used to demonstrate and confirm the role of the viral NA in influenza virus entry/infection, both independently [13, 65] and in collaboration with innate immune proteins [66].

ANTIVIRAL ACTIVITY IN VIVO

As described above, the active NA inhibitor oseltamivir carboxylate has poor oral bioavailability. This deficiency was circumvented by producing an ethyl ester prodrug of the active form. This ethyl ester (oseltamivir) is generally supplied as its phosphate salt (oseltamivir phosphate, Tamiflu). It is important that oseltamivir phosphate, not oseltamivir carboxylate, is used for any in vivo studies. Conversely, oseltamivir carboxylate must be used for in vitro studies.

The antiviral activity and efficacy of oseltamivir phosphate (oseltamivir) against seasonal influenza viruses in vivo has been extensively and most pertinently demonstrated in many double–blind, placebo-controlled clinical trials [67, 68].

Clinical trials against avian influenza viruses causing sporadic outbreaks of infection are very difficult to achieve, and hence in vivo data must come predominantly from animal experiments. While it has been shown above that oseltamivir carboxylate is active against the NAs of all subtypes of influenza viruses, meaning all viruses are intrinsically sensitive to oseltamivir, that alone is not an absolute guarantee of efficacy in vivo. Other factors influencing in vivo activity, particularly pertinent to avian viruses, include the tropism of the virus (i.e., its propensity to replicate in organs other than the respiratory tract) and the effective drug concentration achieved in those tissues; the virulence/replicative capability of the virus (a drug capable of lowering viral load by 1000 times will be effective if the highest virus level reached in vivo is 10^3 EID_{50} but less effective or ineffective if, for example, a level of 10^6 EID$_{50}$ is reached); and finally, there may be a mismatch of HA binding in some organs/tissues/animal species, reflecting the problems with cell culture assays, where viruses with sensitive NAs appear insensitive to the drug. Despite these potential problems, there is a growing body of evidence to suggest that oseltamivir is active against a range of avian viruses in animal/bird models at drug doses that result in exposures to oseltamivir carboxylate similar to those achieved in man by the recommended dose of 75 mg b.i.d. for treatment of adults and 75 mg q.d. for prophylaxis.

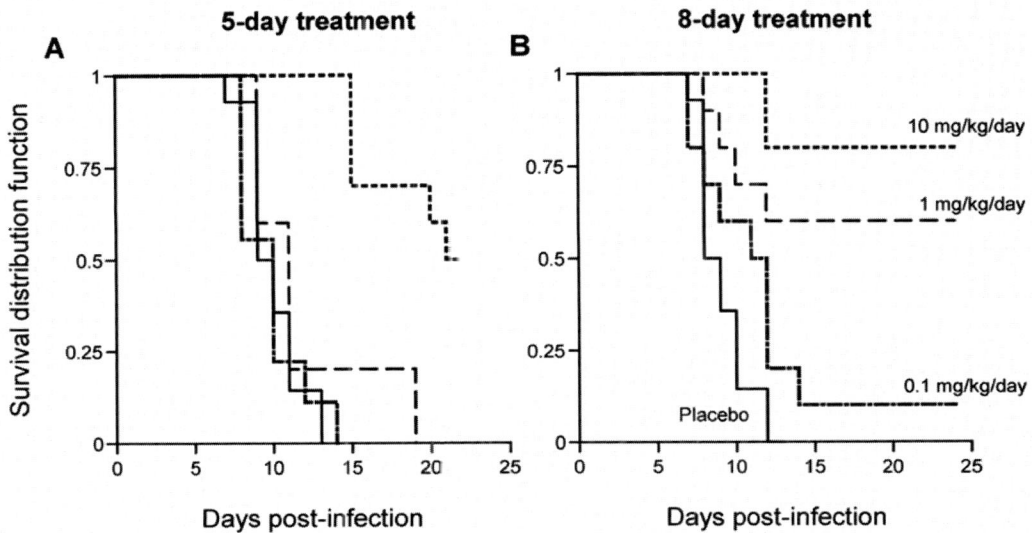

Figure 5. Effect of 5-day and 8-day oseltamivir regimens on survival of mice inoculated with A/Vietnam/1203/04 (H5N1) influenza virus. Six-week-old BALB/c mice were treated with 0.1, 1, or 10 mg/kg/day of oseltamivir twice daily for 5 days (A) or 8 days (B), beginning 4 hours before virus exposure. The Kaplan-Meier method was used to estimate the probability of survival. Results were reported in [70].

The efficacy of oseltamivir against infection caused by highly pathogenic avian influenza viruses has been tested in mammalian (mouse and ferret) models and in avian species. Early studies showed that orally administered oseltamivir is an effective treatment for H5N1 and H9N2 influenza virus infections in mice [36, 69]. Administration twice daily for 5 days of oseltamivir at a dosage of 1 (0.5 mg/kg b.i.d.) and 10 mg/kg/day completely protected mice against lethal infection with the highly pathogenic A/Hong Kong/156/97 (H5N1) and A/quail/Hong Kong/G1/97 (H9N2) influenza viruses that were transmitted from birds to humans in Hong Kong. Oseltamivir at 10 mg/kg/day markedly reduced virus titers in the lungs of mice infected with H9N2 virus and completely eliminated virus in the lungs of mice infected with H5N1 virus [36]. The H5N1 and H9N2 viruses were undetectable in the brains of mice after treatment with oseltamivir at a dosage of 1 mg/kg/day. When treatment with oseltamivir was given as late as 60 hours after virus inoculation, oseltamivir protected more than 65% of mice from lethal infection with A/Hong Kong/156/97 (H5N1) virus. More recent studies showed that the new antigenic variant A/Vietnam/1203/04 (H5N1) virus was more pathogenic in mice than A/Hong Kong/156/97 (H5N1) virus [70]. Higher brain and blood titers of the mice infected with the A/Vietnam/1203/04 (H5N1) virus indicated a greater propensity for systemic spread. Oseltamivir administered twice daily for 5 days at 10 mg/kg/day significantly reduced A/Vietnam/1203/04 (H5N1) virus titers in the lungs (P<0.05) and provided a 50% survival rate. A major improvement in the antiviral effect against lethal infection was achieved with the 8-day schedule: oseltamivir at 1.0 and 10 mg/kg/day significantly reduced virus titers in lungs and brain and resulted in 60% and 80% survival rates, respectively (Figure 5) (P<0.05). Therefore, the significantly higher virulence of the A/Vietnam/1203/04 (H5N1) virus may be a factor that resulted in the different prophylactic efficacy of oseltamivir in mice against the two virus strains, and prolonged and higher-dose oseltamivir regimens may be required for the most beneficial antiviral effect [70].

Ferrets are naturally susceptible to infection with influenza viruses including highly pathogenic viruses of H5N1 and H7N7 subtypes. Moreover, manifestation of clinical symptoms of infection, receptor distribution in the airway epithelium [71], immune response, and histopathologic changes [72, 73] are similar in ferrets and in humans. The use of oseltamivir for early post-exposure prophylaxis and for treatment in ferrets exposed to representatives of two clades of H5N1 virus with markedly different pathogenicity was recently evaluated [74]. Oral administration of oseltamivir at a dose of 5 mg/kg/day for 5 days twice daily initiated 4 hours after inoculation with 10^2 EID$_{50}$/ferret of A/Vietnam/1203/04 (H5N1) virus inhibited the febrile response, reduced weight changes, and, most important, completely protected ferrets from lethal H5N1 infection (Table 3). In the treatment groups, virus replication in the upper respiratory tract of ferrets was prevented, whereas untreated animals shed virus at titers of 2.8-6.5 log$_{10}$EID$_{50}$/mL on days 3, 5, and 7 post-infection (p.i.). Systemic spread of the H5N1 virus was observed in untreated ferrets: virus was detected in multiple internal organs, including the brain. Treatment with oseltamivir resulted in complete inhibition of virus replication in the lungs and small intestine on day 5 p.i. In the brains of treated animals, virus was detected in one of the two animals tested with >99% reduction of titer. When treatment was delayed 24 hours p.i., ferrets administered a higher oseltamivir dosage of 25 mg/kg/day survived lethal challenge [74]. For the treatment of ferrets inoculated with the less pathogenic A/Turkey/15/06 (H5N1) virus, 10 mg/kg/day of oseltamivir was sufficient to reduce the lethargy of the animals, significantly inhibit inflammation in the upper respiratory tract, and block virus spread to the internal organs (Table 3) [74]. These results suggest that earlier treatment with oseltamivir and probably higher dosages can prevent H5N1 mortality in ferrets. However, further studies are needed to investigate optimal doses and treatment durations required to achieve protection against infection with highly pathogenic influenza viruses.

To prepare for a potential pandemic of H5N1 influenza virus, it is necessary to determine a prophylaxis regimen that will protect those in close contact with infected individuals. In a ferret model, the effectiveness of four different oseltamivir prophylaxis regimens against highly pathogenic A/Vietnam/1203/04 (H5N1) influenza virus was evaluated [75]. Oseltamivir was administered to ferrets at dosages of 5 or 10 mg/kg/day as a single application or given in two daily applications over 10 days initiated one day before challenge with a lethal dose (10^2 EID$_{50}$/ferret) of A/Vietnam/1203/04 (H5N1) virus. Control untreated ferrets all had fever, lost >25% of their initial body weight, and were lethargic with neurologic symptoms; these animals died between days 7 and 10 p.i. Prophylaxis with oseltamivir at 5 and 10 mg/kg/day administered once daily prevented death of animals but did not completely prevent development of clinical signs of infection. Marked improvement in

Table 3. Effect of post-exposure oseltamivir treatment on survival of ferrets challenged with H5N1 influenza viruses of clade 1 and clade 2

H5N1 virus	Initiation of treatment	Oseltamivir dose (mg/kg/day)[a]	No. survived/ total no.	Mean day to death ± SD[b]	Clinical signs of disease (no. showing sign/total no.)				Relative inactivity index[f]
					Weight loss[c]	Temperature increase[c]	Respiratory signs[d]	Neurologic signs[e]	
A/Vietnam/1203/04	4 hours after virus inoculation	5	3/3	>21*	3/3 (20.4 ± 1.9)*	1/3 (3.4)*[g]	0/3	0/3	0.34
		0	0/3	7.7 ± 0.7	3/3 (25.2 ± 1.4)	3/3 (7.6 ± 1.4)	1/3	2/3	1.25
A/Vietnam/1203/04	24 hours after virus inoculation	25	3/3	>21*	3/3 (13.4 ± 1.7)*	3/3 (6.0 ± 0.4)	0/3	2/3	0.30
		10	0/3	7.3 ± 0.3	3/3 (22.1 ± 2.9)	3/3 (5.7 ± 1.4)	0/3	2/3	1.05
		0	0/3	6.7 ± 0.4	3/3 (27.8 ± 2.4)	3/3 (6.9 ± 1.4)	1/3	3/3	1.21
A/Turkey/15/06	24 hours after virus inoculation	10	3/3	>21	3/3 (17.9 ± 2.8)	3/3 (6.0 ± 0.9)	2/3	0/3	0.15
		0	3/3	>21	3/3 (19.0 ± 1.8)	3/3 (5.7 ± 0.4)	1/3	0/3	0.46

[a] Young adult male ferrets 4-5 months of age were inoculated with either A/Vietnam/1203/04 (H5N1) virus (clade 1) at a dose of 10^2 EID_{50}/ferret or A/Turkey/15/06 (H5N1) virus (clade 2) at a dose of 10^6 EID_{50}/ferret. Starting either 4 or 24 hours after virus inoculation, oseltamivir or sterile PBS (control animals) was given orally to young adult ferrets twice daily for 5 days. 50% egg infectious dose (EID). Results were reported in [74].

[b] Mean day to death of ferrets was determined by Kaplan-Meier method.

[c] Maximal change in mean value (%) ± SD is shown in parentheses.

[d] Respiratory signs were sneezing, wheezing, and nasal discharge.

[e] Neurologic signs were hind-limb paresis, ataxia, torticollis, and tremors.

[f] Determined by 14-day observation. Because of mortality, control ferrets were observed for only 9 days (10^2 EID_{50}).

[g] Results obtained from 1 ferret.

* P < 0.05, unpaired t-test.

the drug efficacy was observed when the oseltamivir dosage was increased to 10 mg/kg/day in a single application. Prophylaxis with oseltamivir at 5 and 10 mg/kg/day twice daily for 10 days resulted in 100% survival and inhibition of systemic spread of the virus. Notably, all ferrets that survived initial infection when rechallenged with a lethal virus dose 21 days p.i. were completely protected from infection. These data indicated that higher dosages or twice daily oseltamivir administration may be more effective for prophylaxis against highly pathogenic H5N1 influenza viruses.

In an avian model, oseltamivir administered 24 hours and 3 hours prior to infection with highly pathogenic avian influenza A/Chick/Victoria/1/85 (H7N7) virus and administered for 5 days twice daily p.i. at 100 mg/kg p.o. protected 3/5 chickens from death despite their being given a very high challenge dose (100 LD_{50}) of this virus [76]. Two of the three birds exhibited no signs of illness. The survival time of two birds that did die was longer than that of untreated controls. Viral titers in trachea and cloaca were lower in all five birds than in controls (Table 4). The three surviving birds also survived re-challenge with the same virus without antiviral treatment. Pharmacokinetic studies showed that, in contrast to man, oseltamivir phosphate prodrug was poorly converted to oseltamivir carboxylate in chickens such that the oral bioavailability of the active metabolite was only 6.4%. Thus higher drug doses are likely to be required to treat influenza infection in chickens successfully than in mice, ferrets or humans.

Table 4. Tracheal and cloacal titers of A/Chick/Victoria/1/85 (H7N7) influenza virus in chickens treated with oseltamivir

Oseltamivir dose (mg/kg/day) [a]	Bird no.	Day of death	Virus titer on day post challenge [b]			
			3 day		5 day	
			Trachea	Cloaca	Trachea	Cloaca
100	1	6	< [c]	<	4.5	5.5
	2	7	<	<	4.6	5.5
	3	S [d]	<	<	5.0	4.5
	4	S	<	<	5.4	5.4
	5	S	<	<	<	<
0	1	5	3.5	2.4	---- [e]	----
	2	7	<	4.4	> 6.0	> 6.0
	3	4	4.5	2.5	----	----
	4	6	> 5.0	0	5.0	> 6.0
	5	5	> 5.0	2.4	----	----

[a] Three- to 5-week-old specific-pathogen free white leghorn chickens were inoculated intranasally with 100 LD_{50} (50% lethal dose) of influenza A/Chick/Victoria/1/85 (H7N7) virus. Oseltamivir or sterile PBS (control birds) was administered orally 24 hours and 3 hours prior to virus challenge and then twice daily for 5 days after infection. Birds were monitored for up to 10 days after infection for signs of disease.

[b] Virus titers were determined in embryonated chicken eggs and expressed as $\log_{10}EID_{50}$/mL (50% egg infectious dose, EID).

[c] <, the titer was below the limit of detection (<0.75 $\log_{10}EID_{50}$/ml).

[d] S, the bird survived the infection.

[e] ----, samples were not collected from dead bird.

Similarly, Meijer et al. [77] tested oseltamivir in chickens at an oral dose of 120 mg/kg b.i.d. against the highly pathogenic A/Chicken/Pennsylvania/1370/83 (H5N2) influenza virus and showed it to be effective both as prophylaxis and to limit virus transmission to uninfected birds. Dosing with oseltamivir was for 8 days and started one day prior to intra-tracheal inoculation of the birds with 10^5 EID_{50} of virus. One day p.i., each inoculated bird was housed with 5 contact chickens (un-inoculated but dosed with oseltamivir in the same way as the infected birds). Swabs were taken daily from the cloaca and trachea and tested for virus. In the inoculated birds, oseltamivir markedly inhibited spread of virus to the cloaca and reduced the death rate from 4/5 to 1/5. Oseltamivir also markedly inhibited transmission of infection from inoculated birds to their contacts. In particular, there was no transmission of virus until after dosing with oseltamivir had stopped on day 7 p.i.

Treatment with two or more drugs that target different influenza virus proteins or act at different stages of the virus life cycle may offer several advantages, such as greater potency and cost-effectiveness, reduction of the dosages needed, reduction of the risk of respiratory complications, and a potential reduction in the risk of emergence of resistant variants. The effectiveness of combination chemotherapy against highly pathogenic influenza viruses was evaluated in vitro and in vivo. Oseltamivir carboxylate used in combination with amantadine markedly reduced the extracellular virus yield of H5N1 virus in MDCK cells compared with that obtained after treatment with the individual drugs [78]. Moreover, no amino acid substitutions in the HA, NA, or M genes were detected when the combination of amantadine with low doses of NA inhibitor was used (0.001 μM). In a mouse model, oseltamivir combined with amantadine or rimantadine was more effective than oseltamivir used singly in preventing the death of mice infected with H5N1 or H9N2 viruses [69, 79]. Treatment of mice with combinations of oseltamivir and amantadine completely inhibited virus replication in the animals infected with H5N1 virus, whereas it was only partially effective with single-drug usage. Importantly, combination therapy prevented H5N1 virus spread to the brain of the mice: virus was not detected in the brain of treated animals on days 3, 6, and 9 after inoculation, and neurologic symptoms were not observed [79]. Oseltamivir and ribavirin showed principally additive efficacy against both clade 1 and clade 2 H5N1 influenza viruses, although clear differences were seen between the efficacy of drug combinations against two H5N1 viruses: higher doses were required for the protection of mice against A/Turkey/15/06 virus than for A/Vietnam/1203/04 virus [80]. Combination therapy consisting of specific anti-influenza drugs and inhibitors of inflammation, such as celecoxib and mesalazine, was recently reported to be a promising approach to control of H5N1 infection in mice [81]. These observations highlight the need for additional antiviral agents that can be used in combination with oseltamivir for the appropriate management of H5N1 influenza virus infections.

As with all drug efficacy data in animal models, caution must be exercised in its extrapolation to potential efficacy in humans. In the experiments cited here, potential differences between animal and human efficacy will likely be due to differences between animals and humans in the pharmacokinetics and tissue distribution of the drug, the different pathophysiology and tropism of virus infection, and the difference in virus–receptor binding, which all will influence NA inhibitor sensitivity in vivo. Nevertheless, positive efficacy data in animals is a strong pointer to potential efficacy in man but not necessarily to the dosing regimen required to achieve it.

Human Experience

Very substantial clinical data support the prophylactic and therapeutic antiviral activity of oseltamivir against seasonal influenza viruses of H1N1 and H3N2 subtypes and influenza B viruses [67, 68]. In recent years, an increasing body of information has been gathered in support of the efficacy of oseltamivir against highly pathogenic influenza viruses. Oseltamivir was used to control the transmission of H7N7 avian influenza virus to humans during the outbreak of this virus in chickens in The Netherlands in 2003. Oseltamivir treatment twice daily at 75 mg was provided to all new clinical cases, and a prophylactic regimen (75 mg daily) was offered to protect all poultry workers and their families. Prophylaxis started late in the outbreak, and uptake of drug increased toward the end of the infection. Protection against virus transmission was observed, with avian influenza infection being found in 5/52 (9.6%) untreated subjects compared with 1/38 (2.4%) of those who took oseltamivir (protective efficacy 75%). However, the difference was not statistically significant, possibly due to the small numbers [41].

There was an outbreak of avian influenza A (H7N3) in poultry in British Columbia, Canada, in 2004 [82]. Federal workers involved in the cull of infected birds had been advised to wear protective equipment and to take oseltamivir at 75 mg per day as prophylaxis. Despite these protective measures, two federal workers were found to have conjunctivitis, and influenza H7N3 infection was confirmed. Neither had been taking the oseltamivir prophylaxis. Both were then treated with oseltamivir and symptoms resolved fully.

Because of the sporadic nature of outbreaks of H5N1 infection and the high virulence of the virus, there have been no formal clinical trials of antiviral agents against the infection. However, treatment with oseltamivir has been recommended and given to about 200 patients infected with H5N1 virus [3]. Retrospective survival analysis of data from several clinical reports has been complied by a writing committee from the second World Health Oranization consultation on clinical aspects of H5N1 virus infections [3]. They found evidence of a statistically significant survival benefit for subjects treated with oseltamivir for both infections suspected to be H5N1 clade 1 and clade 2 analyzed independently or collectively. For the collective data, clade 1 plus clade 2, the survival rate was 88/188 (47%) of treated subjects and 7/56 (12%, P<0.001) for untreated subjects. Several other observations can be made from these data. First, very few subjects were treated within 48 hours of onset of symptoms as specified for the use of oseltamivir for the treatment of seasonal influenza. Time of onset of treatment has a marked effect on treatment outcome in seasonal influenza, with early treatment being significantly more effective [83]. This is supported by the observation in the treatment of subjects infected with clade 2.2 influenza H5N1 in Egypt. All 34 subjects presenting with H5N1 infection were given oseltamivir, and 20 survived (59%). There was a significantly shorter time from onset of illness to oseltamivir treatment among patients who survived than among those who died (P=0.001). However, late treatment may still be of some benefit. Data from Northern Vietnam showed a significant treatment benefit for subjects infected with clade 1 virus when 73% of subjects started treatment 4 days after onset of illness. Despite the fact that clade 1 H5N1 NAs appear about 15-30 times more sensitive to inhibition than H5N1 clade 2 NAs, as described above [43, 46], there was no evidence from these data that survival was any worse for subjects infected with clade 2 viruses than for those infected with clade 1. In the report on treatment of H5N1 infections in Egypt, two subjects carrying clade 2.2 virus with the N294S NA mutation, which produces a 12-15 fold increase in IC_{50} value were identified. They did not survive the infection but, as in most cases of H5N1 infection, treatment with oseltamivir did not start within the recommended 48 hours of onset of symptoms.

FACTORS THAT MAY AFFECT DRUG DOSING REGIMENS

For the effective treatment of influenza infection in humans oseltamivir dosing should commence within 48 hours of onset of symptoms. Efficacy is improved the earlier treatment is started within this 48 hour window [83]. All available data on treatment of H5N1 infection strongly supports the hypothesis that early treatment start after infection is the major predictor of treatment success [3].

More speculatively, as discussed above, antiviral assays in cell culture systems for oseltamivir carboxylate in particular and NA inhibitors in general are prone to giving variable and often erroneous results. For example, low-passage H3N2 clinical isolates with oseltamivir-sensitive NAs and against which oseltamivir has been proven to be clinically effective can appear completely insensitive to oseltamivir carboxylate when tested in MDCK cells [54]. This appears to be the result of a mismatch between the sialyl receptors on the cells and the binding specificity of the HA of the virus, in this case α-2,3-linked sialyl receptors on the cell and a viral HA specificity for binding to α-2,6-linked sialyl receptors. If binding of the viral HA to the cell receptor is tight, then the viral NA activity is critical to release nascent virus particles and hence spread the infection. In these circumstances, viral replication and spread of infection is critically sensitive to NA inhibition. However, if HA binding is weak, nascent virus particles may detach from the cell surface without need for NA activity, and virus spread and replication will be relatively insensitive to, or even independent of, NA activity. In these circumstances, NA inhibitors (as a class) will have little or diminished effect on influenza virus replication.

This problem could potentially occur in vivo when humans are infected with avian viruses whose HA has a binding specificity for α-2,3-linked sialyl receptors but the predominant receptors in the human respiratory tract are α-2,6-linked sialyl receptors. This could render the avian virus in humans less responsive to NA inhibitors as a class than the sensitivity of their NAs might suggest and less sensitive than seasonal human influenza viruses that have NAs of similar sensitivity. For those avian viruses that replicate outside of the respiratory tract (as H5N1 viruses appear to do), the receptor and binding specificities relating to systemic organs and tissues may also be important. These considerations may, at least in part, explain the relatively poor response of subjects infected with H5N1 virus to oseltamivir treatment. Late start of dosing as described above may be the most important factor, as also may be the occasional emergence of a resistant virus [12, 84, 85]. However, if H5N1 influenza virus, or indeed any other avian virus, were to achieve the ability to readily transmit directly from human to human, which would be required for that virus to initiate a pandemic, one would expect some change in HA binding specificity to allow better binding to human α-2,6-linked sialyl respiratory tract receptors. This adaptation would be expected to reverse the receptor binding mismatch and increase sensitivity to oseltamivir and NA inhibitors in general. Thus, while H5N1 remains an avian virus infecting humans, the efficacy of oseltamivir may be relatively poor compared with the activity that may be realized should H5N1 become a pandemic virus with the ability to transmit between humans.

Nevertheless, it still cannot be assumed that the dose required to successfully treat pandemic influenza will be the same as that required to treat a seasonal influenza virus infection. Other factors that may be pertinent to establishing the correct therapeutic dose include the ability of the virus to cause systemic infection, the distribution of the drug to the systemic sites of viral replication, and the replicative ability of the virus in the respiratory tract or at other systemic sites of replication (the dose to effectively treat a virus reaching 10^6 EID_{50} of viral load may need to be greater than that to treat a virus reaching a 10^3 EID_{50} viral load). The dose of oseltamivr required to achieve a given efficacy is likely to be reduced if the drug is used in combination with other anti-influenza agents. Resistance may be less of a problem when the correct therapeutic dose and timing of dose is applied and when combination treatment regimens are employed.

CONCLUSION

Both NA enzyme inhibition data and x-ray crystallography studies confirm that the strategy of designing an inhibitor of influenza NA that binds to the highly conserved active site of the NA achieves the desired goal of activity against all influenza NA subtypes, N1-N9, and influenza B viruses. Potent NA inhibition by oseltamivir carboxylate in the low nanomolar range is seen with all types of influenza NA. Thus, these data suggest that oseltamivir carboxylate, administered orally as its prodrug oseltamivir phosphate, should potentially be active against all influenza viruses with any combination of H1-H16 and N1-N9 that may arise to give isolated human infections or a human epidemic or pandemic. There are strong clinical data to support the activity of oseltamivir for the treatment and prophylaxis of the common seasonal influenza viruses. For viruses that are currently found predominantly in the avian population with some sporadic infection of man, in vivo antiviral data from animal experiments and some limited data from treatment of human infections confirm the potential efficacy of oseltamivir but suggest there may be factors other than NA sensitivity alone that will determine the dose of oseltamivir required for optimal antiviral efficacy.

Thus, it is reassuring to know that oseltamivir will almost certainly have intrinsic activity against any potential influenza virus and hence any influenza pandemic virus. The correct dosage and usage of the drug will have to be determined urgently on emergence of a pandemic, both to save lives and to ensure optimal use of precious drug. It may well be that countries whose general practitioners have had significant experience in of the use of oseltamivir prior to the emergence of a pandemic will be best placed to make sound front-line judgments on its use in a pandemic environment.

ACKNOWLEDGEMENTS

We thank Dr. Robert G. Webster for valuable suggestions and critical reading of the manuscript. We are also grateful to F. Hoffmann La-Roche and Gilead Sciences for permission to use some of their unpublished data.

REFERENCES

[1] Palmer A and Chambers S. Disease overview – Influenza. *Drugs in Context*, 2006, 2: 601-648.

[2] Wright RF, Neumann G, and Kawaoka Y. Influenza in humans – Past pandemics and the H5N1 epidemic. In: Knipe DM and Howley PM, editors, *Fields Virology*, Fifth edition, Philadelphia, Lippincott Williams and Wilkins Publishers, 2007, 48: 1697-1701.

[3] Writing Committee of the Second World Health Organization Consultation on Clinical Aspects of Human Infections with Avian Influenza A (H5N1) Virus. *New England J. Med.*, 2008, 358: 261-273.

[4] Palese P and Shaw ML. Orthomyxoviridae: The viruses and their replication. In: Knipe DM and Howley PM, editors, *Fields Virology*, Fifth edition, Philadelphia, Lippincott Williams and Wilkins Publishers, 2007, 47: 1647-1689.

[5] Webster RG, Bean WJ, Gorman CT, Chambers TM, and Kawaoka Y. Evolution and ecology of influenza A viruses. *Microbiol Rev.*, 1992, 56 (1): 152-179.

[6] Palese P, Zheng H, Engelhardt OG, Pleschka S, and Garcia-Sastre A. Negative-strand RNA viruses: genetic engineering and applications. *Proc. Natl. Acad. Sci. USA*, 1996, 93: 11354–11358.

[7] Fodor E, Devenish L, Engelhardt OG, Palese P, Brownlee GG, and García-Sastre A. Rescue of influenza A virus from recombinant DNA. *J. Virol.*. 1999, 73: 9679-9682.

[8] Claas EC, Osterhaus AD, van Beek R, De Jong J C, Rimmelzwaan GF, Senne D A, Krauss S, Shortridge K F and Webster RG. Human influenza A H5N1 virus related to a highly pathogenic avian influenza virus. *Lancet*, 1998, 351: 472–477.

[9] Peiris M, Yuen KY, Leung CW, Chan KH, Ip PL, Lai RW, Orr WK, and Shortridge KF. Human infection with influenza H9N2. *Lancet*, 1999, 354: 916-917.

[10] Fouchier RAM, Scneeburger PM, Rozendaal FW, Broekman JM, Kemink SA, Munster V, Kuiken T, Rimmelzwaan GF, Schutten M, Van Doornum GJ, Koch G, Bosman A, Koopmans M, and Osterhaus AD. Avian influenza A virus (H7N7) associated with conjunctivitis and a fatal case of acute respiratory distress syndrome. *Proc. Natl. Acad. Sci. USA*, 2004, 101: 1356-1361.

[11] McKimm-Breschkin JL. Management of influenza virus infections with neuraminidase inhibitors: detection, incidence, and implications of drug resistance. *Treat Respir. Med.*, 2005, 4(2): 107-116.

[12] Aoki FY, Boivin G, Roberts NA. Influenza virus susceptibility and resistance to oseltamivir. *Antiviral Therapy,* 2007, 12: 603-616.

[13] Matrosovich MN, Matrosovich TY, Gray T, Roberts NA, and Klenk H-D. Neuraminidase is important for the initiation of influenza infection in human airway epithelium. *J. Virol.*, 2004, 78: 12665-12667.

[14] Liu C and Air GM. Selection and characterization of a neuraminidase-minus mutant of influenza virus and its rescue by cloned neuraminidase genes. *Virology*, 1993, 194(1): 403-407.

[15] Hughes MT, Matrosovich M, Rodgers ME, McGregor M, and Kawaoka Y. Influenza A viruses lacking sialidase activity can undergo multiple cycles of replication in cell culture, eggs, or mice. *J. Virol.,* 2000, 74: 5206-5212.

[16] Coleman PM. Influenza virus neuraminidase: Structure, antibodies, and inhibitors. *Protein Science,* 1994, 3: 1687-1696.

[17] Russell RJ, Haire LF, Stevens DJ, Collins PJ, Lin YP, Blackburn MG, Hay AJ, Gamblin SJ, and Skehel JJ. The structure of H5N1 avian influenza neuraminidase suggests new opportunities for drug design. *Nature,* 2006, 443: 45-49.

[18] Colman, PM, Varghese JN, and Laver WG. Structure of the catalytic and antigenic sites in influenza virus neuraminidase. *Nature,* 1983, 303: 41-44.

[19] Gubareva LV, Robinson MJ, Bethell RC, and Webster RG. Catalytic and framework mutations in the neuraminidase active site of influenza viruses that are resistant to 4-guanidino-Neu5Ac2en. *J. Virol.,* 1997, 71: 3385-3390.

[20] Chong AKJ, Peggs MS, Taylor NR, and von Itzstein M. Evidence for a sialosyl cation transition-state complex in the reaction of sialidase from influenza virus. *Eur. J. Biochem.,* 1992, 207: 335-343.

[21] Taylor NR and von Itzstein M. Molecular modelling studies on ligand binding to sialidase from influenza virus and the mechanism of catalysis. *J. Med. Chem.,* 1994, 37: 616-624.

[22] Meindl P, Bodo G, Palese P, Schulman J, and Tuppy H. Inhibition of neuraminidase activity by derivatives of 2-Deoxy-2, 3-Dehydro-N-Acetylneuraminic Acid. *Virology,* 1974, 58: 457-463.

[23] von Itzstein M, Wu WY, Kok GB, Pegg MS, Dyason JC, Jin B, Van Phan T, Smythe ML, White HF, Oliver SW, Colman PM, Varghese JN, Ryan DM, Woods JM, Bethell RC, Hotham VJ, Cameron JM, and Penn CR. Rational design of potent sialidase-based inhibitors of influenza virus replication. *Nature,* 1993, 363: 418-423.

[24] Palese P and Schulman JL. Inhibitors of viral neuraminidase as potential antiviral drugs. In: Oxford JS, editor. *Chemoprophylaxis and Virus Infections of the Respiratory Tract,* CRC Press, Cleveland, 1977, 6: 189-205.

[25] Varghese JN. The structure of the complex between influenza virus neuraminidase and sialic acid, the viral receptor. *Proteins: Structure, Function, and Genetics*, 1992, 14: 327-332.

[26] Woods JM, Bethell RC, Coates JAV, Healy N, Hiscox SA, Pearson BA, Ryan DM, Ticehurst J, Tilling J, Walcott SM, and Penn CR. 4-Guanidino-2, 4-Dideoxy-2, 3-Dehydro-N-Acetylneuraminic Acid is a highly effective inhibitor both of the sialidase (neuraminidase) and of growth of a wide range of influenza A and B viruses in vitro. *Antimicrob. Agents Chemother.,* 1993, 37: 1473-1479.

[27] Ryan DM, Ticehurst J, Dempsey MH, and Penn CR. Inhibition of influenza virus replication in mice by GG167 (4-Guanidino-2, 4-Dideoxy-2, 3-Dehydro-N-Acetylneuraminic Acid) is consistent with extracellular activity of viral neuraminidase (sialidase). *Antimicrob. Agents Chemother.,* 1994, 38: 2270-2275.

[28] Ryan DM, Ticehurst J, and Dempsey MH. GG167 (4-Guanidino-2, 4-Dideoxy-2, 3-Dehydro-N-Acetylneuraminic Acid) is a potent inhibitor of influenza virus in ferrets. *Antimicrob. Agents Chemother.,* 1995, 39: 2583-2584.

[29] de Jong M, Thanh TT, Khanh TH, Hien VM, Smith GJD, Chau NV, Cam BV, Qui PT, Ha DQ, Guan Y, Peiris JSM, Hien TT, and Farrar J. Fatal avian influenza A (H5N1) in a child presenting with diarrhea followed by coma. *N. Engl. J. Med.,* 2005, 352: 686-691.

[30] Kim CU, Lew W, Williams MA, Liu H, Swaminathan S, Bischofberger N, Chen MS, Mendel DB, Tai CY, Laver WG, and Stevens RC. Influenza neuraminidase inhibitors possessing a novel hydrophobic interaction in the enzyme active site: Design, synthesis, and structural analysis of carbocyclic sialic acid analogues with potent anti-influenza activity. *J. Amer. Chem. Soc.*, 1997, 119: 681-690.

[31] Li W, Escarpe PA, Eisenberg EJ, Cundy KC, Sweet C, Jakeman KJ, Merson J, Lew W, Williams M, Zhang L, Kim CU, Bischofberger N, Chen MS, and Mendel DB. Identification of GS 4104 as an orally bioavailable prodrug of the influenza virus neuraminidase inhibitor GS 4071. *Antimicrob. Agents Chemother.*, 1998, 42: 647-653.

[32] Mendel DB, Tai CY, Escarpe PA, Li W, Sidwell RW, Huffman JH, Sweet C, Jakeman KJ, Merson J, Lacy SA, Lew W, Williams MA, Zhang L, Chen MS, Bischofberger N, and Kim CU. Oral administration of a prodrug of the influenza virus neuraminidase inhibitor GS 4071 protects mice and ferrets against influenza infection. *Antimicrob. Agents Chemother.*, 1998, 42: 640-646.

[33] He G, Massarella J, and Ward P. Clinical pharmacokinetics of the prodrug oseltamivir and its active metabolite Ro 64-0802. *Clin. Pharmacokinet.*, 1999, 37: 471-484.

[34] Eisenberg EJ, Bidgood A, and Cundy KC. Penetration of GS4071, a novel influenza neuraminidase inhibitor, into rat bronchoalveolar lining fluid following oral administration of the prodrug GS4104. *Antimicrob. Agents Chemother.*, 1997, 41: 1949-1952.

[35] Roberts NA, Wiltshire HR, Mendel DB, and Webster RG. Oseltamivir carboxylate is effective against all subtypes of influenza neuraminidase. Poster 135, ASM Biodefence Research Meeting, Baltimore, March 2003, http://www.asmbiodefence.org/tuepos.asp.

[36] Govorkova EA, Leneva IA, Goloubeva OG, Bush K, and Webster RG. Comparison of efficacies of RWJ-270201, zanamivir and oseltamivir against H5N1, H9N2 and other avian influenza viruses. *Antimicrob. Agents Chemother.*, 2001, 45: 2723-2732.

[37] McKimm-Breshkin J, Trivedi T, Hampson A, Hay A, Klimov A, Tashiro M, Hayden F, and Zambon M. Neuraminidase sequence analysis and susceptibilities of influenza virus clinical isloates to zanamivir and oseltamivir. *Antimicrob. Agents Chemother.*, 2003, 47: 2264-2272.

[38] Hurt AC, Barr IG, Durrant CJ, Shaw RP, Sjogren HM, and Hampson AW. Surveillance for neuraminidase inhibitor resistance in influenza viruses from Australia. *Commun. Dis. Intell.* 2003, 27: 542-547.

[39] World Health Organization. September 2008. Updates on avian influenza A (H5N1) infections in man. http://www.who.int/csr/disease/avian_influenza/country cases_table_2008_09_10/en/index.html.

[40] Tumpey TM, Garcia-Sastre A, Mikulasova A, Taubenberger JK, Swayne DE, Palese P, and Basler CF. Existing antivirals are effective against influenza viruses with genes from the 1918 pandemic virus. *Proc. Natl. Acad. Sci. USA*, 2002, 99: 13849-13854.

[41] Koopmans M, Wilbrink B, Conyn M, Natrop G, van der Nat H, Vennema H, Meijer A, van Steenbergen J, Fouchier R, and Osterhaus A. Transmission of H7N7 avian influenza A virus to human beings during a large outbreak in commercial poultry farms in the Netherlands. *Lancet,* 2004, 363: 587-593.

[42] Meijer A, van de Kamp EEHM, Koch G, and Kimman TG. Cell-ELISA for antiviral susceptibility testing of influenza virus: performance depends on the compatibility of virus strain and type of MDCK cells. *Inter. Congr. Series*, 2004, 1263: 491-494.

[43]   Rameix-Welti MA, Agou F, Buchy P, Mardy S, Aubin JT, Veron M, van der Verf S, and Naffakh N. Natural variation can significantly alter sensitivity to oseltamivir of influenza A (H5N1) viruses. *Antimicrob. Agents Chemother.*, 2006, 50: 3809-3815.

[44]   Saad MD, Boynton BR, Earhart KC, Mansour MM, Niman HL, Elsayed NM, Nayel AL, Abdelghani AS, Essmat HM, Labib EM Ayoub EA, and Monteville MR. Detection of oseltamivir resistance mutations N294S in humans with influenza A H5N1. Options for the Control of Influenza VI, 2007, Toronto, Canada, 228.

[45]   Kiso M, Mitamura K, Sakai-Tagawa Y, Shiraishi K, Kawakami C, Kimura K, Hayden FG, Sugaya N, and Kawaoka Y. Resistant influenza A viruses in children treated with oseltamivir: descriptive study. *Lancet,* 2004, 364: 759-765.

[46]   McKimm-Breschkin JL, Selleck PW, Usman TB, and Johnson MA. Reduced sensitivity of influenza A (H5N1) viruses. *Emerg. Infect. Dis.*, 2007, 9: 1354-1357.

[47]   Monto AS, McKimm-Breschkin JL, Macken C, Hampson AW, Hay A, Klimov A, Tashiro M, Webster RG, Aymard M, Hayden FG, and Zambon M. Detection of influenza viruses resistant to neuraminidase inhibitors in global surveillance during the first 3 years of their use. *Antimicrobial Agents Chemother.*, 2006, 50: 2395-2402.

[48]   Sedyaningsih ER, Isfandari S, Setyaway V, Hendroputranto R, and Soendoro T. Clinical features of avian influenza A (H5N1) infections in Indonesia July 2005-April 2007. Options for the Control of Influenza, 2007, Toronto, Canada, 329.

[49]   Hurt AC, Selleck P, Komadina N, Shaw R, Brown L, and Barr IG. Susceptibility of highly pathogenic A (H5N1) avain influenza viruses to the neuraminidase inhibitors and adamantanes. *Antiviral Res.,* 2007, 73: 228-231.

[50]   Moscona A. Oseltamivir resistance – Disabling our influenza defenses. *New Eng. J. Med.,* 2005, 353: 2633-2636.

[51]   Gubareva LV, Matrosovich MN, Brenner MK, Bethell RC, and Webster RG. Evidence for zanamivir resistance in an immunocompromised child infected with influenza B virus. *J Infect. Dis.,* 1998, 178: 1257-1262.

[52]   Tisdale M. Monitoring of viral susceptibility: new challenges with the development of influenza NA inhibitors. *Rev. Med. Virol.,* 2000, 10: 45-55.

[53]   Zambon M and Hayden FG. Position statement: global neuraminidase inhibitor susceptibility network. *Antiviral Res.,* 2001, 49: 147-156.

[54]   Matrosovich M, Matrosovich T, Carr J, Roberts NA, and Klenk HD. Overexpression of the α-2,6-sialyltransferase in MDCK cells increases influenza sensitivity to neuraminidase inhibitors. *J. Virol.,* 2003, 77: 8418-8425.

[55]   Hatakeyama S, Sakai-Tagawa Y Kiso M, Goto H, Kawakami C, Mitamura K, Sugaya Y, and Kawaoka Y. Enhanced expression of an α2,6-linked sialic acid on MDCK cells improves isolation of human influenza viruses and evaluation of their sensitivity to a neuraminidase inhibitor. *J. Clin. Microbiol.,* 2005, 43: 4139-4146.

[56]   Yen HL, Herlocher L, Hoffmann E, Matrosovich MN, Monto AS, Webster RG, and Govorkova EA. Neuraminidase inhibitor-resistant influenza viruses differ substantially in fitness and transmissibility. *Antimicrob. Agents Chemother.,* 2005, 49: 4075-4084.

[57]   Matrosovich MN, Matrosovich TY, Gray T, Roberts NA, and Klenk HD. Human and avian influenza viruses target different cell types in cultures of human airway epithelium. *Proc. Nat. Acad. Sci. USA,* 2004, 101: 4620-4624.

[58] Ilyushina NA, Govorkova EA, Gray TE, Bovin NV, and Webster RG. Human-like receptor specificity does not affect the neuraminidase-inhibitor susceptibility of H5N1 influenza viruses. *PLoS Pathogens,* 2008, 4(4): e1000043.

[59] Yamanaka T, Tsujimura K, Kondo T, and Matsumura T. In Vitro efficacies of oseltamivir carboxylate and zanamivir against equine influenza viruses. *J. Vet. Med. Sci.,* 2006, 68: 405-408.

[60] Scholtissek C, Bürger H, Kistner O, and Shortridge KF. The nucleoprotein as a possible major factor in determining host specificity of influenza H3N2 viruses. *Virology,* 1985, 147: 287-294.

[61] Bauer K, Schrader C, Suess J, Wutzler P, and Schmidtke M. Neuraminidase inhibitor susceptibility of porcine H3N2 influenza viruses isolated in Germany between 1982 and 1999. *Antiviral Res.,* 2007, 75: 219-226.

[62] Liu C, Eichelberger MC, Compans RW, and Air GM. Influenza type A virus neuraminidase does not play a role in viral entry, replication, assembly, or budding. *J. Virol.,* 1995, 69: 1099-1106.

[63] Palese P, Tobita K, and Ueda M, Compans RW. Characterization of temperature sensitive influenza virus mutants defective in neuraminidase. *Virology,* 1974, 61: 397-410.

[64] Palese P and Compans RW. Inhibition of influenza virus replication in tissue culture by 2-deoxy-2,3-dehydro-N-trifluoro-acetyl-neuraminic acid (FANA): mechanism of action. *J. Gen. Virol.,* 1976, 33: 159-63.

[65] Ohuchi M, Asaoka N, Sakai T, and Ohuchi R. Roles of neuraminidase in the initial stage of influenza virus infection. *Microbes Infect.,* 2006, 8: 1287-1293.

[66] White MR, Crouch E, van Eijk M, Hartshorn M, Pemberton L, Tornoe I, Holmskov U, and Hartshorn KL. Cooperative anti-influenza activities of respiratory innate immune proteins and neuranimidase inhibitor. *Am. J. Physiol. Lung Cell Mol. Physiol.,* 2005, 288: L831-L840.

[67] Singh S, Barghoom J, Bagdonas A, Adler J, Treanor J, Kinnersley N, and Ward P. Clinical benefits with oseltamivir in treating influenza in adult populations. *Clin. Drug Invest.,* 2003, 23: 561-569.

[68] Ward P, Small I, Smith J, Suter P, and Dutkowski R. Oseltamivir (Tamiflu^R) and its potential for use in the event of an influenza pandemic. *J. Antimicrob. Chemother.,* 2005, 55: 5-21.

[69] Leneva IA, Roberts N, Govorkova EA, Goloubeva OG, and Webster RG. The neuraminidase inhibitor GS4104 (oseltamivir phosphate) is efficacious against A/Hong Kong/156/97 (H5N1) and A/Hong Kong/1074/99 (H9N2) influenza viruses. *Antiviral Res.,* 2000, 48 (2): 101-115.

[70] Yen HL, Monto AS, Webster RG, and Govorkova EA. Virulence may determine the necessary duration and dosage of oseltamivir treatment for highly pathogenic A/Vietnam/1203/04 influenza virus in mice. *J. Infect. Dis.,* 2005, 192 (4): 665-672.

[71] Leigh MW, Connor RJ, Kelm S, Baum LG, and Paulson JC. Receptor specificity of influenza virus influences severity of illness in ferrets. *Vaccine,* 1995, 13: 1468-1473.

[72] Zitzow LA, Rowe T, Morken T, Shieh WJ, Zaki S, and Katz JM. Pathogenesis of avian influenza A (H5N1) viruses in ferrets. *J. Virol.,* 2002, 76: 4420-4429.

[73] Govorkova EA, Rehg JE, Krauss S, Yen HL, Guan Y, Peiris M, Nguyen TD, Hanh TH, Puthavathana P, Long HT, Buranathai C, Lim W, Webster RG, and Hoffmann E.

Lethality to ferrets of H5N1 influenza viruses isolated from humans and poultry in 2004. *J. Virol.*, 2005, 79: 2191-2198.

[74] Govorkova EA, Ilyushina NA, Boltz DA, Douglas A, Yilmaz N, and Webster RG. Efficacy of oseltamivir therapy in ferrets inoculated with different clades of H5N1 influenza virus. *Antimicrob. Agents Chemother.*, 2007, 51: 1414-1424.

[75] Boltz DA, Rehg JE, McClaren JL, Webster RG, and Govorkova EA. Oseltamivir prophylactic regimens prevent H5N1 influenza morbidity and mortality in a ferret model. *J. Infect. Dis.*, 2008, 197: 1315–1323.

[76] Gubareva LV, Penn CR, and Webster RG. Inhibition of replication of avian influenza viruses by the neuraminidase inhibitor 4-Guanidino-2,4-dideoxy-2,3-dehydro-*N*-acetylneuraminic acid. *Virology*, 1995, 212 (2): 323-330.

[77] Meijer A, van der Goot JA, Koch G, van Boven M, and Kimman TG. Oseltamivir reduces transmission, morbidity and mortality of highly pathogenic avian influenza in chickens. *Inter. Congr. Series*, 2004, 1263: 495-498.

[78] Ilyushina NA, Bovin NV, Webster RG, and Govorkova EA. Combination chemotherapy, a potential strategy for reducing the emergence of drug-resistant influenza A variants. *Antiviral Res.*, 2006, 70 (3): 121-131.

[79] Ilyushina NA, Hoffmann E, Salomon R, Webster RG, and Govorkova EA. Amantadine-oseltamivir combination therapy for H5N1 influenza virus infection in mice. *Antiviral Therapy*, 2007, 12: 363-370.

[80] Ilyushina NA, Hay A, Yilmaz N, Boon ACM, Webster RG, and Govorkova EA. Oseltamivir-ribavirin combination therapy for highly pathogenic H5N1 influenza virus infection in mice. *Antimicrob. Agents Chemother.*, 2008, 52: 3889-3897.

[81] Zheng B-J, Chan K-W, Lin Y-P, Zhao G-Y, Chan C, Zhang H-J, Chen H-L, Wong SSY, Lau SKP, Woo PCY, Chan K-H, Jin D-Y, and Yuen K-Y. Delayed antiviral plus immunomodulator treatment still reduces mortality in mice infected by high inoculum of influenza A/H5N1 virus. *Proc. Natl. Acad. Sci. USA*, 2008, 105: 8091-8096.

[82] Tweed AS, Skowronski DM, David ST, Larder A, Petric M, Lees W, Li Y, Katz J, Krajden M, Tellier R, Halpert C, Hirst M, Astell, C, Lawrence D, and Mak A. Human illness from avian influenza H7N3, British Columbia. *Emerg. Infect. Dis.*, 2004, 10: 2196-2199.

[83] Aoki FY, Macleod MD, Paggiaro P, Carewicz O, El Sawy A, Wat C, Griffiths M, Waalberg E, and Ward P. Early administration of oral oseltamivir increases the benefits of influenza treatment. *J. Antimicrob. Chemother.*, 2003, 51: 123-129.

[84] de Jong MD, Thanh TT, Khanh TH, Hien VM, Smith GJD, Chau NV, Cam BV, Qui PT, Ha DQ, Guan Y, Peiris JSM, Hien TT, and Farrar J. Oseltamivir resistance during treatment of influenza A (H5N1) infection. *New Engl. J. Med.*, 2005, 353: 2667-2672.

[85] Le QM, Kiso M, Someya K, Sakai YT, Nguyen TH, Nguyen KHL, Pham ND, Ngyen HH, Yamada S, Muramoto Y, Horimoto T, Takada A, Goto H, Suzuki T, Suzuki Y, and Kawaoka Y. Avian flu: isolation of drug-resistant H5N1 virus. *Nature*, 2005, 437: 1108.

[86] Yen HL, Ilyushina NA, Salomon R, Hoffmann E, Webster RG, and Govorkova EA. Neuraminidase inhibitor-resistant recombinant A/Vietnam/1203/04 (H5N1) influenza viruses retain their replication efficiency and pathogenesis in vitro and in vivo. *J. Virol.*, 2007, 81: 12418-12426.

In: Global View of Fight against Influenza
Editor: Petar M. Mitrasinovic

ISBN: 978-1-60741-952-5
© 2009 Nova Science Publishers, Inc.

Chapter 8

Computational Investigations of the Binding Mechanism of Current Influenza Virus Neuraminidase Inhibitors: Correlation with Experiment

Marija L. Mihajlovic and Petar M. Mitrasinovic[*]

Center for Multidisciplinary Studies, University of Belgrade, Serbia

Abstract

In the context of the recent pandemic threat by the worldwide spread of H5N1 avian influenza, novel insights into the mechanisms of ligand binding and interaction between various inhibitors (zanamivir-ZMV, oseltamivir-OTV, DANA, peramivir-PMV) and neuraminidases (NAs) are of vital importance for the structure-based design of new anti-viral drugs. Computational methods are herein shown to be a viable partner to experiment in the investigation of the binding modes of known NA inhibitors. Using the crystal structures of inhibitors bound to either group-2 or group-1 NAs, the AScore/ShapeDock-scoring was shown to identify the binding modes in agreement with the experiment for all inhibitors docked in their own NA/inhibitor crystal structures. To investigate the effect of small changes in protein structure on predicted binding modes, in a set of 132 docking experiments (11 inhibitors docked in 12 group-2 NA structures) AScore/ShapeDock identified the correct binding modes of 116 complexes. In a total of 88 docking experiments (8 inhibitors docked in 11 group-1 NA structures) AScore/ShapeDock predicted 80 binding modes correctly. A small vHTS experiment, reflected by mixing the known activity molecules to a set of randomly selected molecules, confirmed the ability of the AScore/ShapeDock approach to extract biologically active molecules from inactive ones. By both outperforming other docking methods used previously in the literature and being quite reproducible, the AScore/ShapeDock protocol is suggested to be convenient for designing novel H5N1-NA inhibitors. To shed more light on the high resistance of H5N1 strains to various NA inhibitors, the three-dimensional models of H5N1-NA and

---

[*] Correspondence to: petar.mitrasinovic@gmail.com.

N9-NA were generated by homology modeling. Traditional residues within the active site throughout the family of NA protein structures were found to be highly conserved in H5N1-NA, and a subtle variation between lipophilic and hydrophilic environments in H5N1-NA with respect to N9-NA was observed. Besides, molecular bases of the mechanism of H5N1-NA resistance to oseltamivir were elucidated in a systematic fashion. Using the crystal structure of the complex of H5N1-NA with OTV (PDB ID: 2hu0) as the starting point, the following question was addressed and correlated with the experimental data: How mutations at His274 by both smaller side chain (Gly, Ser, Asn, Gln) and larger side chain (Phe, Tyr) residues influence the sensitivity of N1 to oseltamivir? The smaller side chain residue mutations of His274 resulted in slightly enhanced or unchanged NA sensitivity to OTV, while His274Phe and His274Tyr reduced the susceptibility of OTV to N1. In contrast to the binding free energies, the net charges of Glu276 and Arg224, making charge-charge interactions with Glu276, were established to be more sensitive to detecting subtle conformational differences induced at the key residue Glu276 by the His274X mutations. Thus, deeper insights into the possibility of developing viable drug-resistant mutants were possible.

1. INTRODUCTION

Two glycoproteins, haemagglutinin and neuraminidase, are contained in influenza virus membranes with their specific functions. While cell-surface sialic acid receptor binding is mediated by haemagglutinin in order to trigger virus infection, neuraminidase removes sialic acid from virus and cellular glycoproteins after virus replication, thus facilitating virus release and the spread of infection to new cells [1]. Based on different antigenic properties of various glycoprotein molecules, influenza type A viruses are classified into the following subtypes: 16 for haemagglutinin (H1-H16) and 9 for neuraminidase (N1-N9) [2]. Two phylogenetically distinct groups, group-1 (N1, N4, N5, N8) and group-2 (N2, N3, N6, N7, N9), contain N1 and N2 NAs of viruses that currently circulate in humans [3]. One of such viruses is H5N1 avian influenza threatening a new pandemic [4,5]. Because vaccines are not yet available and a number of drugs are undergoing testing, infected patients are currently treated by two approved anti-influenza drugs: oseltamivir (Tamiflu) [6] and zanamivir (Relenza) [7] (Figure 1), targeting NA enzyme of virus. The fact that several tens of different crystal structures of NAs are available in the Protein Data Bank (PDB) [8] has enabled extensive investigations of the effect of small changes in protein structure on predicted binding modes of known inhibitors by means of knowledge-based scoring functions [9-13]. Hence, computational methods are a viable partner to experiment in predicting binding modes of NA inhibitors [14].

The ultimate goals of the docking and scoring technology applications at different stages of the drug discovery process are (1) predicting the binding mode of a known active ligand, (2) identifying new ligands by means of virtual screening, and (3) predicting the binding affinities of related compounds from a known active series [15]. Successful prediction of a ligand binding mode in a protein active site is the area where the most substantial progress has been achieved [16,17]. Docking studies, demonstrating that particular techniques can reproduce observed results in a published data set, represent the first step for evaluating the

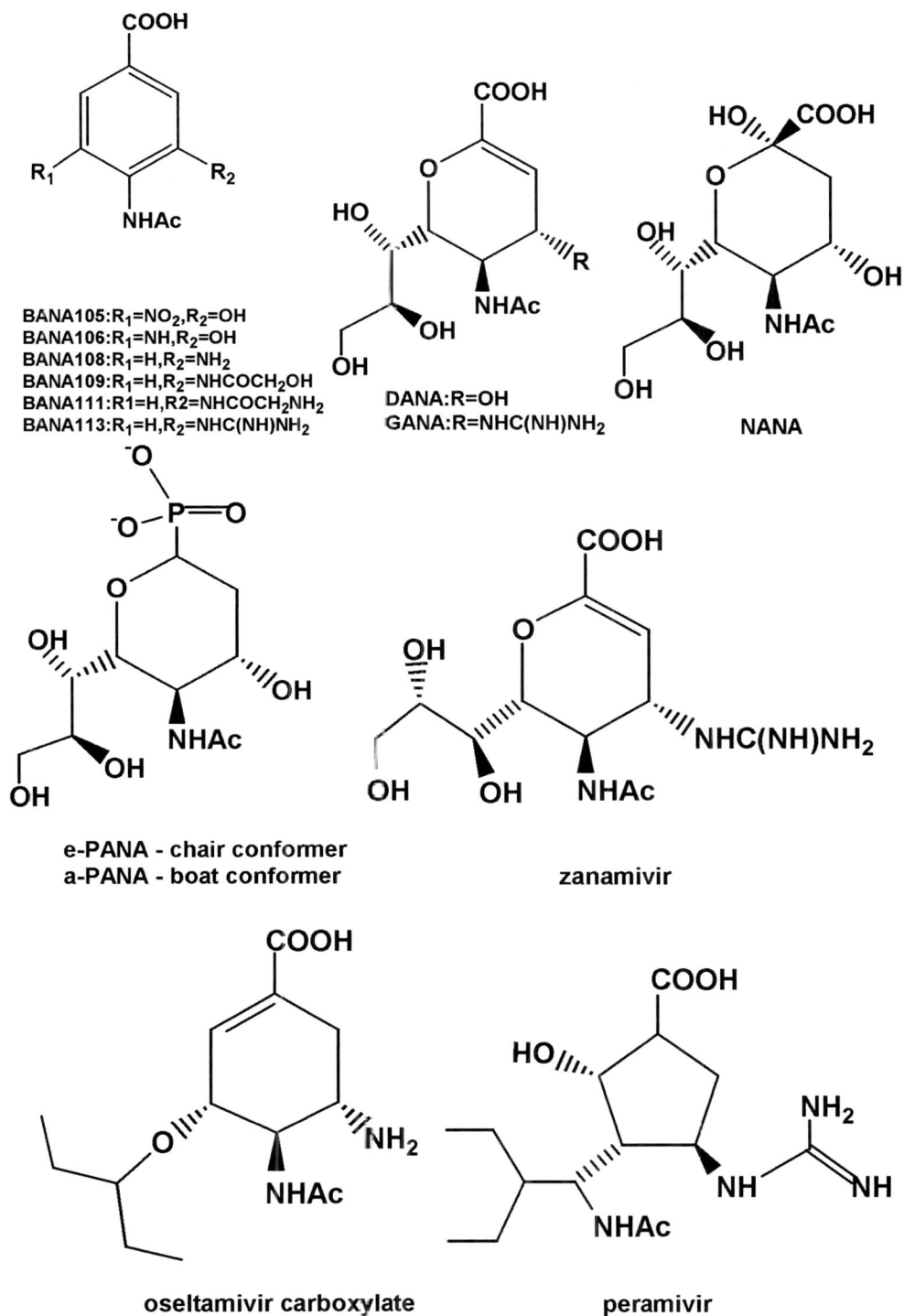

Figure 1. The chemical structures of known influenza virus neuraminidase inhibitors [21].

accuracy of newly developed or improved algorithms. As a consequence of the successful first step, the following step is based on prospective studies, particularly from industry where the opportunity for such work is the greatest [15]. In light of the previous results [9], the first objective of the present chapter is to explore the ability of ArgusLab 4.0, a recently introduced molecular modeling package in which molecular docking is implemented [18], to reproduce crystallographic binding orientations of various inhibitors bound to group-2 NAs, and to compare its accuracy with that of the QuantumLead program [19]. Since the structure of H5N1 suggests a wide spectrum of new opportunities for drug design in the context of a current pandemic threat by the worldwide spread of H5N1 avian influenza [20], the second objective herein is to estimate the accuracy of the same method to predict the binding modes of known inhibitors of group-1 NAs.

2. COMPUTATIONAL METHODS

2.1 Databases

The investigated structures are denoted throughout the paper by their Protein Data Bank codes. The PDB IDs of group-2 NA structures are: 1ivd, 1ivc, 1ive, 1ing, 1inh, 1inf, 2bat, 1ivf, 1nnc, 1inw, 1inx, and 1ivg. The N2 A/Tokyo/3/67 subtypes are: 1ivd (complex with guanidinobenzoic acid inhibitor – BANA105), 1ivc (with BANA106), 1ive (with BANA108), 1ing (with BANA109), 1inh (with BANA111), 2bat (with *N*-acetylneuraminic acid - NANA), 1ivf (with NeuAc2en, 2-deoxy-2,3-didehydro-*N*-acetylneuraminic acid – DANA), 1inx (with (4-acetamido-2,4-dideoxy-*D*-glycero-alpha-*D*-galacto-1-octopyranosyl) phosphonic acid - ePANA), 1inw (with (4-acetamido-2,4-dideoxy-*D*-glycero-*D*-galacto-β-octopyranosyl) phosphonic acid - aPANA), and 1ivg (no inhibitor). The N9 (Tern) subtype is 1nnc (with 4-guanidino-NeuAc2en – GANA), while the only one of type B/Lee/40 is 1inf (with BANA113). The PDB IDs of group-1 NA structures are: 2hty, 2hu0, 2hu4, 2ht5, 2htr, 2ht7, 2ht8, 2htq, 2htu, 2htv, and 2htw. The N1 subtypes are: 2hty (no inhibitor), 2hu0 (with oseltamivir, 20 μM), and 2hu4 (with oseltamivir, 0.5 mM). The N8 subtypes are: 2ht5 (no inhibitor), 2htr (with DANA), 2ht7 (with oseltamivir, 30 min soak), 2ht8 (with oseltamivir, 3 day soak), 2htq (with zanamivir), and 2htu (with peramivir). The N4 subtypes are: 2htv (no inhibitor) and 2htw (with DANA). The chemical structures of various influenza virus neuraminidase inhibitors are schematically shown in Figure 1.

2.2 Molecular Docking with ArgusLab 4.0

The docking problem is conceivable as a complicated optimization or an exhaustive search problem involving many degrees of freedom, and the development of efficient docking algorithms would be of vital importance for the design of new drugs. The ultimate goal is to find the optimal ligand/protein configurations, and accurately as well as consistently predict their binding free energy without relying on formal statistical mechanics approaches. To computationally accomplish the key objective within a reasonable time framework, an empirical scoring function (AScore) and a docking engine (ShapeDock) were developed in ArgusLab 4.0 [18].

2.2.1 Fundamental Idea Behind Empirical Scoring

Since a remarkable work of Böhm [22], a variety of scoring functions have appeared in the literature. All of the approaches share the same assumption that the overall receptor-ligand binding free energy can be conceptually represented by a sum of some basic components:

$$\Delta G_{binding} = \Delta G_{motion} + \Delta G_{interaction} + \Delta G_{desolvation} + \Delta G_{configuration} \tag{1}$$

The separated terms account for the protein-ligand motion (ΔG_{motion}), the hydrogen bond, ionic, aromatic, or lipophilic protein-ligand interaction ($\Delta G_{interaction}$), the desolvation-mediated protein-ligand binding ($\Delta G_{desolvation}$), and the binding free energy for a particular protein-ligand. configuration ($\Delta G_{configuration}$), respectively. In contrast to force fields, empirical scoring functions are not derived from "first principle". Based on a set of protein-ligand complexes with experimentally determined structures and binding affinities, scoring functions are calibrated using multivariate regression analysis. The final form of a scoring function is affected by both the size and the quality of the training set. There are several principal features of various scoring approaches. Since they are derived from diverse protein-ligand complexes, their applications are not restricted to a particular series of ligands or a specific target receptor. Because each of the summing terms in an empirical scoring function is known to be important for the binding processes (eq. 1), it is associated with a clear physical meaning. Most importantly, a characteristic accuracy level of about 2 kcal/mol achieved in binding affinity predictions makes empirical scoring functions acceptable for the structure-based drug design purposes, such as virtual database screening and *de novo* ligand generation.

2.2.2 The AScore Scoring Function

The AScore [18] scoring function extends the previously reported XScore [23]. The total protein-ligand binding free energy is decomposed into several distinct components:

$$\Delta G_{binding} = \Delta G_{vdw} + \Delta G_{hydrophobic} + \Delta G_{H-bond} + \Delta G_{H-bond(chg)} + \Delta G_{deformation} + \Delta G_0. \tag{2}$$

The dissected terms account for the van der Waals interaction between the ligand and the protein (ΔG_{vdw}), the hydrophobic effect ($\Delta G_{hydrophobic}$), the hydrogen bonding between ligand and the protein (ΔG_{H-bond}), the hydrogen bonding involving charged donor and/or acceptor groups ($\Delta G_{H-bond(chg)}$), the deformation effect ($\Delta G_{deformation}$), and the effects of the translational and rotational entropy loss in the binding process (ΔG_0), respectively. The separate $\Delta G_{H-bond(chg)}$ term (eq. 2) is the only addition to the XScore binding free energy of Wang and coworkers [23]. In contrast to XScore, the intra-ligand van der Waals energy is also included in the overall VDW term.

These contributions can be conveniently written as the following products:

$$\Delta G_{vdw} = C_{vdw} \cdot VDW, \Delta G_{hydrophobic} = C_{hydrophobic} \cdot HP \; \Delta G_{H-bond} = C_{H-bond} \cdot HB,$$

$$\Delta G_{H-bond(chg)} = C_{H-bond(chg)} \cdot HB(chg), \Delta G_{deformation} = C_{rotor} \cdot RT, \; \Delta G_0 = C_{regression}.$$

Each of the contributions possesses a specific regression coefficient multiplying a term that has a physical meaning. Investigating the regression coefficients enables more profound insights into the receptor-ligand binding process. The physical definitions of the *VDW, HP, HB,* and *RT* terms are given by the following four equations.

$$VDW = \sum_{i}^{ligand} \sum_{j}^{protein} \left[\left(\frac{d_{ij,0}}{r_{ij}}\right)^8 - 2\left(\frac{d_{ij,0}}{r_{ij}}\right)^4 \right] + \sum_{i}^{ligand} \sum_{j>i}^{ligand} \left[\left(\frac{d_{ij,0}}{r_{ij}}\right)^8 - 2\left(\frac{d_{ij,0}}{r_{ij}}\right)^4 \right], \qquad (3)$$

where $d_{ij,0}$ is the sum of van der Waals radii of atoms i,j, while the intra-ligand *VDW* portion of this term excludes *1,2* and *1,3* bonded pairs.

$$HP = \sum_{i}^{ligand} \sum_{j}^{protein} f(d_{ij}), \qquad (4)$$

where the sum is over hydrophobic ligand-protein atom pairs, and

$$f(d_{ij}) = \begin{cases} 1.0 \;\; for \; d < d_{ij,0} + 0.5 \, \overset{o}{A} \\ 2/3 \cdot (d_0 + 2 - d) \; for \; d_{ij,0} + 0.5 \, \overset{o}{A} < d \le d_{ij,0} + 2.0 \, \overset{o}{A} . \\ 0 \; for \; d > d_{ij,0} + 2.0 \, \overset{o}{A} \end{cases}$$

$$HB = \sum_{i}^{ligand} \sum_{j}^{protein} HB_{ij}, \qquad (5)$$

where $HB_{ij} = f(r_{ij}) f(\theta_{1,ij}) f(\theta_{2,ij})$. r_{ij} is distance between donor/acceptor atoms, $\theta_{1,ij}$ is angle between donor root-donor-acceptor, and $\theta_{2,ij}$ is angle between donor-acceptor-acceptor root. Each term in the sum varies between 1.0 and 0.0, depending on how close to ideal value.

$$RT = \sum_{i}^{ligand} RT_i, \qquad (6)$$

with $RT_i = 0$ if atom i is not involved in any torsion, $RT_i = 0.5$ if atom i is involved in 1 torsion, $RT_i = 1.0$ if atom i is involved in 2 torsions, and $RT_i = 0.5$ if atom i is involved in more than 2 torsions.

2.2.3 The ShapeDock Docking Engine

The ShapeDock docking engine approximates a complicated search problem. Flexible ligand docking is available by describing the ligand as a torsion tree. Groups of bonded atoms that do not have rotatable bonds are nodes, while torsions are connections between the nodes. Topology of the torsion tree is a determinative factor influencing efficient docking. A balanced tree with a large central node is presumably the favorite case. Two grids, overlaying the binding site, distinguish grid points with respect to the free volume of binding site. Fine grid is used to examine whether atoms of a pose fragment are inside or outside the binding site, while coarse grid is used to establish the search points inside the binding site. A set of energetically favorable rotations is generated by placing the root node of a ligand on a search point in the binding site. The torsion search of poses is defined by constructing torsions in breadth-first order for each rotation. Of the survived poses candidates, the N-lowest energy poses (N usually 50–150) makes the final set of poses undergoing coarse minimization, re-clustering and ranking. The AScore/ShapeDock docking protocol is fast, reproducible, and formally explores all energy minima. To illustrate this standpoint, typical ShapeDock times for ligands with 10–15 torsions are shorter than 30 seconds on a 2.4 GHz Pentium computer.

2.3 Homology Modeling of H5N1 and N9 Neuraminidases

Comparative modeling is quite a useful means of predicting unknown 3D protein structures by both starting from a known primary structure and relying on known 3D structures of homologous proteins. Sequentially related proteins are assumed to adopt similar conformations, atomic positions in homologous regions are borrowed from known protein structures, while non-homologous portions are predicted in various ways including potential energy minimization, molecular dynamics, and simulated annealing. Two most convenient criteria for similarity are: (a) an identity of at least 25% for a sequence size > 100 amino acids and (b) an expectation (E) < 10^{-4}, which gives likelihood that similarities are due to chance. The NA protein, containing 449 amino acids from the highly pathogenic chicken H5N1 A viruses isolated during the 2003-2004 influenza outbreaks in Japan (Accession No. Q5H895), was chosen to be modeled [24]. The sequence of N9-NA (Accession No. Q84070), which contains 470 amino acids, was also selected for modeling [25]. SWISS-MODEL [26,27], an automated comparative modeling approach accessible via the ExPASy web server [28], was employed for the prediction of 3D NA structures. The H5N1-NA model was based on the template with a resolution of 2.5 Å (PDB ID: 2htyG) [20], while the N9-NA model was based on the template crystal structure having the 1.4 Å resolution (PDB ID: 1f8dA) [29]. These two crystal structures were identified as the best templates in terms of both sequence identity and E value. To drive generated coordinates toward optimal geometry, energy minimization on the constructed structures was done using the NEWTON subroutine within the TINKER suite of programs known as the Software Tools for Molecular Design running under the Windows operating system [30]. Running the modeling tools was facilitated by the Force Field Explorer 4.2, a graphical user interface to TINKER [31]. The AMBER force field parameter set (AMBER99.PRM), as implemented in the TINKER distribution, was used [32]. The NEWTON algorithm is usually the best choice for minimizations to the 0.01 to 0.000001 kcal mole^{-1} Å^{-1} level of root-mean-square (RMS) gradient convergence. The 0.0001 criterion was chosen in the computations. To evaluate the stereochemical quality of the optimized protein structures by considering their G-factors, the final structures were analyzed by the PROCHECK program [33,34]. The G-factor provides a measure of how "normal", or alternatively how "unusual", a given stereochemical property is. In PROCHECK it is computed for both various combinations of torsion angles and covalent geometry taking into account main-chain bond lengths and main-chain bond angles. The G-factor is a score based on the observed distributions of these stereochemical parameters. When applied to a given residue, a low G-factor indicates that the property corresponds to a low-probability conformation. For example, residues falling in the disallowed regions of the Ramachandran plot will have a low (or very negative) G-factor. Ideally, the scores should be above -0.5. Values below -1.0 may need investigation. For the H5N1-NA and N9-NA optimized models, estimated G factors were -0.5 and -0.48 respectively. Figure 9 shows that the generated model and the template structure of H5N1-NA nicely overlap to a great extent, except in the loop regions due to the sequence alignment.

Table 1. Root mean square deviations (RMSDs) of overlaid Cα and backbone atoms in the binding sites and of docked group-2 NA inhibitors in their top ranked binding mode using AScore/ShapeDock [21]

PDB ID	Inhibitor	$\log IC_{50}$ [a]	$RMSD$ [b] $(Å)$	$RMSD$ [c] $(Å)$	$RMSD$ [d] $(Å)$	$<RMSD>$ [e] $(Å)$
1ivd	BANA105	-3.1	0.34	0.49	2.28	4.33
1ivc	BANA106	-1.7	0.26	0.46	1.01	1.72
1ive	BANA108	-1.7	0.32	0.46	1.58	2.47
1ing	BANA109	-2.4	-	-	0.74	1.49
1inh	BANA111	-2.3	0.32	0.53	1.81	1.42
1inf	BANA113	-5.0	0.45	0.56	1.04	1.47
2bat	NANA	-2.7	0.31	0.47	1.10	1.40
1ivf	DANA	-4.8	0.31	0.51	1.80	1.84
1nnc	GANA	-9.0	0.40	0.54	1.25	1.57
1inw	aPANA	-2.7	0.31	0.48	2.28	1.79
1inx	ePANA	-3.7	0.32	0.48	1.89	2.07
1ivg	none	-	0.32	0.49	-	-
average	-	-	0.33	0.50	1.53	1.96

[a] Experimental values of IC_{50} for all BANAs were taken from [35], for NANA, DANA, and GANA from [36], and for aPANA and ePANA from [37].

[b] RMSD of Cα atoms in the binding site after overlay. The reference structure is 1ing.

[c] RMSD of backbone atoms in the binding site relative to 1ing.

[d] RMSD of the highest ranked binding mode of the inhibitor docked into its crystal structure.

[e] Average RMSD of the highest ranked binding mode of the inhibitor over all 12 crystal structures.

3. BINDING MODE PREDICTION OF NEURAMINIDASE INHIBITORS: CORRELATION WITH EXPERIMENT [1]

In this section, the efficiency of the ArgusLab4/AScore approach, in combination with the ShapeDock search engine is examined for known inhibitors bound to group-2 NAs. A correlation of these results with those obtained by the QunatumLead program is expressed

---

[1] Much of the material contained in this section is taken from our previous paper with the kind permission from Taylor & Francis [21], as specifically acknowledged in the reference list.

quantitatively using the Pearson correlation coefficient (r) approach too. Consequently, the ArgusLab4/AScore/ShapeDock binding modes of group-1 NA inhibitors are explored.

3.1 The AScore/ShapeDock binding affinities of group-2 NA inhibitors

To compare the binding sites of docked inhibitors in their highest ranked binding mode, root mean square deviations (RMSDs) of overlaid Cα and backbone atoms relative to 1ing are given in table 1. The RMSD ranges for these overlays are between 0.26 and 0.45 Å for all Cα atoms, and between 0.47 and 0.56 Å for backbone atoms. The RMSD range between 0.35 and 0.52 Å, which was previously reported for all Cα atoms of residues with heavy atoms closer than 5 Å to BANA109 in 1ing as well as for all Cζ atoms of the arginine residues [9], is correctly between these two for Cα and backbone atoms (Table 1). Figure 2 shows the AScore scoring results for the 11 inhibitors in their own crystal structures. The correlation (r = 0.74, Figure 2a) with the experiment improves to an r of 0.77 if ePANA is removed (Figure 2b), but if two outliers (BANA109 and ePANA) are removed the correlation improves to an r of 0.80 (Figure 2c). In accordance with the experiment, GANA was predicted to be the best binder (Figure 2a). The resulting overlay of 12 NA protein structures with docked GANAs is shown schematically in Figure 3.

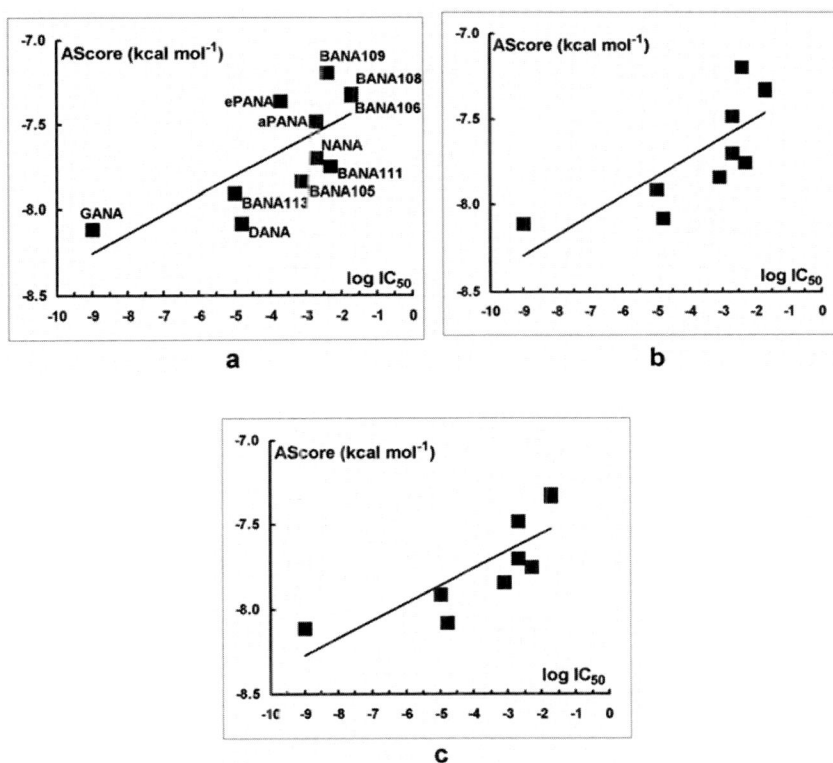

Figure 2. Correlation of the predicted AScore/ShapeDock binding affinities with measured ones for 11 (**a**, r = 0.74), 10 (**b**, ePANA removed, r = 0.77), and 9 (**c**, ePANA and BANA109 removed, r = 0.80) protein/ligand complexes of NA [21].

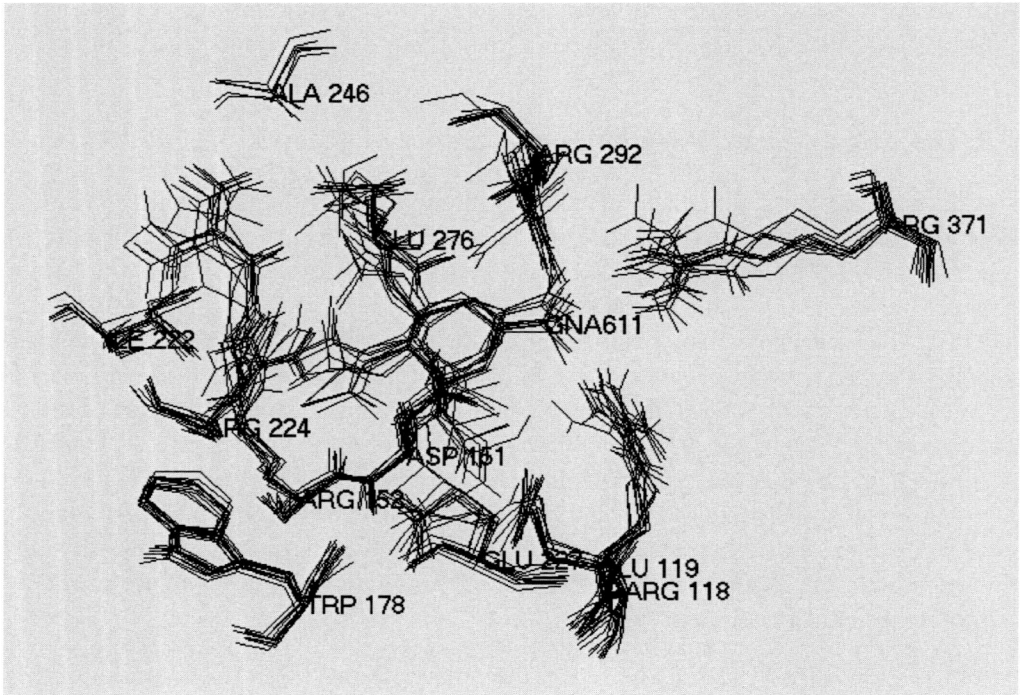

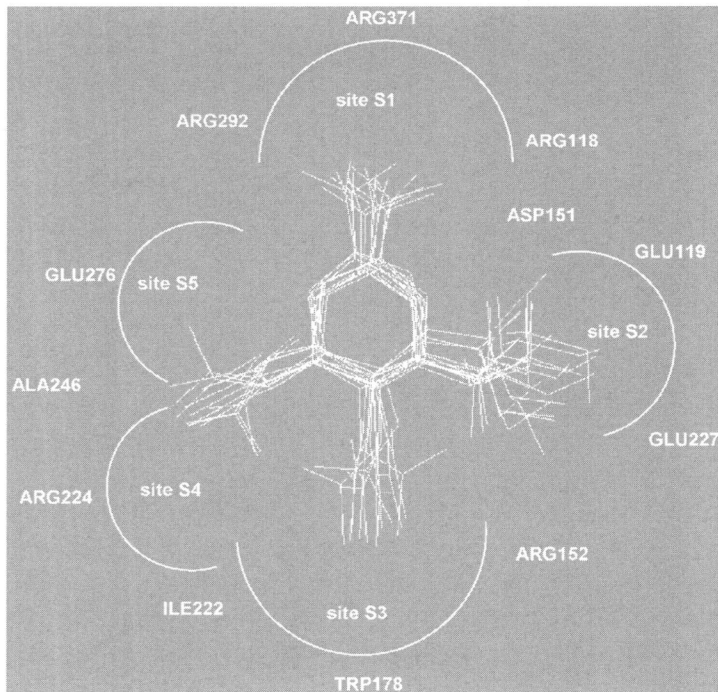

Figure 3. Overlay of 12 group-2 NA protein structures and GANA (denoted by GNA611) inhibitors (top). Overlay of GANA inhibitors with the general locations of important nearby residues (bottom) [21].

Table 2. RMSDs (in Å) of group-2 NA inhibitors docked in their highest ranked binding mode using AScore/ShapeDock [21]

Inhibitor	1ivd	1ivc	1ive	1ing	1irh	1inf	2bat	1ivf	1nnc	1inw	1inx	1ivg
BANA105	2.28	2.11	2.49	5.76	5.79	2.22	6.05	6.08	6.12	1.33	6.05	5.70
BANA106	1.11	1.01	2.46	0.57	2.82	2.18	0.47	2.85	1.19	1.47	1.47	2.98
BANA108	2.34	2.74	1.58	2.62	3.72	2.34	2.49	3.08	1.37	2.31	3.75	1.34
BANA109	1.38	1.84	1.96	0.74	1.34	1.52	1.05	1.55	1.88	1.65	1.66	1.26
BANA111	1.24	1.58	1.16	0.89	1.81	1.24	1.25	1.82	1.65	1.38	1.35	1.70
BANA113	1.59	1.89	0.46	1.04	1.59	1.04	1.97	1.16	1.82	1.41	1.99	1.58
NANA	1.47	1.85	1.66	1.34	1.73	1.32	1.10	1.25	0.81	1.31	1.39	1.60
DANA	2.09	2.65	2.15	2.19	2.24	2.28	0.74	1.80	0.97	1.66	2.25	1.12
GANA	1.90	1.84	1.00	1.51	1.27	2.06	1.67	1.55	1.25	1.15	2.22	1.37
aPANA	1.77	2.10	2.27	1.26	2.37	1.96	1.58	1.32	1.28	2.28	2.06	1.18
ePANA	2.25	1.74	1.78	1.85	2.74	2.25	2.15	2.26	2.03	1.84	1.89	2.07
average	1.76	1.94	1.73	1.80	2.50	1.86	1.86	2.25	1.85	1.62	2.37	1.99

Since RMSD of the top-ranked binding mode of each inhibitor docked into its crystal structure is below 2.5 Å (Table 1), all the inhibitors could thus be docked correctly into their crystal structures. To explore the sensitivity of the docking protocol to changes in the substrate structure, all 11 inhibitors were docked in all 12 NA crystal structures, and computed RMSDs are given in table 2. 88% (70%) of the docked complexes is associated with RMSD between the docked and crystallographic binding modes of less than 2.5 (2.0) Å. This percentage is higher than that of 82% (64%) previously reported [9]. Besides, RMSD for each inhibitor averaged over all crystal structures is given in the last column of table 1. With the exception of BANA105, the average RMSD of each ligand over all crystal structures is below 2.5 Å in the highest ranked binding mode (Table 1). The average RMSD for all inhibitors docked into the same crystal structure is shown on the bottom line of table 2. All the inhibitors could be docked correctly into 4 (1 ivd, 1ive, 1inf, and 1inw) of the 12 crystal structures and for 9 structures the average RMSD of the docked inhibitors is below 2.0 Å (Table 2). In contrast to this observation, it was previously shown that all the inhibitors could be docked correctly into 2 of the 12 protein structures and for 5 structures the average RMSD of the docked inhibitors was found to be less than 2.0 Å [9]. Although some poses exhibit a low RMSD value (below 2.0 Å), it does not mean that they must exhibit the correct binding pattern and vice versa. Hence, to further assess the validity of the docking approach, the binding modes/orientations are analyzed.

The highest ranked binding modes of the NA inhibitors docked in their own crystal structures are depicted in Figure 4. Note that the NH_2 group position of BANA108 was predicted accurately (Figure 4), in contrast to that previously placed in an incorrect pocket [9]. The N-acetyl group locations (Figure 4) were identified much more accurately than those reported earlier [9]. A key reason for it was the previous neglect of a water molecule mediating the interaction between the N-acetyl group and the NA protein (Figure 5).

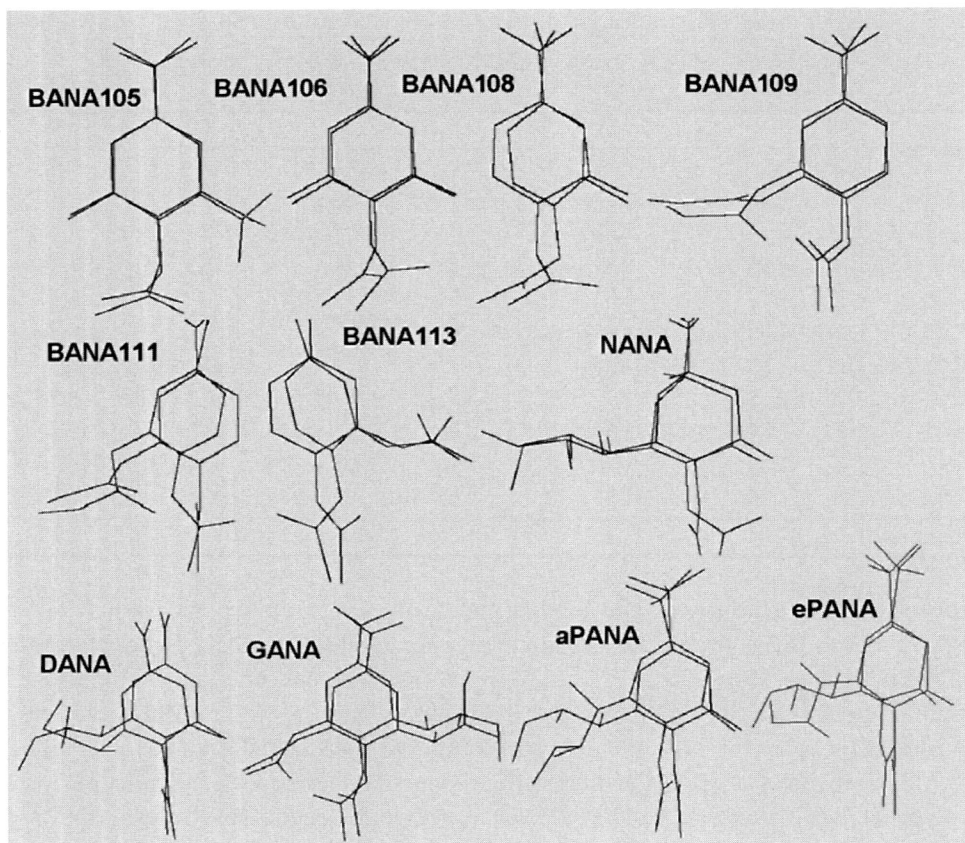

Figure 4. Superposition of crystallographic and the highest ranked binding modes of group-2 NA inhibitors [21].

An unexpected binding orientation of the guanidinobenzoic acid inhibitor BANA113 in its crystal structure (PDB ID: 1inf) was very puzzled, because the guanidino group was established to bind to a different pocket than that of GANA [36]. BANA113 was indeed rotated by 180 degrees relative to GANA, thus enabling the N-acetyl and carboxylate groups to make the same interactions with the NA protein as GANA. The sudden flips in orientation of inhibitors are presumably unique for charged and highly polar pockets [35,36]. Having two similar inhibitors with guanidino-groups placed in different pockets was treated as a good example of investigating the robustness of a docking approach [38,39]. Table 2 shows that BANA113 was docked correctly in all of the 12 protein structures, while it was previously docked correctly in 8 of the 12 NA crystal structures [9]. Noteworthy is GANA docked correctly in all of the 12 crystal structures (Table 2), while it could not be previously docked correctly in 7 of the 12 protein structures [9]. Therefore, a preference for the guanidino-group of GANA to be placed in an incorrect pocket containing Glu275 rather than in a correct one in the proximity of Glu117 and Glu226 [40] is not supported herein.

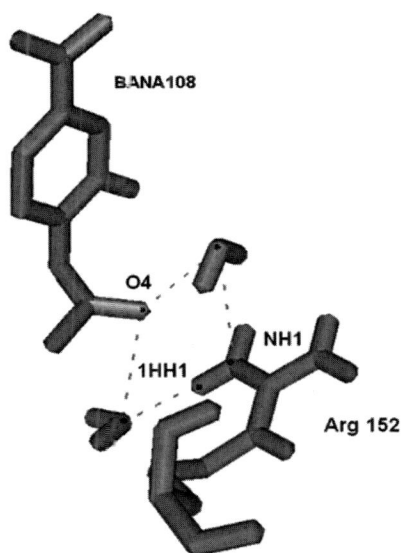

Figure 5. The water molecule-mediated interaction between the N-acetyl group in BANA108 and the NA protein [21].

Based on these results for inhibitors bound to group-2 NAs, the AScore/ShapeDock approach substantially outperforms the PMF-score/docking approach. In contrast to AScore taking into account the separate contributions of the protein-ligand and intra-ligand van der Waals interactions as well as the hydrogen bonding involving charged donor and/or acceptor groups (eq. 2), PMF-scoring, rooted in the sum over all protein-ligand atom pair potentials as a function of the atom pair distance [38,39], underestimates electrostatic contributions to a great extent.

3.2 Comparison between the ArgusLab and QuantumLead programs for group-2 NA inhibitors

To investigate the quality of the above-presented docking results obtained by ArgusLab 4.0 [18], the binding affinities of all 11 inhibitors docked in their own NA crystal structures were determined using QuantumLead [19]. Figure 6 shows the correlation of IC_{50} calculated by QuantumLead with experimental IC_{50}. In agreement with the experiment, GANA was predicted to be the best binder (Figure 6a). The correlation (r = 0.65, Figure 6a) with the experiment improves to an r of 0.75 by removing BANA113 (Figure 6b), while it further improves to an r of 0.82 by removing NANA and aPANA (Figure 6c). Also an r of 0.74 given in Figure 2a for ArgusLab/AScore/ShapeDock clearly shows a better correlation than that (r = 0.65, Figure 6a) accomplished by QuantumLead. This quite satisfactory agreement of the ArgusLab-based results with those generated by QuantumLead is rooted in the composition of the QuantumLead binding free energy [19]. The free energy of non-covalent binding includes the hydrophobic and polar contributions, in addition to other two separate components corresponding to the rotational-translational entropy and the suppression of rotamer degrees of freedom respectively [22].

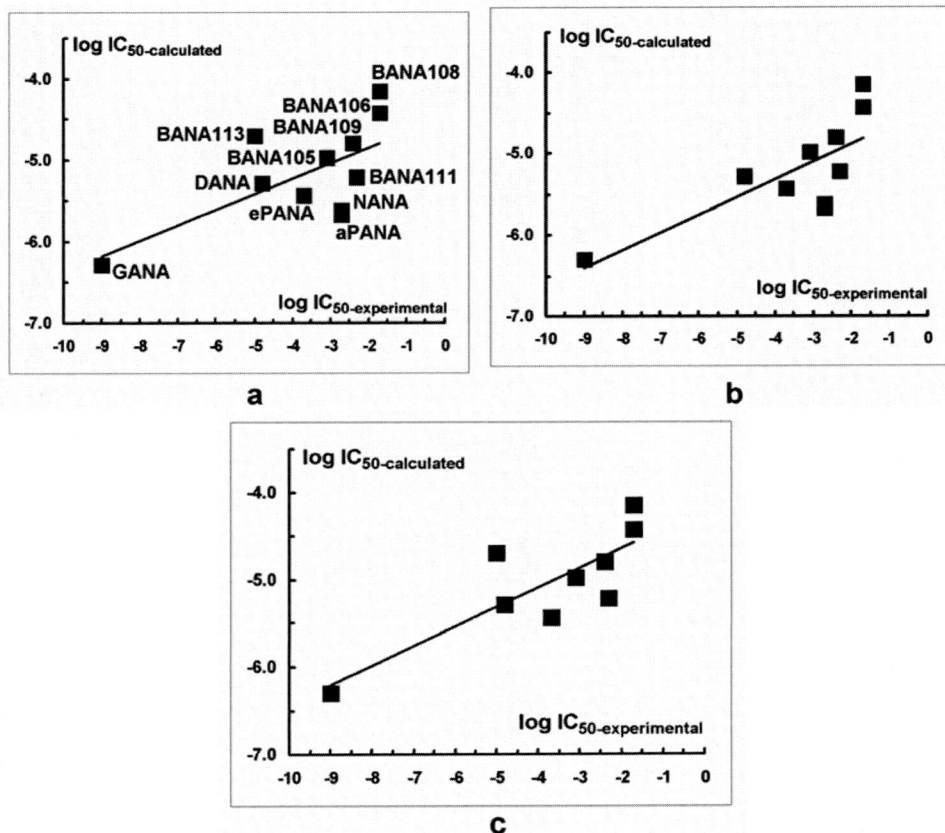

Figure 6. Correlation of the QuantumLead binding affinities with experimental ones for 11 (**a**, r = 0.65), 10 (**b**, BANA113 removed, r = 0.75), and 9 (**c**, NANA and aPANA removed, r = 0.82) protein/ligand complexes of NA [21].

3.2 Comparison between the ArgusLab and QuantumLead programs for group-2 NA inhibitors

To investigate the quality of the above-presented docking results obtained by ArgusLab 4.0 [18], the binding affinities of all 11 inhibitors docked in their own NA crystal structures were determined using QuantumLead [19]. Figure 6 shows the correlation of IC_{50} calculated by QuantumLead with experimental IC_{50}. In agreement with the experiment, GANA was predicted to be the best binder (Figure 6a). The correlation (r = 0.65, Figure 6a) with the experiment improves to an r of 0.75 by removing BANA113 (Figure 6b), while it further improves to an r of 0.82 by removing NANA and aPANA (Figure 6c). Also an r of 0.74 given in Figure 2a for ArgusLab/AScore/ShapeDock clearly shows a better correlation than that (r = 0.65, Figure 6a) accomplished by QuantumLead. This quite satisfactory agreement of the ArgusLab-based results with those generated by QuantumLead is rooted in the composition of the QuantumLead binding free energy [19]. The free energy of non-covalent binding includes the hydrophobic and polar contributions, in addition to other two separate components corresponding to the rotational-translational entropy and the suppression of rotamer degrees of freedom respectively [22].

3.3 The AScore/ShapeDock binding affinities of group-1 NA inhibitors

Since the ArgusLab/AScore/ShapeDock protocol was established as a consistent and easily reproducible algorithm for group-2 NA inhibitors, we employed it to predict the binding affinities of various group-1 NA inhibitors. Table 3 shows RMSDs of overlaid Cα and backbone atoms in the protein active sites relative to 2htu. The RMSD ranges for these superpositions are between 0.22 Å and 0.66 Å for all Cα atoms, and between 0.25 Å and 0.79 Å for backbone atoms, thus being in agreement with those previously estimated for group-1 NA binding sites [20]. As peramivir was predicted to be the best binder, the resulting overlay of 11 NA protein structures with docked peramivir is given in figure 7. In this particular situation, RMSDs of less than 2.5 Å for the highest ranked binding mode (Table 3) indicate the correct docking of each inhibitor into its crystal structure. The highest ranked binding modes/orientations are shown in figure 8.

Table 3. RMSDs (in Å) of overlaid Cα and backbone atoms in the binding sites and of docked group-1 NA inhibitors in their highest ranked binding mode using AScore/ShapeDock [21]

PDB ID	Inhibitor	log IC$_{50}$ [a]	RMSD [b]	RMSD [c]	RMSD [d]	<RMSD> [e]
2hty	-	-	0.53	0.62	-	-
2hu0	Oseltamivir	-5.7	0.60	0.68	1.66	1.83
2hu4	Oseltamivir	-5.4	0.24	0.27	0.92	1.69
2ht5	-	-	0.50	0.61	-	-
2htr	Dana	-5.8	0.22	0.25	1.37	1.75
2ht7	Oseltamivir	-5.7	0.66	0.79	0.73	1.70
2ht8	Oseltamivir	-5.8	0.29	0.33	1.04	1.68
2htq	Zanamivir	-5.6	0.33	0.38	2.45	3.13
2htu	Peramivir	-6.4	-	-	2.38	2.12
2htv	-	-	0.51	0.58	-	-
2htw	Dana	-4.7	0.43	0.63	1.41	1.56
average			0.43	0.51	1.50	1.93

[a] Estimated value of IC$_{50}$ (Mol/L) using the QuantumLead program [30] for the inhibitor in its crystal structure.

[b] RMSD of Cα atoms in the binding site after overlay. The reference structure is 2htu.

[c] RMSD of backbone atoms in the binding site relative to 2htu.

[d] RMSD of the highest ranked binding mode of the inhibitor docked into its crystal structure.

[e] Average RMSD of the highest ranked binding mode of the inhibitor over all 11 crystal structures.

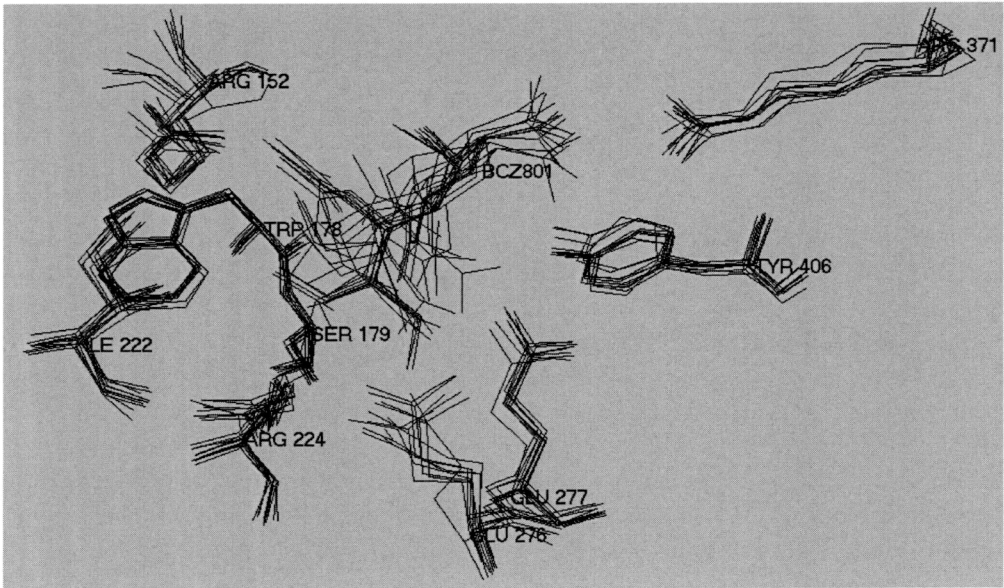

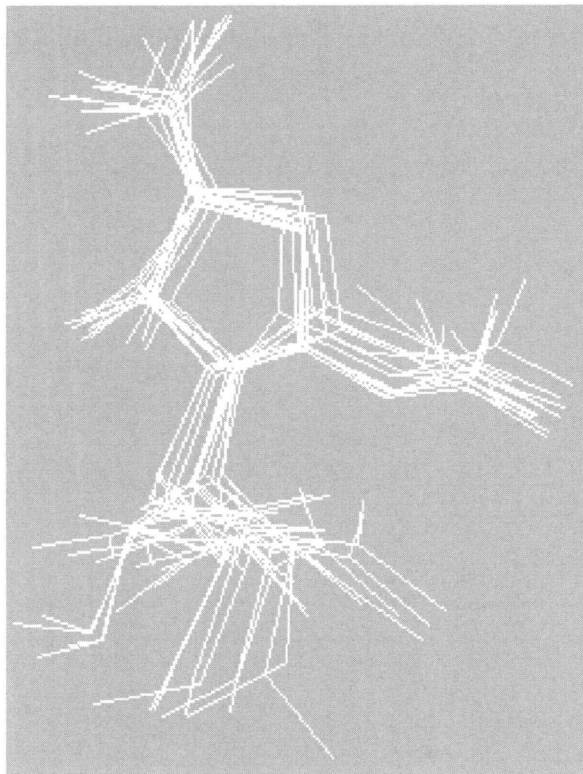

Figure 7. Overlay of 11 group-1 NA protein structures and peramivir (denoted by BCZ801) inhibitors (top). Overlay of peramivir inhibitors (bottom) [21].

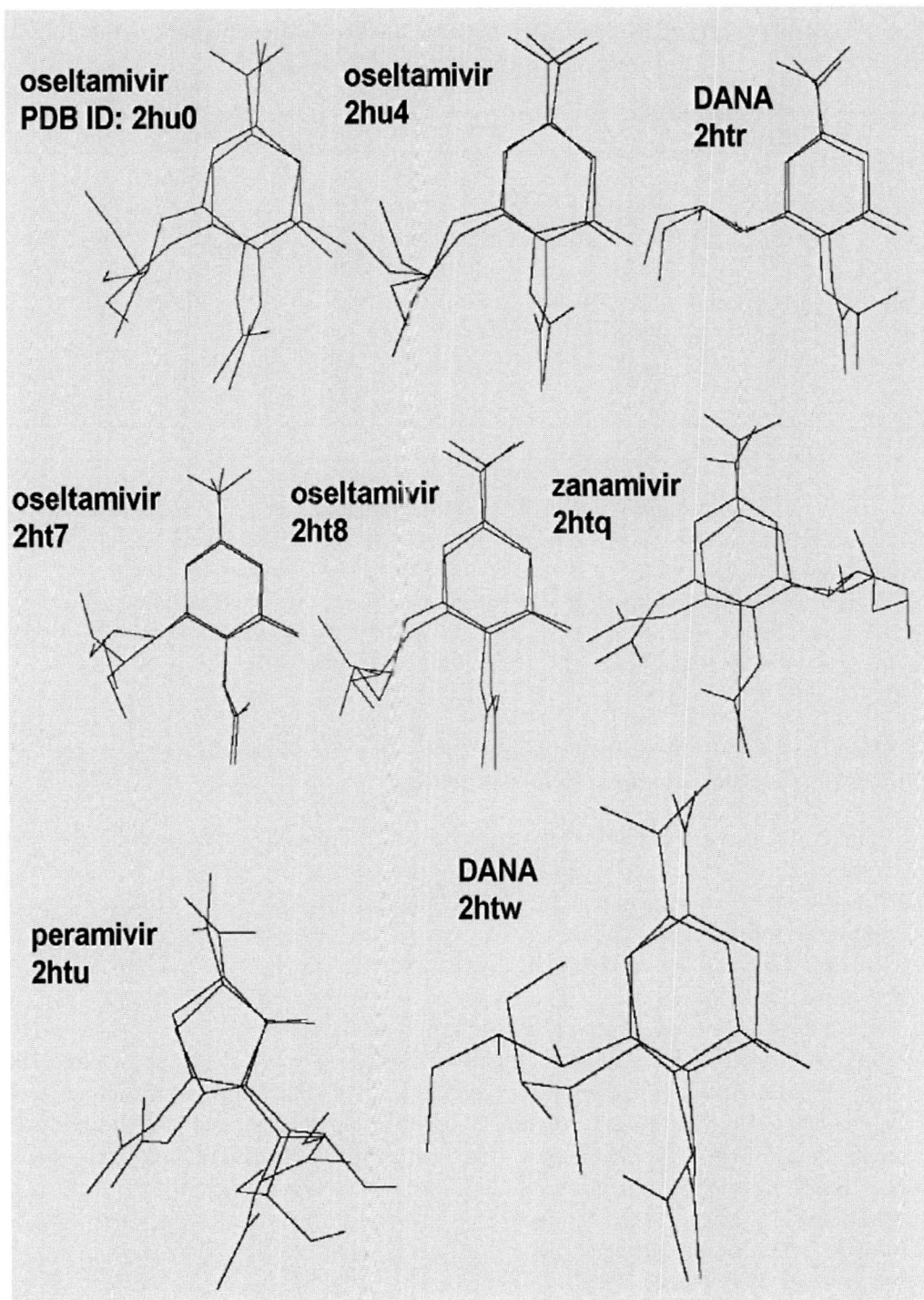

Figure 8. Superposition of crystallographic and the highest ranked binding modes of group-1 NA inhibitors [21].

Table 4. RMSDs (in Å) of group-1 NA inhibitors docked in their highest ranked binding mode using AScore/ShapeDock [21]

Inhibitor	2HTY	2HU0	2HU4	2HT5	2HTR	2HT7	2HT8	2HTQ	2HTU	2HTV	2HTW
Oseltamivir	1.18	1.66	2.12	2.15	1.57	1.66	1.91	2.47	1.83	1.72	1.83
Oseltamivir	2.28	1.57	0.92	1.35	1.46	0.99	1.98	1.56	2.06	2.38	2.03
Dana	1.32	2.31	1.76	1.87	1.37	2.07	1.09	1.47	1.61	2.36	2.04
Oseltamivir	1.85	1.42	1.60	1.84	1.86	0.73	1.09	1.60	2.08	2.40	2.22
Oseltamivir	1.00	1.25	0.93	1.89	1.79	2.40	1.04	1.57	2.19	2.24	2.17
Zanamivir	3.18	4.92	1.43	1.14	5.25	1.26	3.17	2.45	1.23	5.39	5.01
Peramivir	1.18	2.16	2.48	1.70	1.36	2.40	2.82	2.50	2.38	1.37	2.97
Dana	1.64	2.43	1.37	1.87	1.45	2.19	0.98	1.47	1.64	0.69	1.41
average	1.70	2.22	1.58	1.73	2.01	1.71	1.76	1.89	1.88	2.32	2.46

To find out how changes in protein structure affect the quality of docking results, 8 inhibitors were docked in 11 NA crystal structures. 80 of the 88 protein/ligand complexes (91%) have RMSDs below 2.5 Å, while 59 of a total of 88 docked structures (67%) have RMSDs below 2.0 Å (Table 4). With the exception of zanamivir (PDB ID: 2htq), the average RMSD of each ligand over all crystal structures is below 2.5 Å (Table 3). Moreover, for 8 NA structures the average RMSD of the docked inhibitors is below or about 2.0 Å (Table 4).

3.4 The mixing of known activity inhibitors to a set of randomly selected molecules of similar physicochemical profile

While it is important to verify the correctness of the binding mode and the ranking of molecules of known activities, it is as important to validate the approach by conducting a small virtual screening experiment by mixing the known activity molecules to a set of randomly selected molecules (Table 5). The ranking of poses based on AScore speaks in favor of the ability of the AScore/ShapeDock approach to extract active molecules from inactive molecules.

For a published data set of structures composed of various inhibitors docked in group-2 (N2, N9) NA structures, the ArgusLab4/AScore/ShapeDock protocol was shown to identify the binding modes in agreement with the experiment. It is important to note that the correct binding modes and affinities were shown to be both very consistent and easily reproducible. Consequently, an excellent performance of the same docking protocol was established for various inhibitors docked in group-1 (N1, N4, N8) NA structures. Therefore, the ArgusLab4/AScore/ShapeDock approach is believed to be a valuable means of both investigating the binding mechanisms of influenza virus neuraminidase inhibitors, and designing novel, more potent, H5N1-NA inhibitors.

Table 5. The AScore/ShapeDock binding free energies ($kcal\,mol^{-1}$) of known activity inhibitors mixed to a set of randomly selected molecules of similar physicochemical profile [21]

Inhibitor	AScore
3B [c]	-6.68
6B [c]	-6.72
5A [c]	-6.90
ZANAMIVIR [a]	-6.90
7A [c]	-6.98
BANA108 [b]	-7.32
8C [c]	-7.36
OSELTAMIVIR [a]	-7.41
10B [c]	-7.52
OSELTAMIVIR [a]	-7.52
16B [c]	-7.84
OSELTAMIVIR [a]	-7.87
11C [c]	-7.90
OSELTAMIVIR [a]	-7.99
DANA [b]	-8.08
GANA [b]	-8.11
8A [c]	-8.14
12A [c]	-8.24
DANA [a]	-8.31
13B [c]	-8.34
PERAMIVIR [a]	-8.39
DANA [a]	-9.12

[a] The chosen inhibitors of known activity are all group-1 NA inhibitors (Table 3).

[b] The chosen inhibitors of known activity are 3 (DANA, GANA, BANA108) group-2 NA inhibitors (Table 1).

[c] The randomly chosen molecules of similar physicochemical profile are the oseltamivir structure-based analogues (3B, 5A, 6B, 7A, 8A, 8C, 10B, 11C, 12A, 13B, 16B) that were previously reported [41].

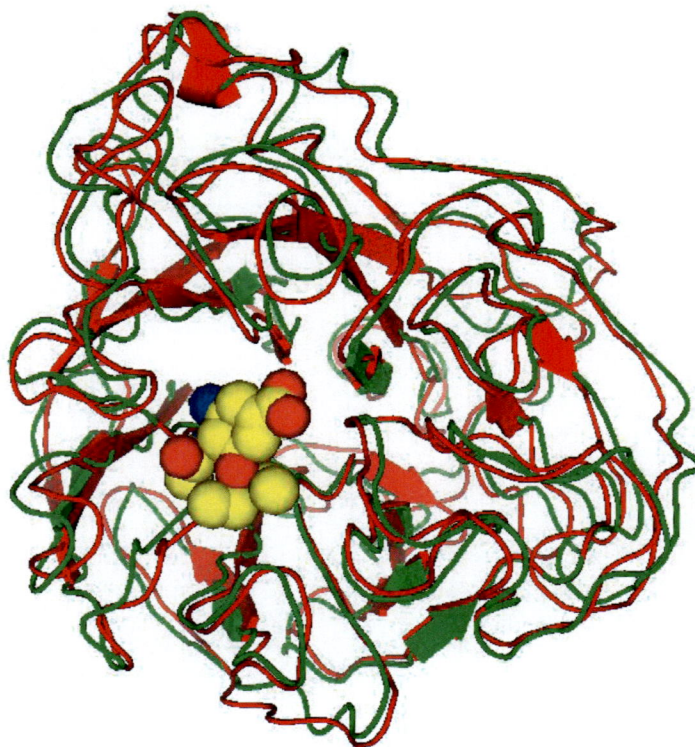

Figure 9. A cartoon representation of the 3D-structural model of H5N1 superimposed on the 2htyG template and complexed with oseltamivir. The model is colored in red, the template is given in green, and the ligand is rendered in space-filling representation.

4. DIFFERENCES BETWEEN ACTIVE CAVITIES OF H5N1 AND N9 NEURAMINIDASES

On the basis of different antigenic properties of various glycoprotein molecules, influenza type A viruses are classified into the following subtypes: 16 for haemagglutinin (H1-H16) and 9 for neuraminidase (N1-N9). Two phylogenetically distinct groups of NAs, group-1 (N1, N4, N5, N8) and group-2 (N2, N3, N6, N7, N9), contain N1 and N9 of viruses that currently circulate in humans. There have also been indications that inhibitor structure/activity relationships do not apply across subtypes [42]. To learn more on subtle differences between active cavities of two subtypes, it is necessary to explore hydrophobic effects, as they are a key factor underlying drug design. To address this issue, the H5N1-NA and N9-NA optimized models of good stereo chemical quality, generated by homology modeling as described in the section 2.3, were employed. Figure 9 illustrates that the generated model of H5N1-NA and its template structure overlap to a great extent, except in the loop regions for the reasons of the deviations caused by the sequence alignment.

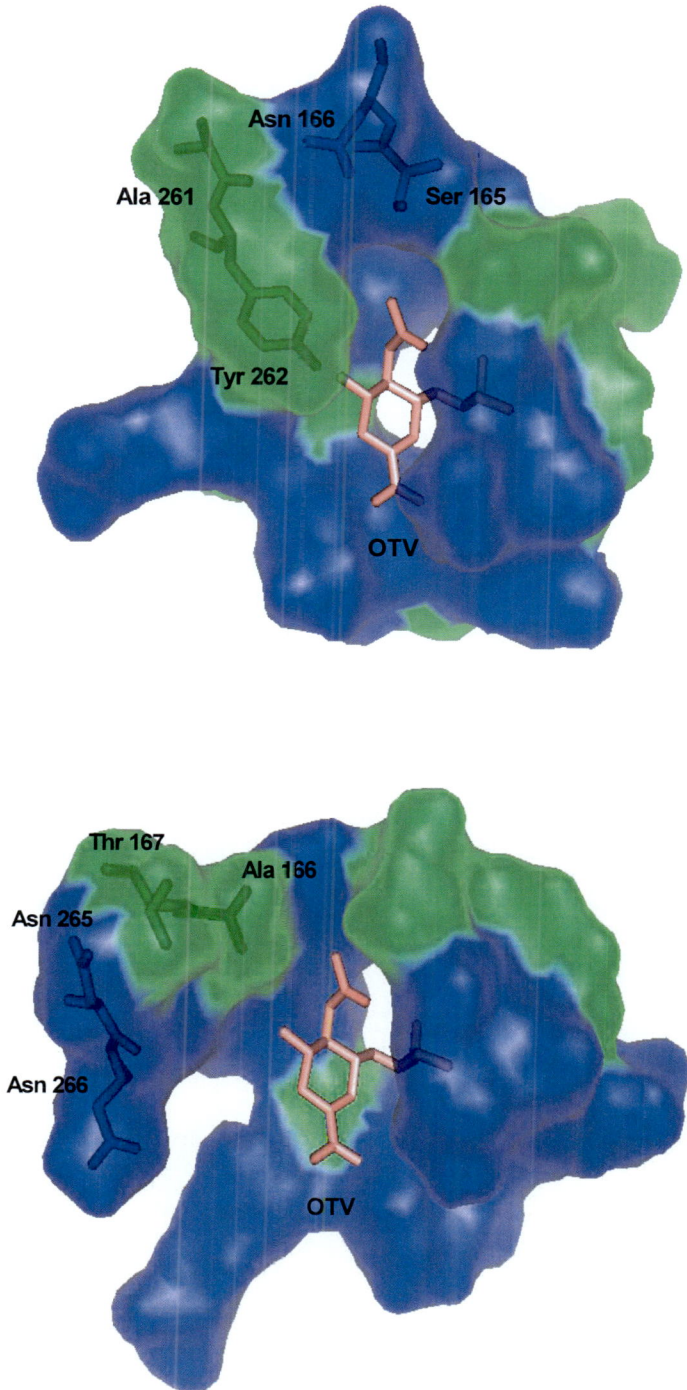

Figure 10. Lipophilic (green) and hydrophilic (blue) environments (residues) near or in the active site of H5N1-NA (top) N9-NA (bottom).

Even though well established residues in the active sites are highly conserved across influenza A NA subtypes, NA inhibitors tend to show different affinities for two influenza subtypes, such as N1 and N9. The different activities are presumably due to a small, but significant, difference between two lipophilic environments. Thus, the lipophilic and hydrophilic surfaces of H5N1-NA and N9-NA are shown in figure 10. Note a subtle variation between lipophilic and hydrophilic environments in H5N1-NA with respect to N9-NA. A partially lipophilic pocket containing Ala261 and Tyr262 in H5N1-NA is lined up by two hydrophilic residues, Asn265 and Asn266, in N9-NA. A partially hydrophilic pocket containing Ser165 and Asn166 in H5N1-NA is lined up with two lipophilic residues, Ala166 and Thr167, in N9-NA. The particular mutations within the H5N1-NA protein structure might be correlated with the high resistance to oseltamivir [43].

5. MOLECULAR MECHANISM OF H5N1 NEURAMINIDASE RESISTANCE TO OSELTAMIVIR[2]

A key reason underlying the OTV-resistance was ascribed to different hydrophobic interactions of lipophilic side chains with influenza A and B NAs having a complete homology in active site [44]. In the context of the resistance of H5N1 to some existing NA inhibitors, the same reason was considered using homology modeling [43]. The oseltamivir-resistance of H5N1-NA was suggested to be caused by the mutations of residues at the positions 119, 152, 274, and 292 [45]. The Tyr252His mutation in H5N1-NA with the His274Tyr substitution was hypothesized to be responsible for an increased affinity of NA for oseltamivir [46]. The only molecular mechanism helping to understand the N1-NA resistance to OTV was proposed by Moscona [47]. This proposal indicated that the N1 active site must reorient itself in order to accommodate the bulky side chain of OTV, whereas such a change is not needed for zanamivir. This reorientation is reflected through the rotation of Glu276 and its bonding to Arg224. The proposed rearrangement of N1 active site was based on the X-ray structure of OTV with N9-NA [47]. Hence, a need for a better understanding of the OTV-resistance of H5N1 virus through a systematic structure-activity relationship study was recognized [48]. This need was satisfied by our more recent study [49] in which molecular bases of the H5N1-NA resistance to oseltamivir were explored using contemporary principles of conformational analysis.

5.1 Oseltamivir-resistant influenza virus neuraminidase mutants: Correlation with experiment

Since two approved anti-influenza drugs, oseltamivir and zanamivir, have come to market, clinically relevant resistance development and possible unknown side effects have become the topics of vital importance. A clinical experience of more than 8 years has not provided evidence that the use of zanamivir would result in viable mutants [50]. This indication may be a consequence of the limited use of ZMV. A much wider use of OTV has

---

[2] Much of the material contained in this section is taken from our previous paper with the kind permission from Elsevier [49], as specifically acknowledged in the reference list.

provided evidence that a viable resistant mutant has emerged [51]. There is a serious indication that mutations at position 274 in H5N1-NA may give rise to the OTV-resistance of H5N1 [45]. To shed more light on the mechanism by which mutations at His274 in the crystal structure of the H5N1-NA/OTV complex (PDB ID: 2hu0) alter the sensitivity of N1-NA to OTV, His274 was mutated by both smaller side chain (Gly, Ser, Asn, Gln) and larger side chain (Phe, Tyr) amino acid residues. The substitutions of His274 were carried out by the Mutate subroutine that was implemented in the HyperChem 5.02 program [52].

Table 6. Binding free energies (ΔG), 50% inhibition concentrations (IC_{50}), and inhibition constants (K_i) for various N1-NA mutants in the complex with oseltamivir [49]

PDB ID: NA Subtype Inhibitor	Residue 274	$\Delta G_{binding}$ [kcal/mol]	IC_{50} [a] [nm]	K_i [b] [nm]	net charge (e)		
					Arg224	Glu276	Glu276 side chain
	His274 (2hu0)	-9.57	90.0	0.3(wt)	+9	-14	-18
	His274Gly	-9.66	82.2	0.2	+4	-14	-18
	His274Ser	-9.60	87.4	0.1	+1	-17	-18
2hu0: N1 Oseltamivir	His274Asn	-9.60	87.4	0.1	+1	-17	-18
	His274Gln	-9.60	87.4	0.3	+1	-17	-18
	His274Phe	-8.69	165	86	-27	-27	-20
	His274Tyr	-8.84	152	105	-26	-31	-20
	His274Tyr Tyr252His [c]	-8.84	152	-	-22	-31	-20

[a] Estimated values on the basis of the correspondence between the experimentally determined ranges of binding free energies and 50% inhibition concentrations [53].

[b] Experimental values for wild type (wt) and mutant influenza A/WS/33 (H1N1) NA [45].

[c] There is a hypothesis that the Tyr252His mutation in H5N1-NA with the His274Tyr substitution could be responsible for an increased NA affinity for oseltamivir [46].

Traditional residues within the active site throughout the family of NA protein structures are highly conserved in all the H5N1-NA mutants, with the only exception that His274Phe and His274Tyr cause to have the bulky Phe and Tyr present in their NA active sites (see the Supplementary Material of ref. 49). All the binding free energies are within 1 $kcal\ mol^{-1}$ (Table 6). For the smaller side chain residue mutations, the energies are about -9.6 $kcal\ mol^{-1}$ and correspond to an estimated IC_{50} of about 85 nM. Thus, the substitution of His274 by Gly, Ser, Asn, and Gln resulted in slightly enhanced or essentially unchanged the NA sensitivity to OTV. For the larger side chain residue mutations, the energies are roughly -8.8 $kcal\ mol^{-1}$ and correspond to an estimated IC_{50} of approximately 158 nM. Therefore, the replacement of His274 with Phe or Tyr reduced the NA sensitivity to OTV. An IC_{50} of 152 nM for the His274Tyr NA mutant (Table 6) is in satisfactory agreement with an experimental value of 200 nM [45]. The trend of both the binding free energies and the corresponding IC_{50} values is in accordance with that of the experimentally determined inhibition constants K_i (Table 6).

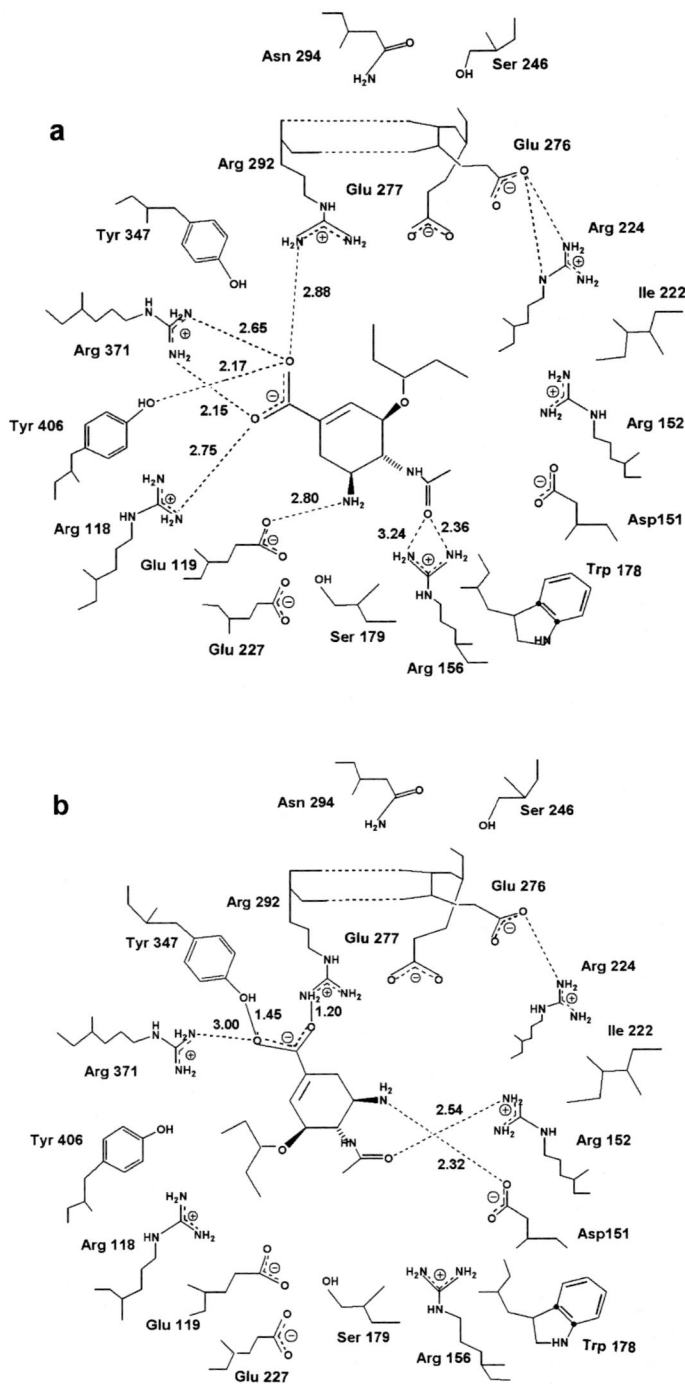

Figure 11. The interactions (in Å) of oseltamivir with the residues in the active site of N1-NA with His274 (**a**) and His274Ser (**b**). Ser is a smaller side chain amino acid residue [49].

In the original complex there are 8 electrostatic interactions between OTV and the active site residues (Figure 11a). The interactions of oseltamivir with the active site residues of each N1 mutants are available as part B of the Supplementary Material of [49]. Since detected interactions of OTV with the His274X (X = Gly, Ser, Asn, Gln) mutants are similar, a representative case is shown in Figure 11b. Due to its capability to rotate around the single bond between oxygen and alkyl chain R, the –O-R group of OTV is able to take a comfortable position relative to its environment. By focusing on the position of the –O-R group, the substitution of His274 by a smaller side chain residue, such as Ser, causes a flip of OTV by 180 degrees (Figure 11). In the complex of N1 with His274Ser, OTV makes 3 electrostatic interactions with Asp151, Arg152, and Arg371 respectively, besides 2 strong interactions (1.20 and 1.45 Å) with Arg292 and Tyr347 respectively (Figure 11b). These two strong interactions of OTV are in common for all the complexes of OTV with the N1 mutants containing His274X (X = Gly, Ser, Asn, Gln) (part B, Supplementary Material of ref. 49). The strong interactions can be viewed as a compensation for fewer electrostatic interactions of OTV with the His274X (X = Gly, Ser, Asn, Gln) NA mutants than with the His274 NA, thus helping to rationalize essentially unchanged the NA sensitivity to OTV (Table 6).

The OTV's particular rotation around the –O-R single bond was established to affect the orientation of the nearest amino acid residues, Trp178, Arg224, Glu227, Glu276, and Arg292 [54]. Glu276 plays a key role by adopting an alternative conformation, which is stabilized by an electrostatic interaction with Arg224 [50,51]. To further investigate the sensitivity of N1-NA to OTV, it is useful to analyze how various side chain volumes of amino acid residues at position 274 affect distinct conformations adopted by Glu276. There are always two electrostatic contacts between Glu276 and Arg292 regardless of the particular mutations at position 274 (parts B and C of Supplementary Material of ref. 49). Figure 12 displays the spatial orientation of Glu276 relative to both oseltamivir and the nearest residues (Arg224, Glu277, Arg292) in the NA active site with His274 and with His274Ser, respectively. There are two electrostatic contacts between Glu276 and Arg224 in the original N1-NA (Figure 12a), while only one is present in the mutated N1-NA (Figure 12b). The sole Arg224-Glu276 contact is in common for all the smaller side chain residue substitutions at position 274 (Supplementary Material of ref. 49, Figures S10-S13). The difference relative to the original complex is visible in the trend of the net charges of Glu276 and Arg224 (Table 6). More negative Glu276 and less positive Arg224, as well as unchanged charge on the side chain of Glu276 are the consequences of the His274X (X = Gly, Ser, Asn, Gln) mutations. Note in Figure 12 that OTV is clearly behind Glu276 in the mutated complex and is shifted more towards Arg292 by making a strong interaction of 1.20 Å in length. The spatial orientation of Glu276 is unique for all the mutants having the smaller side chain amino acid residues at position 274 (Supplementary Material of ref. 49, Figures S10-S13). This conformation adopted by Glu276 is in agreement, to some extent, with the previously proposed mechanism of the OTV-resistance of N1-NA [47].

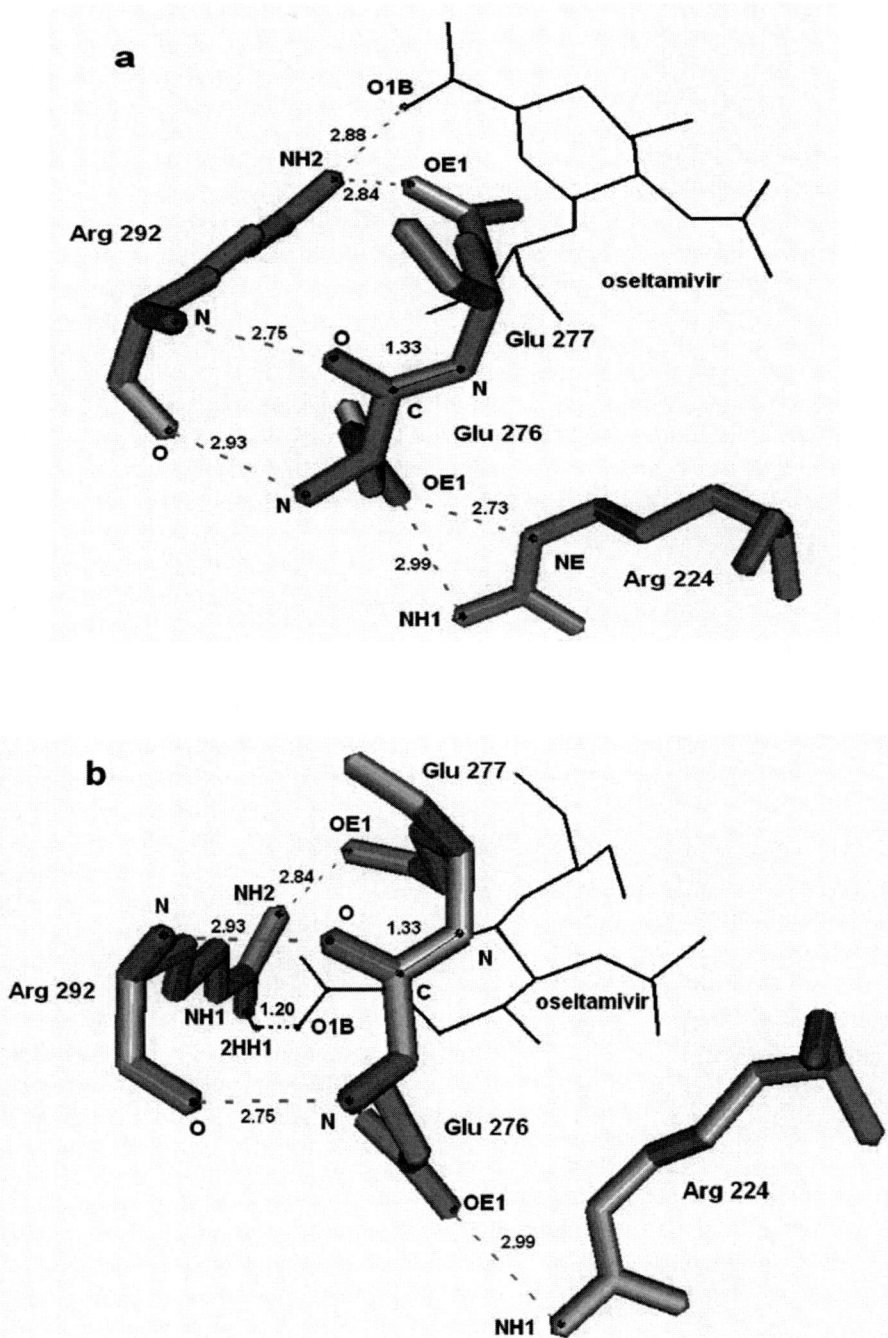

Figure 12. The spatial orientation of Glu276 relative to both oseltamivir and the nearest amino acid residues (Arg224, Glu277, Arg292) in the active site of N1-NA with His274 (**a**) and His274Ser (**b**) [49]. The particular orientation (**b**) of Glu276 is in common for all N1-NAs with the smaller side chain residue (Gly, Ser, Asn, Gln) mutations at position 274 (Supplementary Material of ref. 49, Figures S10-S13).

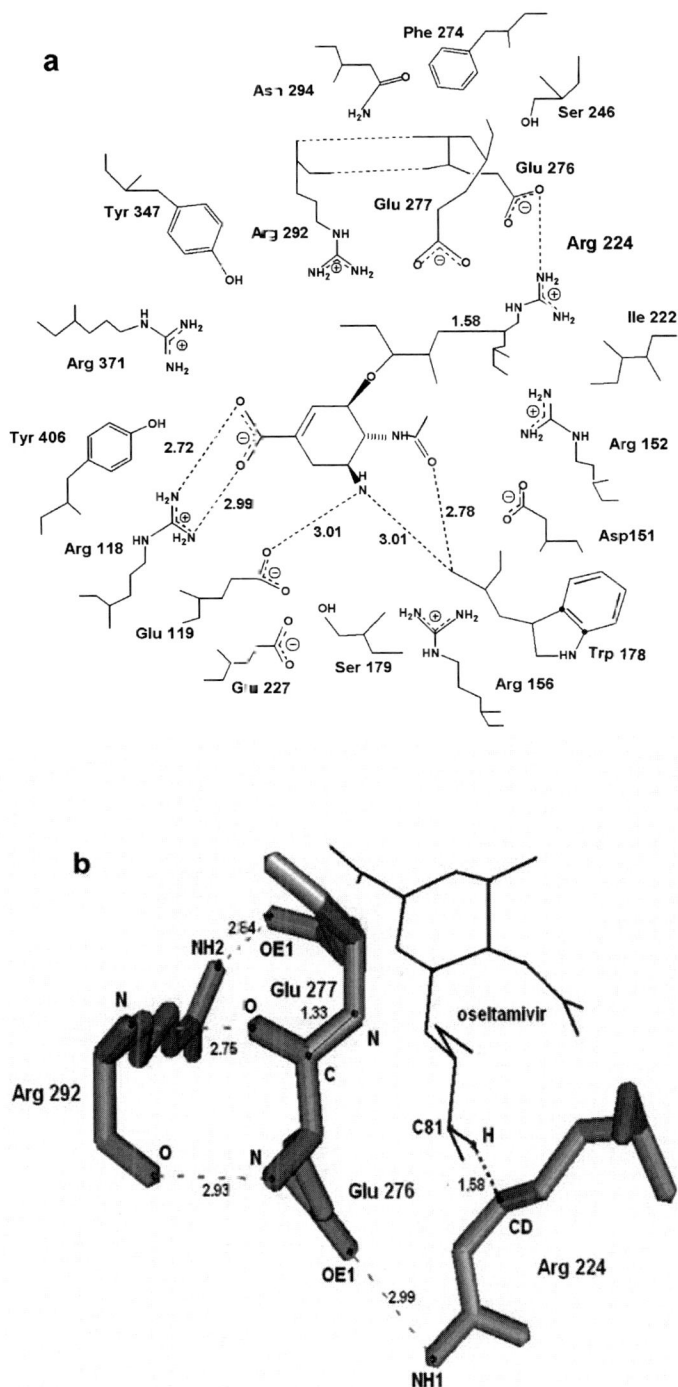

Figure 13. (a) The interactions (in Å) of oseltamivir with the residues in the active site of N1-NA with His274Phe. Phe is a larger side chain amino acid residue. (b) The spatial orientation of Glu276 relative to both oseltamivir and the nearest amino acid residues (Arg224, Glu277, Arg292) [49].

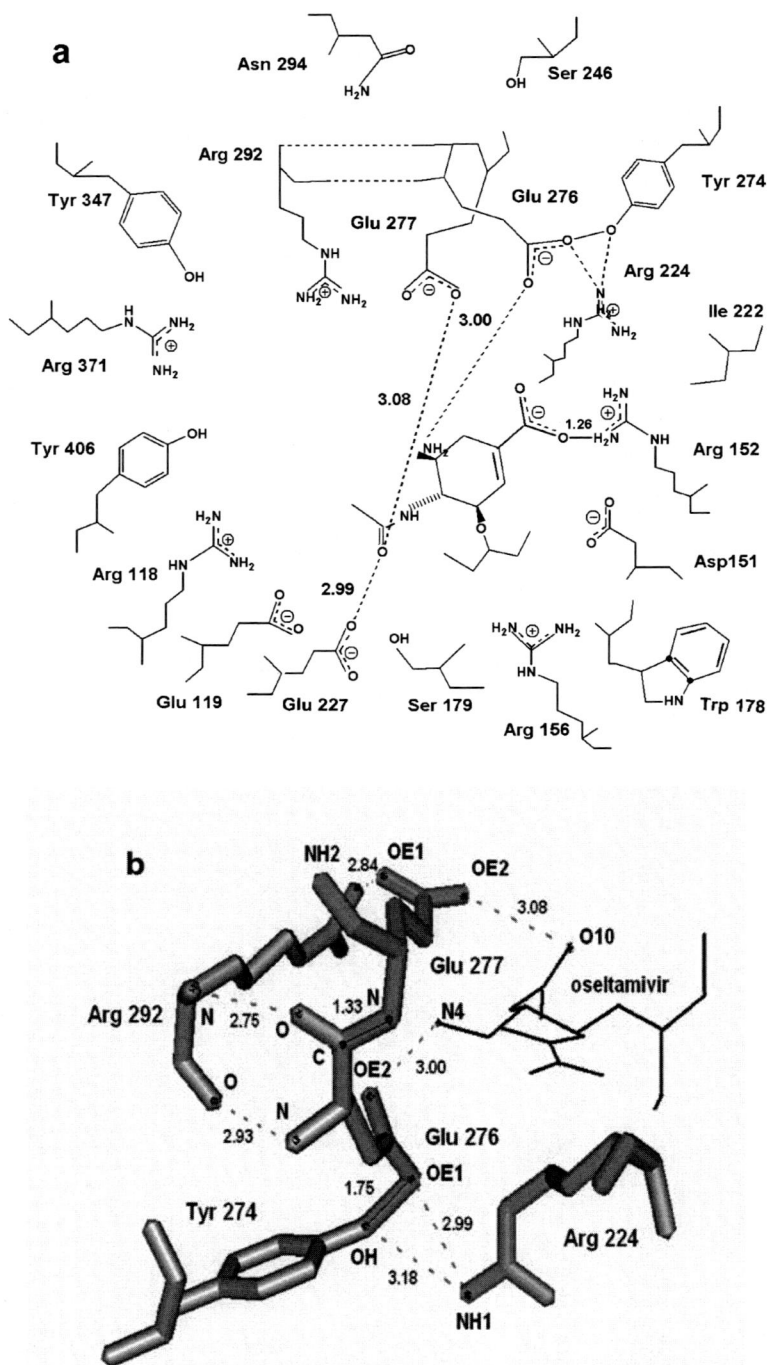

Figure 14. (a) The interactions (in Å) of oseltamivir with the residues in the active site of N1 NA with His274Tyr. Tyr is a larger side chain amino acid residue. (b) The spatial orientation of Glu276 relative to both oseltamivir and the nearest amino acid residues (Arg224, Glu277, Arg292) [49].

His274Phe causes to have Phe involved in the NA active site (Figure 13a). OTV is rotated a bit more towards left with respect to OTV in the original complex (Figure 1a), and its –O-R group makes a strong interaction (1.58 Å) with Arg224, besides other 5 electrostatic contacts with Arg118, Glu119, and Trp178. Although Phe274 does not make interactions with Glu276, it most likely influences Glu276 by being in the immediate vicinity (Figure 13a). Glu276 makes a charge-charge interaction with Arg224 (Figure 13b). The conformational change of Glu276 is reflected through a substantial negative charge (-27 e) of Glu276 and of Arg224 (Table 6). His274Tyr causes to have Tyr involved in the NA active site (Figure 14a). By focusing on the -O-R group, OTV is rotated to right by about 90 degrees (Figure 14a) and is flipped in a horizontal position (Figure 14b) with respect to OTV in the original complex (Figures 11a and 12a). There is a strong Glu276-Tyr274 bond (1.75 Å), besides two Glu276...Arg224 and Tyr274...Arg224 electrostatic interactions (Figure 14a). The conformational change of Glu276, due to the His274Tyr mutation, is visible through substantial negative charges (-31 and -26 e) of Glu276 and Arg224 (Table 6). Note that net charge of the Glu276 side chain does not reflect to a great extent the conformational change of Glu276 due to the His274Phe and His274Tyr mutations (Table 6).

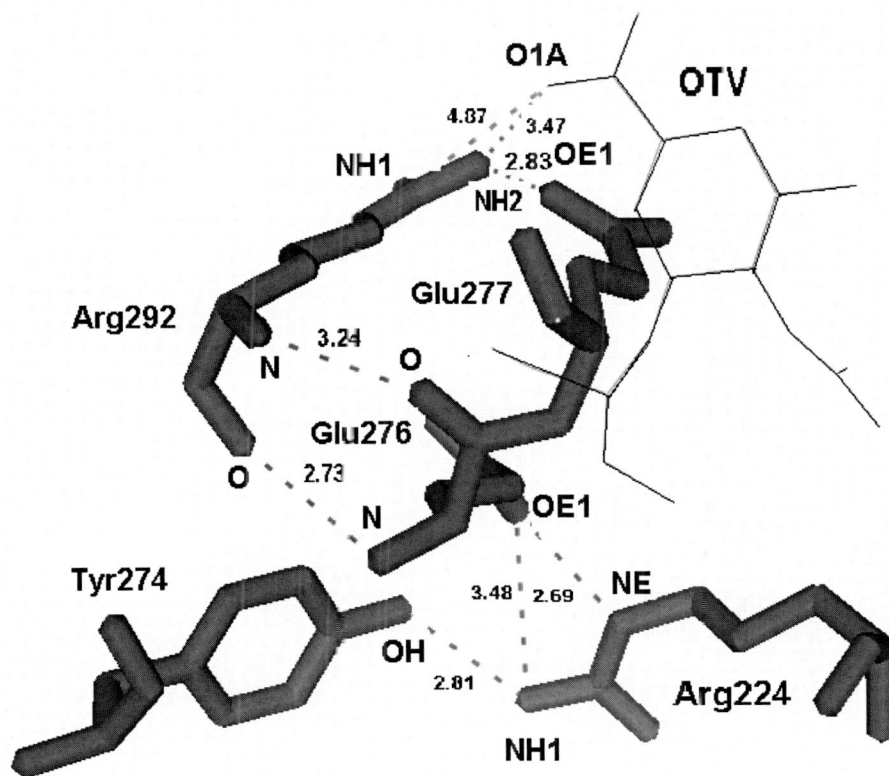

Figure 15. The experimentally determined binding mode of oseltamivir (PDB ID: 3cl0) relative to the nearest residues of the mutant His274Tyr [49].

The crystal structures of oseltamivir-resistant influenza virus neuraminidase mutants were recently reported by Collins et al. [55]. The structure of the H5N1 mutant His274Tyr-oseltamivir complex (PDB ID: 3cl0) showed that substitution of His by the bulkier Tyr pushes the carboxyl group of Glu276 2 Å farther into the binding site. In this position the charged group disrupts the otherwise hydrophobic pocket that normally accommodates the 3-pentyloxy substituent of oseltamivir and causes a change in the conformation of the inhibitor such that its C9 and C91 carbons move about 2.5 Å from the wild-type NA-bound position. The experimentally determined binding mode of oseltamivir relative to the nearest residues of the mutant His274Tyr is shown in Figure 15. Interestingly, the particular binding mode is substantially different from the computationally predicted one (Figure 14b). To rationalize this standpoint, note that the crystal structure of the complex of H5N1 NA with OTV (PDB ID: 2hu0) was the starting point for identifying the active site amino acid residues (Supplementary Material of ref. 49, Table S1). His274Tyr caused to have the bulkier and hydrophobic Tyr involved in the N1 active site, thus making Tyr274 able to directly influence the Glu276 conformation (Figure 14b). In contrast to this, the present computational approach, if applied onto the crystal structure of the H5N1 mutant His274Tyr-oseltamivir complex (PDB ID: 3cl0) reported by Collins et al. [55], properly identifies all the active site amino acid residues, except Tyr274. The experimental binding mode of OTV given in figure 15 is thus more similar with that shown in figure 12a. Also it is important to note that the experimental binding mode of OTV in the original crystal structure of the H5N1 His274-oseltamivir complex (PDB ID: 3cl2F), reported by Collins et al. [55], is quite similar to that shown in Figure 15.

Rungrotmongkol et al. [56] have noted the discrepancies between the theoretical and experimental structures of NA:OTV protein:ligand complexes used in our work [49], and have questioned the relevance of such modeling. We would like to point out that these discrepancies were known to us at the time and, indeed, were commented upon in the original publication (pp. 156-158, Figure 5) [49]. The interest here is that, despite these discrepancies, the binding free energies reported agree with the experimental values of K_i [57]. It is for this reason that we chose to entitle our paper [49] "*Another look at* the molecular mechanism…". Hence, the comment of Rungrotmongkol et al. [56], observed as a whole, on our previous publication [49] is scientifically incorrect [57]. We have extensively (220 docking experiments using all NA subtypes) verified the applicability of the docking algorithms [21] and have also included protein flexibility to account for any incorrect choice of starting structure [58]. This has allowed us to confirm that the correct ligand orientations are obtained in these docking procedures [57].

The Tyr252His mutation in H5N1 NA with the His274Tyr substitution was hypothesized to be responsible for an increased NA affinity for oseltamivir [46]. However, additional mutation Tyr252His does not make any difference in both the binding free energy of OTV (Table 6) and the interaction of OTV with N1-NA (Supplementary Material of ref. 49, Figures S8 and S16).

6. Summary

For a published data set of structures composed of various inhibitors docked in group-2 (N2, N9) NA structures, the ArgusLab4/AScore/ShapeDock protocol has been shown to identify the binding modes in agreement with the experiment. The composition of the AScore scoring function is a key reason for these successful performances. In contrast to XScore [23] form which AScore has been derived, AScore takes into account the separate contributions of the protein-ligand and intra-ligand van der Waals interactions as well as the hydrogen bonding involving charged donor and/or acceptor groups [18]. Besides, the docking results generated by the ArgusLab4/AScore/ShapeDock protocol have been demonstrated to be in agreement with those obtained by QuantumLead [19]. It is important to note that the correct binding modes and affinities for the complexes of group-2 NAs obtained by ArgusLab4/AScore/ShapeDock have been shown to be both very consistent and easily reproducible. Consequently, an excellent performance of the same docking protocol has been established for various inhibitors docked in group-1 (N1, N4, N8) NA structures.

Due to the recent pandemic threat by the worldwide spread of H5N1 avian influenza, the World Health Organization has shown its profound concern regarding the possibility of having the virus spread among humans. Reports on the virus resistance to two approved anti-influenza drugs, oseltamivir (Tamiflu) and zanamivir (Relenza), as well as the lack of adequate vaccine have raised the urgent question of developing new anti-viral drugs. In this context, the ArgusLab4/AScore/ShapeDock approach is believed to be a valuable means for the structure-based design of novel, more potent, H5N1-NA inhibitors.

The resolved question on the way in which volumes occupied by the side chains of various amino acid residues at position 274 influence NA sensitivity to oseltamivir has provided several novel insights into the OTV-resistance of H5N1 NA. The smaller side chain residue (Gly, Ser, Asn, Gln) mutations of His274 have resulted in slightly enhanced or unchanged NA sensitivity to OTV, while His274Phe and His274Tyr have reduced the susceptibility of OTV to N1 NA. The key difference is due to the fact that His274Phe and His274Tyr have caused to have the bulky and hydrophobic residues (Phe, Tyr) involved in the N1 NA active sites, thus directly affecting conformations adopted by Glu276. Hence, OTV-resistance may be ascribed to different hydrophobic interactions of lipophilic side chains with influenza NA. A previous hypothesis [46] that the Tyr252His mutation in H5N1-NA with His274Tyr could be responsible for an increased NA affinity for oseltamivir has not been found to hold. Since the binding of OTV appears to be more dependent on interactions with the active site amino acids than on the active site amino acid reorientation, the possibility of escaping H5N1 mutants might be increased by maintaining a clear resemblance to sialic acid Neu5Ac, a natural substrate from which zanamivir is directly derived with minimal functional modifications.

Computational methods are herein shown to be a viable partner to experiment in investigating binding mechanisms of various influenza virus neuraminidase inhibitors.

REFERENCES

[1]   Murphy, B. R. & Webster, R. G. (1996). Orthomyxoviruses. In B. N. Fields, M. Knipe & P. Howley (Eds.), *Fields Virology* (pp. 1397-1445). Philadelphia, PA: Lippincott-Raven Publishers.

[2]   World Health Organization (1980). A revision of the system of nomenclature for influenza viruses: a WHO memorandum. *Bull. World Health Organ., 58,* 585-591.

[3]   Thompson, J. D.; Higgins, D. G. & Gibson, T. J. (1994). Improved sensitivity of profile searches through the use of sequence weights and gap excision. *Comput. Appl. Biosci., 10,* 19-29.

[4]   Bender, C.; Hall, H.; Huang, J.; Klimov, A.; Cox, N.; Hay, A.; Gregory, V.; Cameron, K.; Lim, W.; & Subbarao, K. (1999). Characterization of the surface proteins of influenza A (H5N1) viruses isolated from humans in 1997–1998. *Virology, 254,* 115-123.

[5]   World Health Organization (2005). Global influenza program surveillance network.evolution of H5N1 avian influenza viruses in Asia. *Emerg. Infect. Dis., 11,* 1515-1521.

[6]   Kim, C.; Lew, W.; Williams, M.; Liu, H.; Zhang, L.; Swaminathan, S.; Bischofberger, N.; Chen, M.; Mendel, D.; Tai, C.; Laver, W.; & Stevens, R. (1997). Influenza neuraminidase inhibitors possessing a novel hydrophobic interaction in the enzyme active site: design, synthesis, and structural analysis of carbocyclic sialic acid analogues with potent antiinfluenza activity. *J. Am. Chem. Soc., 119,* 681-690.

[7]   von Itzstein, M.; Wu, W.; Pegg, M.; Dyason, J.; Jin, B.; Phan, T.; Smythe, M.; White, H.; Oliver, S.; Colman, P.; Varghese, J.; Ryan, M.; Woods, J.; Bethell, R.; Hotham, V.; Camerom, J.; & Penn, C. (1993). Rational design of potent sialidase-based inhibitors of influenza virus replication. *Nature, 363,* 418-423.

[8]   Berman, H.; Westbrook, J.; Feng, Z.; Gilliland, G.; Bhat, T.; Weissig, H.; Shindyalov, I.; & Bourne, P. (2000). The protein data bank. *Nucleic Acids Res., 28,* 235-242.

[9]   Muegge, I. (1999). The effects of small changes in protein structure on predicted binding modes of known inhibitors of influenza virus neuraminidase: PMF-scoring in DOCK4. *Med. Chem. Res., 9,* 490-500.

[10]   Abu Hammada, A.; Afifia, F. & Taha, M. (2007). Combining docking, scoring and molecular field analyses to probe influenza neuraminidase–ligand interactions. *Journal of Molecular Graphics and Modelling, 26,* 443-456.

[11]   Birch, L.; Murray, C.; Hartshorn, M.; Tickle, I.; & Verdonk, M. (2002). Sensitivity of molecular docking to induced fit effects in influenza virus neuraminidase. *Journal of Computer-Aided Molecular Design, 16,* 855-869.

[12]   Murray, C.; Baxter, C. & Frenkel, A. (1999). The sensitivity of the results of molecular docking to induced fit effects: application to thrombin, thermolysin and neuraminidase. *Journal of Computer-Aided Molecular Design, 13,* 547-562.

[13]   Landon, M.; Amaro, R.; Baron, R.; Ngan, C.; Ozonoff, D.; McCammon, J.; & Vajda, S. (2008). Novel druggable hot spots in avian influenza neuraminidase H5N1 revealed by computational solvent mapping of a reduced and representative receptor ensemble. *Chem. Biol. Drug. Des., 71,* 106-116.

[14]   Sangma, C. & Hannongbua, S. (2007). Structural information and computational

methods used in design of neuraminidase inhibitors. *Current Computer-Aided Drug Design, 3,* 113-132.

[15] Leach, A.; Shoichet, B. & Peishoff, C. (2006). Prediction of protein-ligand interactions. Docking and scoring: successes and gaps. *J. Med. Chem., 49,* 5851-5855.

[16] Krovat, E.; Steindl, T. & Langer, T. (2005). Recent advances in docking and scoring. *Current Computer-Aided Drug Design, 1,* 93-102.

[17] Mohan, V.; Gibbs, A.; Cummings, M.; Jaeger, E.; & DesJarlais, R. (2005). Docking: successes and challenges. *Current Pharmaceutical Design, 11,* 323-333.

[18] Thompson, M. (2004). ArgusLab 4.0.1. Seattle, WA: Planaria Software LLC, http://www.arguslab.com.

[19] QuantumLead 3.3.0. Moscow, Russia: Quantum Pharmaceuticals, http://q-pharm.com.

[20] Russell, R.; Haire, L.; Stevens, D.; Collins, P.; Lin, Y.; Blackburn, G.; Hay, A.; Gamblin, S., & Skehel, J. (2006). The structure of H5N1 avian influenza neuraminidase suggests new opportunities for drug design. *Nature, 443,* 45-49.

[21] Reprinted from Molecular Simulation, Vol. 35/Issue 4, Marija L. Mihajlovic and Petar M. Mitrasinovic, Applications of the ArgusLab4/AScore protocol in the structure-based binding affinity prediction of various inhibitors of group-1 and group-2 influenza virus neuraminidases (NAs), 311-324, © 2009 Taylor & Francis. All rights reserved, with permission (2134450480067) from Taylor & Francis.

[22] Böhm, H. (1994). The development of a simple empirical scoring function to estimate the binding constant for a protein-ligand complex of known three dimensional structure. *J. Comput. Aid. Mol. Des., 8,* 243-256.

[23] Wang, R.; Lai, L. & Wang, S. (2002). Further development and validation of empirical scoring functions for structure-based binding affinity prediction. *J. Comput. Aid. Mol. Des., 16,* 11-26.

[24] Mase, M.; Tsukamoto, K.; Imada, T.; Imai, K.; Tanimura, N.; Nakamura, K.; Yamamoto, Y.; Hitomi, T.; Kira, T.; Nakai, T.; Kiso, M.; Horimoto, T.; Kawaoka, Y.; & Yamaguchi, S. (2005). Characterization of H5N1 influenza A viruses isolated during the 2003-2004 influenza outbreaks in Japan. *Virology, 332,* 167-176.

[25] Air, G. M.; Webster, R. G.; Colman, P. M.; & Laver, W. G. (1987). Distribution of sequence differences in influenza N9 neuraminidase of tern and whale viruses and crystallization of the whale neuraminidase complexed with antibodies. *Virology, 160,* 346-354.

[26] Guex, N. & Peitsch, M. C. (1997). SWISS-MODEL and the Swiss-PdbViewer: an environment for comparative protein modeling. *Electrophoresis, 18,* 2714-2723.

[27] Schwede, T.; Kopp, J.; Guex, N.; & Peitsch, M. C. (2003). SWISS-MODEL: an automated protein homology-modeling server. *Nucleic Acids Res., 31,* 3381-3385;

[28] Guex, N.; Diemand, A.; Schwede, T.; & Peitsch, M. C. (2003). SWISS-MODEL 3.5: an uutomated comparative protein modeling server. http://www.expasy.org/swissmod/SWISS-MODEL.html.

[29] Smith, B. J.; Colman, P. M.; von Itzstein, M.; Danylec, B.; & Varghese, J. N. (2001). Analysis of inhibitor binding in influenza virus neuraminidase. *Protein Sci., 10,* 689-696.

[30] Ponder, J. W. (2004). TINKER Molecular Modeling Package.http://dasher.wustl.edu/tinker.

[31] Ponder, J. W. (2004). Force Field Explorer 4.2: A Graphical User Interface to TINKER,

http://dasher.wustl.edu/tinker.

[32] Wang, J.; Cieplak, P.; & Kollman, P. A. (2000). How well does a restrained electrostatic potential (RESP) model perform in calculating conformational energies of organic and biological molecules? *J. Comput. Chem., 21,* 1049-1074.

[33] Laskowski, R. A.; MacArthur, M. W.; Moss, D. S.; & Thornton, J. M. (1993). PROCHECK: a program to check the stereochemical quality of protein structures. *J. Appl. Cryst., 26,* 283-291.

[34] Morris, A. L.; MacArthur, M. W.; Hutchinson, E. G.; & Thornton, J. M. (1992). Stereochemical quality of protein structure coordinates. *Proteins: Structure, Function and Genetics, 12,* 345-364.

[35] Singh, S.; Jedrzejas, M.; Air, G.; Luo, M.; Laver, W.; & Brouillette, W. (1995). Structure-based inhibitors of influenza virus sialidase. A benzoic acid lead with novel interaction. *J. Med. Chem., 38,* 3217-3225.

[36] Sudbeck, E.; Jedrzejas, M.; Singh, S.; Brouillette, W. J.; Air, G.; Laver, W.; Babu, Y.; Bantia, S.; Chand, P.; Chu, N.; Montgomery, J.; Walsh, D.; & Luo, M. (1997). Guanidinobenzoic acid inhibitors of influenza virus neuraminidase. *J. Mol. Biol., 267,* 584-594.

[37] White, C.; Janakiraman, M.; Laver, W.; Philippon, C.; Vasella, A.; Air, G.; & Luo, M. (1995). A sialic acid-derived phosphonate analog inhibits different strains of influenza virus neuraminidase with different efficiencies. *J. Mol. Biol., 245,* 623-634.

[38] Muegge, I. & Martin, Y. (1999). A general and fast scoring function for protein-ligand interactions: a simplified potential approach. *J. Med. Chem., 42,* 791-804.

[39] Muegge, I.; Martin, Y.; Hajduk, P.; & Fesik, S. (1999). Evaluation of PMF scoring in docking weak ligands to the FK506 binding protein. *J. Med. Chem., 42,* 2498-2503.

[40] Jedrzejas, M.; Singh, S.; Brouillette, W.; Air, G.; & Luo, M. (1995). A strategy for theoretical binding constant, Ki, calculations for neuraminidase aromatic inhibitors designed on the basis of the active site structure of influenza virus neuraminidase. *Proteins, 23,* 264-277.

[41] Du, Q-S.; Wang, S-Q. & Chou, K-C. (2007). Analogue inhibitors by modifying oseltamivir based on the crystal neuraminidase structure for treating drug-resistant H5N1 virus. *Biochem. Biophys. Res. Commun., 362,* 525-531.

[42] Brouillette, W. J.; Bajpai, S.; Ali, S.; Velu, S.; Atigadda, V.; Lommer, B.; Finley, J.; Luo, M.; & Air, G. (2003). Pyrrolidinobenzoic acid inhibitors of influenza virus neuraminidase: modifications of essential pyrrolidinone ring substituents. *Bioorg. Med. Chem., 11,* 2739-2749.

[43] Wei, D-K.; Du, Q-S.; Sun, H.; & Chou, K-C. (2006). Insights from modeling the 3D structure of H5N1 influenza virus neuraminidase and its binding interactions with ligands. *Biochem. Biophys. Res. Commun., 344,* 1048-1055.

[44] Kim, C. U.; Lew, W.; Williams, M. A.; Wu, H.; Zhang, L.; Chen, X.; Escarpe, P. A.; Mendel, D. B.; Laver, W. G.; & Stevens, R. C. (1998). Structure-activity relationship studies of novel carbocyclic influenza neuraminidase inhibitors. *J. Med. Chem., 41,* 2451-2460.

[45] Wang, M. Z.; Tai, C. Y. & Mendel, D. B. (2002). Mechanism by which mutations at His274 alter sensitivity of influenza A virus N1 neuraminidase to oseltamivir carboxylate and zanamivir. *Antimicrobial Agents and Chemotherapy, 46,* 3809-3816.

[46] Rameix-Welti, M. A.; Agou, F.; Buchy, P.; Mardy, S.; Aubin, J. T.; Veron, M.; Van der Werf, S., & Naffakh, N. (2006). Natural variation can significantly alter the sensitivity of influenza A (H5N1) viruses to oseltamivir. *Antimicrobial Agents and Chemotherapy, 50*, 3809-3815.

[47] Moscona, A. (2005). Neuraminidase inhibitors for influenza. *N. Engl. J. Med., 353*, 1363-1373.

[48] Liu, Y.; Zhang, J. & Xu, W. (2007). Recent progress in rational drug design of neuraminidase inhibitors. *Current Medicinal Chemistry, 14*, 2872-2891.

[49] Reprinted from Biophysical Chemistry, Vol. 136/Issues 2-3, Marija L. Mihajlovic and Petar M. Mitrasinovic, Another look at the molecular mechanism of the resistance of H5N1 influenza A virus neuraminidase (NA) to oseltamivir (OTV), 152-158, © 2008 Elsevier B.V. All rights reserved, with permission (2035491025627) from Elsevier.

[50] von Itzstein, M. (2007). The war against influenza: discovery and development of sialidase inhibitors. *Nature Reviews Drug Discovery, 6*, 967-974.

[51] Le, Q. M.; Kiso, M.; Someya, K.; Sakai, Y. T.; Nguyen, T. H.; Nguyen, K. H.; Pham, N. D.; Nguyen, H. H.; Yamada, S.; Muramoto, Y.; Horimoto, T.; Takada, A.; Goto, H.; Suzuki, T.; Suzuki, Y.; & Kawaoka, Y. (2005). Avian flu: isolation of drug-resistant

[52] HyperChem™ 5.02. (1997). Molecular Modeling System for Windows/NT. Gainesville, FL: Hypercube, Inc.

[53] Govorkova, E. A.; Leneva, I. A.; Goloubeva, O. G.; Bush, K.; & Webster, R. G. (2001). Comparison of efficacies of RWJ-270201, zanamivir, and oseltamivir against H5N1, H9N2, and other avian influenza viruses. *Antimicrobial Agents and Chemotherapy, 45*, 2723-2732.

[54] Aruksakunwong, O.; Malaisree, M.; Decha, P.; Sompornpisut, P.; Parasuk, V.; Pianwanit, S.; & Hannongbua, S. (2007). On the lower susceptibility of oseltamivir to influenza neuraminidase subtype N1 than those in N2 and N9. *Biophysical Journal, 92*, 798-807.

[55] Collins, P. J.; Haire, L. F.; Lin, Y. P.; Liu, J.; Russell, R. J.; Walker, P. A.; Skehel, J. J.; Martin, S. R.; Hay, A. J.; & Gamblin, S. J. (2008). Crystal structures of oseltamivir-resistant influenza virus neuraminidase mutants. *Nature, 453*, 1258-1261.

[56] Rungrotmongkol, T.; Malaisree, M.; Udommaneethanakit, T.; & Hannongbua, S. (2009). Comment on "Another look at the molecular mechanism of the resistance of H5N1 influenza A virus neuraminidase (NA) to oseltamivir (OTV)". *Biophysical Chemistry, 141*,131-132.

[57] Mitrasinovic, P.M. (2009). Reply to Comment on "Another look at the molecular mechanism of the resistance of H5N1 influenza A virus neuraminidase (NA) to oseltamivir (OTV)". *Biophysical Chemistry, 141*, 133.

[58] Mitrasinovic, P.M. (2009). On the structure-based design of novel inhibitors of H5N1 influenza A virus neuraminidase (NA), *Biophysical Chemistry, 140*, 35-38.

In: Global View of Fight against Influenza
Editor: Petar M. Mitrasinovic

ISBN: 978-1-60741-952-5
© 2009 Nova Science Publishers, Inc.

Chapter 9

THE IMPACT OF STRUCTURAL BIOLOGY ON THE UNDERSTANDING OF THE INFLUENZA VIRUS AND THE RATIONAL DESIGN OF ANTIVIRALS

*Philip S. Kerry and Rupert J. Russell**

Interdisciplinary Centre for Human and Avian Influenza Research, School of Biology,
University of St. Andrews, Fife T, UK

ABSTRACT

In this chapter we will highlight the profound impact that structural biology has had on understanding the influenza virus. In 1981, the way the world visualized part of the influenza virus was transformed by the remarkable publication of the crystal structure of the haemagglutinin (HA) glycoprotein. Shortly afterwards, the crystal structure of neuraminidase (NA) was elucidated, directly leading to the design of Relenza and Tamiflu. Some structural knowledge of all of the influenza proteins is now known, driven by the increased interest owing to the threat of the next pandemic and also due to remarkable advances in crystallographic techniques. We will focus in this chapter on proteins that have the potential to be targets in structure-based drug design programmes.

HAEMAGGLUTININ

The HA glycoprotein attaches the virus to the host cell and is also responsible for triggering the fusion of the viral and host membranes. As such, the ability to block one of these two events would limit virus infection and therefore be potential targets for intervention by a drug. Each monomer of the trimer contains two disulphide-linked polypeptide chains, HA1 and HA2, created by proteolytic cleavage of the precursor protein HA0. The first crystal structure of HA to be determined was from the A/Aichi/2/68 (H3N2) virus [1]. The protein is composed of a membrane-proximal, triple-stranded α-helical stem-like structure, composed

---

* Correspondence to: rjmr@st-andrews.ac.uk.

of residues predominantly from HA2, that supports a membrane-distal globular multi-domain structure, which is composed of residues solely from HA1 (Figure 1). The membrane-distal part of the each monomer can be subdivided into a vestigial esterase domain, an F′ fusion domain and a receptor binding domain. The latter consists of three secondary structure elements — the 190-helix, the 130-loop and the 220-loop — which form the sides of each site, with the base made up of the conserved residues Tyr98, Trp153, His183, and Tyr195 (Figure 2).

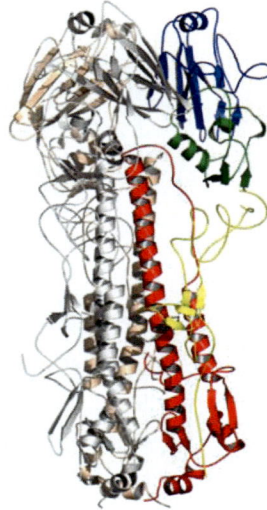

Figure 1. Illustrated representation of the trimer of HA. Monomers 2 and 3 are in silver and gold, respectively, and the featured monomer is colored according to its individual subdomains: receptor binding (RB) in blue, vestigial esterase (E) in green, and fusion subdomains (F′ and F) in yellow and red, respectively.

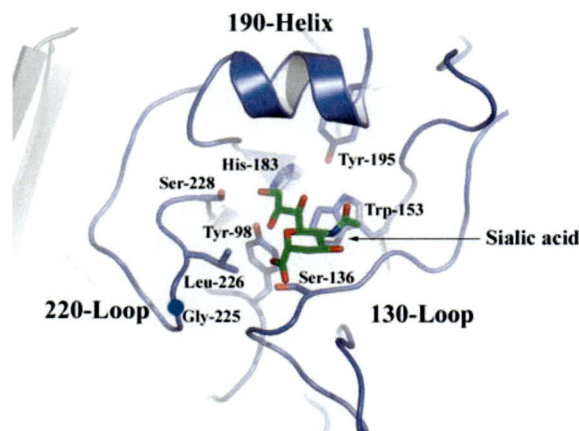

Figure 2. Schematic of the sialic acid binding site of HA. The position of the three secondary structure units making up the site, the 190 helix, and the 130 and 220 loops are indicated. Also shown are the side chains of some residues important for sialic acid binding. Sialic acid is shown in stick representation and coloured green.

There are 16 HA subtypes classified on the basis of their antigenic profiles and amino acid sequence [2]. The crystal structure of HA has been solved from the H1, H3, H5, H7, H9 and H14 subtypes [1, 3-6]. The different subtypes all share the same HA structure but the orientation of the individual domains with respect to each other are characteristic of a particular subtype [5, 7]. The reason for the presence of individual subtypes of Influenza A is not fully understood but is thought to be related to antigenic selection and differences in their fusion characteristics [5].

RECEPTOR BINDING

Crystallographic studies have shown that sialic acid, the terminal sugar of glycoproteins and glycolipids to which HA binds, form specific hydrogen binds to conserved residues in the receptor binding domain (Figure 2). The binding preference of a given influenza virus HA for α2,3- or α2,6- linked Sialic acid correlates with the species specificity for infection, which are the predominant form of the sialosaccharide in avian enteric tracts and human respiratory tracts respectively. Has of all 16 antigenic subtypes (H1-H16) influenza found in avian influenza viruses bind preferentially to sialic acid in α2,3-linkage [8, 9]; swine influenza viruses, are reported to bind sialic acid in either α2,6- or both α2,3- and α2,6- linkages [8, 10] and human viruses of the H1, H2, and H3 subtypes that are known to have caused epidemics, recognize sialic acid in α2,6-linkage [11-13]. As an avian origin is proposed for the Has of swine and human viruses [14], a change in receptor binding specificity is necessary for cross species transfer, and thus the effective infection of humans. The mechanism by which Has of human viruses achieve these changes is different for individual subtypes. For the Has of the H2 and H3 human viruses a minimum of two changes in binding site amino acids, Gln226Leu and Gly228Ser, correlate with the shift in specificity from binding avian to binding human receptors [15, 16]. In contrast, Has of human H1 viruses retain the avian-like Gln226 and Gly228 but can bind to human receptors [10]. This is due to a distinct geometry of the H1 receptor binding site, caused by alterations at other positions in the receptor binding site, which result in the novel positioning of these otherwise avian-specific residues [3]. Similarly, the H5 HA from the currently circulating H5N1 viruses appear to require subtype specific mutations to shift receptor specificity[17]. Thus there seems to be multiple ways to accommodate the human receptor. This is probably due to the apparent flexibility of the human receptor manifested by the different conformations observed when bound to Has of different subtypes [3, 18]. This multiple mode of human receptor binding makes targeting of the receptor binding site for the development of anti-HA drugs extremely difficult, although the design of sialic acid based polymers is being performed [19]. More progress however in designing novel drugs that bind to HA is being made by disrupting the other function of HA; namely the fusion of viral and host membranes (see below).

FUSION

The structure of the HA precursor, HA0, has also been elucidated [20]. In order to prime HA for its fusion capacity, HA0 must be proteolytically cleaved into HA1 and HA2. The structure revealed that the cleavage site (Arg329) is located in a prominent surface loop, which lies adjacent to a cavity that is not present in the cleaved-HA structure and contains three ionisable residues. These residues are buried from solvent after cleavage due the rearrangement and subsequent burial of the nearly formed N-terminal residues of HA2. The first 21 residues of HA2 are referred to as the "fusion peptide" and consist of predominantly hydrophobic amino acids, which are known to insert into the host membrane during the fusion process. Thus it has been proposed that cleavage of HA0 results in a metastable form of the protein in which a low-pH trigger (see below) has been set due to the burial of ionisable residues. A characteristic of highly pathogenic influenza viruses such as the currently circulating H5N1 viruses is an insertion of a number of basic residues amino acids adjacent to the cleavage site. This polybasic insertion is thought to generate a more extended surface loop, which would facilitate more efficient intracellular cleavage.

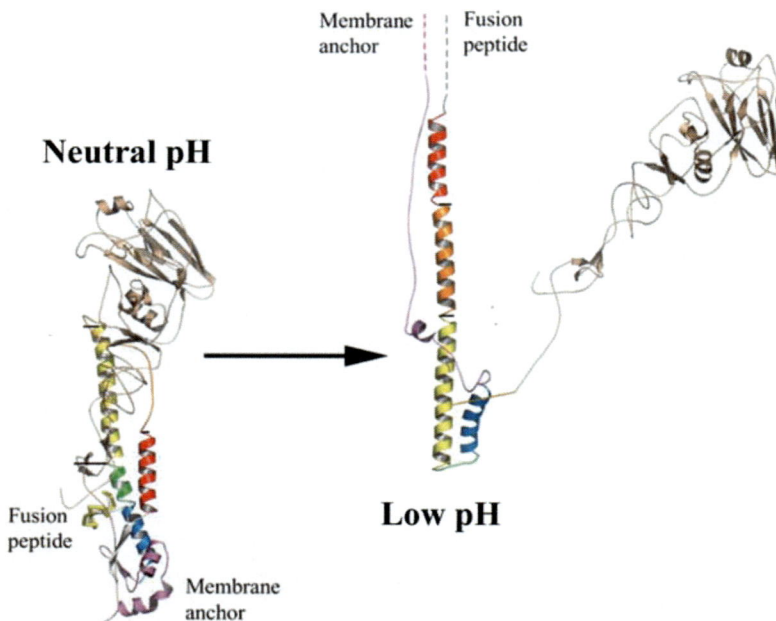

Figure 3. Cartoon representation of the neutral pH and low pH conformations of HA, colour-coded to indicate the re-arrangements and re-folding that occur at fusion pH. HA1 is coloured blue and HA2 coloured as a rainbow from N-terminus to C-terminus. The majority of HA1 is not present in the fusion pH structure and is modelled for completeness since it remains disulfide linked to HA2. Parts of the structures that are not observed or present are shown as discontinuous lines.

Once bound to the receptor on the cell surface, the virus is internalised via endocytosis. The endosome has an acidic pH environment and it is this that acts as the trigger to induce fusion. The HA2 chain contains two membrane-interacting hydrophobic peptide sequences: an N-terminal "fusion peptide" (residues 1-21), which interacts with the target membrane bilayer and a C-terminal transmembrane segment that passes through the viral membrane. In the neutral pH structure the fusion peptide is buried in core of the protein and is distant from the host membrane, and therefore it was unclear from the original HA structure how it could facilitate fusion. Clues were revealed in another landmark publication of the structure HA in its post fusion conformation [21]. Crystallographic studies of HA in the low-pH-induced post-fusion state revealed that there is a dramatic reorganization of HA2, which results in the fusion peptide moving from the interior of the neutral-pH structure approximately 100 Å toward the target membrane in the low-pH structure [1, 21] (Figure 3). At some point along this pathway, the middle of the original long α-helix, of the triple stranded coiled coil, unfolds to form a reverse turn at residue 106 of HA2, jackknifing the C-terminal half of the long α-helix backward toward the N-terminus. Concomitantly the interhelical loop of HA2 converts into a α-helical structure to form part of the stem of a new long coiled coil structure. These molecular rearrangements eventually place the N-terminal fusion peptide and the C-terminal transmembrane anchor at the same end of the rod-shaped HA2 molecule, facilitating membrane fusion by bringing the viral and cellular membranes together. Structural similarities between the low-pH form of HA2 and the post-fusion ectodomains of other viral membrane fusion proteins in their post-fusion states suggest that this juxtaposition of termini is a common mechanism for membrane fusion [22].

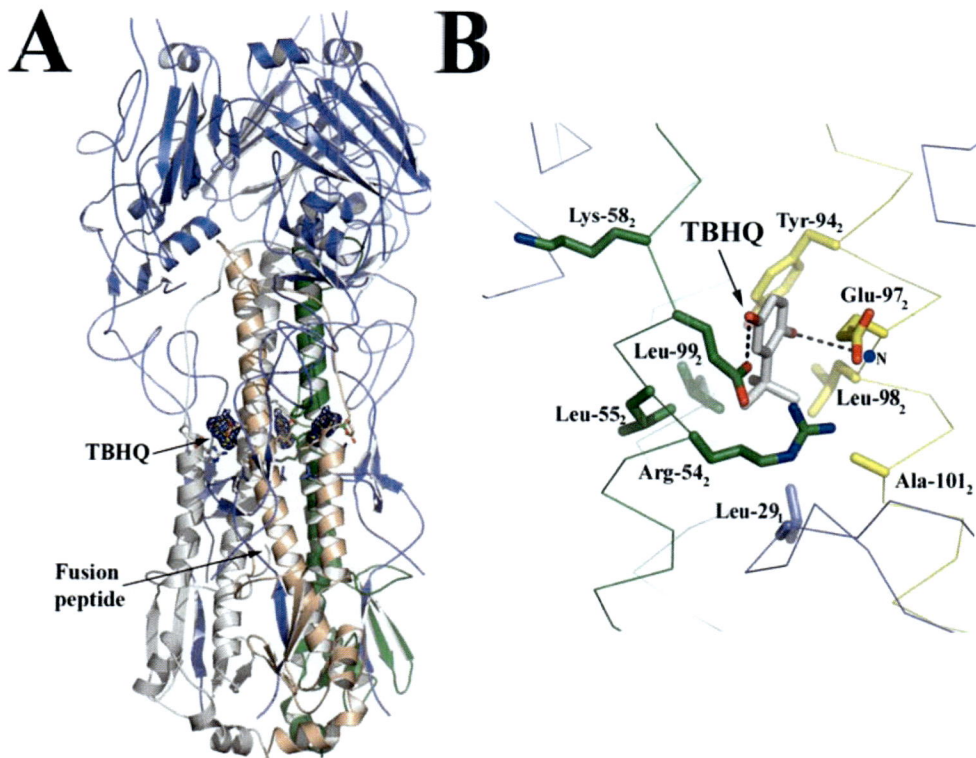

Figure 4. The TBHQ binding site. **A** Cartoon representation of H14 HA trimer in complex with TBHQ. HA1 polypeptides are coloured blue and HA2 polypeptides in yellow, gold and green. TBHQ is shown in mesh and stick representation (dark blue) and the location of the fusion peptide highlighted. B Close-up view of a TBHQ binding site. Selected residues are shown as sticks and potential hydrogen bonds as dashed lines.

INHIBITOR DESIGN

Recently the crystal structure of HA in complex with an inhibitor of fusion, tert-butyl hydroquinone (TBHQ), has been elucidated [6]. The TBHQ binding site is in an interface between monomers and thus there are three binding sites per HA trimer (Figure 4). The site has charged sides ($Arg54_2$, $Glu57_2$ and $Glu97_2$), a highly hydrophobic base into which the tert-butyl group of TBHQ packs and a solvent accessible polar top. The majority of the contacts are to residues of HA2 but hydrophobic interactions are formed to the highly conserved beta-hairpin of HA1 (residues 26-34), which is known to be exposed at fusion pH by the susceptibility of K27 to tryptic digestion. The interactions between TBHQ and HA2 are predominantly hydrophobic. The tert-butyl group packs into the hydrophobic base of the cavity comprising the group-conserved residues $Leu55_2$ and $Leu99_2$, and $Leu29_1$ of one monomer and $Leu98_2$ and $Ala101_2$ of an adjacent monomer. In addition the aliphatic part of the side chain of conserved $Glu-97_2$ of an adjacent monomer packs against the face of the benzene ring of TBHQ. Hydrogen bonds are also observed between O1 of TBHQ and the side chain of $Glu57_2$ and between O2 and the main chain amide of $Leu98_2$ of an adjacent monomer. The compound serves to stabilise the neutral pH conformation of HA preventing fusion of the viral and cellular membranes. Thus this compound has identified a functional site on HA which can be used for the design of more potent inhibitors. However due to structural differences between the two groups, this inhibitor nevertheless is only effective against one of the two phylogenetic groups of HA. Nonetheless compounds that specifically target the other group have been identified that would allow the development of small molecule inhibitors of fusion that could target all HA subtypes [23].

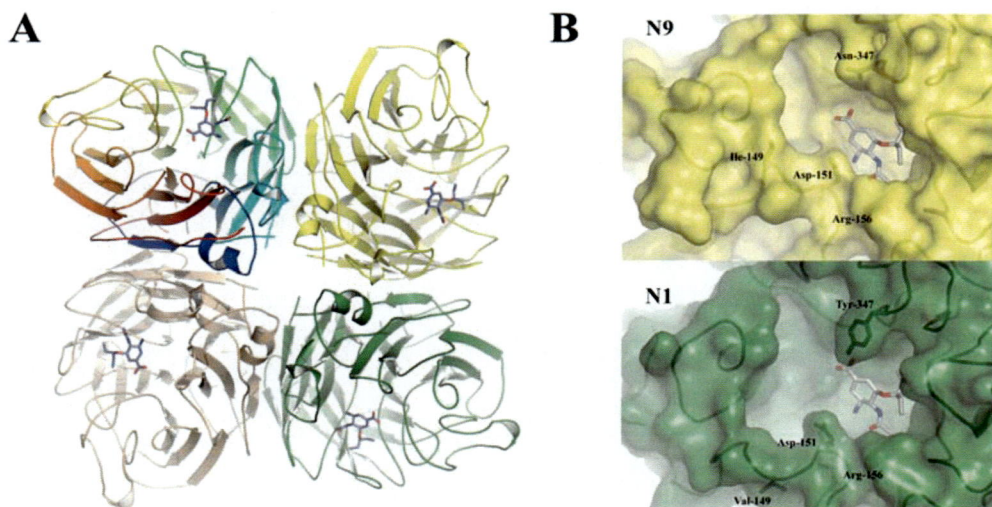

Figure 5. **A** Cartoon representation of the tetramer of NA. Monomers 2,3 and 4 are in yellow, gold and green, and the featured monomer is colored from blue at the amino-terminus to red at the carboxy-terminus. Oseltamivir is shown in stick representation bound to the active site of each monomer and coloured blue. **B** Molecular surfaces of N9 and N1 neuraminidases with bound oseltamivir showing the 150-cavity in the group-1 structure that arises because of the distinct conformation of the 150-loop.

In an alternative approach to designing anti-HA compounds, two groups have recently identified an antibody that exhibits broad neutralizing activity against influenza viruses of one of the two phylogenetic groups of Has [24, 25]. The antibody recognizes a highly conserved region on the viral haemagglutinin located near to the fusion peptide and thus may provide an alternative route to small molecules to prevent infection.

NEURAMINIDASE

The virus neuraminidase (NA) facilitates release of progeny virus particles by the removal of the terminal sialic acid present on cellular receptors, to which the HA binds. In addition, cleavage of sialic acid from mucins in the respiratory tract removes these potential non-specific inhibitors of virus infection. All Influenza neuraminidases are homotetrameric molecules exhibiting fourfold symmetry with each monomer consisting of six topologically identical four-stranded antiparallel β-sheets which are themselves arranged like the blades of a propeller [26, 27] (Figure 5A).

Sialic acid binds in a deep pocket on the surface of the molecule, roughly in the middle of each monomer. The amino acids in this pocket, including Arg118, Asp151, Arg152, Arg224, Glu276, Arg292, Arg371 and Tyr406 (numbered according to N2 sequence), are highly conserved across all NA subtypes. Together these residues form the enzyme active site. The three arginine residues, Arg118, Arg292 and Arg371, interact with the carboxylate of the substrate sialic acid; Arg152 interacts with the acetamido substituent; and Glu276 forms hydrogen bonds with the 8- and 9-hydroxyl groups of the glycerol moiety of the substrate. Other conserved residues provide a framework to maintain the structure of the catalytic site and include Glu119, Arg156, Trp178, Ser179, Asp/Asn198, Ileu222, Glu227, His274, Glu277, Asn294 and Glu425. A feature evident from the initial crystal structure and substrate bound crystal structure is the high level of sequence conservation of the active site across subtypes coupled with an apparent rigidity, both qualities desirable in a structure based drug design programme (see below).

Influenza A NA sequences, however, fall into two distinct phylogenetic groups. Although crystal structures of N1, N4 and N8 of group 1 and N2 and N9 of group 2 all have the same homotetrameric conformation, it has recently been shown that they possess group-specific differences in the active site [28]. The main conformational differences between the two groups are centred on the 150-loop (residues 147-152), adjacent to the active site. The conformation of the 150-loop is such that the α-carbon of valine 149 in group 1 is about 7Å distant from that of the equivalent isoleucine in group 2, and the side chain points away rather than towards the active site. In addition, there is a difference of 1.5Å in the positions of the conserved aspartic acid 151 side chains, and the carboxylate of the nearby conserved glutamic acid 119 points in approximately the opposite direction to that in group 2, such as to increase the width at that point of the active site cavity of group 1 NAs by about 5Å. These features, together with the location of glutamine 136 3.5Å lower at the base of the cavity, produce the 10Å x 5Å x 5Å 150-cavity adjacent to the active site in the group 1 Nas which is not present in group 2 Nas (Figure 5B). The implications of this in terms of retrospective and future drug design strategies are discussed later.

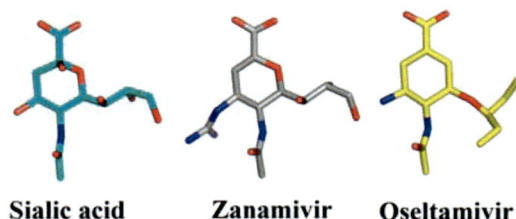

Sialic acid   Zanamivir   Oseltamivir

Figure 6. The structures of sialic acid (carbons coloured blue), zanamivir (carbons coloured grey) and oseltamivir (carbons coloured yellow).

INHIBITOR DESIGN

The first inhibitors were made in the 1960s in an attempt to understand the catalytic mechanism, and resulted in the discovery of 2,3-didehydro-2-deoxy-N-acetylneuraminic acid (DANA) [29, 30], an analogue of sialic acid. This compound has subsequently been shown to be a low μM inhibitor of a wide range of viral and bacterial neuraminidases. Inspection of the crystal structure of Influenza NA in complex with sialic acid or DANA revealed an electronegative cavity adjacent to the O4 position that could be targeted to synthesise an inhibitor with greater potency. Using Neu5Ac2en as an initial scaffold, substitution of O4 with an amino group gained 2 orders of binding over DANA, whereas substitution by a guanidine group (3, 4-guanidino-Neu5Ac2en) gained 5 orders of binding over DANA [31], and thus is a nanomolar inhibitor of influenza NA (Figure 6). In complexes of this compound, known now as Zanamivir/Relenza, with both influenza A and influenza B virus NA (PDB codes 1NNC and 1A4G respectively) [32, 33], the guanidino group interacts almost stereochemically perfectly with Asp151 and Glu227, residues which form part of the electronegative cavity. Relenza is a successful inhibitor of influenza A and B virus Nas, but its highly polar nature requires administration with an inhaler which cause inherent problems of use with regard to correct dosage and use in extremely sick individuals. Thus there was a need to develop an orally available compound, which led to the development and licensing of Oseltamivir/Tamiflu. The starting point for the development of Tamiflu was the use of a cyclohexene moiety instead of the dihydropyran ring of Relenza and DANA. It is chemically more stable and also retains the ability to alter the stereochemistry of ring substituents [34]. Optimal inhibition was observed when there was a double bond in the equivalent position to that in DANA, mimicking the carbonium cation intermediate. The carboxylate and acetamido groups were kept at C1 and C4 respectively, and an amino group at C5 included, in the light of the success of the Relenza development. To improve the lipophilicity and thus oral availability, the glycerol group was substituted by a series of alkyl ethers since the pocket in which this group resided had a significant hydrophobic character. There is a remarkable correlation between the length, geometry and rigidity of the alkyl chains and NA inhibitory activity, suggesting an incremental entropy gain. The crystal structure of the most potent inhibitor, with a 3-pentyl group, showed that Glu276 had rotated away from the active site, adopting a conformation in which the aliphatic side chain of Glu276 packs against the hydrophobic group of the compound. This required conformational change has had recent implications in the development of Tamiflu resistant variants of NA (see below).

Both Relenza and Tamiflu were designed directly through knowledge of the crystal structure of NA of the subtype N2 or N9, which belong to the same phylogenetic group. But as mentioned previously the group-1 and group-2 Nas differ in their active site architectures due to a different conformation of the 150-loop. However both Tamiflu and Relenza are equally effective against both phylogenetic groups. Crystal structures of N1 NA in complex with Relenza or Tamiflu revealed that the 150-loop can undergo a conformational change upon inhibitor binding such that the active site of NA from the two groups is essentially identical when bound to an inhibitor [28]. This explains why all of the inhibitors are effective against both phylogenetic groups despite their unliganded active sites having distinct conformations. Of note regarding the design of the next generation of anti-NA drugs is that Tamiflu can bind to N1 NA without causing the conformational change of the 150-loop [28]. The outcome of this is that this novel cavity can now targeted in new derivatives of Tamiflu or Relenza to try to overcome the problem of resistant viruses (see below).

RESISTANCE MUTATIONS

Despite the current effectiveness of Relenza and Tamiflu, mutations have arisen that result in resistance to one or both inhibitors [35, 36]. A feature of a high number of the resistance mutations is their NA phylogenetic group specificity. The mutation Arg292Lys has a substantial effect on the inhibition of N2-group Nas by Tamiflu [37], but little effect on N1 Nas. A conserved tyrosine residue at position 347 in N1-group Nas makes an additional hydrogen bond to the carboxylate group of the inhibitor that cannot be made by the equivalent residue in N2-group Nas, and which compensates for the loss of the interaction associated with the Arg292Lys mutation.

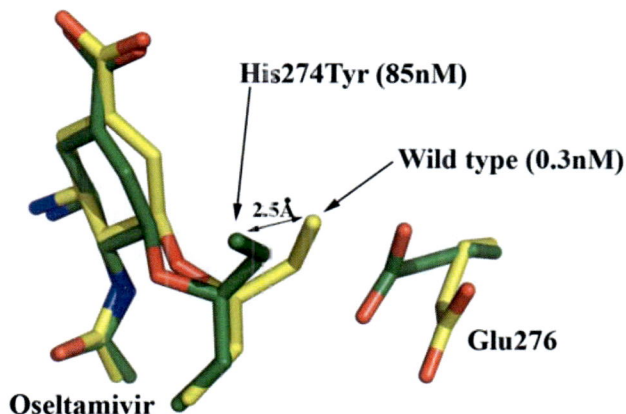

Figure 7. The conformation of oseltamivir and Glu276 from wild type N1 NA and an oseltamivir-resistant N1 NAs; the carbon atoms of the inhibitor from the wild-type complex are coloured yellow and the His274Tyr mutant in dark green.

The mutation His274Tyr leads to high resistance of N1 Nas against Tamiflu but has little effect on N2 Nas [38, 39]. The emergence of an H5N1 virus carrying this mutation has raised concerns about the widespread use of Tamiflu. In addition the sudden emergence of a predominant population of currently circulating H1N1 viruses that carry this resistance mutation but maintain wild type fitness is of major concern. This mutation does not affect the inhibition caused by Relenza. The key structural difference between Tamiflu and Relenza is that the former has a hydrophobic pentyloxy substituent at the C-6 position rather than a polar glycerol group in Zanamivir, as in the sialic acid substrate. For wild-type NA to accommodate Oseltamivir in its active sites requires a rearrangement of the side-chain of Glu276 relative to the ligand-free enzyme. In contrast, the binding of Zanamivir involves hydrogen bond formation between both oxygen atoms of the carboxyl group of Glu276 and the 8- and 9-hydroxyl groups of the glycerol moiety of the inhibitor and requires no change in side-chain conformation. In the structure of the His274Tyr mutant NA in complex with Oseltamivir (Figure 7) the bulkier tyrosine residue causes the side chain of Glu276 to move such that its carboxyl group is about 2Å closer to Tamiflu binding site (40). In this position the charged group disrupts the otherwise hydrophobic pocket that normally accommodates the pentyloxy substituent of Tamiflu and causes the inhibitor to rotate such that the pentyloxy substituent moves about 2Å out of its wild-type NA-bound position. The structure thus provides a direct explanation for the reduction in the binding affinity of the mutant for Tamiflu and consequently the resistance observed. In contrast, Group 2 Nas (N2 & N9), have the smaller threonine residue at position 252, and can accept the His274Tyr substitution, without changing the Oseltamivir binding site.

POLYMERASE

The eight segments of the influenza virus RNA genome are contained within ribonucleoprotein complexes (RNPs). These RNPs are composed of one segment of viral RNA (vRNA) bound at the termini by the influenza RNA-dependent RNA polymerase complex and by multiple copies of the influenza nucleoprotein (NP). The viral RNA polymerase performs the transcription and replication of the RNA segments within the RNP complex. The polymerase complex itself is a heterotrimer of two basic subunits (PB1 and PB2) and one acidic subunit (PA).

Initiation of viral transcription is dependent upon the cleavage of host mRNA molecules for the production of capped RNA primers. Endonuclease cleavage is performed by the viral RNA polymerase 9-15 nucleotides from the 5′ terminus [41, 42]. In contrast, replication of the RNA genome is primer independent and results in RNAs with triphosphorylated 5′ termini [43, 44]. Replication occurs by the production of complimentary copies of the RNA gene segments (cRNA), which are subsequently used as templates for the production of new vRNA.

Although all of the polymerase subunits are required for efficient transcription or replication, roles for each subunit have been established. In particular, the PB1 subunit is known to contain the site of polymerase activity [45], PB2 contains the binding site for capped RNA [46-48] and PA contains the endonuclease active site [49-52]. Currently there is no high-resolution structure of the trimeric polymerase complex, however several low-resolution structures (of both RNPs and free polymerase complexes) have been generated using electron microscopy [53-55]. These indicate the polymerase complex forms a hollow globular structure with an opening facing towards the inside of the RNP complex [55]. Comparison of the RNP-bound and free polymerase complexes indicated that a substantial structural rearrangement occurs upon formation of the RNP complex [55].

Within the last three years high-resolution structures of several domains from polymerase subunits have been solved by X-ray crystallography. These include three domains from PB2 (residues 320-483 [56], 538-693 [57, 58] and 693-741 [58, 59]) and two domains from PA (residues 1-197 [50, 52] and 257-716 [60, 61]). These structures have conclusively identified two sites critical for the process of transcription – the cap binding site (PB2 residues 320-483) and the endonuclease active site (PA residues 1-197). In addition the interface between the C-terminal domain of PA (residues 257-716) and the N-terminus of PB1 was resolved. These sites present a good opportunity for the development of current polymerase inhibitors and the identification of novel antiviral therapies.

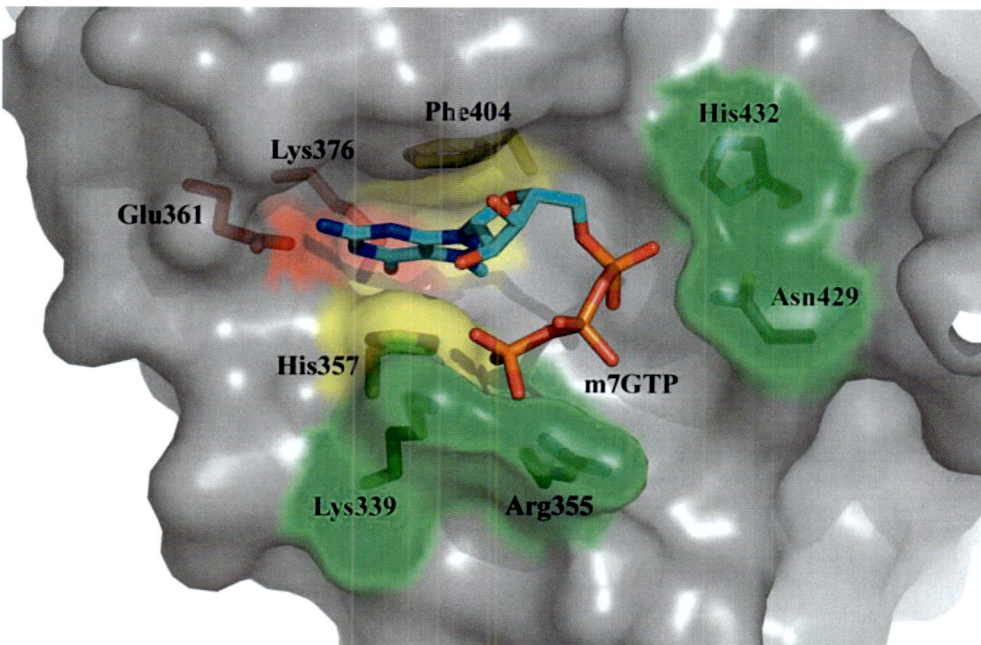

Figure 8. A surface representation of the influenza cap-binding domain. The binding of the cap analogue m^{7}GTP is shown as sticks. Residues involved in interactions with m^{7}GTP are highlighted: (yellow) His357 and Phe404 interact with the m^{7}guanyl ring via an aromatic sandwich, (red) Glu361 and Lys376 form hydrogen bonds with the m^{7}guanyl ring and (green) Lys339, Arg355, His432 and Asn429 form salt bridges and hydrogen bonds with the phosphate groups.

THE CAP-BINDING DOMAIN

The influenza polymerase complex requires short, capped RNA primers for the initiation of viral transcription. These are obtained by the cleavage of host mRNA molecules 9-15 nucleotides from their 5' cap structure in a process known as cap-snatching. For many years it has been known that recognition of capped RNA is mediated by the PB2 subunit of the polymerase complex, although the exact site of cap binding remained controversial [47, 62, 63]. However, recently the three-dimensional structure of a central domain of PB2 was solved in complex with cap-analogue m^7GTP (PDB 2VQZ)(56) (Figure 8). This structure confirmed the prior hypothesis that binding to the methylated guanosine base was via an 'aromatic sandwich' motif characteristic of other known cap-binding proteins [47, 56, 64], including the translation initiation factor eIF4E, the nuclear cap-binding complex (CBC) and vaccinia virus protein VP39. The stacking of three aromatic ring systems leads to a affinity and specificity for the N^7-methylated base, compared to unmethylated analogues, possibly due to the interaction between the delocalised positive charge arising from methylation and the π–electrons of the aromatic side chains. Interestingly the residues of the influenza cap-binding domain involved in this interaction, His357 and Phe404, could be considered somewhat atypical amongst cap-binding proteins, where tryptophan and tyrosine are more common [64]. Indeed, while Phe404 appears to be conserved among influenzas B and C, H357 is substituted with a tryptophan residue [56]. It is likely that the use of histidine contributes to the lower affinity and specificity of PB2 has for m^7GTP is compared to cellular cap-binding proteins. Both eIF4E and CBC have a nanomolar K_D for m^7GTP and are highly selective for the methylated base [65, 66]. In contrast, both cross-linking and SPR data indicate that PB2 binds to m^7GTP with relatively low affinity ($K_d = 170\mu M$) [56, 67] and discriminates between methylated and unmethylated cap analogues poorly (five-fold difference between the inhibition of cap binding by GTP and m^7GTP) [56, 67]. Analysis of polymerase complexes containing a H357W mutation indicate that such a substitution would lead to an increase in affinity for m^7GTP and it is likely that this mutation would also lead to greater specificity [56].

In addition to the aromatic residues that stack above and below the guanine ring, a third face of the cap-binding pocket is formed by Glu361 and Lys376 [56]. These two residues hydrogen bond to the N^1/N^2 and O^6 of the ring structure, respectively, holding it in place. Similar interactions are also observed in other cap-binding proteins, however their relative importance may be greater in this case. Mutation of either of these residues to alanine appears to greatly inhibit the affinity of m^7GTP [56], indicating that these interactions contribute directly substrate binding. In support of this both Glu361 and Lys376 are either conserved or conservatively substituted in influenzas B and C [56].

Supplementing these interactions, the influenza cap-binding domain also interacts with the phosphate groups of the m^7GTP cap analogue via salt bridges with Lys339 and Arg355 and hydrogen bonds to His357, Asn429 and His432 [56]. However, in contrast to the cap-binding sites of eIF4E and CBC, the contribution of interactions with the phosphate groups to the binding affinity is relatively modest [67]. Data from inhibition studies using m^7GTP, m^7GDP, m^7GMP and m^7Guanosine indicate that loss of these phosphate groups only causes a 20-fold decrease in the inhibition of binding to a capped oligonucleotide by RNP complexes, compared to a 2000-fold decrease when binding by eIF4E was investigated [67]. Therefore it appears that the presence of phosphate groups is not essential for interaction between a cap analogue and the influenza cap-binding domain.

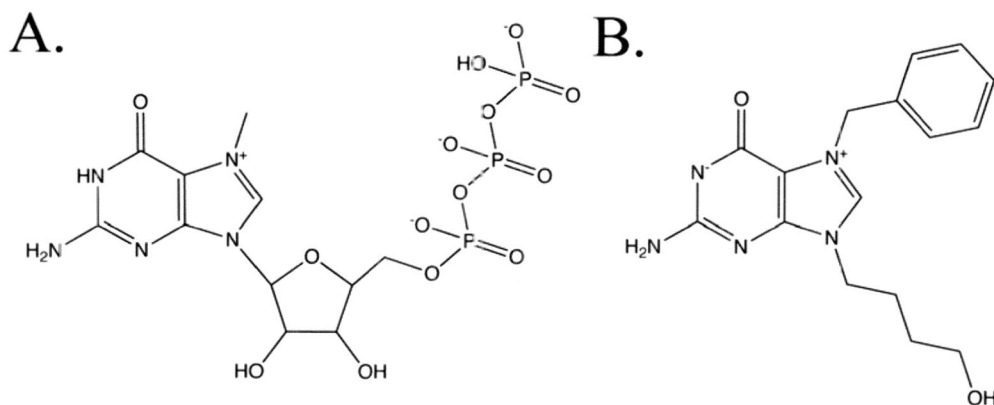

Figure 9. Structures of cap-binding inhibitors: (A) Natural cap analogue m^{7}GTP, (B) Influenza-specific inhibitor of cap binding RO0794238.

The unorthodox nature of the influenza cap-binding site enhances the potential of PB2 as drug target. Comparison with previously characterised cellular cap-binding proteins indicates that while the broad mechanism of interaction with the cap structure may be similar, there are differences in the amino acid residues involved and relative importance of different binding events [56, 64, 67]. In particular, the influenza polymerase has a much weaker selection for methylated and phosphorylated cap analogues, and places much more reliance on hydrogen bonding [56, 67]. These differences have allowed the development of one compound (RO0794238) designed to selectively inhibit the influenza cap-binding site as compared to human eIF4E [67]. RO0794238 was based on the guanine ring structure with aliphatic replacements for the ribose and phosphate moieties and lacks any negative charges, which are essential for binding to eIF4E (Figure 9). The design of this inhibitor was based upon biochemical evidence and was developed prior to the publication of the structure of the cap-binding domain. In the context of this structure, it is now possible to understand more about how this molecule may interact with the influenza cap-binding site. In particular, it is conceivable that the benzyl substitution at N^7 may pack against residues within the hydrophobic rear wall of the binding pocket such as Phe325, Ile352 and Met431. Additionally, the substitution of ribose for an acyclic aliphatic group at position 9 of the guanine may allow greater interaction with Phe323 on the roof of the binding pocket.

However, the structure of the influenza cap-binding domain needs to be considered in the context of the remainder of the PB2 subunit and the polymerase complex as a whole. While this site may explain the interactions with the guanine base of the cap structure, it does not inform us about the specificity of the polymerase for cap1 (m^{7}GpppN$_m$) compared to cap0 (m^{7}GpppN) structures [68]. Cross-linking data using oligonucliotides including a thio-uracil residue at the third position indicate that residues 544-556 of PB2 may be close to this region and could therefore contribute to this specificity 68]. These residues form the first α-helix of the '627 domain', which has also been characterised by X-ray crystallography (PDB 2VY6) [68]. However, it is unclear at present how these two domains interact, and how residues 544-556 may influence this specificity.

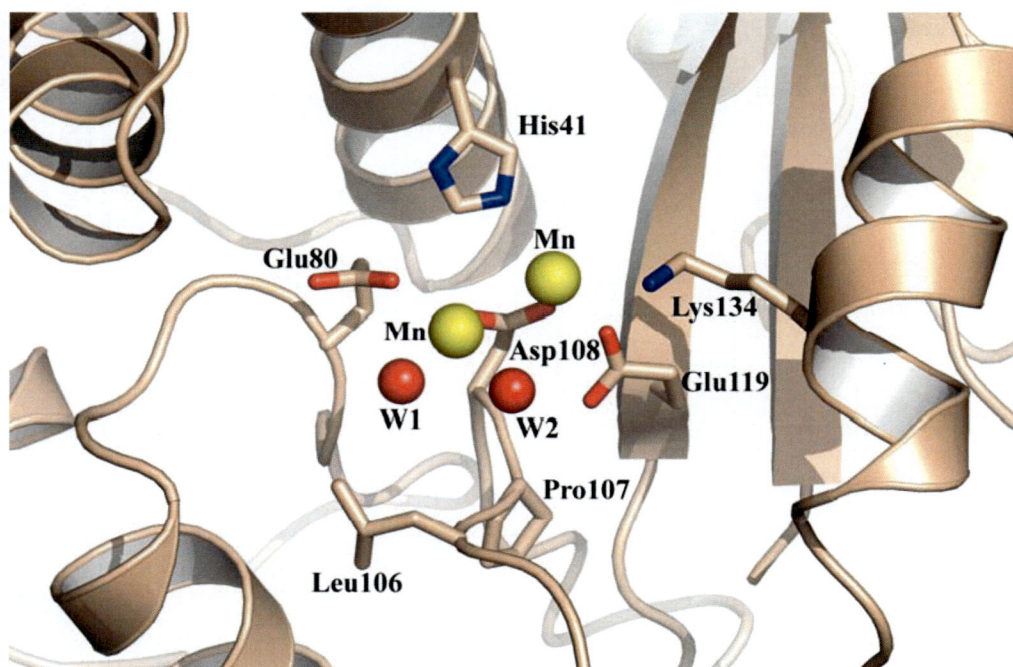

Figure 10. A cartoon representation of the endonuclease binding site. Two Mn^{2+} ions are bound within an acidic pocket. These are co-ordinated by the side chains of Glu80, Asp108, Glu119 and His41 and the carbonyl oxygens of Leu106 and Pro107 (all shown as sticks). Two water molecules (labelled W1 and W2) are also involved in co-ordination. Lys134 is also likely to be involved in a PDXDXK endonuclease motif with Asp108 and Glu119.

THE ENDONUCLEASE DOMAIN

The cleavage of host mRNA molecules for the production of capped RNA primers is essential for the initiation of viral transcription. This cleavage occurs 9-15 nucleotides downstream of the 5' cap structure, with a preference for lysis after a CA sequence [69]. Until recently the site of endonuclease activity was highly controversial. Initially it was believed that the PB2 subunit contained the endonuclease active site in addition to the cap-binding site [48, 70]. Later evidence from cross-linking and mutagenesis studies indicated that residues in the C terminal half of the PB1 subunit may be involved [63, 71], while other mutagenesis studies indicated a role for the PA subunit [49, 51]. However, this dispute now appears to have been resolved by the publication of two high-resolution structures of an N-terminal domain of PA with a putative endonuclease active site (PDB ID: 3EBJ and 2W69) [50, 52]. Both structures contained divalent metal cations and a $(P)DX_N(D/E)XK$ motif characteristic of many endonucleases. In addition, the function of this site was confirmed by both biochemical and mutagenic analysis.

The two structures of the influenza endonuclease domain are very similar, although not identical. Both structures have the same α/β fold with a mixed 5 strand β-sheet surrounded by seven α-helices. These come together to form a negatively charged cleft containing either one or two metal cations (Figure 10). The identity and number of these cations is controversial as one structure shows the presence of one Mg^{2+} ion [53], whereas the other identified two Mn^{2+}

ions (50). In agreement with previous studies, thermal stability assays have indicated that Mn^{2+} ions may be preferred over other divalent cations [50, 72]. However, endonuclease activity does not appear to be contingent upon the presence of manganese, as transcription activity is observed in its absence [52]. Co-ordination of the metal ions is similar in both structures, with the side chains of Glu80 and Asp108 and the carbonyl oxygens of Leu106 and Pro107 directly involved in binding to both Mg^{2+} and Mn^{2+} [50, 52]. Residues His41 and Glu119 are also involved, although co-ordination of Mg^{2+} is mediated indirectly via stabilised water molecules [52]. Comparison of this site with other endonuclease active sites indicates that residues may form a $(P)DX_N(D/E)XK$ motif with Lys134 and are highly likely to constitute the enzyme active site. Mutagenesis of Glu80, Asp108, Glu119 and Lys134 to alanine resulted in the loss of transcriptase activity both in vivo and in vitro, while H41A, L106A and P107A mutations lead to a broader decrease in polymerase activity [51, 52].

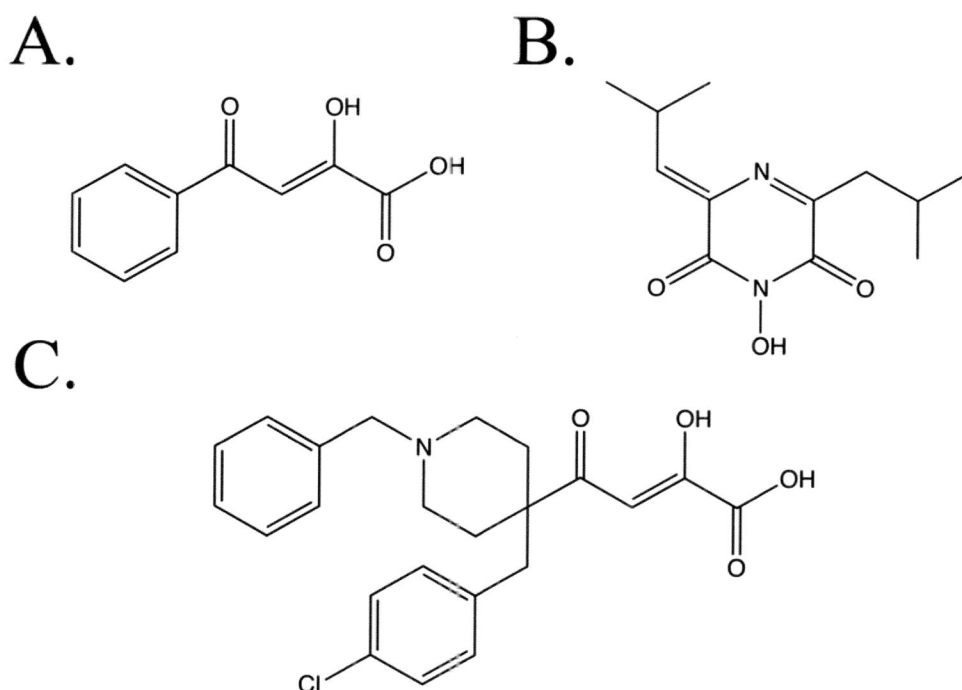

Figure 11. Structures of influenza endonuclease inhibitors: (A) 2,4-dioxo-4-phenylbutanoic acid, (B) Flutimide, (C) L-742,001.

The central role of endonuclease activity in influenza mRNA synthesis makes it a prime target for the design of novel antiviral compounds [73-78]. Analysis of lead compounds has been benefited by the use of in vitro transcription assays using purified RNPs or polymerase complexes and capped RNA substrates. Such assays were used in combination with random screening to identify a class of endonuclease inhibitors based around a 2,4-diketobutanoic acid structure [73, 76] (Figure 11). Later studies identified a second endonuclease inhibitor for fungal extracts. This compound, flutimide, is a substituted 2,6-diketopiperazine with a similar molecular architecture to the 2,4-diketobutanoic acids [75, 77, 78]. It appears likely that these inhibitors bind directly to the endonuclease active site for several reasons. Firstly, binding of 2,4-dioxo-4-phenylbutanoic acid (DPBA) to the endonuclease domain was observed by thermal shift assays [50]. Binding appears to require the presence of metal ions, indicating that it may be involved co-ordination of the cations within the catalytic pocket. Secondly, the endonuclease activity of the residues 1-197 of PA is inhibited by DPBA in a dose dependent manner with an inhibition constant (K_i=26 μM) [50] consistent with the half-maximal inhibitory concentration observed using polymerase complexes (IC_{50} = 21.3 μM) [76]. Thirdly, a recent study identified a mutation within the endonuclease domain (Thr20Ala), which confers weak (three-fold) resistance to another substituted 2,4-diketobutanoic acid (L742,001) [74]. This mutation is found in many influenza strains and is present in both endonuclease domain structures. It is unclear how this residue may influence the binding of endonuclease inhibitors, although it is located close to the active site within the acidic cleft.

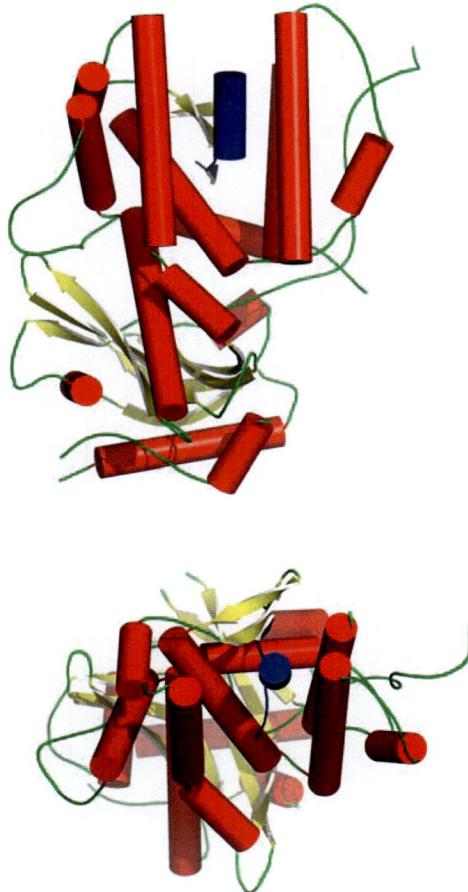

Figure 12. Orthogonal views of a cartoon representation of the C-terminal domain of PA (α-helices, β-strands and loops are coloured red, yellow and green respectively) in complex with the N-terminus of PB1 (blue).

However, as with the cap-binding domain, the structures of the endonuclease domain do not exclude a role for other residues within the polymerase in RNA cleavage. In particular two sites within the PB1 subunit (residues 508-522 and 669-672) have been identified, which also appear to be involved in the initiation of transcription [63, 71]. Mutations within these regions lead to inhibition of cap-dependent RNA synthesis. At present it is unclear whether these residues interact directly with the capped RNA substrate or whether the effects of mutation are more indirect. However, it has been noted that the structures of the endonuclease domain do not appear to contain any obvious RNA binding sites [52]. Additionally, in the context of the trimeric polymerase complex endonuclease activity is dependent upon prior interaction with the termini of the vRNA gene segments, which form the vRNA promoter [79-81]. Currently it is believed that the primary sites of interaction with the vRNA promoter are also located within the PB1 subunit [82, 83]. Until we have a high-resolution structure of the complete polymerase heterotrimer the interactions between these sites remain undetermined.

PA-PB1 SUBUNIT INTERFACE

The three subunits of the polymerase complex are all involved in the process of transcription. Assembly of the trimeric complex is therefore essential for efficient polymerase activity and has been identified as a potential target for the development of novel antiviral inhibitors [84]. Current models of polymerase complex assembly indicate that PB1 forms a central core with which both PA and PB2 interact independently [85-89]. In particular, interactions have been observed between the C-terminal domain of PA and the N-terminus of PB1 and the C-terminal domain of PB1 and an N-terminal domain of PB2. Additional contacts are believed to occur between the subunits, although these remain relatively uncharacterized [90-92].

The absence of any high-resolution structure of the trimeric polymerase has hindered our understanding of complex formation. However recently progress was made by the publication of two independent structures of the C-terminal domain of PA (residues 257-716) in complex with the first 15 residues of PB1 (60, 61) (Figure 12). Both structures are very similar, despite originating from avian (A/goose/Guangdong/1/96 H5N1, PDB ID: 3CM8) [60] and human (A/Puerto Rico/8/1934 H1N1, PDB ID: 2ZNL)(61) viruses. These structures indicate that the C-terminus of PA consists of 13 α-helices and 9 β-strands, with one short 3_{10} helix. The residues 5-11 of the N-terminus of PB1 form a 3_{10} helix, which is held between two sets of α-helices like the jaws of a clamp.

The interactions between PA and PB1 are largely hydrophobic, with some additional contribution from hydrogen bonds [60, 61]. In particular, PB1 residues Pro5, Leu7, Leu8, Phe9 and Leu10 form hydrophobic interactions with residues Phe411, Met595, Trp619, Val636, Leu640, Leu666, Trp706 and Phe710 of PA. The PTLLPL sequence of PB1 is almost completely conserved amongst all isolates of influenza A, with rare variations to Thr6 [61, 84]. Furthermore, mutation of any of these residues to aspartic acid (or mutation of Pro5 to leucine) results a total absence of complex formation [93]. Similarly, mutations to PA residues Val636, Leu640, Leu666 and Trp706 also greatly reduce binding affinity [61]. In addition to these hydrophobic contacts, hydrogen bonds are made between the main chain nitrogens and carbonyls of the PB1 peptide and PA [60, 61]. These interactions are centred on

PB1 residues 2-4 and 9-14 and are supplemented by further hydrogen bonding between the side chains of PB1 residues Asp2, Asn4 and Lys11 with the side chains of PA residues Asn412 and Glu617 and main-chain carbonyls of residues Thr618 and Trp706.

It must be noted that this site is unlikely to be the only point of contact between the PA and PB1 subunits. The current low-resolution images of the polymerase heterotrimer indicate a tight globular complex with no clear subunit boundaries [55]. Additionally, there is evidence that the linker between the endonuclease and C-terminal domains of PA (residues 257-276) may also be involved in binding to the PB1 subunit [91]. At present the importance of this interaction is unclear as disruption of the binding between the N-terminus of PB1 and the C-terminal domain of PA by mutation results in reduction of complex formation to levels below the detection limit [60, 87, 93]. However, these disruptions do not prevent polymerase activity entirely [61] and attenuated viruses containing such mutations have been produced [93]. It is therefore possible that inhibition of this interaction may induce compensatory mutations within PA (or PB1), which increase the role of the linker in binding to the PB1 subunit. Clearly, further work is needed to characterise this interface in more detail.

The potential of the PA-PB1 subunit interface as a target for the design of novel antivirals has recently been explored using a peptide derived from the first 25 amino acids of the PB1 sequence [84]. A version of this peptide was synthesised in fusion with a C-terminal sequence from the Tat protein of human immunodeficiency virus, which is known to mediate cell entry. Application of this peptide to infected cells resulted in a 90% reduction in viral titre and an 80% reduction in expression of the viral nucleoprotein. However, currently no small molecule inhibitors of polymerase complex assembly have been identified.

M2

Influenza A and B viruses each contain a small integral membrane protein, M2 and BM2, respectively, which are minor components of the virus membrane, and form homotetrameric pH-activated proton-selective channels [94, 95] and has two roles in influenza replication [96]; to allow an influx of protons into the infecting virion during virus entry initiating the low pH dissociation of the vRNP from the matrix protein and its release into the cytoplasm for transport into the cell nucleus to initiate replication [97]. Also, in highly pathogenic avian influenza viruses (H5 and H7), M2 acts at a later stage in infection by reducing the pH of the *trans* Golgi Network [98], necessary to prevent exposure of the HA1/HA2 to a pH that could trigger prematurely the low-pH conformational change in HA [99] (see above).

M2 is the molecular target of the aminoadamantanes, amantadine (Symmetrel) and its derivative rimantadine (Flumadine) that represent the first class of antivirals clinically approved for treatment of influenza A infection, and show an efficacy of 70–90% when used prophylactically [100]. However there has been a wide spread emergence of mutations within the M2 proton channel that render the virus resistant to these drugs. The location of amantadine resistance mutations in the transmembrane ™ domain of the M2 protein enabled the identification of both the target and mechanism of action of the drugs [101]. Single substitutions at either of five amino acid positions, 26, 27, 30, 31 or 34 have been shown to confer resistance to amantadine and rimantadine in vitro and/or in vivo, depending on the virus. These mutations tend to cause cross-resistance between amantadine, rimantadine and analogous inhibitors, and attempts to develop alternative, complementary inhibitors of M2, effective against these resistant mutants, have been unsuccessful, probably due to the lack of structural information of M2 itself and the precise mode of binding of the inhibitors.

X-ray

NMR

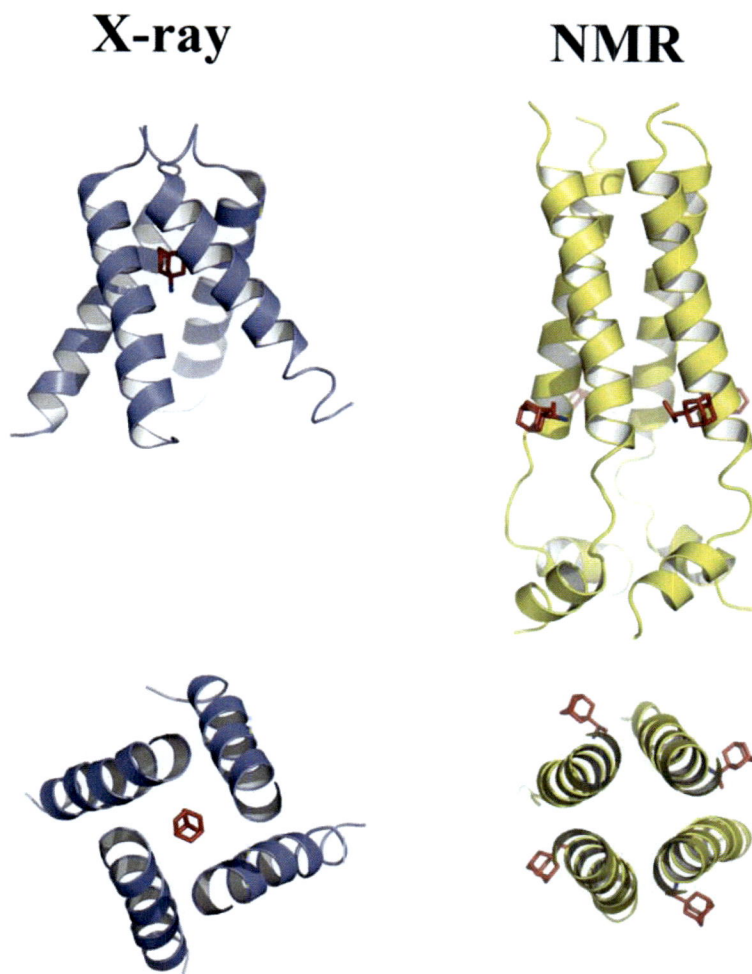

Figure 13. Orthogonal views of a cartoon representation of the M2 protein determined by x-ray crystallography (blue) and NMR (yellow). The proposed binding sites of amantadine (x-ray) and rimantadine (NMR) are highlighted, and each compound shown in stick representation and coloured red.

Low resolution structural studies of a transmembrane peptide of M2 have indicated that the residues that lead to drug resistance probably line the channel of M2 and are consistent with drug binding within the channel in the vicinity of residues 27 to 34 [102, 103]. Other studies have shown that the drug binds to the channel with a stoichiometry of one molecule per channel, but does not act as a simple non-competitive blocker, instead acting allosterically via structural alterations in the channel itself [104, 105]. Whereas most resistance mutations inhibit amantadine binding, mutations at residue 27, appear to permit some level of drug binding, as is the case of various resistance mutations observed in NA [106] (see above).

Recently, two higher resolution structures of M2 have been elucidated, one via x-ray crystallography using a construct that corresponds to the transmembrane section of M2 [107], and one via NMR using a construct that also contains part of the cytoplasmic domain of M2 [108]. Both of the structures reveal as expected a four-helix, cone-shaped bundle with a polar pore formed by all 4 helices that is capped by a constriction that is too narrow for any other type of ion, other than protons, to pass (Figure 13). Additionally both structures show that two residues that have been shown to be functionally important, His37 and Trp41, occur at locations that are appropriate for the suggested roles; Trp41 acting as a gate that opens when the proton sensor (His37) experiences low pH.

Despite these overall similarities, the two structures show considerable differences when bound to an aminoadamantane. The NMR structure is in an apparently closed conformation, with the four Trp41 side chains of the tetramer pointing inwards and sterically blocking the pore of the channel. The X-ray structure in contrast is in an open conformation, with the helices splayed out on the cytoplasmic side of the channel serving to widen the gate formed by Trp41. Even more surprising are differences in the proposed binding site of the drug. The X-ray structure shows a single amantadine molecule plugging the open pore, in accordance with the suggested 1:1 stoichiometry of one molecule per channel. In the NMR structure there is no room is available in the pore for a molecule to bind since it has adopted a closed conformation. Instead four drug molecules are bound at the channel's lipid-exposed outer surface, one at each helix–helix interface (Figure 13). Thus both structures suggest conflicting modes of action. The crystal structure reveals that the drug physically blocks the proton pathway in the open pore. In contrast the NMR structure reveals that the drug binds preferentially to, and thereby stabilizes, the closed state of the M2 proton channel. Further structural and biophysical studies on both wild type and mutant are therefore needed to elucidate the exact inhibitory mechanism of the aminoadamantanes, and to enable structure based drug design programmes to develop this class of antivirals.

NS1

Influenza A virus NS1 protein is a multifunctional virulence factor, contributing to efficient virus replication by participating in multiple protein-RNA and protein-protein interactions. The sequence and structure of the NS1 protein is highly conserved across all Influenza subtypes and therefore is an extremely attractive target to develop new drugs against.

The N-terminal 73 amino-acids of NS1 form a symmetrical homodimeric RNA-binding domain [109], that serves to inhibit both interferon (IFN) induction [110], and the antiviral effects of IFN [111]. The subsequent 157 amino-acids of NS1 (residues 74-230) and is known as the effector domain, and binds to a wide range of host-cell proteins resulting in the specific disruption of normal cellular function: (a) the enhancement of viral mRNA translation [112]; (b) the deregulation of cellular mRNA processing [113]; (c) the inhibition of dsRNA-activated protein kinase (PKR) [114]; and (d) activation of phosphoinositide 3-kinase (PI3K) signalling [115]. Undoubtedly, additional binding partners and functions will be discovered.

STRUCTURAL STUDIES

The influenza NS1 protein is comprised of a RNA-binding domain (residues 1-66) and an effector domain (residues 72-230) that are joined by a flexible linker. Crystallographic analysis has revealed that both domains in isolation form stable dimer. The RNA-binding domain alone is a symmetrical homodimer with each monomer consisting of three α-helices [116, 117], with dimerization being essential for binding dsRNA [118]. Two identical helices from each NS1 monomer contribute towards dsRNA-binding by forming antiparallel 'tracks' on either side of a deep cleft [117]. The crystal structure of NS1 RNA-binding domain bound to a double-stranded RNA (dsRNA) has recently been reported and shows that the homodimer to recognizes the major groove of A-form dsRNA in a length-independent mode via a concave surface formed by dimeric anti-parallel α-helices [119]. dsRNA is anchored by Arg38 from each monomer, forming a network of hydrogen bonds. This Arg38-Arg38 pair and also Arg35-Arg46 pairs are located at the concave surface and are crucial for dsRNA binding, with the former penetrating into the bound dsRNA and the latter probably critical for the stabilization of NS1A RNA binding domain dimer. A dramatic conformational change also occurs upon dsRNA binding resulting in the reorientation of the side chain of Arg38. This Arg38 pair acts as a lid to cover a deep pocket underneath the concave dsRNA-binding. The release of dsRNA causes the breakage of the Arg38 pair opening up a deep pocket, which has the potential to be targeted by small molecules in a drug design programme.

Crystallographic studies has revealed that the C-terminal effector domain of human and avian NS1 proteins homodimerize, with each monomer consisting of seven β-strands and three α-helices [120-122]. Within each monomer, the β-strands form a twisted, crescent-like, anti-parallel β-sheet around a long, central α-helix. Despite being present in the crystallization constructs, the C-terminal ~25 amino acids of NS1, a region which is involved in many strain-specific functions, have not been visible in the electron density maps. It is likely that this stretch of NS1 is intrinsically disordered, and only adopts an ordered structure upon binding the appropriate binding partner.

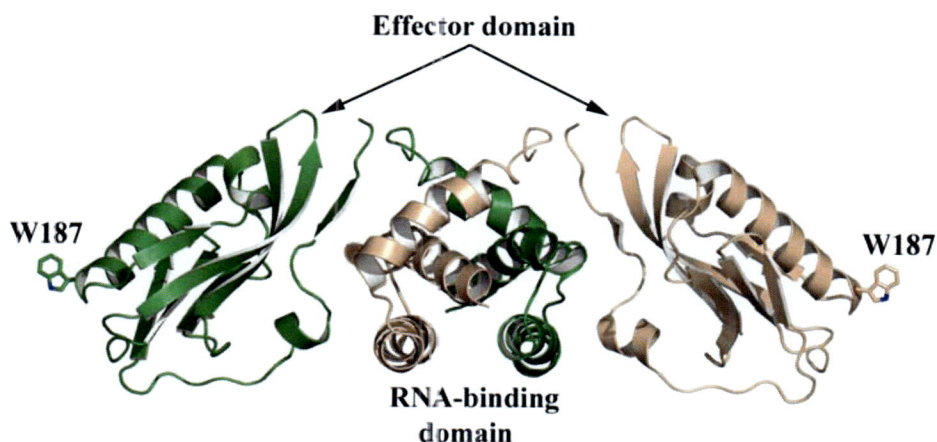

Figure 14. Cartoon representation of the full length H5N1 NS1 dimer. The monomers are coloured gold and green. W187 is highlighted and shown in stick representation.

The precise dimeric assembly of the NS1 effector domain remains a matter of debate, as two distinct dimer conformations have been proposed: a strand–strand dimer [120], and a helix–helix dimer [121]. Despite a high level of amino acid conservation at both dimer interfaces mutagenesis evidence indicates that Trp187 (a residue located at the helix–helix interface and distant from the strand-strand interface) is essential for dimerization of an avian NS1 effector domain in solution [121]. This suggests that the helix–helix dimer, at least for the avian NS1 protein used, is likely to be biologically predominant.

Recently, however, the structure of the full length NS1 from an H5N1 virus was reported which, as expected, showed a dimeric protein with each monomer consisting a RNA-binding domain and an effector domain [123]. An unexpected finding however was the fact that the effector domains do not contribute to the dimer interface (despite being dimeric in the absence of the RNA-binding domain) but instead flank the core RNA-binding domains, creating a "domain-swapped dimer" (Figure 14). The linker between the two domains was not visible, presumably due to inherent flexibility. Further structural studies are needed to determine if the oligomeric plasticity observed is related to its multifunctionality.

NS1-CPSF30 COMPLEX

The NS1 protein of many human influenza A viruses inhibit the production of antiviral mRNAs via binding to the 30-kDa subunit of the cellular cleavage and polyadenylation specificity factor (CPSF30), which is required for the 3' end processing of all cellular pre-mRNAs. A recent crystal structure of the complex formed between the second and third zinc finger domains of CPSF30 and the effector domain of NS1 revealed tetrameric complex, where two F2F3 molecules wrap around two NS1 effector domains (124). From a drug design perspective, the structure revealed a CPSF30 binding pocket on NS1 comprised of amino acid residues that are highly conserved among human influenza A viruses, and is therefore an exciting target for antiviral drug development. The crystal structure also reveals that two amino acids adjacent to this pocket, Phe103 and Met106 participate in key hydrophobic interactions with F2F3. Interestingly, these two residues are highly conserved (>99%) among influenza A viruses isolated from humans but not in avian isolates.

CONCLUSION

In this chapter we have discussed the way structural biology has been used to investigate the fundamental biology of the influenza virus and, through the use of the structures, to design effective anti-influenza agents. The studies on haemagglutinin alone have had a profound impact on the relationship between the structure and function of proteins in general. The use of the structure of neuraminidase in the rational design of novel anti-virals is widely seen as the paradigm of structure-based drug design. However, since the virus is a constantly "shifting target", there is an urgent need to continue the aforementioned structural biology effects. The remarkable progress on the polymerase structure in recent years holds great promise with regard to the design of novel drugs, and while the spectre of the next pandemic looms large, we wait with anticipation the forthcoming years of influenza virus structural biology.

REFERENCES

[1] Wilson IA, Skehel JJ, Wiley DC. Structure of the haemagglutinin membrane glycoprotein of influenza virus at 3Å resolution. *Nature*. 1981 Jan 29;289(5796):366-73.

[2] Fouchier RA, Munster V, Wallensten A, Bestebroer TM, Herfst S, Smith D, et al. Characterization of a novel influenza A virus hemagglutinin subtype (H16) obtained from black-headed gulls. *J Virol*. 2005 Mar;79(5):2814-22.

[3] Gamblin SJ, Haire LF, Russell RJ, Stevens DJ, Xiao B, Ha Y, et al. The structure and receptor binding properties of the 1918 influenza hemagglutinin. *Science*. 2004 Mar 19;303(5665):1838-42.

[4] Ha Y, Stevens DJ, Skehel JJ, Wiley DC. X-ray structures of H5 avian and H9 swine influenza virus hemagglutinins bound to avian and human receptor analogs. *Proc Natl Acad Sci U S A*. 2001 Sep 25;98(20):11181-6.

[5] Russell RJ, Gamblin SJ, Haire LF, Stevens DJ, Xiao B, Ha Y, et al. H1 and H7 influenza haemagglutinin structures extend a structural classification of haemagglutinin subtypes. *Virology*. 2004 Aug 1;325(2):287-96.

[6] Russell RJ, Kerry PS, Stevens DJ, Steinhauer DA, Martin SR, Gamblin SJ, et al. Structure of influenza hemagglutinin in complex with an inhibitor of membrane fusion. *Proc Natl Acad Sci U S A*. 2008 Nov 18;105(46):17736-41.

[7] Ha Y, Stevens DJ, Skehel JJ, Wiley DC. H5 avian and H9 swine influenza virus haemagglutinin structures: possible origin of influenza subtypes. *EMBO J*. 2002 Mar 1;21(5):865-75.

[8] Ito T, Couceiro JN, Kelm S, Baum LG, Krauss S, Castrucci MR, et al. Molecular basis for the generation in pigs of influenza A viruses with pandemic potential. *J Virol*. 1998 Sep;72(9):7367-73.

[9] Nobusawa E, Aoyama T, Kato H, Suzuki Y, Tateno Y, Nakajima K. Comparison of complete amino acid sequences and receptor-binding properties among 13 serotypes of hemagglutinins of influenza A viruses. *Virology*. 1991 Jun;182(2):475-85.

[10] Rogers GN, D'Souza BL. Receptor binding properties of human and animal H1 influenza virus isolates. *Virology*. 1989 Nov;173(1):317-22.

[11] Baum LG, Paulson JC. Sialyloligosaccharides of the respiratory epithelium in the selection of human influenza virus receptor specificity. *Acta Histochem Suppl*. 1990;40:35-8.

[12] Couceiro JN, Paulson JC, Baum LG. Influenza virus strains selectively recognize sialyloligosaccharides on human respiratory epithelium; the role of the host cell in selection of hemagglutinin receptor specificity. *Virus Res*. 1993 Aug;29(2):155-65.

[13] Rogers GN, Paulson JC. Receptor determinants of human and animal influenza virus isolates: differences in receptor specificity of the H3 hemagglutinin based on species of origin. *Virology*. 1983 Jun;127(2):361-73.

[14] Webster RG. 1918 Spanish influenza: the secrets remain elusive. *Proc Natl Acad Sci U S A*. 1999 Feb 16;96(4):1164-6.

[15] Connor RJ, Kawaoka Y, Webster RG, Paulson JC. Receptor specificity in human, avian, and equine H2 and H3 influenza virus isolates. *Virology*. 1994 Nov 15;205(1):17-23.

[16] Naeve CW, Hinshaw VS, Webster RG. Mutations in the hemagglutinin receptor-binding site can change the biological properties of an influenza virus. *J Virol.* 1984 Aug;51(2):567-9.

[17] Stevens J, Blixt O, Chen LM, Donis RO, Paulson JC, Wilson IA. Recent avian H5N1 viruses exhibit increased propensity for acquiring human receptor specificity. *J Mol Biol.* 2008 Sep 19;381(5):1382-94.

[18] Russell RJ, Stevens DJ, Haire LF, Gamblin SJ, Skehel JJ. Avian and human receptor binding by hemagglutinins of influenza A viruses. *Glycoconj J.* 2006 Feb;23(1-2):85-92.

[19] Umemura M, Itoh M, Makimura Y, Yamazaki K, Umekawa M, Masui A, et al. Design of a sialylglycopolymer with a chitosan backbone having efficient inhibitory activity against influenza virus infection. *J Med Chem.* 2008 Aug 14;51(15):4496-503.

[20] Chen J, Lee KH, Steinhauer DA, Stevens DJ, Skehel JJ, Wiley DC. Structure of the hemagglutinin precursor cleavage site, a determinant of influenza pathogenicity and the origin of the labile conformation. *Cell.* 1998 Oct 30;95(3):409-17.

[21] Bullough PA, Hughson FM, Skehel JJ, Wiley DC. Structure of influenza haemagglutinin at the pH of membrane fusion. *Nature.* 1994 Sep 1;371(6492):37-43.

[22] Skehel JJ, Wiley DC. Receptor binding and membrane fusion in virus entry: the influenza hemagglutinin. *Annu Rev Biochem.* 2000;69:531-69.

[23] Hoffman LR, Kuntz ID, White JM. Structure-based identification of an inducer of the low-pH conformational change in the influenza virus hemagglutinin: irreversible inhibition of infectivity. *J Virol.* 1997 Nov;71(11):8808-20.

[24] Ekiert DC, Bhabha G, Elsliger MA, Friesen RH, Jongeneelen M, Throsby M, et al. Antibody recognition of a highly conserved influenza virus epitope. *Science.* 2009 Feb 26.

[25] Sui J, Hwang WC, Perez S, Wei G, Aird D, Chen LM, et al. Structural and functional bases for broad-spectrum neutralization of avian and human influenza A viruses. *Nat Struct Mol Biol.* 2009 Mar;16(3):265-73.

[26] Burmeister WP, Henrissat B, Bosso C, Cusack S, Ruigrok RW. Influenza B virus neuraminidase can synthesize its own inhibitor. *Structure.* 1993 Sep 15;1(1):19-26.

[27] Varghese JN, Laver WG, Colman PM. Structure of the influenza virus glycoprotein antigen neuraminidase at 2.9Å resolution. *Nature.* 1983 May 5-11;303(5912):35-40.

[28] Russell RJ, Haire LF, Stevens DJ, Collins PJ, Lin YP, Blackburn GM, et al. The structure of H5N1 avian influenza neuraminidase suggests new opportunities for drug design. *Nature.* 2006 Sep 7;443(7107):45-9.

[29] Meindl P, Tuppy H. [2-Deoxy-2,3-dehydrosialic acids. II. Competitive inhibition of Vibrio cholerae neuraminidase by 2-deoxy-2,3-dehydro-N-acylneuraminic acids]. *Hoppe Seylers Z Physiol Chem.* 1969 Sep;350(9):1088-92.

[30] Meindl P, Bodo G, Palese P, Schulman J, Tuppy H. Inhibition of neuraminidase activity by derivatives of 2-deoxy-2,3-dehydro-N-acetylneuraminic acid. *Virology.* 1974 Apr;58(2):457-63.

[31] von Itzstein M, Dyason JC, Oliver SW, White HF, Wu WY, Kok GB, et al. A study of the active site of influenza virus sialidase: an approach to the rational design of novel anti-influenza drugs. *J Med Chem.* 1996 Jan 19;39(2):388-91.

[32] Taylor NR, Cleasby A, Singh O, Skarzynski T, Wonacott AJ, Smith PW, et al. Dihydropyrancarboxamides related to zanamivir: a new series of inhibitors of influenza

virus sialidases. 2. Crystallographic and molecular modeling study of complexes of 4-amino-4H-pyran-6-carboxamides and sialidase from influenza virus types A and B. *J Med Chem.* 1998 Mar 12;41(6):798-807.

[33] Varghese JN, Epa VC, Colman PM. Three-dimensional structure of the complex of 4-guanidino-Neu5Ac2en and influenza virus neuraminidase. *Protein Sci.* 1995 Jun;4(6): 1081-7.

[34] Kim CU, Lew W, Williams M, Liu H, Zhang L, Swaminathan S, et al. Influenza Neuraminidase Inhibitors Possessing a Novel Hydrophobic Interaction in the Enzyme Active Site: Design, Synthesis, and Structural Analysis of Carbocyclic Sialic Acid Analogues with potent Anti-influenza Activity. *J Am Chem Soc.* 1997;119:681-90.

[35] de Jong MD, Tran TT, Truong HK, Vo MH, Smith GJ, Nguyen VC, et al. Oseltamivir resistance during treatment of influenza A (H5N1) infection. *N Engl J Med.* 2005 Dec 22;353(25):2667-72.

[36] Kiso M, Mitamura K, Sakai-Tagawa Y, Shiraishi K, Kawakami C, Kimura K, et al. Resistant influenza A viruses in children treated with oseltamivir: descriptive study. *Lancet.* 2004 Aug 28-Sep 3;364(9436):759-65.

[37] Varghese JN, Smith PW, Sollis SL, Blick TJ, Sahasrabudhe A, McKimm-Breschkin JL, et al. Drug design against a shifting target: a structural basis for resistance to inhibitors in a variant of influenza virus neuraminidase. *Structure.* 1998 Jun 15;6(6):735-46.

[38] Wang MZ, Tai CY, Mendel DB. Mechanism by which mutations at his274 alter sensitivity of influenza a virus n1 neuraminidase to oseltamivir carboxylate and zanamivir. *Antimicrob Agents Chemother.* 2002 Dec;46(12):3809-16.

[39] Yen HL, Herlocher LM, Hoffmann E, Matrosovich MN, Monto AS, Webster RG, et al. Neuraminidase inhibitor-resistant influenza viruses may differ substantially in fitness and transmissibility. *Antimicrob Agents Chemother.* 2005 Oct;49(10):4075-84.

[40] Collins PJ, Haire LF, Lin YP, Liu J, Russell RJ, Walker PA, et al. Crystal structures of oseltamivir-resistant influenza virus neuraminidase mutants. *Nature.* 2008 Jun 26;453(7199):1258-61.

[41] Plotch SJ, Bouloy M, Krug RM. Transfer of 5'-terminal cap of globin mRNA to influenza viral complementary RNA during transcription in vitro. *Proc Natl Acad Sci U S A.* 1979 Apr;76(4):1618-22.

[42] Plotch SJ, Bouloy M, Ulmanen I, Krug RM. A unique cap(m7GpppXm)-dependent influenza virion endonuclease cleaves capped RNAs to generate the primers that initiate viral RNA transcription. *Cell.* 1981 Mar;23(3):847-58.

[43] Hay AJ, Abraham G, Skehel JJ, Smith JC, Fellner P. Influenza virus messenger RNAs are incomplete transcripts of the genome RNAs. *Nucleic Acids Res.* 1977 Dec;4(12): 4197-209.

[44] Hay AJ, Skehel JJ, McCauley J. Characterization of influenza virus RNA complete transcripts. *Virology.* 1982 Jan 30;116(2):517-22.

[45] Biswas SK, Nayak DP. Mutational analysis of the conserved motifs of influenza A virus polymerase basic protein 1. *J Virol.* 1994 Mar;68(3):1819-26.

[46] Blaas D, Patzelt E, Kuechler E. Identification of the cap binding protein of influenza virus. *Nucleic Acids Res.* 1982 Aug 11;10(15):4803-12.

[47] Fechter P, Mingay L, Sharps J, Chambers A, Fodor E, Brownlee GG. Two aromatic residues in the PB2 subunit of influenza A RNA polymerase are crucial for cap binding. *J Biol Chem.* 2003 May 30;273(22):20381-8.

[48]   Ulmanen I, Broni BA, Krug RM. Role of two of the influenza virus core P proteins in recognizing cap 1 structures (m7GpppNm) on RNAs and in initiating viral RNA transcription. *Proc Natl Acad Sci U S A*. 1981 Dec;78(12):7355-9.

[49]   Fodor E, Crow M, Mingay LJ, Deng T, Sharps J, Fechter P, et al. A single amino acid mutation in the PA subunit of the influenza virus RNA polymerase inhibits endonucleolytic cleavage of capped RNAs. *J Virol*. 2002 Sep;76(18):8989-9001.

[50]   Dias A, Bouvier D, Crepin T, McCarthy AA, Hart DJ, Baudin F, et al. The cap-snatching endonuclease of influenza virus polymerase resides in the PA subunit. *Nature*. 2009 Feb 4.

[51]   Hara K, Schmidt FI, Crow M, Brownlee GG. Amino acid residues in the N-terminal region of the PA subunit of influenza A virus RNA polymerase play a critical role in protein stability, endonuclease activity, cap binding, and virion RNA promoter binding. *J Virol*. 2006 Aug;80(16):7789-98.

[52]   Yuan P, Bartlam M, Lou Z, Chen S, Zhou J, He X, et al. Crystal structure of an avian influenza polymerase PA(N) reveals an endonuclease active site. *Nature*. 2009 Feb 4.

[53]   Area E, Martin-Benito J, Gastaminza P, Torreira E, Valpuesta JM, Carrascosa JL, et al. 3D structure of the influenza virus polymerase complex: localization of subunit domains. *Proc Natl Acad Sci U S A*. 2004 Jan 6;101(1):308-13.

[54]   Martin-Benito J, Area E, Ortega J, Llorca O, Valpuesta JM, Carrascosa JL, et al. Three-dimensional reconstruction of a recombinant influenza virus ribonucleoprotein particle. *EMBO Rep*. 2001 Apr;2(4):313-7.

[55]   Torreira E, Schoehn G, Fernandez Y, Jorba N, Ruigrok RW, Cusack S, et al. Three-dimensional model for the isolated recombinant influenza virus polymerase heterotrimer. *Nucleic Acids Res*. 2007;35(11):3774-83.

[56]   Guilligay D, Tarendeau F, Resa-Infante P, Coloma R, Crepin T, Sehr P, et al. The structural basis for cap binding by influenza virus polymerase subunit PB2. *Nat Struct Mol Biol*. 2008 May;15(5):500-6.

[57]   Kuzuhara T, Kise D, Yoshida H, Horita T, Murazaki Y, Nishimura A, et al. Structural Basis of the Influenza A Virus RNA Polymerase PB2 RNA-binding Domain Containing the Pathogenicity-determinant Lysine 627 Residue. *J Biol Chem*. 2009 Mar 13;284(11):6855-60.

[58]   Tarendeau F, Crepin T, Guilligay D, Ruigrok RW, Cusack S, Hart DJ. Host determinant residue lysine 627 lies on the surface of a discrete, folded domain of influenza virus polymerase PB2 subunit. *PLoS Pathog*. 2008;4(8):e1000136.

[59]   Tarendeau F, Boudet J, Guilligay D, Mas PJ, Bougault CM, Boulo S, et al. Structure and nuclear import function of the C-terminal domain of influenza virus polymerase PB2 subunit. *Nat Struct Mol Biol*. 2007 Mar;14(3):229-33.

[60]   He X, Zhou J, Bartlam M, Zhang R, Ma J, Lou Z, et al. Crystal structure of the polymerase PA(C)-PB1(N) complex from an avian influenza H5N1 virus. *Nature*. 2008 Aug 28;454(7208):1123-6.

[61]   Obayashi E, Yoshida H, Kawai F, Shibayama N, Kawaguchi A, Nagata K, et al. The structural basis for an essential subunit interaction in influenza virus RNA polymerase. *Nature*. 2008 Aug 28;454(7208):1127-31.

[62]   Honda A, Mizumoto K, Ishihama A. Two separate sequences of PB2 subunit constitute the RNA cap-binding site of influenza virus RNA polymerase. *Genes Cells*. 1999 Aug;4(8):475-85.

[63] Li ML, Rao P, Krug RM. The active sites of the influenza cap-dependent endonuclease are on different polymerase subunits. *EMBO J*. 2001 Apr 17;20(8):2078-86.

[64] Fechter P, Brownlee GG. Recognition of mRNA cap structures by viral and cellular proteins. *J Gen Virol*. 2005 May;86(Pt 5):1239-49.

[65] Niedzwiecka A, Marcotrigiano J, Stepinski J, Jankowska-Anyszka M, Wyslouch-Cieszynska A, Dadlez M, et al. Biophysical studies of eIF4E cap-binding protein: recognition of mRNA 5' cap structure and synthetic fragments of eIF4G and 4E-BP1 proteins. *J Mol Biol*. 2002 Jun 7;319(3):615-35.

[66] Worch R, Niedzwiecka A, Stepinski J, Mazza C, Jankowska-Anyszka M, Darzynkiewicz E, et al. Specificity of recognition of mRNA 5' cap by human nuclear cap-binding complex. *RNA*. 2005 Sep;11(9):1355-63.

[67] Hooker L, Sully R, Handa B, Ono N, Koyano H, Klumpp K. Quantitative analysis of influenza virus RNP interaction with RNA cap structures and comparison to human cap binding protein eIF4E. *Biochemistry*. 2003 May 27;42(20):6234-40.

[68] Bouloy M, Plotch SJ, Krug RM. Both the 7-methyl and the 2'-O-methyl groups in the cap of mRNA strongly influence its ability to act as primer for influenza virus RNA transcription. *Proc Natl Acad Sci U S A*. 1980 Jul;77(7):3952-6.

[69] Rao P, Yuan W, Krug RM. Crucial role of CA cleavage sites in the cap-snatching mechanism for initiating viral mRNA synthesis. *EMBO J*. 2003 Mar 3;22(5):1188-98.

[70] Braam J, Ulmanen I, Krug RM. Molecular model of a eucaryotic transcription complex: functions and movements of influenza P proteins during capped RNA-primed transcription. *Cell*. 1983 Sep;34(2):609-18.

[71] Kerry PS, Willsher N, Fodor E. A cluster of conserved basic amino acids near the C-terminus of the PB1 subunit of the influenza virus RNA polymerase is involved in the regulation of viral transcription. *Virology*. 2008 Mar 30;373(1):202-10.

[72] Doan L, Handa B, Roberts NA, Klumpp K. Metal ion catalysis of RNA cleavage by the influenza virus endonuclease. *Biochemistry*. 1999 Apr 27;38(17):5612-9.

[73] Hastings JC, Selnick H, Wolanski B, Tomassini JE. Anti-influenza virus activities of 4-substituted 2,4-dioxobutanoic acid inhibitors. *Antimicrob Agents Chemother*. 1996 May;40(5):1304-7.

[74] Nakazawa M, Kadowaki SE, Watanabe I, Kadowaki Y, Takei M, Fukuda H. PA subunit of RNA polymerase as a promising target for anti-influenza virus agents. *Antiviral Res*. 2008 Jun;78(3):194-201.

[75] Singh SB, Tomassini JE. Synthesis of natural flutimide and analogous fully substituted pyrazine-2,6-diones, endonuclease inhibitors of influenza virus. *J Org Chem*. 2001 Aug 10;66(16):5504-16.

[76] Tomassini J, Selnick H, Davies ME, Armstrong ME, Baldwin J, Bourgeois M, et al. Inhibition of cap (m7GpppXm)-dependent endonuclease of influenza virus by 4-substituted 2,4-dioxobutanoic acid compounds. *Antimicrob Agents Chemother*. 1994 Dec;38(12):2827-37.

[77] Tomassini JE, Davies ME, Hastings JC, Lingham R, Mojena M, Raghoobar SL, et al. A novel antiviral agent which inhibits the endonuclease of influenza viruses. *Antimicrob Agents Chemother*. 1996 May;40(5):1189-93.

[78] Parkes KE, Ermert P, Fassler J, Ives J, Martin JA, Merrett JH, et al. Use of a pharmacophore model to discover a new class of influenza endonuclease inhibitors. *J Med Chem*. 2003 Mar 27;46(7):1153-64.

[79]   Cianci C, Tiley L, Krystal M. Differential activation of the influenza virus polymerase via template RNA binding. *J Virol*. 1995 Jul;69(7):3995-9.

[80]   Hagen M, Chung TD, Butcher JA, Krystal M. Recombinant influenza virus polymerase: requirement of both 5' and 3' viral ends for endonuclease activity. *J Virol*. 1994 Mar;68(3):1509-15.

[81]   Lee MT, Bishop K, Medcalf L, Elton D, Digard P, Tiley L. Definition of the minimal viral components required for the initiation of unprimed RNA synthesis by influenza virus RNA polymerase. *Nucleic Acids Res*. 2002 Jan 15;30(2):429-38.

[82]   Li ML, Ramirez BC, Krug RM. RNA-dependent activation of primer RNA production by influenza virus polymerase: different regions of the same protein subunit constitute the two required RNA-binding sites. *EMBO J*. 1998 Oct 1;17(19):5844-52.

[83]   Jung TE, Brownlee GG. A new promoter-binding site in the PB1 subunit of the influenza A virus polymerase. *J Gen Virol*. 2006 Mar;87(Pt 3):679-88.

[84]   Ghanem A, Mayer D, Chase G, Tegge W, Frank R, Kochs G, et al. Peptide-mediated interference with influenza A virus polymerase. *J Virol*. 2007 Jul;81(14):7801-4.

[85]   Gonzalez S, Zurcher T, Ortin J. Identification of two separate domains in the influenza virus PB1 protein involved in the interaction with the PB2 and PA subunits: a model for the viral RNA polymerase structure. *Nucleic Acids Res*. 1996 Nov 15;24(22):4456-63.

[86]   Ohtsu Y, Honda Y, Sakata Y, Kato H, Toyoda T. Fine mapping of the subunit binding sites of influenza virus RNA polymerase. *Microbiol Immunol*. 2002;46(3):167-75.

[87]   Perez DR, Donis RO. A 48-amino-acid region of influenza A virus PB1 protein is sufficient for complex formation with PA. *J Virol*. 1995 Nov;69(11):6932-9.

[88]   Poole EL, Medcalf L, Elton D, Digard P. Evidence that the C-terminal PB2-binding region of the influenza A virus PB1 protein is a discrete alpha-helical domain. *FEBS Lett*. 2007 Nov 13;581(27):5300-6.

[89]   Zurcher T, de la Luna S, Sanz-Ezquerro JJ, Nieto A, Ortin J. Mutational analysis of the influenza virus A/Victoria/3/75 PA protein: studies of interaction with PB1 protein and identification of a dominant negative mutant. *J Gen Virol*. 1996 Aug;77 (Pt 8):1745-9.

[90]   Biswas SK, Nayak DP. Influenza virus polymerase basic protein 1 interacts with influenza virus polymerase basic protein 2 at multiple sites. *J Virol*. 1996 Oct;70(10): 6716-22.

[91]   Guu TS, Dong L, Wittung-Stafshede P, Tao YJ. Mapping the domain structure of the influenza A virus polymerase acidic protein (PA) and its interaction with the basic protein 1 (PB1) subunit. *Virology*. 2008 Sep 15;379(1):135-42.

[92]   Poole E, Elton D, Medcalf L, Digard P. Functional domains of the influenza A virus PB2 protein: identification of NP- and PB1-binding sites. *Virology*. 2004 Mar 30;321(1):120-33.

[93]   Perez DR, Donis RO. Functional analysis of PA binding by influenza a virus PB1: effects on polymerase activity and viral infectivity. *J Virol*. 2001 Sep;75(17):8127-36.

[94]   Chizhmakov IV, Geraghty FM, Ogden DC, Hayhurst A, Antoniou M, Hay AJ. Selective proton permeability and pH regulation of the influenza virus M2 channel expressed in mouse erythroleukaemia cells. *J Physiol*. 1996 Jul 15;494 (Pt 2):329-36.

[95]   Mould JA, Paterson RG, Takeda M, Ohigashi Y, Venkataraman P, Lamb RA, et al. Influenza B virus BM2 protein has ion channel activity that conducts protons across membranes. *Dev Cell*. 2003 Jul;5(1):175-84.

[96] Hay AJ. The action of adamantanamines against influenza A viruses: inhibition of the M2 ion channel protein. *Seminars in Virology.* 1992;3:21-30.

[97] Martin K, Helenius A. Nuclear transport of influenza virus ribonucleoproteins: the viral matrix protein (M1) promotes export and inhibits import. *Cell.* 1991 Oct 4;67(1):117-30.

[98] Sugrue RJ, Bahadur G, Zambon MC, Hall-Smith M, Douglas AR, Hay AJ. Specific structural alteration of the influenza haemagglutinin by amantadine. *EMBO J.* 1990 Nov;9(11):3469-76.

[99] Steinhauer DA, Wharton SA, Skehel JJ, Wiley DC, Hay AJ. Amantadine selection of a mutant influenza virus containing an acid-stable hemagglutinin glycoprotein: evidence for virus-specific regulation of the pH of glycoprotein transport vesicles. *Proc Natl Acad Sci U S A.* 1991 Dec 15;88(24):11525-9.

[100] Dolin R, Reichman RC, Madore HP, Maynard R, Linton PN, Webber-Jones J. A controlled trial of amantadine and rimantadine in the prophylaxis of influenza A infection. *N Engl J Med.* 1982 Sep 2;307(10):580-4.

[101] Hay AJ, Wolstenholme AJ, Skehel JJ, Smith MH. The molecular basis of the specific anti-influenza action of amantadine. *EMBO J.* 1985 Nov;4(11):3021-4.

[102] Duff KC, Gilchrist PJ, Saxena AM, Bradshaw JP. Neutron diffraction reveals the site of amantadine blockade in the influenza A M2 ion channel. *Virology.* 1994 Jul;202(1):287-93.

[103] Hu J, Asbury T, Achuthan S, Li C, Bertram R, Quine JR, et al. Backbone structure of the amantadine-blocked trans-membrane domain M2 proton channel from Influenza A virus. *Biophys J.* 2007 Jun 15;92(12):4335-43.

[104] Czabotar PE, Martin SR, Hay AJ. Studies of structural changes in the M2 proton channel of influenza A virus by tryptophan fluorescence. *Virus Res.* 2004 Jan;99(1):57-61.

[105] Okada A, Miura T, Takeuchi H. Protonation of histidine and histidine-tryptophan interaction in the activation of the M2 ion channel from influenza A virus. *Biochemistry.* 2001 May 22;40(20):6053-60.

[106] Astrahan P, Kass I, Cooper MA, Arkin IT. A novel method of resistance for influenza against a channel-blocking antiviral drug. *Proteins.* 2004 May 1;55(2):251-7.

[107] Stouffer AL, Acharya R, Salom D, Levine AS, Di Costanzo L, Soto CS, et al. Structural basis for the function and inhibition of an influenza virus proton channel. *Nature.* 2008 Jan 31;451(7178):596-9.

[108] Schnell JR, Chou JJ. Structure and mechanism of the M2 proton channel of influenza A virus. *Nature.* 2008 Jan 31;451(7178):591-5.

[109] Yin C, Khan JA, Swapna GV, Ertekin A, Krug RM, Tong L, et al. Conserved Surface Features Form the Double-stranded RNA Binding Site of Non-structural Protein 1 (NS1) from Influenza A and B Viruses. *J Biol Chem.* 2007 Jul 13;282(28):20584-92.

[110] Donelan NR, Basler CF, Garcia-Sastre A. A recombinant influenza A virus expressing an RNA-binding-defective NS1 protein induces high levels of beta interferon and is attenuated in mice. *J Virol.* 2003 Dec;77(24):13257-66.

[111] Min JY, Krug RM. The primary function of RNA binding by the influenza A virus NS1 protein in infected cells: Inhibiting the 2'-5' oligo (A) synthetase/RNase L pathway. *Proc Natl Acad Sci U S A.* 2006 May 2;103(18):7100-5.

[112] Burgui I, Aragon T, Ortin J, Nieto A. PABP1 and eIF4GI associate with influenza virus NS1 protein in viral mRNA translation initiation complexes. *J Gen Virol.* 2003 Dec;84(Pt 12):3263-74.

[113] Noah DL, Twu KY, Krug RM. Cellular antiviral responses against influenza A virus are countered at the posttranscriptional level by the viral NS1A protein via its binding to a cellular protein required for the 3' end processing of cellular pre-mRNAS. *Virology.* 2003 Mar 15;307(2):386-95.

[114] Li S, Min JY, Krug RM, Sen GC. Binding of the influenza A virus NS1 protein to PKR mediates the inhibition of its activation by either PACT or double-stranded RNA. *Virology.* 2006 May 25;349(1):13-21.

[115] Hale BG, Jackson D, Chen YH, Lamb RA, Randall RE. Influenza A virus NS1 protein binds p85beta and activates phosphatidylinositol-3-kinase signaling. *Proc Natl Acad Sci U S A.* 2006 Sep 19;103(38):14194-9.

[116] Chien CY, Tejero R, Huang Y, Zimmerman DE, Rios CB, Krug RM, et al. A novel RNA-binding motif in influenza A virus non-structural protein 1. *Nat Struct Biol.* 1997 Nov;4(11):891-5.

[117] Liu J, Lynch PA, Chien CY, Montelione GT, Krug RM, Berman HM. Crystal structure of the unique RNA-binding domain of the influenza virus NS1 protein. *Nat Struct Biol.* 1997 Nov;4(11):896-9.

[118] Wang W, Riedel K, Lynch P, Chien CY, Montelione GT, Krug RM. RNA binding by the novel helical domain of the influenza virus NS1 protein requires its dimer structure and a small number of specific basic amino acids. *RNA.* 1999 Feb;5(2):195-205.

[119] Cheng A, Wong SM, Yuan YA. Structural basis for dsRNA recognition by NS1 protein of influenza A virus. *Cell Res.* 2009 Feb;19(2):187-95.

[120] Bornholdt ZA, Prasad BV. X-ray structure of influenza virus NS1 effector domain. *Nat Struct Mol Biol.* 2006 Jun;13(6):559-60.

[121] Hale BG, Barclay WS, Randall RE, Russell RJ. Structure of an avian influenza A virus NS1 protein effector domain. *Virology.* 2008 Aug 15;378(1):1-5.

[122] Xia S, Monzingo AF, Robertus JD. Structure of NS1A effector domain from the influenza A/Udorn/72 virus. *Acta Crystallogr D Biol Crystallogr.* 2009 Jan;65(Pt 1):11-7.

[123] Bornholdt ZA, Prasad BV. X-ray structure of NS1 from a highly pathogenic H5N1 influenza virus. *Nature.* 2008 Dec 18;456(7224):985-8.

[124] Das K, Ma LC, Xiao R, Radvansky B, Aramini J, Zhao L, et al. Structural basis for suppression of a host antiviral response by influenza A virus. *Proc Natl Acad Sci U S A.* 2008 Sep 2;105(35):13093-8.

Chapter 10

THE STRUCTURE-BASED DESIGN OF NOVEL INHIBITORS OF H5N1 VIRUS NEURAMINIDASE[*]

Petar M. Mitrasinovic[†]

Belgrade Institute of Science and Technology, Belgrade, Serbia

ABSTRACT

In the context of both a recent pandemic threat by the worldwide spread of H5N1 avian influenza and the high resistance of H5N1 virus to the most widely used commercial drug, oseltamivir-OTV (Tamiflu), the structure-based design of novel H5N1 neuraminidase (NA) inhibitors is a research topic of vital importance at this time. Possible structures of more potent H5N1-NA inhibitors are herein examined using contemporary principles of conformational analysis. A specific criterion used for the determination of fully acceptable conformations of potential inhibitors is the previous experimental proposal (ref. 5) of exploiting potential benefits for drug design offered by the "150-cavity" adjacent to the H5N1-NA active site (Figure 1). Using the crystal structure of H5N1-NA (PDB ID: 2hty) as the starting point, in a set of 54 inhibitors that had been proposed by modifying the side chains of oseltamivir (ref. 4), 4 inhibitors were identified using two different computational strategies (ArgusLab4.0.1, FlexX-E3.0.1) both to lower the binding free energy (BFE) of oseltamivir and to have partially acceptable conformations. In agreement with the experimental proposal (ref. 5), these four oseltamivir structure-based analogues were found to adopt the most promising conformations identifying the guanidinium side chain of Arg156 as a prospective partner for making polar contacts. In contrast to the experimental proposal (ref. 5), none of the modified 4-amino groups of oseltamivir in the four favorable conformations was found to make polar contacts with the guanidinium side chain of Arg156. Hence, two novel inhibitor structures were designed and shown to further lower the binding free energy of OTV relative to the previous 54 inhibitors. These two novel structures clearly suggest

---

[*] Much of the material contained in this contribution is taken from our previous paper with the kind permission from Elsevier [1], as specifically acknowledged in the reference list.

[†] Correspondence to: petar.mitrasinovic@gmail.com.

that it may be possible for a new substituent to be developed by functional modifications at position of the 4-amino group of oseltamivir in order to make polar contacts with the guanidinium side chain of Arg156, and thereby enhance the binding of a more potent inhibitor. Several key standpoints for designing novel structures of potentially more effective H5N1-NA inhibitors are discussed.

1. INTRODUCTION

Due to different antigenic properties of various glycoprotein molecules, influenza type A viruses are classified into two phylogenetically distinct groups—group-1 (N1, N4, N5, N8) and group-2 (N2, N3, N6, N7, N9)—which contain N1 and N2 NAs of viruses that currently circulate in humans. One such virus is H5N1 avian influenza NA, threatening a new pandemic. The high resistance of H5N1 virus to oseltamivir makes the structure-based design of novel anti-viral molecules a priority [2-4]. The crystal structure of H5N1-NA offers a wide spectrum of new opportunities for drug design [5,6]. This can be accounted for by structural differences between group-1 (N1, N4, N5, N8) and group-2 (N2, N3, N6, N7, N9) NAs. A major consequence of these differences in structure is the presence of a large cavity, known as the "150-cavity", adjacent to the active site in group-1 but not in group-2 neuraminidases. This cavity is accessible from the N1 active site due to the differences in the position of Asp151 and Glu119. The combined effect of the differences in the position of these two particular residues results in a width increase of the active site cavity by about 5 Å. The conserved Arg156, having the side chain approximately mid-way between Asp151 and Glu119 (Figure 1) and being at the base of the "150-cavity", adopts almost the same position in the group-1 and group-2 NA structures, thus defining the entrance from the N1 active site into the "150-cavity". Tyr347 is also shown in Figure 1 because this particular residue in group-1 NAs makes a hydrogen bond interaction with the C1 carboxylate of oseltamivir [5]. N1 neuraminidase initially binds to OTV in this open conformation, but more likely adopts the higher energy or closed conformation of the 150-loop (residues 147-152) via a relatively slow conformational change. Based on an examination of the crystal structure of OTV/H5N1-NA (PDB ID: 2hu0B), it has been proposed [5] that new, more potent inhibitors may be developed from the 4-amino group of oseltamivir into the "150-cavity", while the prominent guanidinium side chain of Arg156 has been hypothesized as a prospective partner for a salt-bridge or hydrogen bond with a new inhibitor (Figure 1). This proposal is herein explored and rationalized.

2. METHODS

Flexible docking calculations were performed using two different methods: (**I**) the AScore/ShapeDock protocol from the ArgusLab4.0.1 suite of programs [7] and (**II**) the FlexX-E3.0.1 program [8,9].

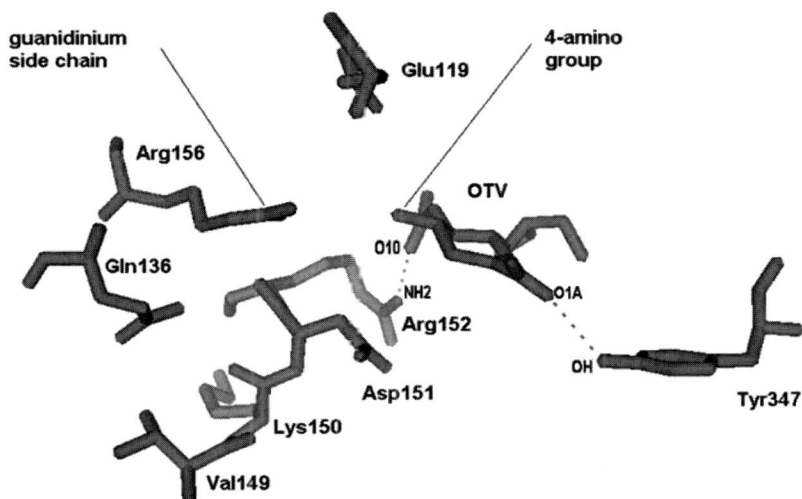

Figure 1. Experimental proposal of the possibility of exploiting the "150-cavity" of H5N1-NA (PDB ID: 2hu0B) by developing a new substituent from the 4-amino group of oseltamivir (OTV) making polar contacts with the guanidinium side chain of Arg156 [1].

I. AScore is based on the decomposition of the total protein-ligand binding free energy, taking into account the following contributions: the van der Waals interaction between the ligand and the protein, the hydrophobic effect, the hydrogen bonding between the ligand and the protein, the hydrogen bonding involving charged donor and/or acceptor groups, the deformation effect, and the effects of the translational and rotational entropy loss in the binding process, respectively. The ShapeDock docking engine approximates a complicated search problem. Flexible ligand docking is available by describing the ligand as a torsion tree. Groups of bonded atoms that do not have rotatable bonds are nodes, while torsions are connections between the nodes. Topology of a torsion tree is a determinative factor influencing efficient docking. The AScore/ShapeDock protocol is fast, reproducible, and formally explores all energy minima [7]. This particular protocol was shown to be very consistent for docking OTV in the crystal structures of H5N1 NAs and thus proposed to have the potential for the successful structure-based design of new anti-viral molecules [2].

II. The FlexX scoring function [10] is an estimate of the free binding energy for an ideal hydrogen bond, ionic, aromatic, or lipophilic protein-ligand interaction, adjusted by a penalty function depending on deviation from the ideal interatomic radius for the two interacting elements [11]. The computational algorithm underlying FlexX is based on the decomposition of a ligand into pieces, which are then flexibly built up in the active site using a variety of placement strategies. To take into account receptor flexibility, the docking experiment also consists of an ensemble-based soft docking procedure using FlexX-Ensemble [12]. At the very end, an effective flexible receptor-ligand complex optimization is accomplished by means of the Yasara program [13]. All the calculations were done using default parameters.

Figures shown in this paper were generated by PyMol [14].

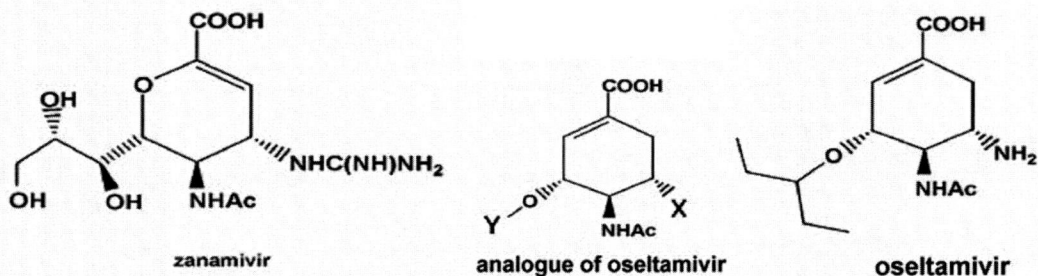

Figure 2. Oseltamivir structure-based analogues [4] that were considered in tables S1 and S2 given in the Supplementary material of [1].

3. STRUCTURE-BASED DESIGN OF
NOVEL H5N1 NEURAMINIDASE INHIBITORS

The binding of the previously proposed [4] structures of 54 oseltamivir analogues (Figure 2) to H5N1-NA (PDB ID: 2hty) was herein investigated using FlexX-E (Table S1, Supplementary material of ref. 1) and ArgusLab (Table S2, Supplementary material of ref. 1). Besides considering the binding free energies of the complexes for identifying the promising candidates for more potent inhibitors, conformational requirement, based on the experimental proposal for exploiting the "150-cavity" of H5N1-NA (Figure 1), was considered too. A most favorable conformation was thus viewed to have a modified 4-amino group of oseltamivir making polar contacts with the guanidinium side chain of Arg156.

Four inhibitors (11 and 12 with X = $NHC(=NH_2^+)NH_2$; 13 and 17 with X = $NHC(=N-CH_4^+)NH_2$) were identified both to lower the binding free energy of oseltamivir (Tables S1 and S2, Supplementary material of ref. 1) and to have partially acceptable conformations. All the spatial orientations of the particular inhibitors (Figure 3) properly make polar contacts with the guanidinium side chain of Arg156, but none of them has its X side chain (modified 4-amino group of OTV) involved in the interactions with Arg156, as experimentally proposed (Figure 1). While the carboxylic group of ligand 11 makes a polar contact with Arg156 (Figure 3a), the –O-Y side chain of ligand 12 makes 2 polar contacts with Arg156 (Figure 3b). Note that the X side chain of ligand 11 (Figure 3a) is not involved in any polar contact, while the X side chain of ligand 12 makes 1 intraligand polar contact with the carboxylic group (Figure 3b), thus accounting for the difference in position of the X group of ligand 11 relative to that of ligand 12. The X side chain of ligand 13 makes 2 polar contacts with Asp151 (Figure 3c), while that of ligand 17 makes 1 polar contact with Asp151 (Figure 3d). At the first look, this might indicate a similar spatial orientation of the ligands 13 and 17. However, it is important to note 1 electrostatic interaction between Tyr347 and the C1 carboxylate of ligand 17 (Figure 3d), which also exists in the case of ligand 12 (Figure 3b). The specific Tyr347-carboxylic group contact is not present in the cases of ligands 11 and 13 (Figures 3a and 3c), thus showing different spatial orientation of the –COOH group in these ligands relative to that in ligands 12 and 17 (Figures 3b and 3d).

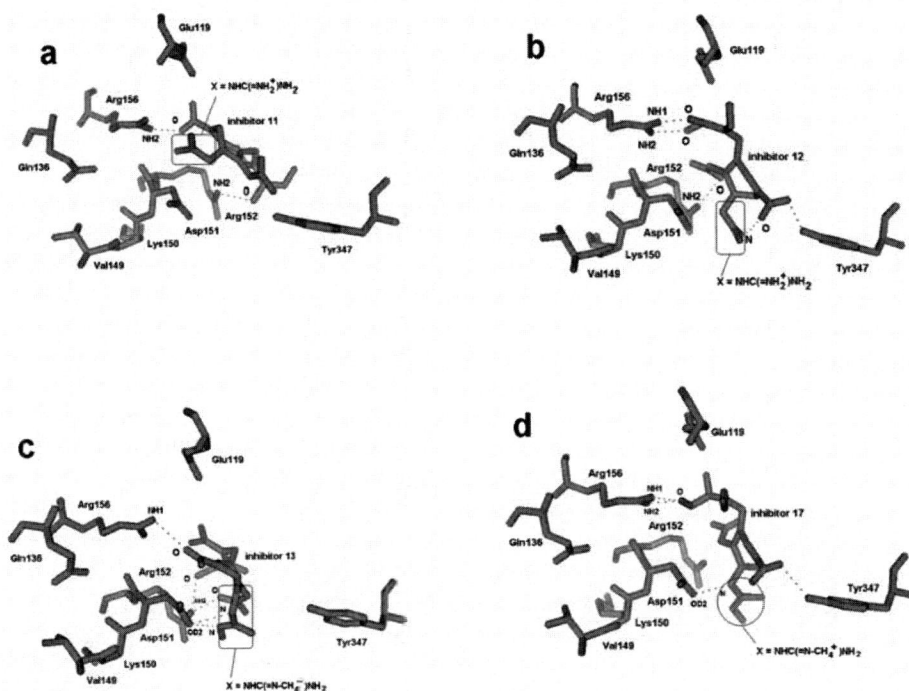

Figure 3. The conformations of (**a**) ligand 11 ($X = NHC(=NH_2^+)NH_2$), (**b**) ligand 12 ($X = NHC(=NH_2^+)NH_2$), (**c**) ligand 13 ($X = NHC(=N-CH_4^+)NH_2$), and (**d**) ligand 17 ($X = NHC(=N-CH_4^+)NH_2$) considered in table S2 (Supplementary material of ref. 1) using AScore.'ShapeDock. All the conformations properly identify the guanidinium side chain of Arg156 as a prospective partner for making polar contacts, but none of the contacts is with the X side chain (modified 4-amino group of OTV) of the inhibitors, as experimentally proposed in Figure 1 [1].

The same set of 54 potential inhibitors (Table S1, Supplementary material of ref. 1) was previously investigated using two different scoring functions, the Amber and Grid scores, implemented in the Dock6.01 program [4]. Of these 54 ligands, the identified inhibitors, having both the better binding affinity with respect to oseltamivir and the most favorable conformations, were: inhibitors 4, 7 and 13 with $X = NHC(=NH_2^+)NH_2$, inhibitor 14 with $X = NH_3^+$, and inhibitor 14 with $X = NHC(=NH_2^+)NH_2$ [4]. Because the conformational requirement for selecting the most favorable conformations in the previous study [4] was substantially different from the experimental proposal shown in Figure 1, these 5 previously identified favorable conformations [4] are distinct from the 4 most promising ones shown in Figure 3.

Since the spatial orientation of the –COOH group is different in the ligands 11, 12, 13, and 17 (Figure 3) as discussed above, and none of the particular conformations was found to fit the "150-cavity" as experimentally proposed (Figure 1), it is therefore difficult to say which one of the 4 favorable conformations would be the most rational choice leading to the structure-based design of more potent inhibitors. It is well established that two or three Arg residues surrounding the carboxylic group of NA inhibitors play a key role in orienting and stabilizing various inhibitors [15,16]. The fact that Arg156 makes 1 polar contact with the – COOH group in the inhibitors 11 and 13 (Figures 3a and 3c) was the first crucial idea for us to attempt to exploit two nearby Arg residues, Arg152 and Arg156, as a predominant factor for orienting and stabilizing novel inhibitors by making electrostatic interactions with the carboxylic group. The second crucial idea was that the X side chain of novel inhibitors needs to be involved in electrostatic contacts with the guanidinium side chain of Arg156, as experimentally proposed (Figure 1). Taking into account the high resistance of H5N1-NA both to oseltamivir and most likely to the OTV analogues [4], the third crucial idea was to increase the probability of escaping viable drug-resistant H5N1 mutants by maintaining a clear resemblance of the structures of more potent inhibitors to sialic acid, a natural substrate from which zanamivir is directly derived with minimal functional modifications (Figure 2), as more recently recommended experimentally [6] and computationally [2]. To reconcile these three standpoints of vital importance for developing novel structures of potentially more effective inhibitors, chemical intuition was employed.

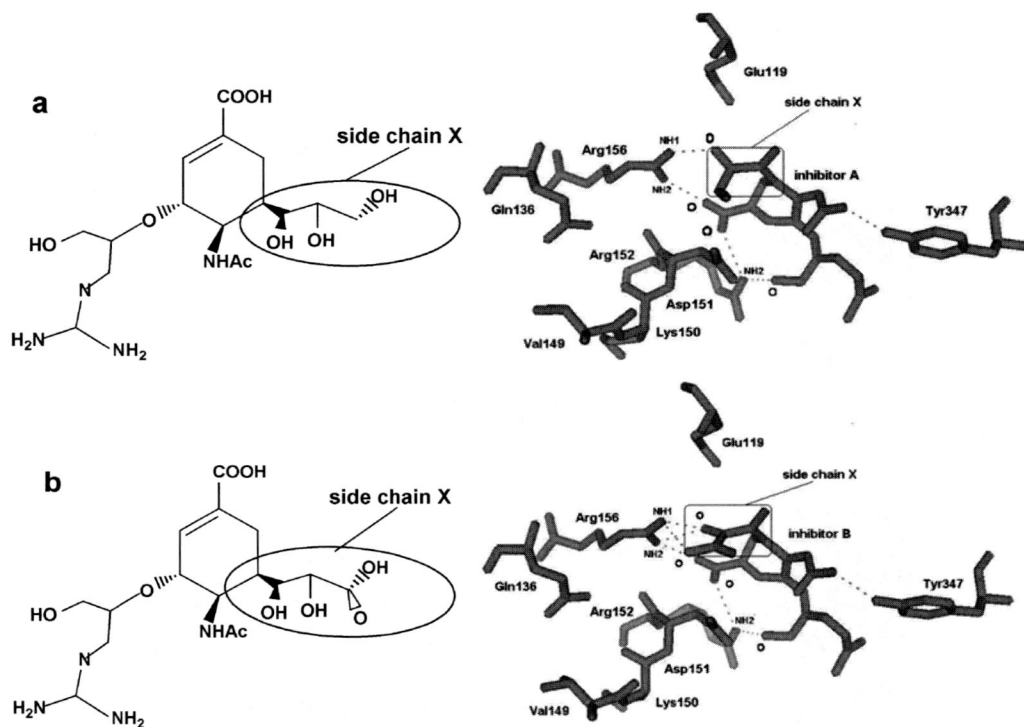

Figure 4. (a) Proposal of chemical structure of new inhibitor A designed by AScore/ShapeDock. The X side chain makes 1 polar contact with Arg156. The BFEs of the H5N1 NA-inhibitor A complex are -9.17 kcal/mol (ArgusLab) and -51.56 kcal/mol (FlexX-E). (b) Proposal of chemical structure of new inhibitor B designed by AScore/ShapeDock. The X side chain makes 3 polar contacts with Arg156. The BFEs of the H5N1 NA-inhibitor B complex are -9.37 kcal/mol (ArgusLab) and -58.78 kcal/mol (FlexX-E). Note that the BFEs of the H5N1 NA-oseltamivir complex are -5.89 kcal/mol (ArgusLab) and -41.06 kcal/mol (FlexX-E) [1].

Oseltamivir, having the –O-Y group instead of the glycerol side chain, is quite a different inhibitor from zanamivir (Figure 2). The key difference is the –O-Y group of OTV that is capable of rotating around the single bond between oxygen and alkyl chain Y, thus adapting itself to a comfortable position relative to its environment. Hence, various modifications (Table S1, Supplementary material of ref. 1) of the 4-amino group of OTV did not establish a consistent spatial orientation of the carboxylic group, which could stabilize the oseltamivir analogues by providing an effective fit of the "150-cavity". Shortly after this indication in our search for more potent inhibitor structures, it became interesting that the nature of the X side chain must be quite different from that of the 4-amino group of OTV in order to have the – COOH group stabilized by the Arg152 and Arg156 amino acid residues. The fact that the X side chains of the oseltamivir derivatives (Table S1, Supplementary material of ref. 1) were not involved in electrostatic interactions with Arg156 indicated that substantial modifications of the 4-amino group are expected to be followed by substantial modifications of the Y side chain of OTV. After examining many different substituents for the alkyl chain Y, it was quite indicative that the particular side chain needs to be primarily based on oxygen and nitrogen atoms that are able to make additional electrostatic interactions. In this context, the first encouraging proposal of a new inhibitor structure was that given in Figure 4a. The binding free energies of the H5N1 NA-inhibitor A complex, determined by FlexX-E and ArgusLab, are -51.56 kcal/mol and -9.17 kcal/mol respectively. The computed energies are lower than those reported in tables S1 and S2 (Supplementary material of ref. 1). The carboxylic group of inhibitor A makes 2 polar contacts, the first with Arg152 and the second with Arg156. In agreement with the experimental proposal (Figure 1), the X side chain of inhibitor A makes 1 polar contact with Arg156 (Figure 4a). A slight modification, reflected by introducing a – COOH group at the very end of the X side chain of inhibitor A, led to the most encouraging chemical structure of inhibitor B shown in Figure 4b. The binding free energies of the H5N1 NA-inhibitor B complex, determined by FlexX-E and ArgusLab, are -58.78 kcal/mol and - 9.37 kcal/mol respectively. The first of the computed energies is significantly lower (by about 7 kcal/mol) than that reported above for inhibitor A. Besides, the carboxylic group of inhibitor B makes 3 polar contacts with Arg residues, 1 with Arg152 and 2 with Arg156. Most importantly, the X side chain of inhibitor B properly identifies the guanidinium side chain of Arg156 as a prospective partner by making 3 polar contacts with Arg156 (Figure 4b). Because the experimental structure of H5N1 avian influenza neuraminidase, in the same way, previously suggested new opportunities for the design of more potent anti-viral molecules [5], the proposed inhibitor structures (Figure 4) are believed to confer specificity for avain flu strain of influenza.

4. SUMMARY

Two novel structures (Figure 4) of possibly more effective H5N1-NA inhibitors suggest that successful modifications of both the -O-Y and 4-amino side chains of oseltamivir are possible in order to exploit experimentally identified potential benefits (Figure 1) offered by the "150-cavity" adjacent to the H5N1-NA active site. Interestingly, a slightly modified Y side chain of zanamivir (Figure 2) may be a promising candidate for the X side chain of novel inhibitors. Two Arg residues, Arg152 from the 150-loop and Arg156, are presumably needed to make electrostatic interactions with the carboxylic group of potential inhibitors, thus being a prevailing factor for orienting and stabilizing more potent candidates.

REFERENCES

[1]   Reprinted from *Biophysical Chemistry*, Vol. 140/Issues 1-3, Petar M. Mitrasinovic, On the structure-based design of novel inhibitors of H5N1 influenza A virus neuraminidase (NA), 35-38, ©2009 Elsevier B.V. All rights reserved, with permission from Elsevier (2116690946828).

[2]   Mihajlovic, M. L. & Mitrasinovic, P. M. (2008). Another look at the molecular mechanism of the resistance of H5N1 influenza A virus neuraminidase (NA) to oseltamivir (OTV). *Biophysical Chemistry, 136,* 152-158.

[3]   von Itzstein, M. (2007). The war against influenza: discovery and development of sialidase inhibitors. *Nature Reviews Drug Discovery, 6,* 967-974.

[4]   Du, Q-S.; Wang, S-Q. & Chou, K-C. (2007). Analogue inhibitors by modifying oseltamivir based on the crystal neuraminidase structure for treating drug-resistant H5N1 virus. *Biochem. Biophys. Res. Commun., 362,* 525-531.

[5]   Russell, R.; Haire, L.; Stevens, D.; Collins, P.; Lin, Y.; Blackburn, G.; Hay, A.; Gamblin, S., & Skehel, J. (2006). The structure of H5N1 avian influenza neuraminidase suggests new opportunities for drug design. *Nature, 443,* 45-49.

[6]   Collins, P. J.; Haire, L. F.; Lin, Y. P.; Liu, J.; Russell, R. J.; Walker, P. A.; Skehel, J. J.; Martin, S. R.; Hay, A. J.; & Gamblin, S. J. (2008). Crystal structures of oseltamivir-resistant influenza virus neuraminidase mutants. *Nature, 453,* 1258-1261.

[7]   Thompson, M. A. (2004). ArgusLab 4.0.1. Planaria Software LLC, Seatle, WA, http://www.arguslab.com.

[8]   Claussen, H.; Buning, C.; Rarey, M.; & Lengauer, T. (2001). FlexE: efficient molecular docking considering protein structure variation. J. Mol. Biol., 308, 377-395.

[9]   Rarey, M. 2008. FlexX 3.0.1. BioSolveIT GmbH, St. Augustin, Germany, http://www.biosolveit.de.

[10]   Gastreich, M.; Lilienthal, M.; Briem, H.; & Claussen, H. (2006). Ultrafast de novo docking combining pharmacophores and combinatorics. *J. Comput. -Aided Mol. Des., 20,* 717-734.

[11]   Böhm, H. –J. (1994). The development of a simple empirical scoring function to estimate the binding constant for a protein-ligand complex of known three-dimensional structure. *J. Comput. -Aided Mol. Des., 8,* 243-256.

[12]   Rarey, M.; Kramer, B.; Lengauer, T.; & Klebe, G. (1996). A fast flexible docking method using an incremental construction algorithm. *J. Mol. Biol., 261,* 470-489.

[13]   Krieger, E. YASARA Biosciences, Graz, Austria, http://www.yasara.org/.

[14]   DeLano, W. L. (2004). PyMol™. Release 0.97. DeLano Scientific LLC, San Carlos, CA.

[15]   Wang, T. & Wade, R. C. (2001). Comparative binding energy (COMBINE) analysis of influenza neuraminidase-inhibitor complexes. *J. Med. Chem., 44,* 961-971.

[16]   Ortiz, A. R.; Pisabarro, M. T.; Gago, F.; & Wade, R. C. (1995). Prediction of drug binding affinities by comparative binding energy analysis. *J. Med. Chem., 38,* 2681-2691.

PART IV:
VACCINES AGAINST INFLUENZA

In: Global View of Fight against Influenza ISBN: 978-1-60741-952-5
Editor: Petar M. Mitrasinovic © 2009 Nova Science Publishers, Inc.

Chapter 11

ON THE DEVELOPMENT OF VACCINES AGAINST PANDEMIC INFLUENZA

*Petar M. Mitrasinovic**

Belgrade Institute of Science and Technology, Belgrade, Serbia

Definition of a pandemic influenza A virus comprises the following: (1) isolation from humans of an influenza A virus with a novel hemagglutinin or a novel hemagglutinin and neuraminidase gene, (2) susceptibility (lack of antibody) to this novel virus in a large proportion of the population, and (3) demonstrated ability of the virus to cause disease and spread from person-to-person [1]. During an influenza pandemic, the immune status of the population would differ from that existing during interpandemic periods. Since its emergence in 1997, the highly pathogenic avian influenza virus (H5N1) has affected wild birds and poultry in more than 10 Asian countries as well as in Europe and Africa. A total of 321 confirmed human cases have occurred since late 2003 resulting in 194 deaths and a fatality rate of approximately 60%. Selected clinical features of H5N1 influenza in humans include the following: (i) an incubation period of 2–8 days, possibly as long as 17 days (versus 2–3 days with seasonal flu); (ii) initial symptoms such as high fever (usually > 38°C) and influenza-like symptoms—diarrhea, vomiting, abdominal pain, chest pain, and bleeding from the nose and gums; (iii) early involvement of lower respiratory tract; and (iv) atypical presentations with no respiratory symptoms—acute encephalitis, diarrhea [2]. Although there are currently some antiviral drugs available for treatment of influenza virus infection, H5N1 has proven resistant to most, therefore emphasizing the need for an effective vaccine.

Universal flu vaccines have been proposed, but none currently exists on the market. There is a fundamental problem associated with the development of a vaccine that has not been solved so far. The more the pandemic virus differs antigenically from the vaccine virus, the less effective the vaccine will be. If the pandemic is caused by a virus of a different subtype, the vaccine will be no good at all [3]. The fact that many manufacturers are making a split H5N1 influenza virus or "subunit" vaccine, when they should be making a whole, inactivated virus vaccine, is closely related to its dose-dependent effectiveness. At low doses,

---

* Correspondence to: petar.mitrasinovic@gmail.com.

the whole virus vaccine is very much better at inducing an antibody response than the split virus vaccine, while at high doses, there is little difference between the two [4]. The whole virus vaccine can cause some unwanted side reactions, worse in some people than in others, but it is unlikely that any H5N1 vaccine would be used for mass immunization before a pandemic. The advantage of making a whole virus vaccine is that in an emergency the lower dose required means there would be much more vaccine to go around for everyone [3].

According to the Federal Drug Administration (FDA), influenza vaccine production timeline include: virus selection (January–May), testing and licensure (June, July), filling and packaging (August), product release and shipping (September), and beginning of vaccination (Oct, Nov). Immunity usually develops approximately two weeks after vaccination. Selected strategies for influenza vaccines are (a) inactivated or "killed" vaccines; (b) live, attenuated vaccines; (c) DNA vaccines; (d) recombinant subunit vaccines; (e) recombinant vector vaccines; and (f) synthetic peptide vaccines [1]. The manufacture of vaccines from pathogenic avian influenza viruses by traditional methods is not feasible for safety reasons as well as technical issues, which need solving beforehand [5].

The highly pathogenic H5N1 viruses are too dangerous to use by vaccine manufacturers. This problem has been solved by the use of reverse genetics to attenuate the H5N1 viruses, followed by a series of safety tests to demonstrate safety before shipment to vaccine manufacturers [6].

It appears that an H5N1 vaccine must be formulated in a different way from seasonal vaccines, in order to stimulate robust immune responses. This in turn requires re-licensing of candidate pandemic vaccines. There has been a lot of regulatory activity in the European Union (EU) and the United States of America to provide guidance to vaccine manufacturers. Much of the pandemic vaccine preparation in the EU is now directed toward obtaining an EU pandemic vaccine license [6].

In clinical trials, conventional surface-antigen influenza virus vaccines produced from avian viruses have proved poorly immunogenic in immunologically naive populations. Adjuvant or whole-virus preparations may improve immunogenicity and allow sparing of antigen [5].

The occurrence of antigenic variant H5N1 viruses in birds and man has an impact on vaccine development and attempts to stockpile vaccines. In the short term, new vaccine viruses must be developed and made available to vaccine manufacturers, but in the long term it is necessary to explore alternative vaccination strategies, including those based on conserved regions of the virus [6].

Since vaccination is the principal means to combat the impact of influenza, an emerging pandemic virus will create a surge in worldwide vaccine demand and new approaches in immunization strategies may be needed to ensure optimum protection of unprimed individuals when vaccine antigen may be limited. Therefore, major challenges to pandemic vaccine development and availability are to (a) expand production of current (egg-based) vaccine, (b) accelerate development of modern (non-egg) vaccines, (c) evaluate dose-sparing technology (adjuvant, intramuscular vs. intradermal route), and (d) target new antigens [1].

REFERENCES

[1]   Lambert, L. (2006) Pandemic threats and security: research in action. *31st Annual AAAS Forum on Science and Technology Policy*, Washington, DC, 20-26 April.

[2]   Beigel, J. H. et al. (2005) Avian influenza A (H5N1) infection in humans. *The New England Journal of Medicine, 353,* 1374-1385.

[3]   Laver, G. W. (2006) Submission to the Royal Society and Academy of Medical Sciences' call for evidence on pandemic influenza. March 1, http://royalsociety.org/page.asp?id=5573&tip=1.

[4]   Webster, R. G. & Laver, W. G. (1966) Influenza virus subunit vaccines: immunogenicity and lack of toxicity for rabbits of ether and detergent-disrupted virus. *J. Immunology, 96,* 596-605.

[5]   Stephenson, I. et al. (2004) Confronting the avian influenza threat: vaccine development for a potential pandemic. *Lancet Infect. Dis., 4,* 499-509.

[6]   Wood, J. & Robertson, J. (2006) Development of vaccines against pandemic influenza. *Journal of Clinical Virology, 36 (suppl 2),* S4.

In: Global View of Fight against Influenza
Editor: Petar M. Mitrasinovic

ISBN: 978-1-60741-952-5
© 2009 Nova Science Publishers, Inc.

Chapter 12

ALTERNATIVE STRATEGIES FOR VACCINE DEVELOPMENT AGAINST AVIAN FLU

Michele A. Zacks[1] and Slobodan Paessler[1,2,]*

[1] Galveston National Laboratory and Institute for Human Infections and Immunity, Department of Pathology, University of Texas Medical Branch (UTMB), Galveston, USA

[2] Sealy Center for Vaccine Development, Department of Pediatrics, UTMB, Galveston, USA

ABSTRACT

Intense focus has been placed on investigation of vaccine strategies that provide cross-protection against H5N1. In April of 2007, an inactivated influenza A/Vietnam/1203/04 (H5N1) vaccine developed by Sanofi-Aventi was approved by the U.S. Food and Drug Administration, despite its suboptimal efficacy profile. Nonetheless, other approaches to vaccine development are being tested, including recombinant subunit, viral vectored and plasmid DNA (pDNA) vaccines. This chapter will focus on several alternative H5N1 vaccines and therapeutic antibody approaches not covered in previous reviews: linear DNA vaccines, protein-based flagellin conjugate vaccines, and an alphavirus based vaccine approach. In addition, we describe some of the animal models potentially useful for testing the efficacy of the vaccine candidates against avian influenza.

* Corresponding author: Slobodan Paessler, Department of Pathology, Galveston National Laboratory, UTMB, 301 University Boulevard, Galveston, TX 77555-1019. Phone (409) 747-0764. Fax: (409) 747-0762. E-mail: slpaessl@utmb.edu

INTRODUCTION

Overview

Several comprehensive reviews on the status of the development of effective prophylactics, particularly on vaccines against highly pathogenic avian influenza A (H5N1), have been published recently [1-6]. Intense focus has been placed on investigation of vaccine strategies that provide cross-protection against H5N1. In April of 2007, an inactivated influenza A/Vietnam/1203/04 (H5N1) vaccine developed by Sanofi-Aventi was approved by the U.S. Food and Drug Administration, despite its suboptimal efficacy profile [7-10]. Nonetheless, other approaches to vaccine development are being tested, including recombinant subunit, viral vectored and plasmid DNA (pDNA) vaccines. These studies have shown some promise in preclinical as well as clinical studies. Manufacturing of influenza vaccines remains an important limitation to the timely production of vaccine stocks for use in avian influenza outbreaks.

This chapter will focus on several alternative H5N1 vaccines and therapeutic antibody approaches not covered in these reviews: linear DNA vaccines [11, 12], protein-based flagellin conjugate vaccines [13], and an alphavirus based vaccine approach [14].

Animal Model of HPAI

The inbred mouse (female BALB/c strain) is a widely-accepted animal model for the study of influenza A and for drug/vaccine efficacy testing [15]. The studies described in this review have utilized an influenza A/Vietnam/1203/04 (H5N1, VN04)-BALB/c challenge model for preclinical studies. The rationale for use of VN04 among other H5N1 isolates was the suggestion by several studies that VN04, isolated from a fatal human case in 2004, may be more virulent than certain 1997 Hong Kong isolates and that rapid infection of and replication in the central nervous system may account for this difference [16-18]. Survival studies have shown that doses in the range of 1.8 PFU to 1.8×10^3 PFU per animal will infect the lungs and brain, result in encephalitis, and are lethal in six-week-old female Balb/c mice ([19] and Paessler, unpublished data). These outcomes occur without prior adaptation of the virus, unlike the adapted H1N1 virus, PR8 [20], which is used for evaluation of seasonal influenza vaccines. Clinical disease is associated with hypothermia and loss of body weight.

The target challenge dose for vaccine and antiviral studies was initially selected based upon a limited fifty percent lethal dose study [19] and was subsequently verified in numerous replicate studies. For mice inoculated with H5N1 doses of $>2 \times 10^3$ $TCID_{50}$ per mouse, 100% develop paralysis or died between day 7 and 10 post-infection. To date, we have conducted H5N1 studies in the mouse model that includes a cumulative total of >2000 mice, confirming this dose selection. A representative selection of these dose-response studies is shown in Figure 1.

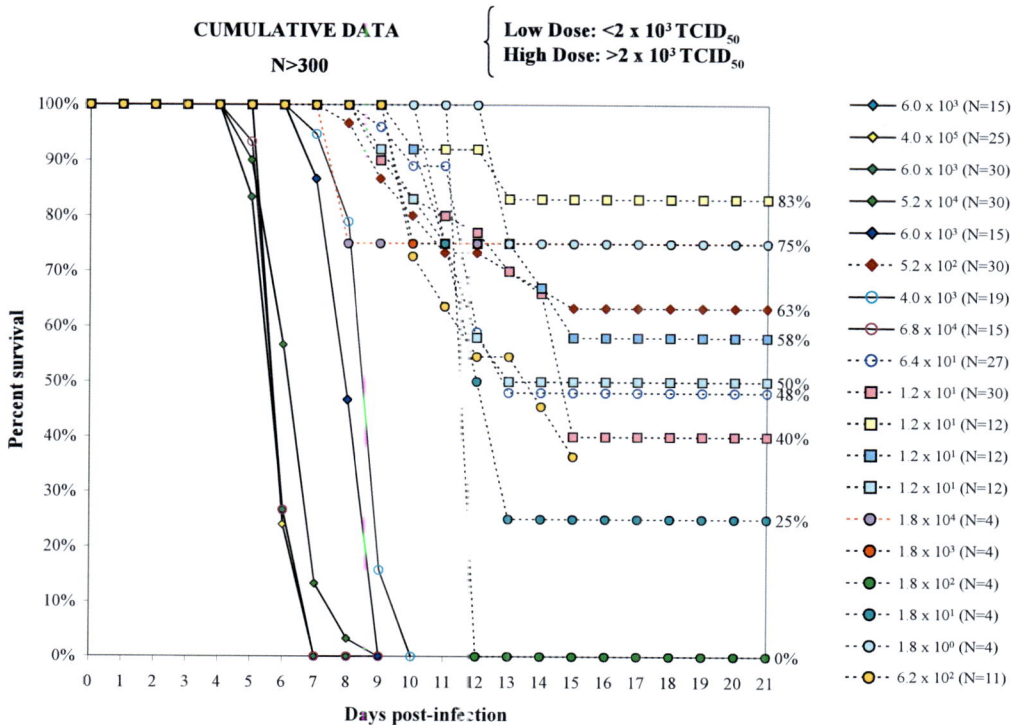

Figure 1. H5N1 dose-response in the mouse model. Data compiled from several independent intranasal infection studies is shown. Survival represents non-paralyzed animals. The fifty percent tissue culture infective ($TCID_{50}$) dose of influenza delivered per mouse and the number of animals per group (N, in parentheses) is indicated in the legend.

SYNDNA™ VACCINE

Background

The traditional approach to DNA vaccination has been to utilize plasmid-driven gene expression (pDNA) to elicit an immune response to defined proteins or their subunits (antigens or epitopes). To date, although there are no approved pDNA vaccine products for humans, three therapies for non-infectious diseases are in phase III clinical trials [21], and a variety of therapies are in phase I or II trials [22]. Four pDNA vaccines have been approved, two for antiviral and one for anticancer applications for veterinary and fishery use [23, 24].

However, pDNA vaccines have several drawbacks. First, production of pDNA in bacteria results in the presence of contaminants, e.g., antibiotics or bacterial byproducts such as endotoxin, and cell culture media components such as animal serum, some of which may cause toxicity [25, 26]. These impurities require extensive purification to minimize or eliminate and residual toxins, and subsequent screening for bacterial lipopolysaccharide. In addition, scaling up production for vaccination studies may prove challenging [21]. Secondly, the pDNA backbone may elicit an immune response against the pDNA backbone [27, 28], may result in gene silencing [29], or may down regulate gene expression [30]. Thus, efforts have been made to produce DNA that does not contain these backbone sequences [31-34].

The anti-influenza therapeutic efficacy of single stranded DNA has been evaluated for 1) the homologous H3 or H1 from influenza A/Puerto Rico/8/34 H1N1 against the mouse adapted influenza A/HK/8/68 (H3N2) virus [11], and 2) the homologous HA, NA and combined HA and NA from influenza A/Vietnam/1203/04 H5N1 [12].

Technology

synDNA™ is a novel, cell-free DNA manufacturing process that produces linear DNA using a process which does not require bacterial fermentation [12], unlike traditional DNA vaccine approaches [22]. This provides an advantage to other described DNA vaccines since its manufacture circumvents the use of antibiotic resistance genes and inclusion of other nucleic acid sequences unrelated to the antigen gene expression in the actual therapeutic DNA construct.

Preclinical Studies

The immunogenicity and efficacy of synDNA™ constructs as vaccines against influenza A/H5N1 were evaluated in the BALB/c-VN04 mouse model [12]. The vaccines were designed to express both the hemagglutinin (HA) and neuraminidase (NA) proteins (H5N1 synDNA™), HA alone (H5 synDNA™) or NA alone (N1 synDNA™). HA and/or NA expression were verified by Western blot analysis.

Two independent efficacy trials using two intramuscular doses of each synDNA vaccine against a high dose VN04 challenge were performed. Daily survival outcomes as well as disease symptoms were assessed over a 21-day period [12]. The immunogenicity of the vaccines was determined using H5 ELISA. Protection was enhanced for H5N1 synDNA™ and H5 synDNA™ vaccinated mice in comparison with the placebo (synDNA™ control). The N1 synDNA™ vaccine did not provide protection, although protein expression in transfected cells could be detected via Western blot. In both trials, the majority of H5N1 synDNA™-immunized animals remained asymptomatic after challenge. However, many of the vaccinated animals that were initially symptomatic (i.e., exhibiting hypothermia and clinical encephalitis) recovered, demonstrated by survival to the end of the monitoring period and recovery of body weight and normal body temperature. The level of protection of the synDNA™ H5N1 vaccine was better than that of the H5 alone and was comparable (up to 93%) to that achievable by pDNA vaccines. H5 ELISA titer levels at two weeks following the last booster dose were correlated with survival in mice immunized with the synDNA™ -HA vaccine. In both trials, all animals that survived the lethal influenza A/H5N1 virus challenge, whether immunized with the H5N1 or the H5 synDNA™ vaccine, had high anti-H5 antibody titer prior to challenge. Mice that succumbed to infection had low anti-H5 antibody titers.

FLAGELLIN CONJUGATE VACCINE

Background

Toll-like receptors (TLRs) are expressed on the cell surface of professional antigen presenting and other cells, where they act as primary sensors of microbial infection and then activate signaling cascade that lead to the induction of immune responses [35, 36]. Prior studies have shown that antigenicity can be enhanced by physical linkage of TLR ligands to a variety of viral, bacterial and parasite antigens (reviewed in [37]). These fusion proteins are immunologically potent vaccines that can be efficiently manufactured at scales to meet global needs using standard *E.coli* fermentation systems.

A flagellin-based HA vaccine approach was initiated to address significant barriers to HPAI vaccine development, namely: 1) the low immunogenicity of pandemic influenza strains relative to the seasonal human influenza strains [38, 39], 2) challenges in the influenza manufacturing processes, i.e., inefficiency of production in eggs or eukaryotic cell culture [2, 40, 41].

Technology

This approach utilizes the toll-like receptor (TLR) 5 agonist, flagellin, linked to a subunit of influenza HA to augment the immune response to influenza [13, 42-44]. Recently this approach was used to generate novel influenza vaccines that fuse flagellin with the globular head of the HA molecules of influenza A/Vietnam/1203/04 H5N1. The majority of neutralizing epitopes are within the HA globular head domain [37, 45].

Preclinical Studies

The immunogenicity and efficacy of the HA-flagellin protein were evaluated in the BALB/c-VN04 mouse model [46]. Purified HA-flagellin protein was detected in Western blot both by influenza A/Vietnam/1203/04 convalescence sera as well as a monoclonal anti-flagellin antibody. ELISA-based detection was also positive. Six-week-old female BALB/c mice (Harlan) were vaccinated subcutaneously (s.c.) with two or three doses of the HA-flagellin vaccine (day -28, -14) or (-42, -28, -14) in 40 µl of vehicle (DPBS). The animals were bled 7 or 12 days following the last vaccination. Seroconversion was then evaluated via hemagglutination inhibition assay. Challenge with VN04 was subsequently performed. Clinical observations of disease development and mortality were monitored daily following vaccination and following challenge.

H5-specific (IgG) ELISA was performed to determine the antibody titer of serum samples obtained 7 days following the booster immunization. All animals in all dose groups (0.3 to 30 µg) seroconverted following immunization and the geometric mean endpoint titers exhibited a dose dependent increase. HAI was evaluated for 1 and 10 mg doses and titers were overall low, but showed four-fold or greater rises in the geometric mean HAI titers for both dose groups.

Preclinical trials with two immunizations with doses of 1, 3, or 10 µg of the HA-flagellin vaccine delivered subcutaneously resulted in a dose-dependent decrease in severe disease and death relative to the placebo control group, with survival rates of 18, 40, and 73% of mice respectively. Increasing the vaccine dose to 30 µg in the second trial, however, did not improve the survival outcome. Addition of a third immunization at doses of 1, 3, and 10 µg of HA-flagellin increased survival rates to 87%, 93%, and 100%, respectively. Immunogenicity experiments performed in tandem with the efficacy studies indicated that the H5-ELISA showed seroconversion for all immunized mice. Endpoint titers for the 3- and 10-µg dose groups were comparable to each other and higher than those for the 1 µg dose group.

The survival pattern was consistent in repeat trials and organ viral loads were examined via fifty percent tissue culture infective dose ($TCID_{50}$) assay in this subsequent trial. Differences between vaccinated and placebo groups were detected irrespective of the vaccine dose (1, 3 or 10 µg). In the brains of all vaccinated animals, virus was below the limit of detection ($<1 \times 10^4$ $TCID_{50}$/g of tissue), whereas for the placebo group, the average titer was ~5 $\log_{10}$ $TCID_{50}$/g. In the lungs, a titer difference of ~2-3 $\log_{10}$ was detected; for vaccinated animals the average titer was between ~4-5 $\log_{10}$ $TCID_{50}$/g, whereas the placebo average was 7.6 $\log_{10}$ $TCID_{50}$/g. Virus was undetectable in 60% of the lungs of those vaccinated with 1 µg and 80% of those vaccinated with 3 or 10 µg vaccine doses. In contrast, virus could be detected in 100% of the lungs and brains of the placebo animals. Thus, both improved survival outcomes and reduced brain/lung viral loads indicate that the HA-flagellin vaccine is efficacious in the murine model. Refinements in the design of the globular head construct and additional preclinical testing suggests that the immunogenicity (HAI titer) and efficacy can be further increased.

ALPHAVIRUS-BASED VACCINES

Background

Recombinant live-attenuated vaccines and, in particular, an alphavirus-based approach reviewed in [14]), represent a viable approach to the production of safe, immunogenic and efficacious vaccines against the encephalitis alphaviruses (e.g., Venezuelan equine encephalitis virus, VEEV), as well as the bunyavirus, Rift Valley fever virus (RVFV). The advantage of this approach is that alphavirus genomes are relatively easy to manipulate, and infectious clones are available for construction and in vitro transcription of recombinant viruses for vaccine production by cell transfection. Previously Sindbis virus (SINV), a relatively nonpathogenic alphavirus in humans, has been used to engineer a series of chimeric viruses that express heterologous viral antigens of VEEV and RVFV. These viruses have been shown to elicit a high level of neutralizing antibody in a variety of inbred and outbred mouse strains.

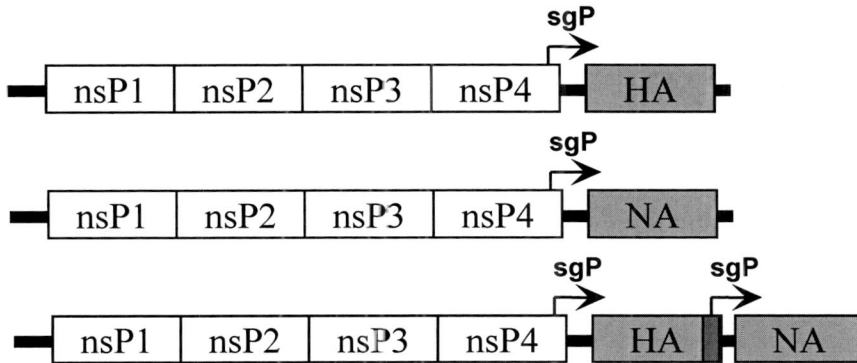

Figure 2. Alphavirus-H5N1 vaccine candidates. Schematic representation of the alphavirus vaccine constructs designed for alphavirus driven expression of heterologous genes, e.g., HA and/or NA from influenza A/Vietnam/1203/04 (H5N1). The alphavirus replicons with codon-optimized HA or NA are designed for expression under the subgenomic (SG) promoter and utilize a two helper packaging system. Abbreviations: nsP, alphavirus nonstructural protein.

TECHNOLOGY

H5N1 candidate vaccines were developed based on the HA (TC83-H5) or both HA and NA (TC83-H5N1) of VN04 (Paessler, unpublished). These alphavirus based constructs contain the cis-acting RNA elements and non-structural protein genes of the TC83 (VEEV IND vaccine strain) genome, which are required for replication and transcription of the subgenomic RNA, e.g., 5' untranslated region (UTR), 3' UTR, and the subgenomic promoter. The promoter element, located upstream of the subgenomic RNA transcription start, and the four 5' terminal nucleotides of the subgenomic RNA encompass the end of nsP4 and the termination codon of the nsP-coding open reading frame. These constructs are schematically depicted in Figure 2.

PRECLINICAL STUDIES

The immunogenicity and efficacy of the HA-flagellin protein were evaluated in the BALB/c-VN04 mouse model. Protein expression for the TC83-H5 and TC83-H5N1 constructs was confirmed by Western blot using H5N1 convalescent serum. Two efficacy trials were performed using a single dose of 10^6 plaque forming units per animal of the live-attenuated candidate vaccine delivered subcutaneously either 33 days (trial 1) or 21 days (trial 2) prior to VN04 challenge. Daily survival outcomes as well as disease symptoms were assessed over a 21-day period. The immunogenicity of the vaccines was determined using H5 ELISA.

In the first trial, protection of 100% and 56% was provided by the TC83-H5 and TC83-H5N1 in comparison to 0% for placebo. All of the animals in the TC83-HA group seroconverted, whereas the TC83-H5N1 group had low to moderate titers. In the second trial (TC83-HA only), survival was 81% for vaccinated animals (0% for placebo). The majority of the TC83-HA immunized animals seroconverted, whereas the range of titers was more varied in this trial (from negative for one animal to high).

CONCLUSION

A variety of alternative vaccination approaches targeting the known influenza A/Vietnam/1203/04 H5N1 antigens, HA and NA, show promise in preclinical (mouse) efficacy trials. These include synDNA™ linear DNA, protein-based HA-flagellin and live attenuated alphavirus based vaccines. H5 ELISA can be used to assess immunogenicity in an effort to circumvent the low predictive value of the HAI assay due to the overall low HAI titers of H5N1-challenged animals, irrespective of vaccination status. Further studies are ongoing using these approaches, with a focus on improvement of formulations that augment immunogenicity. The results presented here warrant further testing in a second small animal model, the outbred ferret. H5N1 challenge studies in ferrets present additional limitations in terms of space for housing of increased animal numbers for these efficacy trials but nonetheless will provide additional disease and survival data for evaluating H5N1 vaccines.

REFERENCES

[1] Stephenson, I., et al., Confronting the avian influenza threat: vaccine development for a potential pandemic. *Lancet Infect Dis*, 2004. **4**(8): p. 499-509.

[2] Cox, M.M., Cell-based protein vaccines for influenza. *Curr Opin Mol Ther*, 2005. **7**(1): p. 24-9.

[3] Subbarao, K. and T. Joseph, Scientific barriers to developing vaccines against avian influenza viruses. *Nat Rev Immunol*, 2007. **7**(4): p. 267-78.

[4] Subbarao, K. and C. Luke, H5N1 Viruses and Vaccines. *PLoS Pathog*, 2007. **3**(3): p. e40.

[5] Hoelscher, M., et al., Vaccines against epidemic and pandemic influenza. *Expert Opin Drug Deliv*, 2008. **5**(10): p. 1139-57.

[6] Kreijtz, J.H., A.D. Osterhaus, and G.F. Rimmelzwaan, Vaccination strategies and vaccine formulations for epidemic and pandemic influenza control. *Hum Vaccin*, 2009. **5**(3).

[7] Bresson, J.L., et al., Safety and immunogenicity of an inactivated split-virion influenza A/Vietnam/1194/2004 (H5N1) vaccine: phase I randomised trial. *Lancet*, 2006. **367**(9523): p. 1657-64.

[8] Lin, J., et al., Safety and immunogenicity of an inactivated adjuvanted whole-virion influenza A (H5N1) vaccine: a phase I randomised controlled trial. *Lancet*, 2006. **368**(9540): p. 991-7.

[9] Treanor, J.J., et al., Safety and immunogenicity of an inactivated subvirion influenza A (H5N1) vaccine. *N Engl J Med*, 2006. **354**(13): p. 1343-51.

[10] Carter, N.J. and G.L. Plosker, Prepandemic influenza vaccine H5N1 (split virion, inactivated, adjuvanted) [Prepandrix]: a review of its use as an active immunization against influenza A subtype H5N1 virus. *BioDrugs*, 2008. **22**(5): p. 279-92.

[11] Vilalta, A., et al., Vaccination with polymerase chain reaction-generated linear expression cassettes protects mice against lethal influenza a challenge. *Hum Gene Ther*, 2007. **18**(8): p. 763-71.

[12] Kendirgi, F., et al., Novel linear DNA vaccines induce protective immune responses against lethal infection with influenza virus type A/H5N1. *Hum Vaccin*, 2008. **4**(6): p. 410-9.

[13] Song, L., et al., Efficacious recombinant influenza vaccines produced by high yield bacterial expression: a solution to global pandemic and seasonal needs. *PLoS ONE*, 2008. **3**(5): p. e2257.

[14] Zacks, M.A. and S. Paessler, Alphavirus virus-based chimeric vaccines against encephalitic alphaviruses. *Croatian Journal of Infection*, 2007. **27**(4): p. 155-160.

[15] van der Laan, J.W., et al., Animal models in influenza vaccine testing. *Expert Rev Vaccines*, 2008. **7**(6): p. 783-93.

[16] Zitzow, L.A., et al., Pathogenesis of avian influenza A (H5N1) viruses in ferrets. *J Virol*, 2002. **76**(9): p. 4420-9.

[17] Gao, P., et al., Biological heterogeneity, including systemic replication in mice, of H5N1 influenza A virus isolates from humans in Hong Kong. *J Virol*, 1999. **73**(4): p. 3184-9.

[18] Katz, J.M., et al., Pathogenesis of and immunity to avian influenza A H5 viruses. *Biomed Pharmacother*, 2000. **54**(4): p. 178-87.

[19] Yun, N.E., et al., Injectable peramivir mitigates disease and promotes survival in ferrets and mice infected with the highly virulent influenza virus, A/Vietnam/1203/04 (H5N1). *Virology*, 2008. **374**(1): p. 198-209.

[20] Fields, S., G. Winter, and G.G. Brownlee, Structure of the neuraminidase gene in human influenza virus A/FR/8/34. *Nature*, 1981. **290**(5803): p. 213-7.

[21] Bower, D.M. and K.L. Prather, Engineering of bacterial strains and vectors for the production of plasmid DNA. *Appl Microbiol Biotechnol*, 2009.

[22] Kutzler, M.A. and D.B. Weiner, DNA vaccines: ready for prime time? *Nat Rev Genet*, 2008. **9**(10): p. 776-88.

[23] Weiner, D.B., Introduction to DNA vaccines issue. *Vaccine*, 2006. **24**(21): p. 4459-60.

[24] Bergman, P.J., et al., Development of a xenogeneic DNA vaccine program for canine malignant melanoma at the Animal Medical Center. *Vaccine*, 2006. **24**(21): p. 4582-5.

[25] Listner, K., L.K. Bentley, and M. Chartrain, A simple method for the production of plasmid DNA in bioreactors. *Methods Mol Med*, 2006. **127**: p. 295-309.

[26] Boyle, J.S., et al., Inhibitory effect of lipopolysaccharide on immune response after DNA immunization is route dependent. *DNA Cell Biol*, 1998. **17**(4): p. 343-8.

[27] Liu, L., et al., CpG motif acts as a 'danger signal' and provides a T helper type 1-biased microenvironment for DNA vaccination. *Immunology*, 2005. **115**(2): p. 223-30.

[28] Vabulas, R.M., et al., CpG-DNA activates in vivo T cell epitope presenting dendritic cells to trigger protective antiviral cytotoxic T cell responses. *J Immunol*, 2000. **164**(5): p. 2372-8.

[29] Paillard, F., CpG: the double-edged sword. *Hum Gene Ther*, 1999. **10**(13): p. 2089-90.

[30] Chen, Z.Y., et al., Silencing of episomal transgene expression by plasmid bacterial DNA elements in vivo. *Gene Ther*, 2004. **11**(10): p. 856-64.

[31] Chen, Z.Y., et al., Minicircle DNA vectors devoid of bacterial DNA result in persistent and high-level transgene expression in vivo. *Mol Ther*, 2003. **8**(3): p. 495-500.

[32] Moreno, S., et al., DNA immunisation with minimalistic expression constructs. *Vaccine*, 2004. **22**(13-14): p. 1709-16.

[33] Leutenegger, C.M., et al., Immunization of cats against feline immunodeficiency virus (FIV) infection by using minimalistic immunogenic defined gene expression vector vaccines expressing FIV gp140 alone or with feline interleukin-12 (IL-12), IL-16, or a CpG motif. *J Virol*, 2000. **74**(22): p. 10447-57.

[34] Schakowski, F., et al., A novel minimal-size vector (MIDGE) improves transgene expression in colon carcinoma cells and avoids transfection of undesired DNA. *Mol Ther*, 2001. **3**(5 Pt 1): p. 793-800.

[35] Akira, S., K. Takeda, and T. Kaisho, Toll-like receptors: critical proteins linking innate and acquired immunity. *Nat Immunol*, 2001. **2**(8): p. 675-80.

[36] Takeda, K., T. Kaisho, and S. Akira, Toll-like receptors. *Annu Rev Immunol*, 2003. **21**: p. 335-76.

[37] Ben-Yedidia, T. and R. Arnon, Epitope-based vaccine against influenza. *Expert Rev Vaccines*, 2007. **6**(6): p. 939-48.

[38] Rowe, T., et al., Detection of antibody to avian influenza A (H5N1) virus in human serum by using a combination of serologic assays. *J Clin Microbiol*, 1999. **37**(4): p. 937-43.

[39] Katz, J.M., et al., Antibody response in individuals infected with avian influenza A (H5N1) viruses and detection of anti-H5 antibody among household and social contacts. *J Infect Dis*, 1999. **180**(6): p. 1763-70.

[40] Hampson, A.W., Ferrets and the challenges of H5N1 vaccine formulation. *J Infect Dis*, 2006. **194**(2): p. 143-5.

[41] Gerdil, C., The annual production cycle for influenza vaccine. Vaccine, 2003. **21**(16): p. 1776-9.

[42] Huleatt, J.W., et al., Vaccination with recombinant fusion proteins incorporating Toll-like receptor ligands induces rapid cellular and humoral immunity. *Vaccine*, 2007. **25**(4): p. 763-75.

[43] McDonald, W.F., et al., A West Nile virus recombinant protein vaccine that coactivates innate and adaptive immunity. *J Infect Dis*, 2007. **195**(11): p. 1607-17.

[44] Huleatt, J.W., et al., Potent immunogenicity and efficacy of a universal influenza vaccine candidate comprising a recombinant fusion protein linking influenza M2e to the TLR5 ligand flagellin. *Vaccine*, 2008. **26**(2): p. 201-14.

[45] Ben-Yedidia, T. and R. Arnon, Towards an epitope-based human vaccine for influenza. *Hum Vaccin*, 2005. **1**(3): p. 95-101.

[46] Song, L., et al., Superior efficacy of a recombinant flagellin:H5N1 HA globular head vaccine is determined by the placement of the globular head within flagellin. (Submitted to *Vaccine*, Jan 2009), 2009.

Chapter 13

Advances in Quantitative Analyses of the Hemagglutinin of Influenza A Viruses and Vaccines

Xuguang Li[a,e,], Terry D. Cyr[a], Michel Girard[a], Changgui Li[b], Junzi Wang[b], Gary Van Domselaar[d], Aaron Farnsworth[a], Helen MacDonald-Piquard[c] and Runtao He[d]*

[a]Centre for Biologics Research, Biologics and Genetic Therapies Directorate, Health Products and Food Branch, Health Canada, Ottawa, ON, Canada
[b]National Institute for the Control of Pharmaceutical and Biological Products, Beijing, PR China
[c]Centre for Biologics Evaluation, Biologics and Genetic Therapies Directorate, HPFB, Health Canada, Ottawa, ON, Canada
[d]National Microbiology Laboratory, Public Health Agency of Canada, Winnipeg, MB, Canada
[e]Department of Biochemistry, Microbiology and Immunology, University of Ottawa, Ottawa, ON, Canada

Abstract

The surface proteins of the influenza A viruses are hemagglutinins and neuraminidases, which are known to induce immune protection in a variety of hosts. The major viral surface protein that induces protective immune responses, which is a hemagglutinin, is currently the sole marker of vaccine potency. Single radial immunodiffusion is the standard method for quantifying this hemagglutinin, because of its simplicity and its ability to identify hemagglutinin subtypes. However, this method depends on the availability of reference materials, specifically reference antigens and

---

[*] Corresponding author: Dr. Xuguang (Sean) Li, Centre for Biologics Research, Biologics and Genetic Therapies Directorate, Health Canada, Sir F.G. Banting Research Centre, A/L 2201E, 251 Sir Frederick Banting Driveway, Ottawa, ON K1A 0K9, Canada. Tel: 613 941 6149; Fax: 613 941 8933; E-mail: Sean_Li@hc-sc.gc.ca

corresponding antisera. In addition, it is an insensitive, labor-intensive method. In recent years, other analytical methods, such as reversed-phase high-performance liquid chromatography in conjunction with mass spectrometry, have been developed to separate and identify individual viral proteins in vaccine preparations. Yet challenges remain, including lack of methods for quantifying these proteins, determining their three-dimensional structure and analyzing elusive components of the vaccines; the need to develop subtype-specific protein standards; high equipment costs; the need for highly trained staff; and the demand for high through-put. Availability of antibodies against the universally conserved sequence (fusion peptides) of the hemagglutinins of influenza A and B would not only facilitate timely release of influenza virus vaccines in the event of a pandemic but also represent a versatile research tool for investigating conformational epitopes and virus entry and for molecular studies of the immune complexes, all of which are pertinent to the formulation of new antiviral strategies. Yet, the universal antibody assay is not intended to identify the hemagglutinin subtypes and would benefit from being used in conjunction with physicochemical methods. Clearly, the application of all these emerging methods to routine testing of vaccine potency still requires vigorous international validation. Here, we discuss new analytical and immunological tools for the qualitative and quantitative analysis of viral hemagglutinins, with a focus on the underlying principles and the strengths and weaknesses of these new methods.

1. INTRODUCTION

Influenza infection occurs in as many as 5%–15% of the world's population, resulting in 3 to 5 million cases of severe illness and up to 500,000 deaths annually [1,2]. Seasonal influenza vaccines are produced about six to eight months ahead of the targeted season using the strains recommended by the World Health Organization (WHO) [3]. These vaccines typically contain two subtypes of influenza virus type A and one of influenza virus type B, all derived from the strains predicted to circulate in the coming year. The inherent disadvantages associated with preparing conventional influenza vaccines include uncertainty about the strains that will be circulating, need for annual updates of the manufacturing process and the time required to prepare reagents before vaccine lots are released. In particular, any mismatch between the strains selected for the vaccine and those circulating in the population can severely limit vaccine efficacy [4,5]. In the event of a pandemic influenza outbreak, these shortcomings would be dramatically amplified, in terms of increased morbidity and mortality, given the much-shortened timeframe for producing the vaccines that would be required for global needs. All of these problems can be attributed to a single biological characteristic of the influenza virus itself: the rate of mutation of the viral surface proteins. The major viral surface protein that induces protective immune responses, which is a hemagglutinin (HA), is currently the sole marker of vaccine potency. It is assayed by single radial immunodiffusion (SRID) [6].

SRID depends on the availability of reference HA antigens and corresponding antisera, which are updated and distributed annually by WHO collaborating centers. Once a new viral strain has been recommended for inclusion in the seasonal vaccine, a period of two to three months is needed to prepare these reagents, a process that involves injecting purified antigens into sheep to produce polyclonal antibodies. In the case of an influenza pandemic, the necessary reference materials would not be available for timely release of vaccine lots.

Although this represents in part a regulatory hurdle, it also means that the amount of antigen per dose would be unknown. Therefore, the WHO has been encouraging manufacturers to develop alternative methods of determining the potency of vaccines in the event of a pandemic outbreak [7]. Alternative methods that have been recommended by the WHO include determination of total protein and SDS-PAGE scanning [7]. However, the combination of SDS-PAGE with total protein determination may yield inaccurate results because the extent of glycolsylation modification varies among viral strains, as does the ratio of HA to total proteins [8]. In addition, the WHO has recommended that the reference library of vaccine strains and potency reagents for different hemagglutinin subtypes be prepared in advance [7]. This task will be difficult, because of the need to prepare all of the reagents and validate the assays before the next pandemic. Furthermore, since it is impossible to predict which influenza subtypes will be involved in such a pandemic, preparing the necessary SRID reagents would require successful guesswork. Clearly, it is of great interest to find alternative approaches that would facilitate more rapid regulatory approval of vaccines that could potentially save millions of human lives. In this chapter, we present an overview of recent developments in physicochemical and immunological methods for the qualitative and quantitative analysis of hemagglutinins, with emphasis on practical applications and mechanistic elucidation.

2. IMMUNOLOGICAL ASSAY TARGETING UNIVERSALLY CONSERVED SEQUENCES OF HEMAGGLUTININS

2.1 Viral Hemagglutinins

To date, influenza A viruses representing 16 HA and 9 neuraminidase (NA) subtypes have been detected in wild birds and poultry throughout the world [9,23]. HA is the receptor-binding and membrane fusion glycoprotein of influenza viruses and the target for infectivity-neutralizing antibodies [9]. It is initially synthesized in the infected cell as a single-chain precursor, termed HA0, which is later cleaved into two subunits (HA1 and HA2) by the host proteases [9,16]. After the cleavage, the HA1 and HA2 subunits are linked by disulfide bonds [9]. Given the importance of neutralizing antibodies against HA in controlling influenza infection, the conserved regions in the HA proteins have received much attention in recent years. The HA1/HA2-HA1–HA2 joint region is the most widely conserved, the HA2 N-terminal 11 amino acid being conserved among all influenza A subtypes [15].

2.2 Antibodies against the Universally Conserved Sequence

Several groups have reported the generation of antibodies against the HA1/HA2 joint region with the use of branched peptides or peptide–carrier conjugate [11-14], but attempts to generate antibodies against the more universally conserved N-terminus of HA2 (the fusion peptide) have been unsuccessful [11-14]. Recently, using a novel approach, Chun et al. [15] succeeded in generating antibodies exclusively targeted to the HA2 fusion peptide and analysis of the binding characteristics of these antibodies to the diverse subtypes of HA proteins, in terms of quantification, specificity and detection of conformational epitopes. In this study, generating and characterizing universal antibodies against the most highly conserved sequences consisted of three steps: (1) comprehensive bioinformatics analyses of a public database to select viral sequences that would represent the totality of sequence variation among the fusion peptides of different HA proteins, (2) modification and conjugation of the selected peptides to the carrier protein (Keyhole Limpet Hemocyanin [KLH]) and (3) determination of antibody binding to the fusion peptide epitope of diverse strains of influenza A viruses or vaccines, both on solid phase and in solution.

Identification of conserved regions of the HA proteins by bioinformatics analyses

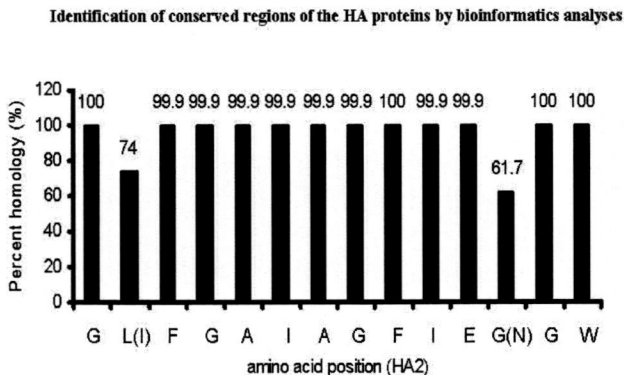

Identification of conserved regions of hemagglutinin (HA) proteins by bioinformatics analysis. A total of 3896 sequences were analyzed separately for each subtype of influenza A. Shannon's entropy was calculated for each amino acid position of the identified consensus sequences to determine the degree of variation. The sequence shown along the horizontal axis represents the 14 N-terminal amino acids of the HA2 polypeptide. Only two positions had noticeable substitutions: position 2, from L to I, and position 12, from G to N. The consensus sequence for the fusion peptide of 250 influenza B viruses differed from that of influenza A viruses, with a substitution of the amino acid at position 2, from L(I) to F (not shown in the figure) [15].

Figure 1.

Through extensive analyses of all HA sequences in the public domain, Chun et al. confirmed that the fusion peptide is conserved across all known subtypes of influenza viruses with only minor substitutions (Figure 1), in agreement with other investigators [11-14]. They then took a different approach in the selection of the peptides for immunization and epitope mapping since previous attempts using peptides or peptide-conjugates to generate antibodies against the same sequence were not been successful [11-14], suggesting the immunogenicity of this region is very weak. To overcome these hurdles, they first linked the identified peptide to a spacer, 6-aminocaproic acid in hope of improving immunogenicity and followed this with the addition of a tripeptide KKC to enable solubilization of the peptides, and conjugation of the modified peptide to the carrier protein (KLH). Through these necessary modifications, i.e., the insertion of the 6-aminocaproic acid and the tripeptide KKC, these investigators were successful in generating specific antibodies against the fusion peptide [15]. Importantly, these antibodies demonstrated remarkable specificity against the influenza HAs of diverse influenza strains as no cross-reactivity to the proteins derived from allantoic fluids was detected.

2.3 Exposure of Fusion Peptide after Denaturation

Previous data from crystallographic studies revealed that the fusion peptide is partially exposed as a surface loop in HA0, but after cleavage into the HA1 and H2 subunits, the fusion peptide becomes buried inside the trimer at the interface of the two long alpha helices [9,17,18]. Acidic treatment (pH 5.0) of the HA proteins resulted in irreversible exposure of the C-terminus of the HA1 subunit [10,28], and moderately concentrated urea at neutral pH (pH 4.5) induced conformational changes identical with those induced at low pH [15,18]. Chun et al. then used indirect ELISA to determine how the fusion peptide epitope was exposed to the antibodies under various conditions. Urea treatment promoted greater binding between antibodies and antigens than occurred with acidic treatment, whereas only minimal interaction between the antigen and antibodies was observed with native HA antigens (PBS). These results suggest that urea treatment drastically destabilized the HA2 proteins, allowing the fusion peptide to be exposed on the surface. The same was true for the exposure of fusion peptides in solution, as revealed by antibody binding results from competitive ELISA [15]. Taken together, these results suggest that the fusogenic state of HA induced by either acidic pH or moderately concentrated urea involves exposure of the fusion peptide to the surface of the proteins, making it readily accessible to the antibodies. However, during the course of infection, exposure of the fusion peptide is insufficient to allow binding to whole IgG antibody molecules. It is unclear whether the smaller antibody fragment (Fab or scFv) could inhibit entry of the virus into susceptible cells[1].

2.4 Quantitative Determination of Influenza Viral HAs in Vaccine Preparations

In addition to serving as a research tool, these antibodies could be used to quantify the HA content in vaccine preparations [15]. The discovery of a single fusion peptide sequence in the HA protein led to development of competitive ELISA using the same HA protein antigen for both the plate coating and the competitive antigens. The concentrations of competing antigens (HA recombinant proteins) in solution were inversely proportional to the optical density values. The widely accepted four-parameter logistic model for immunoassay fitted the curve very well ($R = 0.99$). In comparative experiments, the quantities of diverse subtypes of recombinant HAs, as determined by competitive ELISA, were largely in agreement with the expected values, as determined by standard assays for recombinant HA proteins [15]. Furthermore, the amounts of human vaccine samples detected by competitive ELISA were also close to those determined by SRID.

3. CHROMATOGRAPHIC ANALYSES OF VIRAL COMPONENTS IN INFLUENZA VACCINES

3.1 High-Performance Liquid Chromatography

In a pioneering study of influenza vaccine preparations, Bucher et al. [29] reported the potential of high-performance liquid chromatography (HPLC) as a method of separating influenza virus components. Despite low yields, these researchers found that the use of size-exclusion HPLC (SE-HPLC) with SDS-containing mobile phases for elution enabled them to

---

[1] Farnsworth A, Li X, unpublished observations.

isolate the HA1 and HA2 subunits from vaccine preparations containing HA0. A few years later, Calam and Davidson [30)] reported the usefulness of detergent-containing mobile phases in SE-HPLC to isolate viral proteins from whole-virus extracts. In particular, they found that the HA retained its immunological activity despite the use of detergents. However, attempts to separate viral proteins by ion-exchange HPLC were unsuccessful because of very low recoveries and lack of selectivity. More recently, Garcia-Cañas and Girard studied the influence of several factors, including use of detergents, pH and ionic strength, on the reproducibility and selectivity of protein profiles obtained by SE-HPLC. They reported the optimization of conditions as the first step in a process involving one-dimensional (1D) gel electrophoresis and mass spectrometry for characterizing influenza vaccines. They suggested that this methodology might be useful to manufacturers wishing to verify protein profiles in both monovalent strain preparations and trivalent vaccines[2].

Phelan and Cohen [31] were the first to demonstrate the use of reversed-phase HPLC (RP-HPLC) for separating the components of influenza viruses. Using a C8-bonded silica column of medium hydrophobicity and wide pores, they separated the components of a virus preparation treated with 8 M guanidine hydrochloride and 2 mM dithiothreitol (DTT) with a gradient eluent of acetonitrile containing trifluoroacetic acid. Under these conditions, the HA0 was reduced into its subunits, and the HA1 co-eluted with NP. However, the yields of the separated proteins were less than optimal [31]. Recently, two independent groups [32,33] reported quantification of HA by RP-HPLC using similar approaches based on the selective detection of the hydrophilic HA1 subunit, separated from the more hydrophobic viral and matrix components. Notably, both methods featured separation of the HA1 subunits of the 3 strains contained in trivalent vaccines. Kapteyn et al. [32] used a linear gradient elution with acetonitrile containing 0.1% trifluoroacetic acid on poly(styrene-divinylbenzene) POROS columns. This type of polymeric support generally provides binding strength similar to low-hydrophobicity, C4-bonded silica columns. Before being separated by RP-HPLC, the purified virus preparations were subjected to several treatments. First, trypsin was applied, to ensure cleavage of the HA0 into the HA1 and HA2 subunits (the subunits remained linked by disulfide bonds). The samples were reduced by DTT at 90°C for 10 min. The reduced samples were then alkylated by incubation with 50 mM iodoacetamide at 30°C for 45 min in the dark, to prevent formation of an aberrant complex through the free reactive sulfhydryl groups of the viral HA or NA. Finally, DTT was added to neutralize the residual iodoacetamide. The authors found that these extra steps were critical; without them, the separation peaks became deformed [32]. They found good correlation between the HPLC method and SRID for quantification of HA in monovalent preparations obtained at various steps of the manufacturing process. The reported linear range was between 8 and 62 µg/mL, with a lower limit of 0.4 µg injected on the column. The assay was found to be precise, as demonstrated by the relative standard deviation (between 5% and 7%). As mentioned above, the method also provided very good selectivity by enabling separation of the HA1 subunits from the three monovalent strains in a trivalent vaccine. In their most recent report, Kapteyn et al. [34] demonstrated that this RP-HPLC method is also suitable for HA quantification of active beta-propiolactone or formaldehyde-inactivated egg-based and MDCK cell-based whole-virus samples, as well as final (monovalent) subunit vaccines. In addition, the RP-HPLC assay was shown to be useful in the early stages of production of seasonal influenza

---

[2] Garcia-Cañas V, Girard M, unpublished observations.

vaccine, when SRID reagents are not yet available, thus enabling fast and reliable viral growth studies in eggs, which in turn would allow selection of the best-growing viral strains or reassortants for production of the seasonal trivalent influenza vaccine. Finally, the authors discussed the observed differences between HA1 molecules from various HA subtypes (in terms of ultraviolet absorbance, FLD response and retention times during RP-HPLC) in relation to the primary structure of the HA1 molecules.

Garcia-Cañas et al. [33] described RP-HPLC conditions leading to the rapid separation of influenza proteins on C18-bonded, nonporous silica columns. Although hydrophobic proteins such as those found in influenza viruses would not be expected to elute from such highly hydrophobic columns, the combination of the absence of pores on the silica particles, reducing the surface area for C18 bonding, and fast mass transfer, which mitigates the strong retention of the C18 bonded phase, enabled efficient elution. In addition, the use of a nonporous silica stationary phase minimized the carry-over and nonspecific adsorption that are observed with conventional columns. Before the separation step, a concentration step was necessary, and the authors showed that solubilization of influenza components in the concentrated preparations was critical to obtaining quantitative and reproducible results. The optimal procedure for concentration and solubilization involved a combination of detergents and a reduction step with DTT to release the HA1 and HA2 subunits. RP-HPLC analysis allowed separation of the influenza proteins HA1, NP (nucleoprotein) and MP (matrix protein) and other constituents in both monovalent bulk preparations and trivalent vaccines. As mentioned previously, the HA1 subunits of the 3 influenza strains present in vaccines were resolved from each other and eluted in the following order, according to increasing retention time: HA1 of B, HA1 of A/H3N2 and HA1 of H1N1. Using standard HA antigen reagents, the authors demonstrated the quantitative nature of the method. Good linearity was achieved for the detection of HA1 from the A/H1N1 and B subtypes in the range of 50 to 300 µg/mL, with limits of detection of 443 ng and 327 ng, respectively. The precision of the method was also very good, with percent RSD (relative standard deviation) values for peak areas of 4.86% to 6.46% for same-day and different-day experiments, respectively.

3.2 Two-Dimensional High-Performance Liquid Chromatography

In a continuing effort to improve the characterization of vaccines, Garcia-Cañas et al. [35] used the greater resolving power of two-dimensional HPLC (2D-HPLC) to circumvent the interference of excipients that may occur in the detection of HA1 by RP-HPLC. The reported method used size-based separation by SE-HPLC in the first dimension and an orthogonal separation mode, RP-HPLC, in the second dimension. Despite the availability of 1D chromatographic methods for the chosen separation modes, direct coupling of these modes into a 2D system necessitated modifications to ensure compatibility. Fluorescence detection was also introduced in the RP-HPLC, which resulted in significantly improved sensitivity, with limits of detection for HA reference antigens of 105 ng/mL for the influenza A/New Caledonia/20/99 strain and 172 ng/mL for the B/Jiangsu/10/ 2003 strain. A notable feature of the 2D-HPLC methodology was that it required no prior concentration and solubilization of the sample, as was required for one-dimensional procedures. Furthermore, quantification of HA by this method correlated very well with the nominal HA content as determined by conventional SRID. The precision of the assay was better than 2% and 3%, respectively, for calculated antigen concentrations in commercial vaccines for samples from the same lot and from different lots. A comparative analysis of commercial vaccines from three different manufacturers showed that the method was highly selective, reproducibly providing a characteristic chromatographic profile for each vaccine.

4. CHROMATOGRAPHIC SEPARATION / MASS SPECTROMETRY METHODS

4.1 Liquid Chromatography Combined with Tandem Mass Spectrometry

Williams et al. [36] reported a method based on liquid chromatography combined with tandem mass spectrometry for quantifying viral proteins in a complex mixture. Using an isotope dilution approach, these authors determined HA from viral subtypes of H1, H3, H5 and B strains. Quantification was based on a standard curve, using short peptides that stoichiometrically represented the conserved sequences of HAs following trypsin digestion. These peptides contained stable carbon 13 or nitrogen 15 isotopes, which resulted in a mass difference but not a shift in chromatographic retention time. The accuracy of the method depended largely on the integrity of tryptic digestion of the HA samples, in terms of degree of completeness and fidelity of cleavage sites, as well as the purity and concentration of the labelled peptides. One drawback of this method is the lack of peptide standards for these HAs makes it difficult for other investigators to directly compare their results with those from SRID. Regardless, this method allowed simultaneous quantification of HAs from three influenza subtypes in commercial vaccines in the presence of residual detergents and other vaccine components [36].

4.2 Ultra-Performance Liquid Chromatography Combined with Isotope Dilution Tandem Mass Spectrometry

The principle of ultra-performance liquid chromatography combined with isotope dilution tandem mass spectrometry is very similar to that of liquid chromatography combined with tandem mass spectrometry, described above [36]. For ultra-performance liquid chromatography, the stationary-phase particles are of diameter 1.7 μm instead of 3.5 μm. This smaller particle size leads to a corresponding increase in back pressure. An ultra-performance liquid chromatography was used because it can function at pressures up to 15,000 psi, well beyond the usual maximum of about 6,000 psi. This method was reported to allow simultaneous quantification of multiple peptides and proteins in commercial influenza vaccine preparations [37]. In that study, linear calibration curves for tryptic peptides corresponding to HA digestion sequences were obtained in a range of 10–90 fmol/μL. The reproducibility of this chromatographic method was also comparable to that of conventional chromatography, as demonstrated by relative standard deviation values below 6.5%. The authors made a concerted effort to develop a rapid method by using an accelerated tryptic digestion procedure and a rapid HPLC gradient. Although the through-put was not as high as that achieved by ELISA methods, which can process hundreds of samples per day, the ultra-performance liquid chromatographic method is quite fast and allows analysis of more than 100 samples per day.

5. CONCLUSION

Conventional SIRD has been used for more than 20 years to quantify HA in influenza vaccines. SRID, the only approved assay for influenza vaccine potency in most (if not all) jurisdictions around the globe, is relatively simple and reproducible. However, it requires subtype-specific antisera, which must be generated annually. For unknown reasons, the generation of such antisera has proven very difficult for certain avian strains. SRID is also labor-intensive and has far lower through-put than ELISA. The development of alternative assays for the quantification of influenza viral HAs could shorten the time required to produce vaccines and facilitate more rapid release of vaccines for human immunization, which would be urgently required in the event of a pandemic influenza outbreak. Such alternative methods might also allow rapid quantification of vaccine seeds (required for initiation of vaccine production), thus substantially reducing manufacturing costs [38,39]. The newly reported methods that have been described in this chapter are complementary, with each having its own strengths and weaknesses. A coordinated effort to combine these assays should be encouraged. Specifically, the ELISA method based on universal antibodies is the simplest of all new methods and has high through-put, but it is not intended to distinguish HA subtypes in vaccine preparations. This shortcoming can be overcome by using chromatography and mass spectrometry, which are more complex and slower but which can identify HA subtypes and separate multiple components in a mixture of viral strains. One important question that remains unanswered is whether exposure of samples to organic solvents, denaturants or trypsin prevents observation of the "antigenic structure" of the native proteins. Furthermore, it is unknown whether vaccine-induced protection correlates better with the results reported by SRID or those generated by these emerging methods. Finally, we do not know the extent to which the "native" structure of the antigens should be maintained in potency assays. The scientific knowledge that has been gathered to date does not provide definite answers to these questions, given that the proteins must be processed into small peptides by the antigen-presenting cells, and denatured (or aggregated) forms of proteins are often more immunogenic than the corresponding native forms [40,41,42].

ACKNOWLEDGMENTS

Research on the development of an alternative assay for influenza viruses and vaccines was supported by the Canadian Regulatory Strategy for Biotechnology and Pandemic Preparedness Funds of Health Canada (to X.L., T.D.C., M.G.), the Ministry of Science and Technology, P.R. China (2004BA519A69 to J.W., C.L.) and Public Health Agency of Canada research funds (to G.V.D., R.H.). We thank Drs. Shiv Prasad and Michael Rosu-Myles for their critical review of the manuscript. Peggy Robinson is acknowledged for her excellent editorial job.

REFERENCES

[1] Poland, GA; Rottinghaus, ST; Jacobson, RM. Influenza vaccines: a review and rationale for use in developed and underdeveloped countries. *Vaccine*, 2001 19, 2216-2220.

[2] Simonsen, L; Taylor, RJ; Viboud, C; Miller, MA; Jackson, LA. Mortality benefits of influenza vaccination in elderly people: an ongoing controversy. *Lancet Infect Dis*, 2007 7, 658-666.

[3] Carrat, F; Flahault, A. Influenza vaccine: the challenge of antigenic drift. *Vaccine*, 2007 25, 6852-6862.

[4] Bridges, CB; Thompson, WW; Meltzer, MI; Reeve, GR; Talamonti, WJ; Cox, NJ; *et al.* Effectiveness and cost-benefit of influenza vaccination of healthy working adults: a randomized controlled trial. *JAMA*, 2000 284, 1655-1663.

[5] De Filette, M; Min Jou, W; Birkett, A; Lyons, K; Schultz, B; Tonkyro, A; *et al.* Universal influenza A vaccine: optimization of M2-based constructs. *Virology*, 2005 337, 149-161.

[6] Wood, JM; Dunleavy, U; Newman, RW; Riley, AM; Robertson, JS; Minor, PD. The influence of the host cell on standardisation of influenza vaccine potency. *Dev Biol Stand*, 1999 98, 183-188.

[7] World Health Organization Expert Committee on Biological Standardization. Proposed guidelines on regulatory preparedness for human pandemic influenza vaccines [online]. 2007 Available from: http://www.who.int/vaccine_research/diseases/influenza/ Guidelines_regulatory_preparedness_pandemic_influenza_vaccines.pdf ([accessed on Feb. 19, 2009].

[8] Harvey, R; Wheeler, JX; Wallis, CL; Robertson, JS; Engelhardt, OG. Quantitation of haemagglutinin in H5N1 influenza viruses reveals low haemagglutinin content of vaccine virus NIBRG-14 (H5N1). *Vaccine*, 2008 Oct 7 [Epub ahead of print].

[9] Skehel, JJ; Wiley, DC. Receptor binding and membrane fusion in virus entry: the influenza hemagglutinin. *Annu Rev Biochem*, 2000 69, 531-569.

[10] Horváth, A; Tóth, GK; Gogolák, P; Nagy, Z; Kurucz, I; Pecht I; *et al.* A hemagglutinin-based multipeptide construct elicits enhanced protective immune response in mice against influenza A virus infection. *Immunol Lett*, 1998 60, 127-136.

[11] Bianchi, E; Liang, X; Ingallinella, P; Finotto, M; Chastain, MA; Fan, J; *et al.* Universal influenza B vaccine based on the maturational cleavage site of the hemagglutinin precursor. *J Virol*, 2005 79, 7380-7388.

[12] Nestorowicz, A; Tregear, GW; Southwell, CN; Martyn, J; Murray, JM; White, DO; *et al.* Antibodies elicited by influenza virus hemagglutinin fail to bind to synthetic peptides representing putative antigenic sites. *Mol Immunol*, 1985 22, 145-154.

[13] Schoofs, PG; Geysen, HM; Jackson, DC; Brown, LE; Tang, XL; White, DO. Epitopes of an influenza viral peptide recognized by antibody at single amino acid resolution. *J Immunol*, 1988 140, 611-616.

[14] Jackson, DC; Brown, LE. A synthetic peptide of influenza virus hemagglutinin as a model antigen and immunogen. *Pept Res,* 1991 4, 114-124.

[15] Chun, S; Li, C; Van Domselaar, G; Wang, J; Farnsworth, A; Cui, X; et al. Universal antibodies and their applications to the quantitative determination of virtually all subtypes of the influenza A viral hemagglutinins. *Vaccine*, 2008 26, 6068-6076.

[16] Scott, D; Nitecki, DE; Kindler, H; Goodman, JW. Immunogenicity of biotinylated hapten-avidin complexes. *Mol Immunol*, 1984 21, 1055-1060.

[17] Stevens, J; Blixt, O; Tumpey, TM; Taubenberger, JK; Paulson, JC; Wilson, IA. Structure and receptor specificity of the hemagglutinin from an H5N1 influenza virus. *Science*, 2006 312, 404-410.

[18] Carr, CM; Chaudhry, C; Kim, PS. Influenza hemagglutinin is spring-loaded by a metastable native conformation. *Proc Natl Acad Sci U S A*, 1997 94, 14306-14313.

[19] Das Sarma, J; Duttagupta, C; Ali, E; Dhar, TK. Antibody to folic acid: increased specificity and sensitivity in ELISA by using epsilon-aminocaproic acid modified BSA as the carrier protein. *J Immunol Methods*, 1995 184, 1-6.

[20] Okawa, Y; Howard, CR; Steward, MW. Production of anti-peptide specific antibody in mice following immunization with peptides conjugated to mannan. *J Immunol Methods*, 1992, 149, 127-131.

[21] Chen, J; Lee, KH; Steinhauer, DA; Stevens, DJ; Skehel, JJ; Wiley, DC. Structure of the hemagglutinin precursor cleavage site, a determinant of influenza pathogenicity and the origin of the labile conformation. *Cell*, 1998 95, 409-417.

[22] Atherton, E; Sheppard, RC. *Solid-Phase Peptide Synthesis: A Practical Approach.* Oxford, England: IRL Press; 1989.

[23] Röhm, C; Zhou, N; Süss, J; Mackenzie, J; Webster, RG. Characterization of a novel influenza hemagglutinin, H15: criteria for determination of influenza A subtypes. *Virology*, 1996 217, 508-516.

[24] Fouchier, RA; Munster, V; Wallensten, A; Bestebroer, TM; Herfst, S; Smith, D. Characterization of a novel influenza A virus hemagglutinin subtype (H16) obtained from black-headed gulls. *J Virol*, 2005 79, 2814-2222.

[25] Huang, D; Pereboev, AV; Korokhov, N; He, R; Larocque, L; Gravel C; et al. Significant alterations of biodistribution and immune responses in Balb/c mice administered with adenovirus targeted to CD40(+) cells. *Gene Ther*, 2008 15, 298-308.

[26] Li, KB. ClustalW-MPI: ClustalW analysis using distributed and parallel computing. *Bioinformatics*, 2003 19, 1585-1586.

[27] Nagy, Z; Rajnavölgyi, E; Hollósi, M; Tóth, GK; Váradi, G; Penke, B; et al. The intersubunit region of the influenza virus haemagglutinin is recognized by antibodies during infection. *Scand J Immunol*, 1994 40, 281-291.

[28] White, JM; Wilson, IA. Anti-peptide antibodies detect steps in a protein conformational change: low-pH activation of the influenza virus hemagglutinin. *J Cell Biol*, 1987 105, 2887-2896.

[29] Bucher, DJ; Li, SSL; Kehoe JM; Kilbourne, ED. Chromatographic isolation of the hemagglutinin polypeptides from influenza virus vaccine and determination of their amino-terminal sequences. *Proc Nat Acad Sci U S A*, 1976 73, 238-242.

[30] Calam, DH; Davidson, J. Isolation of influenza viral proteins by size-exclusion and ion-exchange high-performance liquid chromatography: the influence of conditions on separation. *J Chromatogr*, 1984 296, 285-292.

[31] Phelan, MA; Cohen, KA. Gradient optimization principles in reversed-phase high-performance liquid chromatography and the separation of influenza virus components. *J Chromatogr,* 1983 266, 55-66.

[32] Kapteyn, JC; Saidi, MD; Dijkstra, R; Kars, C; Tjon, JC; Weverling, GJ; *et al.* Haemagglutinin quantification and identification of influenza A&B strains propagated in PER.C6 cells: a novel RP-HPLC method. *Vaccine,* 2006 24, 3137-3144.

[33] Garcia-Cañas, V; Lorbetskie, B; Girard, M. Rapid and selective characterization of influenza virus constituents in monovalent and multivalent preparations using non-porous reversed-phase high performance liquid chromatography columns. *J Chromatogr A,* 2006 Aug 11 1123, 225-232.

[34] Kapteyn, JC; Porre, AM; de Rond, EJ; Hessels, WB; Tijms, MA; Kessen, H; *et al.* HPLC-based quantification of haemagglutinin in the production of egg- and MDCK cell-derived influenza virus seasonal and pandemic vaccines. *Vaccine,* 2009 27, 1468-1477.

[35] García-Cañas, V; Lorbetskie, B; Bertrand, D; Cyr, TD; Girard, M. Selective and quantitative detection of influenza virus proteins in commercial vaccines using two-dimensional high-performance liquid chromatography and fluorescence detection. *Anal Chem,* 2007 79, 3164-3172.

[36] Williams, TL; Luna, L; Guo, Z; Cox, NJ; Pirkle, JL; Donis, RO; *et al.* Quantification of influenza virus hemagglutinins in complex mixtures using isotope dilution tandem mass spectrometry. *Vaccine,* 2008 26, 2510-2520.

[37] Luna, LG; Williams, TL; Pirkle, JL; Barr, JR. Ultra performance liquid chromatography isotope dilution tandem mass spectrometry for the absolute quantification of proteins and peptides. *Anal Chem,* 2008 80, 2688-2693.

[38] Kitler, ME; Gavinio, P; Lavanchy, D. Influenza and the work of the World Health Organization. *Vaccine,* 2002 20 Suppl 2, S5-S14.

[39] Gerdil, C. The annual production cycle for influenza vaccine. *Vaccine,* 2003 21, 1776-1779.

[40] Rocha, N; Neefjes, J. MHC class II molecules on the move for successful antigen presentation. *EMBO J,* 2008 27, 1-5.

[41] Jackson, DC; Purcell, AW; Fitzmaurice, CJ; Zeng, W; Hart, DN. The central role played by peptides in the immune response and the design of peptide-based vaccines against infectious diseases and cancer. *Curr Drug Targets,* 2002 175-196.

[42] Blanchard, N; Shastri, N. Coping with loss of perfection in the MHC class I peptide repertoire. *Curr Opin Immunol,* 2008 Feb 20, 82-88.

PART V:
RESOURCES FOR DEVELOPMENT OF NEW INFLUENZA THERAPEUTICS

In: Global View of Fight against Influenza
Editor: Petar M. Mitrasinovic

ISBN: 978-1-60741-952-5
© 2009 Nova Science Publishers, Inc.

Chapter 14

NIAID RESOURCES FOR THE GLOBAL RESEARCH COMMUNITY TO SUPPORT DEVELOPMENT OF NEW INFLUENZA THERAPEUTICS

Amy Krafft, Rachelle Salomon and Martin Crumrine
Division of Microbiology and Infectious Diseases
National Institute of Allergy and Infectious Diseases
National Institutes of Health, Department of Health and Human Services,
Bethesda, MD, USA

ABSTRACT

With the threat of pandemic influenza still looming, preparedness efforts to develop new diagnostics, vaccines, and therapeutics have expanded to help control the persistent threat of seasonal and novel influenza viruses. The National Institute of Allergy and Infectious Diseases (NIAID), part of the National Institutes of Health (NIH), has issued solicitations for proposals to fund development of new influenza therapeutics and optimization of existing antivirals. NIAID has also implemented programs designed to support qualified researchers worldwide who may not be funded by NIAID but who are engaged in discovery, early development, and evaluation of new influenza therapeutics. These programs are designed to foster development of antivirals with novel mechanisms of action and immunotherapeutics to prevent or treat influenza. These support services are also part of a larger NIAID effort to build a comprehensive set of research resources to facilitate efforts to develop the next generation of vaccines, diagnostics, and therapeutics.

Resources available to influenza researchers at different stages of the product development path include support of the following:

- Early development of new therapeutic compounds ranging from monoclonal antibodies to novel small molecules with antiviral or immunomodulatory activity against influenza infection;

- Preclinical evaluation services, for example, *in vitro* assessment of antiviral activity, followed by *in vivo* efficacy testing in animal models;
- Advanced preclinical services, if warranted, to provide data to inform regulatory review and approval processes;
- Clinical testing units for Phase I studies, for the most promising therapeutic candidates.

NIAID's research resources are intended to help researchers navigate the various complexities and challenges inherent in the scientific and regulatory process of discovery and early development of new influenza therapeutics. This chapter will also illustrate how these resources have been used for the early development of peramivir and T-705, two promising new drugs that are currently in clinical trials. For more information on NIAID's research resources, including eligibility requirements and contact information, visit www.niaid.nih.gov/research/resources.

INTRODUCTION

The recent widespread emergence of antiviral-resistant seasonal influenza A strains, combined with the continuing threat of a potential pandemic outbreak, has generated new urgency for the development of safe and effective antivirals with novel mechanisms of action and broad spectrum activity against a myriad of influenza viruses.

New drug development is an expensive, lengthy, and complicated process with a low likelihood of success in bringing a new drug or biologic product to market. Challenges may continue to rise with the global economic downturn resulting in more limited financing for the drug discovery and development process. The National Institute of Allergy and Infectious Diseases (NIAID), part of the National Institutes of Health (NIH), supports a comprehensive set of research services to facilitate the transition from early discovery into translational research needed to advance product development. These resources have been created to support development of the next generation of vaccines, diagnostics, and therapeutics for diseases caused by biodefense agents classified as NIAID Category A-C priority pathogens and emerging and re-emerging infectious disease agents [1]. Recently, broad-based platform approaches to drug development, rather than the traditional one-bug, one-drug approach, have been supported to advance the next generation of vaccines, diagnostics, and therapeutics. NIAID resources for developing new therapeutics for severe viral infections, including influenza, have been recently reviewed [2].

A major priority of NIAID's research resources is to facilitate development of therapeutics for treating and preventing influenza, a NIAID Category C priority pathogen. During the 2008–09 flu season, antiviral treatment of seasonal influenza was restricted by widespread circulation of antiviral-resistant influenza strains. Currently, two classes of influenza antivirals are approved for use in the United States: the adamantanes and neuraminidase inhibitors. The adamantanes—amantadine and rimantadine—are active against influenza A virus only and the neuraminidase inhibitors—zanamivir and oseltamivir phosphate—are active against influenza type A and B viruses. Widespread circulation of oseltamivir-resistant H1N1 strains and amantadine-resistant H3N2 have limited the use of available antivirals. On December 19, 2008, the U.S. Centers for Disease Control and

Prevention (CDC) issued a Health Network Advisory to health care professionals (HCP) on recommended antiviral treatment options for the remainder of the 2008–09 flu season [3]. In the absence of rapid, sensitive diagnostic tests to determine which viruses are circulating, CDC recommended to HCPs that they use an alternative antiviral—inhaled zanamivir—or dual therapy of oral oseltamivir phosphate and rimantadine, which should provide effective treatment against all known circulating influenza viruses.

NIAID's research resources and services are available to qualified researchers in academia, not-for-profit organizations, industry, and government institutions worldwide. Priority for access is based on public health impact, scientific merit, likelihood that the service will contribute to further development of the product, and the overall cost and availability of the resource. These resources are intended to lower the barriers for those who undertake the difficult challenge of drug discovery and early development of new therapeutics.

This review will first examine the numerous challenges that exist in the influenza therapeutics development field. While the need for new therapeutics has increased in the face of widespread antiviral resistance, the challenges of testing drugs for influenza, especially against the highly pathogenic avian influenza viruses with pandemic potential, have increased. All work with these lethal influenza viruses, now designated as select biological agents for both humans and animals, requires high level biocontainment facilities. We will then describe the various programs NIAID has implemented to help bridge gaps at different stages of the drug development process. Finally, we will illustrate how NIAID resources have been used for the development of peramivir and T-705, two new antiviral drugs currently in clinical trials.

I. Challenges Facing Influenza Therapeutics Development

A. Outbreaks of Highly Pathogenic Avian Influenza Viruses Raise Spectre of the Next Pandemic

Influenza experts have long predicted that a novel influenza subtype to which there is little or no preexisting immunity in the human population, will emerge and cause the next influenza pandemic. In 1997, two remarkable events occurred that changed basic understanding of influenza biology at the human-animal interface. In May 1997, public health officials in Hong Kong reported the first human death caused by a highly pathogenic avian influenza A virus, which is thought to be the first time a lethal avian influenza A virus (H5N1) crossed the avian-human species barrier [4,5]. Avian influenza A (H5N1) viruses that emerged in Hong Kong in 1997 and again in late 2003 continue to spread today and have caused unprecedented epizootic disease in wild birds and domestic poultry in 50 countries across Asia, parts of Europe, the Near East, and Africa. Since 2003, the increasing numbers of human H5N1 infections transmitted directly from domestic poultry have a lethality rate in humans of more than 60 percent. As a result, many experts believe that the next pandemic strain will be related to emergence of a highly pathogenic avian influenza virus (HPAIV). The potential for such highly virulent, lethal viruses to spread globally, as in the 1918 "Spanish flu" pandemic, is alarming and has turned international attention to the need to prepare for the next influenza pandemic [6].

In March 1997, *Science* published a report of the RNA sequence of the first gene from the highly lethal "Spanish influenza" pandemic virus recovered from archival lung tissue of a U.S. Army private who died during the 1918 pandemic [7]. Eight years later, the arduous task of sequencing all eight RNA segments of the 1918 influenza A (H1N1) virus recovered from preserved lung tissues of three victims of the pandemic was completed by scientists at the Armed Forces Institute of Pathology in Washington, DC. Phylogenetic analysis would reveal that the highly lethal 1918 pandemic strain was avian-like and not swine-like, suggesting that avian influenza viruses could infect humans without prior adaptation in a susceptible intermediate mammalian host [8]. The 1918 virus was reconstructed in 2005 and subsequent experimental studies in animal models have shown a pattern of immunopathology and high lethality similar to recent HPAIV infections [9-14]. Efforts to better understand the pathogenesis of highly lethal influenza infections may help researchers to develop and test improved and more effective diagnostics, vaccines, and therapeutics.

B. Biocontainment of Select Agents

Work with HPAIV has become highly restricted in recent years in an effort to increase global biosafety and biosecurity against influenza viruses with pandemic potential. In response to the 2001 anthrax attacks on civilians in the United States, Congress enacted the Public Health Security and Bioterrorism Preparedness and Response Act of 2002. The Act requires the United States Department of Health and Human Services (DHHS) and the United States Department of Agriculture (USDA) to establish regulations and security requirements for possession, use, and transfer of select biological agents and toxins and impose significant criminal and civil penalties for inappropriate use. While this Act was initially focused on protecting against the intentional use of biological agents in acts of bioterrorism, HPAIVs with pandemic potential were soon added to the select agent list.

Contemporary influenza A viruses with pandemic potential are recognized as posing a significant threat to both human and animal public health and safety. These include HPAIVs (H5 and H7 subtypes) responsible for recent epizootics in birds and poultry and more than 400 human deaths since 1997. In March 2005, HPAIV was declared a select agent. It is regulated as a human select agent by the DHHS and as an agricultural select agent by the USDA. In October 2005, the reconstructed influenza A (H1N1) virus responsible for the 1918 "Spanish flu" pandemic was added to the list of DHHS select agents and toxins [15].

The CDC and the USDA Animal and Plant Health Inspection Service (APHIS) Select Agent Programs oversee the possession, use, and transfer of HPAIV with pandemic potential, and register all U.S. laboratories, scientists, and researchers engaged in these activities. The select agent approval process for work with human isolates of HPAIV requires a site inspection and clearance by the CDC. Work with swine and avian influenza viruses requires APHIS permits. Security risk assessments, including background checks and fingerprinting, are conducted by the Federal Bureau of Investigation (FBI) for those having access to select agents, and access is restricted for selected categories of individuals [16-19]. Additionally, all foreign entities working on HPAIV that receive funding from NIH must have their systems evaluated by CDC and they will receive recommendations from CDC. Laboratories generating recombinant or reassortant influenza viruses are also subject to the NIH Guidelines for Research Involving Recombinant DNA Molecules [20].

Laboratory researchers and institutions working with influenza A select agents or with exotic low pathogenic avian influenza viruses must obtain Select Agent approval and meet laboratory requirements detailed in the 2006 HHS publication "Biosafety in Microbiological and Biomedical Laboratories (BMBL), 5th edition" [20]. The BSL-3 rules were amended to enhance protection of laboratory workers and the environment by requiring "showering out" of personnel before they leave the laboratory. All BSL-3 requirements must be followed, including controlled access double-door entry with change room; use of negative-pressure and HEPA-filtered respirators or positive air-purifying respirators (PAPRs); decontamination of all wastes; and maintenance of records in a national select agent database. These stringent biosafety and biosecurity precautions are necessary to protect laboratory workers and the environment from possible exposure to HPAIV.

Eligible academic researchers and institutions seeking to conduct research on avian influenza viruses or to develop new diagnostic tests, novel vaccines, or therapeutics may request virus isolates from the Global Influenza Surveillance Network (GISN). The GISN, which is coordinated by the World Health Organization (WHO), was established in 1952 to select the candidate strains of influenza A and B for yearly production of influenza vaccine in northern and southern hemispheres. The network has four WHO Global Collaborating Centers (CC) that work primarily on human influenza and a fifth CC for Studies on the Ecology of Influenza in Animals. The network characterizes the antigenic properties of a select number of influenza strains using hemagglutinin inhibition assays and sequencing of the hemagglutinin (HA) glycoprotein HA1 domain forming the globular head [21,22]. Antigenic, genetic, and epidemiologic data are then examined to make recommendations of candidate strains for seasonal influenza vaccines, known as reference viruses. Since 2004, the five WHO CC's have also served as the WHO H5 Reference Laboratory Network, established in response to the major public health needs arising from avian influenza A (H5N1) infection in humans.

Following the global health crisis precipitated by the emergence of the SARS coronavirus for nine months in 2002–03, new International Health Regulations were established in 2005 to coordinate the management of events that may constitute a public health emergency of international concern, and to improve the capacity of all countries to detect, assess, notify, and respond to public health threats [23]. The new global public health order for obtaining emerging viruses for risk-assessment and vaccine development from Member states was temporary. In 2007, the GISN framework for sharing highly pathogenic avian influenza A (H5N1) viruses was challenged [24]. A new framework is now being developed for sharing virus strains and data, which takes into account the needs and interests of countries affected by H5N1. The new system is expected to require commercial users of a virus to obtain prior informed consent from the originating country and negotiate the terms of use.

In response to challenges raised by Member states, in November 2007 WHO implemented an electronic system to track receipt and distribution of all influenza A (H5) viruses shared with the GISN and also H5 viruses that have been developed into reassortant viruses as potential vaccine candidates [25]. Several H5N1 reference viruses are available from the CDC, the National Institute for Biological Standards and Control (NIBSC), the U.S. Food and Drug Administration (FDA), or NIAID and can be requested for use by the broader influenza research community outside the GISN. The HPAIV strains are lethal for embryonated chicken eggs, the traditional strategy for vaccine production, thus influenza reverse genetics (rg) methods have been used to remove the polybasic amino acids from the

HA cleavage site associated with high virulence for chickens and ferrets [26]. Many candidate reference viruses are available and can be manipulated in lower level biocontainment facilities, including representatives of the major highly pathogenic H5N1 clades in circulation. Although recent circulating influenza viruses are distributed freely among WHO CCs and reference laboratories, access to viruses by external laboratories conducting important influenza research on HPAIV pathogenesis and product development can be a lengthy process. To obtain HPAIV isolates, investigators and institutions must meet country-specific requirements for permits, obtain consent from the originating country, and have full access to appropriate biocontainment facilities. In the U.S., the select agent security process depends on the host range and pathogenicity of the virus in question, requiring USDA and/or U.S. Public Health Service import permits for animal and human HPAIV strains, respectively. Separate biocontainment facilities are required for animal and human influenza viruses to prevent generation of influenza reassortants.

C. Natural History of Influenza Infection in Humans

Influenza A virus strains undergo continuous genetic change, especially in the major surface glycoprotein genes, hemagglutinin (H) and neuraminidase (N). Variations in these genes are the basis for classifying influenza A viruses into 16 HA and 9 NA antigenic subtypes. The changing surface proteins present a constant challenge, not only for developing rapid and sensitive laboratory and point-of-care diagnostics, but also for developing safe and effective vaccines and therapeutics for preventing and treating influenza. Clinical diagnosis of seasonal influenza can also be challenging because of the wide range of clinical symptoms and variable manifestations of the disease. In cases with no other health complications, seasonal influenza is usually an acute illness restricted to the upper respiratory tract and lasting three to five days. More typically, influenza disease involves a rhinitis that can progress to tracheobronchitis, or rarely, a severe interstitial pneumonitis or acute respiratory distress syndrome (ARDS) [27].

Influenza infections in infants, the elderly, and immunocompromised individuals have high morbidity and can be fatal. Pulmonary complications include primary viral pneumonia, secondary bacterial pneumonia, and combined bacterial and viral pneumonia. Serious influenza with bacterial superinfection leading to pneumonia and sepsis was responsible for the majority of deaths during the 1918-19 pandemic [28]. In recent years, secondary bacterial pneumonia during seasonal influenza outbreaks is most often associated with influenza H3N2 virus infections. In the U.S., a number of fatalities due to community-associated pneumonia (CAP) have been attributed to methicillin-resistant Staphylococcus aureus (MRSA), which is often associated with influenza virus infection or influenza-like illness (ILI) [29,30].

The illness caused by HPAIV ranges in severity. An outbreak of an H7 influenza virus in humans in the Netherlands predominantly caused mild conjunctivitis; however, there was one death [31-34]. Serious disease caused by highly pathogenic H5N1 influenza is characterized by a severe, rapidly progressive diffuse interstitial pneumonitis with a mortality rate of greater than 60 percent since 2003 [35-37].

D. Mouse and Ferret Models of Influenza

The mouse and ferret are the most common animal models for research on seasonal and HPAIV but other animals, including non-human primates, guinea pigs, cotton rats, chinchillas, hedgehogs, chickens, and rats, have been used [38]. Although not a natural host to influenza infection, the inbred laboratory mouse (*Mus musculus*) is the primary small animal model of influenza pneumonia caused by severe seasonal influenza strains (H1 and H3 subtypes) and is frequently used to study pathogenesis and evaluate new anti-influenza therapies and vaccines for HPAIV [39]. The mouse model has also proven useful for evaluating immunomodulator compounds to reduce immunopathology and pulmonary inflammation accompanying influenza pneumonia [40].

Like any other animal model, the mouse model has drawbacks, but their small size, low cost, and availability of reagents allow researchers to conduct studies on a larger scale than possible with other available animal models. Experimental infections with seasonal influenza A and B virus strains in mice or rats require adaptation by multiple lung passage before they can replicate and/or cause disease. Strikingly, a highly pathogenic H5N1 virus and the reconstructed 1918 (H1N1) pandemic influenza virus did not require prior adaptation and were lethal for inbred laboratory mice strains [41]. Research on the interferon response system to viral infection helps explain this puzzling finding. Inbred mice used in research laboratories have genetic defects and lack the Mx1 gene, an important mediator of the host innate immune response to viral infections. Transgenic mice expressing the Mx1 protein (found in wild mice) are protected against lethal challenges of both HPAIV (H5N1) influenza virus and the 1918 pandemic virus [42,43]. Nevertheless, our knowledge of and ability to manipulate the mouse genome has provided valuable information about host factors important in influenza pathogenicity, virulence, and transmission. Recently, a variety of antiviral treatments have conferred protection in a mouse lethality model of influenza. These treatments included defective-interfering viruses [44]; MegaRibavirin aerosol [45]; long chain pentraxin PTX3 [46]; cyanovirin-N [47]; M2 monoclonal antibody [48]; and HA monoclonal antibodies [49-52].

The ferret (*Mustela putorius furo*) has demonstrated a number of advantages for studying influenza. Both influenza A and B viruses can naturally infect the ferret. Furthermore, influenza infection in the ferret closely resembles the human illness in terms of pathogenesis, transmission, clinical signs of disease, immunologic response, and localization in the upper and/or lower respiratory tract [53,54]. Ferrets, like humans, differ in their susceptibility to influenza strains and infection can cause asymptomatic, mild, moderate, severe, or lethal disease [55].

Over the last several years, NIAID has supported several contracts to develop ferret models for seasonal and HPAI infection. Challenges have included obtaining a ready supply of pathogen-free animals. Since ferrets are naturally susceptible to influenza, it is important to obtain animals with no previous exposure to influenza. Ferrets are tested serologically for prior exposure to currently circulating strains of influenza virus by the breeder and prior to use to ensure that they have not been infected by contact with humans infected with influenza. Additionally, it can be difficult to conduct large studies due to biocontainment requirements for HPAIV. There is limited availability of ferret-specific reagents necessary for advancing this model for influenza. NIAID support of these efforts is discussed later.

Efforts to control the type of experimental HPAIV disease induced in mouse and ferret models has been confounded by numerous variables, including virulence of the virus, infectious or lethal challenge dose, route of inoculation, type of anesthesia used, the rapid clinical course, and the age and immune status of the animal. Because ferrets have diverse genetic backgrounds, they do not all respond the same way to a particular strain of virus, increasing the range of variables in the study [56,57]. The increasing number of studies comparing influenza infection in both mice and ferrets are shedding valuable light on the strengths and differences of the models. Consistent, reproducible, and interpretable results in animal models are needed to evaluate the effects of new therapeutics and guide the drug development process. A variety of treatments with antiviral activity against seasonal influenza infection have recently been evaluated in ferrets, including injectable peramivir [58]; cyanovirin-N [47]; QR-435 [59]; Low pH gel intranasal sprays [60]; and defective-interfering viruses [61].

The critical need for influenza vaccines and therapeutics to prevent or treat HPAIV has created an enormous demand for efficacy testing in a robust ferret model of HPAIV infection. A well-characterized ferret model of HPAIV may be used in the future for evaluation, development and licensure of new HPAIV treatments under the Animal Rule. The Rule, officially known as the "Approval of Biological Products/New Drugs when Human Efficacy Studies are not Ethical or Feasible," is a counterterrorism measure that has been in effect since 2002 [62]. The Animal Rule allows the FDA to approve specific biologics and drugs when adequate and well-controlled efficacy studies in humans are not ethical or feasible.

E. Human Influenza Challenge Studies

Experimental infection using seasonal influenza strains in healthy human volunteers has been conducted to better understand the human immune response and evaluate the efficacy of vaccines and therapeutics. The currently licensed neuraminidase inhibitors (NAI) [63-65] and an orally administered form of the experimental NAI, peramivir, have been tested in experimental human challenge studies [66-67]. In general, the symptoms and course of disease elicited in human challenge studies are mild and self-limited. In most experimental infections, the influenza virus inoculum is administered into the nasopharynx of the volunteer. Viral shedding is monitored over several days to a week and typically peaks approximately 48 h after inoculation, with little or no infectious virus shed after six days [68]. These experiments are challenging to conduct for a number of reasons that include appropriate but significant safety precautions and assessments required prior to, during, and following the administration of challenge virus to the volunteer. Challenges for conducting experimental influenza infection in the U.S. include rigorous cardiac monitoring, the availability of an influenza virus challenge "pool" that has been produced under current Good Manufacturing Practice (cGMP) and meets regulatory standards, and the need to screen large numbers of volunteers for susceptibility to that challenge virus. Despite these challenges, efforts continue to develop challenge strains of influenza A virus that meet the criteria needed for experimental use in humans.

II. NIAID Resources Available to the Scientific Research Community for Discovery and Development of New Therapeutics

Through its Division of Microbiology and Infectious Diseases (DMID), NIAID supports a comprehensive set of community resources and services for researchers to facilitate translational research needed to develop the next generation of safe and effective drugs, vaccines, and diagnostics to control and prevent infectious diseases from natural outbreaks or terrorist attacks. The following is an overview of the various resources available from NIAID to support discovery, evaluation, and early development of new influenza therapeutic candidates and to advance them along the product development pipeline towards regulatory approval. Investigators interested in any of the services described below can visit the Research Resources section of the NIAID website: www.niaid.nih.gov/research/resources. Those needing additional information about influenza resources beyond what is included on the Web site can contact the NIAID DMID influenza program.

A. NIAID Biocontainment Facilities and Core Services

Access to high-level BSL-3+ biocontainment facilities is required for research and development work with HPAIV with pandemic potential and the reconstructed 1918 pandemic influenza (H1N1) virus. These viruses are currently classified as indigenous or exotic agents that may cause serious or potentially lethal disease as a result of exposure by inhalation [20]. This enhanced biosafety requirement has resulted in the construction of new BSL-3/BSL-4 facilities and upgrading of BSL-2 to BSL-3/BSL-3+ at many academic centers and research institutions in the U.S. and elsewhere. Researchers may contact the individual influenza investigators at the NIAID supported Centers for collaborative opportunities.

As part of our nation's biodefense preparedness efforts, the U.S. Congress substantially increased funding for infectious diseases. NIAID responded by establishing a solid infrastructure to facilitate high priority infectious disease research on lethal agents. This is helping to elucidate the basic biology of bacterial and viral agents considered to be potential agents of bioterrorism and to rapidly accelerate efforts to develop effective countermeasures. The infrastructure includes a network of secure high-level biocontainment facilities needed to support civilian research and training focused on these rare, but highly lethal pathogens, as well as emerging and re-emerging infectious diseases. The new NIAID Biodefense Network is made up 13 Regional Biocontainment Laboratories (RBLs) and two National Biocontainment Laboratories (NBLs) to provide BSL-2/3 facilities and maximum BSL-2/3/4 containment, respectively. For more information on the NIAID Biodefense Network, visit www.niaid.nih.gov/research/resources/dmid/NBL_RBL.

Of the 15 RBL and NBL biocontainment facilities, nine have select agent clearance (or are in the clearance process) for HPAIV, a NIAID Category C priority pathogen (Table 1). The University of Medicine and Dentistry of New Jersey has served as the regional small animal core for the past five years and supports studies of H5N1 influenza in the mouse model. The University of Pittsburgh RBL researchers focus on pathogenesis and lung infections caused by more than a dozen select agents and emerging pathogens, including

HPAIV. The four independent ABSL3 suites that are available at the University of Pittsburgh RBL can house large colonies of nonhuman primates, ferrets, and mice for proof of principle studies by IM, IV, intranasal, and aerosol delivery methods. The two NBLs at the Center for Biodefense and Emerging Infectious Diseases (CBEID) at the Galveston National Laboratory (GNL) University of Texas Medical Branch and at Boston University Medical Campus (BUMC) - National Emerging Infectious Diseases Laboratories (NEIDL) are under construction but anticipate having mice and ferret models for avian influenza and the reconstructed 1918 influenza virus, and Good Laboratory Practice (GLP) / cGMP capacity in the near future.

Table 1. Biocontainment Laboratories in the United States with Select Agent Clearance* for Highly Pathogenic Avian Influenza Virus (HPAIV)

Regional (RBL) or National Biocontainment Laboratory	GLP/cGMP compliant	Animal models	Regional Center of Excellence (RCE) Association
University of Pittsburgh	No	mice ferrets NHP	Mid-Atlantic
University of Medicine & Dentistry of New Jersey (Newark)	Yes	mice	Northeast
Colorado State University (Fort Collins)	Yes	mice ferrets	Rocky Mountain
University of Alabama	Yes	mice ferrets	Southeast
Tulane University*	No	NHP ferrets	Southeast & Western
Duke University*	Future	mice	Southeast
University of Louisville	No	mice ferrets	Southeast
University of Texas Medical Branch– Galveston National Lab*	2009-10	mice ferrets	Western
Boston University Medical Campus*	Future	mice ferrets	Northeast

Legend: Abbreviations: NHP, non-human primates; *Facilities in process of CDC select agent approval process

NIAID's Regional Centers of Excellence for Biodefense and Emerging Infectious Diseases (RCEs) are a consortium of universities and research institutions that provide state-of-the-art core facilities and services to promote discovery and translational research capacity for developing the next generation of vaccines, drugs, and diagnostics focused on NIAID Category A-C Priority Pathogens [2]. RCEs support researchers involved in discovery and early development of influenza therapeutics at academic, private, and government institutions, globally, on a fee-for-service basis. Core services vary at each Center, and may include high throughput small molecule screening, genomic-scale proteomics, large-scale biological molecule production, preclinical development activities, BSL-3+ animal model support, immunologic techniques, microscopy, aerobiology, and clinical investigations of vaccines, therapeutics, and diagnostics. For more information about NIAID's RCEs, visit www.niaid.nih.gov/research/resources/rce.

B. Biological Research Repositories

Strains of seasonal influenza A (H1N1 and H3N2) viruses, HPAIV strains, and influenza B viruses are necessary to evaluate new antiviral compounds for efficacy, toxicity, and spectrum of antiviral activity by non-clinical *in vitro* assays and *in vivo* animal models of influenza infection. NIAID established the Biodefense and Emerging Infections Research Resources Repository (BEI) through a contract to the American Type Culture Collection (ATCC) in September 2003 to acquire, authenticate, produce, store, and distribute reagents for the global research community. The BEI has a large inventory of influenza virus strains and reagents, which has dramatically increased in recent years. Viruses and other reagents are available free to eligible global academic, private, and government researchers conducting basic or translational research on influenza. Registration is required before investigators can order materials through an online catalog. Investigators are also encouraged to deposit into BEI reagents that are frequently requested or would like to have made widely available. This eases the burden on investigators of maintaining and distributing these reagents. BEI also actively solicits suggestions for reagents that are of broad interest to a scientific community so that it can make those available. Investigators are encouraged to make suggestions directly to BEI for reagents needed to advance specific areas of research.

Many of the materials recently deposited in BEI were produced by researchers in the six NIAID Centers of Excellence for Influenza Research and Surveillance (CEIRS) program, awarded in 2007. The CEIRS investigators conduct research on animal influenza surveillance, pathogenesis, and host response. Many of the reference reagents to HPAIV strains are prepared at St. Jude Children's Research Hospital. The BEI also contains inactivated H5N1 vaccines for use in *in vitro* and *in vivo* studies, human H5 sera from volunteers who participated in NIAID clinical trials, monoclonal antibody and polyclonal antisera panels, as well as recombinant proteins and overlapping peptide arrays of influenza HA and NA proteins. Monoclonal antibodies and polyclonal antisera raised in different animal species (goat, rabbit, rooster, guinea pig, and chicken) against many of the 16 HA and 9 NA subtypes of low-pathogenic and recent HPAIVstrains are available. Currently BEI has numerous polymerase chain reaction (PCR) primer sets for the detection of ferret host genes and a monoclonal antibody to measure ferret interferon-gamma [69]. NIAID is also supporting the development of ferret reagents to more fully evaluate the ferret immune response during treatment with therapeutic candidates. Some ferret reagents are currently in BEI and others still in production will be deposited shortly.

The BEI has a collection of historical and contemporary influenza A and B vaccine strains produced over many decades by Dr. Edwin M. Kilbourne, viral RNA, recombinant vaccine reference viruses, and is in the process of obtaining influenza A viruses of the 16 HA and 9 NA subtypes. Recombinant vaccine reference viruses to HPAIV in BEI have been exempted from the select agent list based on results from *in vitro* and *in vivo* studies indicating that these strains are not pathogenic in avian species. These strains can be used to evaluate new therapeutic candidates for efficacy, toxicity, and the spectrum of antiviral activity by *in vitro* assays and *in vivo* animal models of influenza infection in BSL-2 biocontainment facilities. HPAIV strains are not currently available through BEI, though renovations for BSL-3 facilities are underway to accommodate them. For more information, visit www.beiresources.org.

C. Viral Genome Sequencing and Analysis Tools

Many of the barriers to study influenza genetics and evolution have fallen since the Human Genome Project was completed in 2003 at an estimated cost of **one dollar** per base pair. Rapid advances in inexpensive sequencing chemistries and automated genome sequencing platforms have stimulated the recent growth of genomics, proteomics, and bioinformatics and transformed biomedical research. Not long ago, the majority of influenza sequences available were partial sequences encoding the antigenic variable regions of the genes encoding the HA and NA proteins used for evaluating risk-assessments and annual vaccine composition. The first public Influenza Sequence Database at the Los Alamos National Laboratory (LANL) created in the post-World War II era to house the GISN influenza sequences used by influenza researchers has recently closed.

Since 2001, influenza researchers have been calling for a global lab to study influenza with automated high-throughput genome sequencing platforms. This would facilitate sequencing of the whole genome of a greater variety of human and animal influenza viruses than commonly done by the GISN for determining risk-assessment and vaccine composition [21]. NIAID responded in 2004 by launching the collaborative Influenza Genome Sequencing Project [70] to improve the availability of influenza type A and B sequences in the public domain. As of January 28, 2009, the complete genomes of 3338 human and avian influenza A isolates from samples collected all over the world have been sequenced at the J.Craig Venter Institute (JCVI), annotated at the National Center for Biotechnology Information (NCBI), and deposited in GenBank. Potential collaborators with an influenza virus sequencing project should visit the Research Resources section of the NIAID Web site at www.niaid.nih.gov/research/resources.

The free, user-friendly genomic database tools for sequence analysis from the Influenza Sequence Database at LANL have been updated and moved to the BioHealthBase Influenza Virus Bioinformatics Resource Center (BRC) [71]. The BioHealthBase (BHB) comprehensive Web-based resource was launched in 2004 to integrate diverse data sets imported from public databases, information extracted from the scientific literature, and more recently, experimental data from NIAID-supported researchers. The influenza virus sequence database contains all influenza sequence data obtained from the NIAID Influenza Genome Sequencing Project as well as from GenBank. Individualized work spaces are provided as well as a simplified on-line interface to facilitate submission of influenza sequences directly to GenBank. BHB also provides a centralized Web-accessible repository of surveillance and experimental research data. Analysis tools are integrated with the database to allow phylogenetic analyses. The BHB Influenza Virus BRC is supported by a multi-disciplinary team consisting of microbiologists, bioinformaticians, and computer scientists at Northrop Grumman, University of Texas Southwestern Medical Center (UTSMC), and Vecna Technologies. The team is complemented by consultants with influenza virus expertise who provide advice for new developments and test BHB features. BHB's potential to support and advance the influenza field is manifold. It can be used to support basic research in influenza virus molecular evolution, surveillance, pathogenicity, drug resistance, disease transmission, host response, and to facilitate influenza product development. The BHB is available to all eligible members of the global public health and influenza research communities. NIAID is seeking feedback from researchers on improvements for the database as well as collaborators. For more information, visit www.biohealthbase.org/GSearch/home.do?decorator=influenza

D. *In vitro* Testing

The *in vitro* Antiviral Screening Program was established by NIAID in 1989 and is the oldest and one of the most popular research resources available that is free to eligible scientists. It is designed to screen pure compounds for antiviral activity against influenza viruses and to evaluate cytotoxicity. Occasionally, screening for antiviral activity is also done on biological extracts. The compound supplier is requested to release information about the chemical identity and/or any previous data on the characterization of the compounds to the NIAID project manager, in confidence, prior to screening to avoid the use of resources to screen the same compounds repeatedly. The compound sponsor generally receives data from the *in vitro* screen within two months. Routine assays are performed in the Madin-Darby canine kidney (MDCK) cell line and typically compounds are tested for antiviral activity against several influenza strains, including influenza type A (H1 and H3 subtypes) and B. Additional recombinant reference viruses derived from recent clinical isolates may also be used. The standard assays used for evaluating influenza antiviral activity and cell toxicity are the inhibition of viral cytopathic effect, increase in neutral red dye uptake, and confirmatory testing with decrease in virus yield assays [72]. When relatively large numbers (10 or more) of test compounds are submitted at the same time from a single sponsor, rapid screening assays for influenza antiviral activity are available. Compounds generally need an *in vitro* evaluation prior to consideration of testing in animal models; submitters can give their own *in vitro* data to access *in vivo* testing services.

E. *In vivo* Mice and Ferret Testing

In vivo models are used in early stage preclinical development for proof-of-principle studies to help determine drug candidate efficacy for a specific indication. Animal models of seasonal and HPAIV are available free of charge to scientists who demonstrate eligibility for testing and evaluation of influenza antiviral and immunomodulatory compounds. Different methods of drug delivery, including intraperitoneal, IM, IV, topical inhalation, topical intranasal, or oral may be evaluated, as well as dose-range studies and regimens to determine the therapeutic window. Numerous endpoints can be used to monitor influenza infection, assess the effectiveness of a therapeutic, and determine protection from death and weight loss. Disease-inhibitory effects of experimental therapeutics observed in mice can include reduced spread of virus to various organs, reduced decline of arterial oxygen saturation, inhibition of lung consolidation, reduced rise in serum alpha-1-acid glycoprotein, and lowering of lung virus titers [39,57,73]. Therapeutic combinations can also be evaluated in mice models [74-80]. Chemical assays on animal-derived specimens for product or metabolites and pharmacokinetic and pharmacodynamic (PK and PD) determinations are the responsibility of the compound submitter. The mouse model contractor can harvest tissue/blood samples at appropriate times and store for further testing by the compound submitter [2].

The ferret models for initial proof-of-concept and potential GLP studies with seasonal and HPAIV are in development at three research centers supported by NIAID contracts. The natural history of infection or pathogenesis has been characterized with A/Brisbane/10/07 (H3N2) and A/Vietnam/1203/04 (H5N1) in the ferret model. Infectious and lethal dose studies have been conducted with the H3N2 and H5N1 strains, respectively. Following infection, animals are typically monitored for 21 days for changes in clinical signs, body temperature, and body weight. Other parameters measured for clinical disease include hematology, serum chemistry and viral titers in nasal washes. Full necropsies are conducted post-mortem and different tissue (lung, spleen, liver and brain) sections are examined for histopathology and viral burden (quantified by qPCR and tissue culture infectious dose, $TCID_{50}$). The egg infectious dose, EID_{50} of the influenza challenge viruses has been determined for therapeutic and vaccine studies to evaluate protection in ferret challenge models. Experimental therapeutics are evaluated for protection against fever, weight loss, changes in serum chemistry, and infiltration of inflammatory cells in the ferret model.

To gain access to the animal model testing services, submitters must complete a form providing information on the product being submitted. This is used to select and prioritize compounds for testing. Compounds that are anti-inflammatory or immunomodulatory in nature are considered for direct submission for testing in the mouse model because they would not be expected to show antiviral activity *in vitro*. Typically, compounds must be evaluated in the mouse model prior to consideration for testing in the ferret model due to the significant costs associated with the ferret model.

F. Services for the Preclinical Development of Therapeutic Agents

Because many compound sponsors do not have all of the resources and technologies needed to fully develop a promising drug or biological candidate through the steps of preclinical evaluation, NIAID established the Services for the Preclinical Development of Therapeutic Agents program in November 2006. SRI International, a nonprofit contract research organization located in Menlo Park, California, under contract to NIAID can provide a wide array of preclinical services to fill specific gaps in the overall development plan of a product.

In response to the critical need for new influenza therapeutics, many U.S. and international researchers are now working on diverse therapeutic approaches and products to treat and prevent seasonal and/or HPAIV. Most of the investigators who contact NIAID for information on services to further develop their therapeutic candidate may have demonstrated efficacy *in vitro* and/or limited animal efficacy data and may be seeking information or assistance with the next steps in the development of their product.

To help transition from discovery to a focused product development tract, SRI can prepare planning and evaluation tools, such as a Product Development Plan (PDP) and a Target Product Profile (TPP), along with an outline of the key Investigational New Drug (IND)-enabling studies with appropriate go/no-go decision points. The PDP outlines the specific steps required to complete an IND application to bring a lead candidate to Phase I safety trials in humans. The TPP, is an organized list of key components of a potential product profile—including product indication, patient population, delivery mode, dosage form, regimen, efficacy, safety, storage conditions, and shelf-life stability -- with agreed on criteria for acceptance. SRI prepares these planning tools considering guidance and draft guidance documents from the FDA and the International Conference on Harmonization (ICH).

NIAID encourages product sponsors to establish communications with the FDA early in development. Pre-IND interactions with the FDA should be started prior to initiating definitive GLP animal toxicology studies for input on proposed study design and intended clinical use to obtain some assurance that the agency considers the proposed studies acceptable. For other product development issues, the FDA can provide case-by-case recommendations about the developmental approach of each therapeutic candidate, since the results of preliminary testing may trigger additional testing to assess the safety, toxicity, or manufacturing process for a given compound.

The general process for drug and biologic development is similar for anti-infective products in oral, parental, and topical form. They include clearly prescribed manufacturing, safety, and regulatory activities to obtain evidence of the safety and efficacy of a new product. This evidence is needed for an IND application to FDA for approval to begin human clinical trials. SRI recommends that work proceed in three stages, with a go/no-go decision point at the end of each stage. The first stage is to demonstrate animal efficacy, the second stage consists of toxicopharmacokinetic (t?K)/range-finding studies, and the third stage is the full set of definitive pivotal GLP and cGMP studies required to move the product to a successful IND application.

Examples of the wide array of services available at different stages of the developmental path for therapeutics include:

- Lead identification and development including chemical screening, lead optimization schemes, synthesis or resynthesis of chemical analogues and custom synthesis of radiolabeled compounds
- Manufacture of purified drug substance (DS) batches under non-GMP or "GMP-like" conditions for pilot characterization and stability studies
- Manufacture of purified bulk DS under formal cGMP compliance
- Preformulation studies and formulation development for dosage design
- Analytical and bioanalytical methods development and assay validation for biological samples to support PK, dose range-finding, toxicokinetic (TK), immunogenicity, and tissue cross-reactivity studies
- Metabolic and PK/PD studies including bioavailability and absorption, distribution, metabolism, excretion/elimination and toxicity (ADMET) studies
- Toxicology studies including safety, single- and repeat-dose PK, and toxicity GLP studies in two species
- cGMP manufacture of drug product for clinical trials

The Services for the Preclinical Development of Therapeutic Agents program can offer assistance at any of the steps in the discovery and preclinical development process. Access to these resources is competitive and is based on public health impact, scientific merit, likelihood that the service will contribute to the further development of the product, and the overall cost and availability of the resource.

G. Different Paths to Regulatory Approval of New Therapeutics

NIAID works with drug company sponsors from around the world at different stages of the product development path. These discussions have been beneficial to gain insight into the different challenges facing the drug development community and the complexities of conducting appropriate studies to meet regulatory approval. Companies developing new influenza therapeutics may seek guidance and feedback about the design and conduct of their preclinical, Phase I, and Phase II studies. The NIAID Office of Regulatory Affairs (ORA) within DMID is available to meet with company representatives and principal investigators who conduct clinical trials to discuss preclinical and clinical development plans and the types of studies and data to inform the FDA. With many new therapeutics in early product development, the FDA has released a new Draft Guidance to Industry on Influenza: Developing Drugs for Treatment and/or Prophylaxis (February 2009) which should greatly facilitate the design and conduct of studies needed for new antiviral development programs for seasonal, HPAIV, and novel influenza. This new guidance is available at: www.fda.gov/cder/guidance/7927dft.pdf.

H. Clinical Research in Infectious Diseases

NIAID supports several clinical units around the world that can perform clinical studies and trials on the most promising influenza therapeutics. Because many compound sponsors do not have financial resources for the initial clinical evaluation, drug sponsors can request access to these units. The process for requesting clinical evaluation of a therapeutic agent includes submitting a formal concept to NIAID that describes the study objectives, rationale for the proposed clinical trial, recruitment and site plan, protocol timeline (including specific milestones for protocol development and initiation), requested personnel, and the study budget. For consideration, drug sponsors must have sufficient drug product available. All materials, including Chemistry Manufacturing and Controls (CMC) and an investigator's brochure, required to complete preclinical assessments for an IND for Phase I trials must be accessible in a master file acceptable to the FDA. Submission of a concept is typically followed by detailed discussions about the product, supporting data, the development plan, and the requestor's timelines. Concepts are reviewed according to the following general criteria: public health impact; appropriateness and feasibility of the study design; and availability of resources. Protocols for approved concepts are developed collaboratively by the study protocol team which includes the drug developer, the clinical investigator, and NIAID staff.

Two Phase I Clinical Trial Units for Therapeutics contracts were awarded in 2008 to conduct Phase I safety trials on promising anti-infective products. Services are provided by DynPort Vaccine Company with a clinical site at the Quintiles Phase I Unit in Overland Park, Kansas, and Clinical Research Management with clinical sites at Johns Hopkins University in Baltimore, Maryland, and Case Western Reserve University in Cleveland, Ohio. These clinical research sites perform safety oversight, clinical monitoring, data management and regulatory management of trials with anti-infective products.

The Vaccine and Treatment Evaluation Units (VTEUs) have been supported by NIAID contracts since 1962 and are comprised of a consortium of VTEU sites within academic centers and organizations that provide a ready resource for the conduct of clinical trials to evaluate promising vaccines and treatments for infectious diseases. The VTEUs can conduct a broad range of studies including Phase I–IV clinical trials in people of all ages and risk categories. The VTEUs can also undertake a variety of other studies that support product development such as evaluations of novel product delivery systems and reevaluation of current vaccine formulations and schedules of delivery.

The Collaborative Antiviral Study Group (CASG) is a multi-center clinical trials group that conducts Phase I–IV pediatric and adult research trials to evaluate novel therapeutic regimens for viral infections in over 100 clinical centers across the country and in select international sites. The Central Unit at the University of Alabama at Birmingham (UAB) provides medical, laboratory, biostatistical, and administrative staff to coordinate research design and regulatory affairs for the clinical centers. The CASG undertakes therapeutic intervention trials of promising therapies for unmet medical needs, such as rare viral diseases and other viral illnesses, such as influenza; studies to document the development of resistance to antiviral therapies; studies of rare or emerging viral diseases in special populations such as immunocompromised, pediatric, elderly, and pregnant women; and natural history/pathogenesis studies to support future therapeutic or medical management. For therapeutic trials, investigators must provide an adequate supply of the study product, and matching placebo or comparison therapy as applicable, at no cost.

In January 2009, the South East Asian Influenza Clinical Research Network, which was established in late 2005, expanded its efforts to advance knowledge and clinical research in emerging infectious disease study beyond influenza and changed its name to South East Asian Infectious Disease Clinical Research Network, keeping the SEAICRN acronym [81]. The SEA Network is a five year multilateral, collaborative partnership of hospitals and institutions in Thailand, Indonesia, Vietnam, United Kingdom, and the United States. The Network is financially supported by several donors, including NIAID and the Wellcome Trust. The network has made progress preparing South East Asian clinical research sites to conduct clinical studies. Much effort has been focused on training site staff and putting in place protocols, data management systems, pharmacy support, diagnostic laboratories, and independent oversight groups in advance of when an emerging infection makes a sporadic or unpredictable appearance in any of these countries [82]. For more information, visit www.seaclinicalresearch.org.

I. T-705 and Peramivir

T-705, a novel pyrazine derivative, was discovered by scientists at the Toyama Chemical Co. in 2002 and shown to have potent *in vitro* and *in vivo* activities against influenza [83,84]. Mechanistic studies suggested the compound acts as an RNA Polymerase inhibitor of influenza [85]. It has been suggested that host cell kinases convert T-705 into T-705 ribofuranosyl phosphate (T-705RTP), a form that inhibits viral polymerases without affecting host cell RNA or DNA synthesis. Toyama submited T-705 samples for further testing through the NIAID *in vitro* and *in vivo* antiviral testing programs at the Institute for Antiviral Research at Utah State University, a NIAID contract site. The *in vitro* and *in vivo* studies showed that orally administered T-705 had potent antiviral activity against a range of influenza strains including avian H5N1 viruses [86]. In a lethal mouse model with avian H5N1, T-705 treatment protected all mice from death and subsequent challenge experiments showed that orally administered T-705, given up to 60 h after virus exposure, was still significantly inhibitory to lethal infection. T-705 has also shown activity against other serious viral disease agents, including arenavirus and bunyavirus agents of hemorrhagic fever [87,88]. Toyama Chemical Co. has been supporting clinical trials in the U.S. and Japan and company representatives periodically meet with NIAID staff to review progress and discuss regulatory issues.

Peramivir, a novel neuraminidase inhibitor (NAI) for influenza prophylaxis and treatment, has been tested extensively in preclinical and clinical development studies since its discovery by scientists at the University of Alabama at Birmingham (UAB) and BioCryst Pharmaceuticals, Inc. in 1987 [89]. Peramivir (BCX-1812; RWJ-27021) is a unique NA inhibitor with a cyclopentane ring structure. NIAID has supported preclinical studies of peramivir throughout its development, first as an oral form and then as an injectable form. Like the licensed NAI's, zanamivir and oseltamivir, peramivir was rationally designed using the group 2 NA crystal structure available in the 1980s to have potent and selective activity against both influenza type A and B viruses.

Peramivir has shown comparable or greater potency than zanamivir and oseltamivir against multiple influenza strains, including H1N1 and H3N2 seasonal isolates, oseltamivir-resistant influenza strains, and influenza B viruses by *in vitro* NA inhibition testing [90-92]. Peramivir has shown effective antiviral activity against all nine NA subtypes and inhibited the replication of avian influenza viruses of both Eurasian and American lineages *in vitro* [93]. Orally administered peramivir has protected mice and ferrets against influenza virus challenge with multiple seasonal influenza strains and completely protected mice against lethal challenge with highly pathogenic avian influenza A/Hong Kong/156/97 (H5N1) reducing viral titers in the lungs, and preventing the spread of virus to the brain [94-96].

Oral peramivir has been shown to be safe and well tolerated in humans and advanced to Phase III clinical trials in North America and Europe in February 2000 [97,98]. Despite strong evidence for the antiviral effectiveness of once daily oral administration of peramivir from murine pharmacodynamic and Phase IIa human experimental influenza studies, the Phase III trials with this dosing regimen were unsuccessful [66,67,99,100]. Peramivir failed to show statistically significant improvement of the primary endpoint, the length of time from the first dose to the clinically significant relief of influenza symptoms, compared to oseltamivir treatment in 2002, possibly due to poor oral bioavailability. Peramivir development continued and intravenous and intramuscular injectable formulation are currently in advanced clinical development.

CONCLUSIONS

Discovery and development of new safe and effective antivirals with new molecular targets and novel mechanisms of action against influenza viruses are urgently needed. While this chapter has focused on the substantial array of research resources and services NIAID has developed to help facilitate global efforts to develop new drugs and immunomodulators for influenza, many resources are offered to support broad-based approaches to drug, vaccine and diagnostics development, rather than the traditional one-bug, one-drug approach. Investigators interested in more information about these resources and services should review the information provided at www.niaid.nih.gov/research/resources and contact the influenza program at DMID NIAID.

REFERENCES

[1] U.S. National Institute of Allergy and Infectious Disease. Biodefense and related programs. Bethesda, MD: NIAID online; [cited 2009 Feb 21]. Available from: http://www3.niaid.nih.gov/.

[2] Greenstone H, Spinelli B, Tseng C, Peacock S, Taylor K, Laughlin C. NIAID resources for developing new therapies for severe viral infections. *Antiviral Res*. 2008;78(1):51-9.

[3] U.S. Centers for Disease Control and Prevention. Influenza antiviral resistance and interim recommendations for the use of influenza antiviral medications in the United States [podcast on the Internet]. Atlanta: CDC online; 2008 Dec 19 [cited 2009 Feb 21]. Available from: www2a.cdc.gov/podcasts/download/.

[4] U.S. Centers for Disease Control and Prevention. Isolation of avian influenza A (H5N1) viruses from humans -- Hong Kong, May - December 1997. MMWR. 1997;46:1204-7.

[5] Claas EC, Osterhaus AD, van Beek R, de Jong JC, Rimmelzwaan GF, Senne DA, et al. Human influenza A H5N1 virus related to a highly pathogenic avian influenza virus. *Lancet*. 1998; 351:472-77.

[6] Salomon R, Webster RG. The influenza virus enigma. *Cell*. 2009;136:402-10.

[7] Taubenberger JK, Reid AH, Krafft AE, Bijwaard KE, Fanning TG. Initial genetic characterization of the 1918 "Spanish" influenza virus. *Science*. 1997;275:1793-6.

[8] Taubenberger JK, Reid AH, Lourens RM, Wang R, Jin G, Fanning TG. Characterization of the 1918 influenza virus polymerase genes. *Nature*. 2005;437 (7060):889-93.

[9] Tumpey TM, Basler, CF, Aguilar PV, Zeng H, Solórzano A, Swayne DE, et al. Characterization of the Reconstructed 1918 Spanish Influenza Pandemic Virus. *Science*. 2005;310(5745):77-80.

[10] Cheung CY, Poon LL, Lau AS, Luk W, Lau YL, Shortridge KF, et al. Induction of proinflammatory cytokines in human macrophages by influenza A (H5N1) viruses: a mechanism for the unusual severity of human disease? *Lancet*. 2002;360:1831-7.

[11] Perrone LA, Plowden JK, Garcia-Sastre A, Katz JM, Tumpey TM. H5N1 and 1918 pandemic influenza virus infection results in early and excessive infiltration of macrophages and neutrophils in the lungs of mice. PLoS Pathogens [serial on the Internet]. 2008 [cited 2009 Feb 21];4(8):1-11. Available from: www.plospathogens.org/.

[12] Kash JC, Tumpey TM, Proll SC, Carter V, Perwitasari O, Thomas MJ, et al. Genomic analysis of increased host immune and cell death responses induced by 1918 influenza virus. *Nature*. 2006;443(7111):578-81.

[13] de Jong MD, Simmons CP, Thanh TT, Hien VM, Smith GJ, Chau TN, et al. : Fatal outcome of human influenza A (H5N1) is associated with high viral load and hypercytokinemia. *Nat Med.* 2006;12(10):1203-7.

[14] Kobasa D, Jones SM, Shinya K, Kash JC, Copps J, Ebihara H, et al. Aberrant innate immune response in lethal infection of macaques with the 1918 influenza virus. *Nature.* 2007;445(7125):319-23.

[15] U.S. Centers for Disease Control and Prevention and U.S. Department of Agriculture - Plant Health Inspection Service. National Select Agent Registry. CDC-APHIS online; [document on the Internet] [cited 2009 Feb 21]; Available from: http://www. selectagents.gov/.

[16] U.S. Department of Health and Human Services. "Additional Requirements for Facilities Transferring or Receiving Select Agents," Public Health 42 Federal Register 72 (2005 Mar 18) [document on the Internet] [cited 2009 Feb 21] Available from: http://www.access.gpo.gov/.

[17] U.S. Department of Health and Human Services. "Select Agents and Toxins," Public Health 42 Federal Register 73 (2005 Mar 18) [document on the Internet] [cited 2009 Feb 21] Available from: http://www.access.gpo.gov/.

[18] U.S. Department of Agriculture. "Possession, Use, and Transfer of Select Agents and Toxins," Agriculture: 7 Code of Federal Regulations Part 331 (2005 Dec 30) [document on the Internet] [cited 2009 Feb 21] Available from: http://www.access.gpo.gov/.

[19] U.S. Department of Agriculture. "Possession, Use, and Transfer of Select Agents and Toxins," Animals and Animal Products: 9 Code of Federal Regulations Part 121 (2005 Dec 30) [document on the Internet] [cited 2009 Feb 21] Available from: http://www.access.gpo.gov/.

[20] U.S. Department of Health and Human Services. Biosafety in Microbiological and Biomedical Laboratories (BMBL) 5th edition, 2007 Feb [document on the Internet] [cited 2009 Feb 1] Available from: http://www.cdc.gov/OD/ohs/biosfty/bmbl5/.

[21] Layne SP, Beugelsdijk TJ, Patel CK, Taubenberger JK, Cox NJ. A global lab against influenza. Science. 2001; 293:1729.

[22] Kitler ME, Gavinio P, Lavanchy D. Influenza and the work of the World Health Organization. Vaccine. 2002;20(Suppl 2):S5–S14.

[23] World Health Organization. International Health Regulations (2005) Second edition. [document on the Internet] [cited 2009 Feb 21] Available from: http://www.who.int/csr/ihr/IHR_2005_en/. 82 pages.

[24] Statement by the Minister of Health of the Republic of Indonesia H.E. DR. Dr. Siti Fadilah Supari at the Inter-Governmental Meeting for Pandemic influenza Preparedness Geneva: 2007 Nov 20. [document on the Internet] [cited 2009 Feb 21] Available from: (http://www.ip-watch.org/files/Indonesia_statement_WHO/.

[25] World Health Organization. Influenza Virus Tracking System (interim). Geneva: WHO online. [cited 2009 Feb 21] Available from: https://www.who.int/fluvirus_tracker/.

[26] Webby RJ, Perez DR, Coleman JS, Guan Y, Knight JH, Govorkova EA, et al. Responsiveness to a pandemic alert: use of reverse genetics for rapid development of influenza vaccines. *Lancet.* 2004;363(9415):1099-103.

[27] Wright PF, Webster RG. Orthomyxoviruses. In: Knipe DM, Howley PM, editors. *Fields Virology, 4th edition.* Vol 1. New York: Lippincott Williams & Wilkins; 2001. p. 1158-60.

[28] Morens DM, Taubenberger JK, Fauci AS. Predominant role of bacterial pneumonia as a cause of death in pandemic influenza: implications for pandemic influenza preparedness. *J Infect Dis*. 2008;198(7):962-70.

[29] Jones-Nazar C, Robertson D, Eavey J, Kravel L, Brian F, Mayeux LJ, et al. Severe methicillin-resistant Staphylococcus aureus community-acquired pneumonia associated with influenza--Louisiana and Georgia, December 2006-January 2007. *MMWR Morb Mortal Wkly Rep*. 2007;56:325–9.

[30] Tenover FC, McDougal LK, Goering RV, Killgore G, Projan SJ, Patel JB, et al. Characterization of a strain of community-associated methicillin-resistant Staphylococcus aureus widely disseminated in the United States. *J Clin Microbiol*. 2006;44:108–18.x

[31] Munster VJ, de Wit E, van Riel D, Beyer WE, Rimmelzwaan GF, Osterhaus AD, et al. The molecular basis of the pathogenicity of the Dutch highly pathogenic human influenza A H7N7 viruses. *J Infect Dis*. 2007;196(2):258-65.

[32] Fouchier RA, Schneeberger PM, Rozendaal FW, Broekman JM, Kemink SA, Munster V, et al. Avian influenza A virus (H7N7) associated with human conjunctivitis and a fatal case of acute respiratory distress syndrome. *Proc Natl Acad Sci USA*. 2004;101(5):1356-61.

[33] Koopmans M, Wilbrink B, Conyn M, Natrop G, van der Nat H, Vennema H, et al. Transmission of H7N7 avian influenza A virus to human beings during a large outbreak in commercial poultry farms in the Netherlands. *Lancet*. 2004;363(9409):587-93.

[34] Elbers AR, Fabri TH, de Vries TS, de Wit JJ, Pijpers A, Koch G. The highly pathogenic avian influenza A (H7N7) virus epidemic in The Netherlands in 2003--lessons learned from the first five outbreaks. *Avian Dis*. 2004;48(3):691-705.

[35] de Jong MD. H5N1 transmission and disease: observations from the frontlines. *Pediatr Infect Dis J*. 2008;27(10 Suppl):S54-56.

[36] Writing committee of the Second World Health Organization Consultation on Clinical Aspects of Human Infection with Avian influenza (H5N1) Virus, Abdel-Ghafar AN, Chotpitayasunondh T, Gao Z, Hayden FG, Nguyen DH, et al. Update on avian influenza A (H5N1) virus infection in humans. *N Engl J Med*. 2008;358(3):261-73. Review.

[37] Beigel JH, Farrar J, Han AM, Hayden FG, Hyer R, de Jong MD, et al. Avian influenza A (H5N1) infection in humans. *N Engl J Med*. 2005;353(13):1374-85. Review.

[38] Renegar, KB . Influenza virus infections and immunity: a review of human and animal models. *Lab Anim Sci*. 1992;42:222-32.

[39] Sidwell, RW, Smee DF. In vitro and in vivo assay systems for study of influenza virus inhibitors. *Antiviral Res*. 2000;48:1-16.

[40] Marsolais D, Hahm B, Walsh KB, Edelmann KH, McGavern D, Hatta Y, et al. A critical role for the sphingosine analog AAL-R in dampeing the cytokine response during influenza virus infection. *Proc Natl Acad Sci USA*. 2009;106(5):1560-5.

[41] Tumpey TM, García-Sastre A, Taubenberger JK, Palese P, Swayne DE, Pantin-Jackwood MJ, et al. Pathogenicity of influenza viruses with genes from the 1918 pandemic virus: functional roles of alveolar macrophages and neutrophils in limiting virus replication and mortality in mice. *J Virol*. 2005;79(23):14933-44.

[42] Salomon R, Staeheli P, Kochs G, Yen HL, Franks J, Rehg JE, Webster RG, Hoffmann E. Mx1 gene protects mice against the highly lethal human H5N1 influenza virus. *Cell Cycle*. 2007;6(19):2417-21.

[43] Dittmann J, Stertz S, Grimm D, Steel J, García-Sastre A, Haller O, Kochs G. Influenza A virus strains differ in sensitivity to the antiviral action of Mx-GTPase. *J Virol*. 2008;82(7):3624-31.

[44] Dimmock NJ, Rainsford EW, Scott PD, Marriott AC. Influenza virus protecting RNA: an effective prophylactic and therapeutic antiviral. *J Virol*. 2008;82:8570-8.

[45] Gilbert BE, McLeay MT. MegaRibavirin aerosol for the treatment of influenza A virus infections in mice. *Antiviral Res*. 2008;8:223-9.

[46] Reading PC, Bozza S, Gilbertson B, Tate M, Moretti S, Job ER, et al. Antiviral activity of the long chain pentraxin PTX3 against influenza viruses. *J Immunol*. 2008;80:3391-8.

[47] Smee DF, Bailey KW, Wong MH, O'Keefe BR, Gustafson KR, Mishin VP, et al. Treatment of influenza A (H1N1) virus infections in mice and ferrets with cyanovirin-N. *Antiviral Res*. 2008;80:266-71.

[48] Wang R, Song A, Levin J, Dennis D, Zhang NJ, Yoshida H et al. Therapeutic potential of a fully human monoclonal antibody against influenza A virus M2 protein. *Antiviral Res*. 2008;80:168-77.

[49] Simmons CP, Bernasconi NL, Suguitan AL, Mills K, Ward JM, Chau NV, et al. Prophylactic and therapeutic efficacy of human monoclonal antibodies against H5N1 influenza. PLoS Med [serial on the Internet]. 2007 [cited 2009 Feb 21];4(5)e178. Available from: www.plosjournals.org/.

[50] Kashyap AK, Steel J, Oner AF, Dillon MA, Swale RE, Wall KM, et al. Combinatorial antibody libraries from survivors of the Turkish H5N1 avian influenza outbreak reveal virus neutralization strategies. *Proc Natl Acad Sci USA*. 2008;105(16):5986-91.

[51] Throsby M, van den Brink E, Jongeneelen M, Poon LL, Alard P, Cornelissen L, et al. Heterosubtypic neutralizing monoclonal antibodies cross-protective against H5N1 and H1N1 recovered from human IgM+ memory B cells. PloS One. [serial on the Internet]. 2008 [cited 2009 Feb 21];3(12):e3942. Available from: www.plosone.org/.

[52] Sui J, Hwang WC, Perez S, Wei G, Aird D, Chen LM, et al. Structural and functional bases for broad-spectrum neutralization of avian and human influenza A viruses. *Nat Struct Mol Biol*. 2009 Feb 22. [Epub ahead of print]

[53] Pearson CR and Gorham JR. Ferrets. In: Fox JG, editor. *Biology and Diseases of the Ferret, 2nd edition*. Lippincott Williams and Wilkins, New York, 1998, p 487-97.

[54] Watanabe T, Watanabe S, Shinya K, Kim JH, Hatta M, Kawaoka Y. Viral RNA polymerase complex promotes optimal growth of 1918 virus in the lower respiratory tract of ferrets. *Proc Natl Acad Sci USA*. 2009;106:588-92.

[55] Govorkova EA, Ilyushina NA, Boltz DA, Douglas A, Yilmaz N, Webster RG. Efficacy of oseltamivir therapy in ferrets inoculated with different clades of H5N1 influenza virus. *Antimicrob Agents Chemother*. 2007;51(4):1414-24.

[56] Maher JA and DeStefano . 2004 The ferret: an animal model to study influenza virus. *Lab Animal*. 2004;33:50-3.

[57] Barnard DL. Animal models for the study of influenza pathogenesis and therapy. Antiviral Res. 2009;[25 Jan 2009 Epub ahead of print]

[58] Yun NE, Linde NS, Zacks MA, Barr IG, Hurt AC, Smith JN et al. Injectable peramivir mitigates disease and promotes survival in ferrets and mice infected with the highly virulent influenza virus, A/Vietnam/1203/04 (H5N1). *Virology*. 2008;374(1):198-209.

[59] Oxford JS, Lambkin R, Guralnik M. Rosenbloom RA, Petteruti MP, Digian K et al. In vivo prophylactic activity of QR-435 against H3N2 influenza virus infection. *Am J Ther*. 2007;14:462-8.

[60] Rennie P, Bowtell P, Hull D, Charbonneau D, Lambkin-Williams R, Oxford J. Low pH gel intranasal sprays inactivate influenza viruses in vitro and protect ferrets against influenza infection. *Respir Res*. 2007;8:38.

[61] Mann A, Marriott AC, Balasingam S, Lambkin R, Oxford JS, Dimmock NJ. Interfering vaccine (defective interfering influenza A virus) protects ferrets from influenza, and allows them to develop solid immunity to reinfection. *Vaccine*. 2006;24:4290-6.

[62] Department Of Health And Human Services, Food and Drug Administration. Rules and Regulations. 21 Code of Federal Regulations Part 314.610 and 601.90-95 subpart H31 pages 37988-98. (2002 May 31) [document on the Internet] [cited 2009 Feb 21] Available from: http://www.fda.gov/cber/rules/humeffic.htm.

[63] Calfee DP, Peng AW, Hussey EK, Lobo M, Hayden FG. Safety and efficacy of once daily intranasal zanamivir in preventing experimental human influenza A infection. *Antivir Ther*. 1999;4(3):143-9.

[64] Hayden FG, Treanor JJ, Fritz RS, Lobo M, Betts RF, Miller M et al. Use of the oral neuraminidase inhibitor oseltamivir in experimental human influenza: randomized controlled trials for prevention and treatment. *JAMA*. 1999;282(13):1240-6.

[65] Fritz RS, Hayden FG, Calfee DP, Cass LM, Peng AW, Alvord WG et al. Nasal cytokine and chemokine responses in experimental influenza A virus infection: results of a placebo-controlled trial of intravenous zanamivir treatment. *J Infect Dis*. 1999;180(3):586-93.

[66] Iyer GR, Liao S, Massarella J. Population analysis of the pharmacokinetics and pharmacodynamics of RWJ-270201 (BCX-1812) in treating experimental influenza A and B virus in healthy volunteers. *AAPS PharmSci*. 2002;4(4):1-10.

[67] Barroso L, Treanor J, Gubareva L, Hayden FG. Efficacy and tolerability of the oral neuraminidase inhibitor peramivir in experimental human influenza: randomized, controlled trials for prophylaxis and treatment. *Antivir Ther*. 2005;10(8):901-10.

[68] Baccam P, Beauchemin C, Macken CA, Hayden FG, Perelson AS. Kinetics of influenza A infection in humans. *J Virol*. 2006;80(15):7590-9.

[69] Ochi A, Danesh A, Seneviratne C, Banner D, Devries ME, Rowe T, Xu L, Ran L, Czub M, Bosinger SE, Cameron MJ, Cameron CM, Kelvin DJ. Cloning, expression and immunoassay detection of ferret IFN-gamma. *Dev Comp Immunol*. 2008;32(8):890-7.

[70] Fauci AS. Race against time. *Nature*. 2005;435:423-4.

[71] Squires B, Macken C, Garcia-Sastre A, Godbole S, Noronha J, Hunt V et al. BioHealthBase: informatics support in the elucidation of influenza virus host–pathogen interactions and virulence. *Nucleic Acids Res*. 2008;36(Database issue):D497-503.

[72] Smee DF, Morrison AC, Barnard DL, Sidwell RW. Comparison of colorimetric, fluorometric, and visual methods for determining anti-influenza (H1N1 and H3N2) virus activities and toxicities of compounds. *J Virol Methods*. 2002;106(1):71-9.

[73] Sidwell RW, Wong MH, Bailey KW, Barnard DL, Jackson MK, Smee DF. Utilization of alpha-1-acid glycoprotein levels in the serum as a parameter for in vivo assay of influenza virus inhibitors. *Antivir Chem Chemother.* 2001; 12(6):359-65.

[74] Smee DF, Bailey KW, Morrison AC, Sidwell RW. Combination treatment of influenza A virus infections in cell culture and in mice with the cyclopentane neuraminidase inhibitor RWJ-270201 and ribavirin. *Chemotherapy.* 2002;48(2):88-93.

[75] Smee DF, Wong MH, Bailey KW, Sidwell RW. Activities of oseltamivir and ribavirin used alone and in combination against infections in mice with recent isolates of influenza A (H1N1) and B viruses. *Antivir Chem Chemother.* 2006;17(4):185-92.

[76] Ilyushina NA, Hay A, Yilmaz N, Boon AC, Webster RG, Govorkova EA. Oseltamivir-ribavirin combination therapy for highly pathogenic H5N1 influenza virus infection in mice. *Antimicrob Agents Chemother.* 2008;52(11):3889-97.

[77] Ilyushina NA, Hoffmann E, Salomon R, Webster RG, Govorkova EA. Amantadine-oseltamivir combination therapy for H5N1 influenza virus infection in mice. *Antivir Ther.* 2007;12(3):363-70.

[78] Galabov AS, Simeonova L, Gegova G. Rimantadine and oseltamivir demonstrate synergistic combination effect in an experimental infection with type A (H3N2) influenza virus in mice. *Antivir Chem Chemother.* 2006;17(5):251-8.

[79] Zheng BJ, Chan KW, Lin YP, Zhao GY, Chan C, Zhang HJ, et al. Delayed antiviral plus immunomodulator treatment still reduces mortality in mice infected by high inoculum of influenza A/H5N1 virus. *Proc Natl Acad Sci USA.* 2008;105(23):8091-6.

[80] Wilson SZ, Knight V, Wyde PR, Drake S, Couch RB. Amantadine and ribavirin aerosol treatment of influenza A and B infection in mice. *Antimicrob Agents Chemother.* 1980;17(4):642-8.

[81] The Southeast Asian Influenza Clinical Research Network. [document on the Internet]. SEAICRN online; [cited 2009 Feb 25]. Available from: http://www.seaclinicalresearch. org.

[82] Higgs ES, Hayden FG, Chotpitayasunondh T, Whitworth J, Farrar J. The Southeast Asian Influenza Clinical Research Network: development and challenges for a new multilateral research endeavor. *Antiviral Res.* 2008;78:64-8.

[83] Furuta Y, Takahashi K, Fukuda Y, Kuno M, Kamiyama T, Kozaki K et al. In vitro and in vivo activities of anti-influenza virus compound T-705. *Antimicrob Agents Chemother.* 2002;46(4):977-81.

[84] Takahashi K, Furuta Y, Fukuda Y, Kuno M, Kamiyama T, Kozaki K, et al. In vitro and in vivo activities of T-705 and oseltamivir against influenza virus. *Antivir Chem Chemother.* 2003 Sep;14(5):235-41.

[85] Furuta Y, Takahashi K, Kuno-Maekawa M, Sangawa H, Uehara S, Kozaki K, et al. Mechanism of action of T-705 against influenza virus. *Antimicrob Agents Chemother.* 2005 Mar;49(3):981-6.

[86] Sidwell RW, Barnard DL, Day CW, Smee DF, Bailey KW, Wong MH, et al. Efficacy of orally administered T-705 on lethal avian influenza A (H5N1) virus infections in mice. *Antimicrob Agents Chemother.* 2007 Mar;51(3):845-51.

[87] Gowen BB, Wong MH, Jung KH, Sanders AB, Mendenhall M, Bailey KW, et al. In vitro and in vivo activities of T-705 against arenavirus and bunyavirus infections. *Antimicrob Agents Chemother.* 2007;51(9):3168-76.

[88] Gowen BB, Smee DF, Wong MH, Hall JO, Jung KH, Bailey KW, Stevens JR, Furuta Y, Morrey JD. Treatment of late stage disease in a model of arenaviral hemorrhagic fever: T-705 efficacy and reduced toxicity suggests an alternative to ribavirin. PLoS ONE. 2008;3(11):e3725.

[89] Babu YS, Chand P, Bantia S, Kotian P, Dehghani A, El-Kattan Y, et al. BCX-1812 (RWJ-270201): discovery of a novel, highly potent, orally active, and selective influenza neuraminidase inhibitor through structure-based drug design. *J Med Chem.* 2000;43(19):3482–86.

[90] Smee, DF; Huffman, JH; Morrison, AC; Barnard, DL; Sidwell, RW. Cyclopentane neuraminidase inhibitors with potent in vitro anti-influenza virus activities. *Antimicrob Agents Chemother.* 2001;45(3):743–48.

[91] Gubareva LV, Webster RG, Hayden FG. Comparison of the activities of zanamivir, oseltamivir, and RWJ-270201 against clinical isolates of influenza virus and neuraminidase inhibitor-resistant variants. *Antimicrob Agents Chemother.* 2001;45(12): 3403-8.

[92] Bantia S, Parker CD, Ananth SL, Horn LL, Andries K, Chand P, et al. Comparison of the anti-influenza virus activity of RWJ-270201 with those of oseltamivir and zanamivir. *Antimicrob Agents Chemother.* 2001;45(4):1162–67.

[93] Govorkova EA, Leneva IA, Goloubeva OG, Bush K, Webster, RG. Comparison of efficacies of RWJ-270201, zanamivir, and oseltamivir against H5N1, H9N2, and other avian influenza viruses. *Antimicrob Agents Chemother.* 2001;45(10):2723–32.

[94] Sidwell RW, Smee DF, Huffman JH, Barnard DL, Bailey KW, Morrey JD, et al. In vivo influenza virus-inhibitory effects of the cyclopentane neuraminidase inhibitor RJW-270201. *Antimicrob Agents Chemother.* 2001;45(3):749–57.

[95] Sidwell RW, Smee DF, Huffman JH, Barnard DL, Morrey JD, Bailey KW, Feng WC, Babu YS, Bush K. Influence of virus strain, challenge dose, and time of therapy initiation on the in vivo influenza inhibitory effects of RWJ-270201. *Antiviral Res.* 2001;51(3):179-87.

[96] Sweet C, Jakeman KJ, Bush K, Wagaman PC, McKown LA, Streeter AJ, et al. Oral administration of cyclopentane neuraminidase inhibitors protects ferrets against influenza virus infection. *Antimicrob Agents Chemother.* 2002;46(4):996-1004.

[97] Barnard DL. RWJ-270201 BioCryst Pharmaceuticals/Johnson & Johnson. *Curr Opin Investig Drugs.* 2000;1(4):421-4. Review.

[98] Sidwell RW, Smee DF. Peramivir (BCX-1812, RWJ-270201): potential new therapy for influenza. *Expert Opin Investig Drugs.* 2002;11(6):859-69. Review.

[99] Young D, Fowler C, Bush K. RWJ-270201 (BCX-1812): a novel neuraminidase inhibitor for influenza. *Philos Trans R Soc Lond B Biol Sci.* 2001;356(1416):1905-13. Review.

[100] Drusano GL, Preston SL, Smee D, Bush K, Bailey K, Sidwell RW. Pharmacodynamic evaluation of RWJ-270201, a novel neuraminidase inhibitor, in a lethal murine model of influenza predicts efficacy for once-daily dosing. *Antimicrob Agents Chemother.* 2001;45(7):2115–18.

PART VI:
NATURAL THERAPIES

Chapter 15

MICRONUTRIENTS IN THE GLOBAL FIGHT AGAINST INFLUENZA

R.J. Jariwalla, M.W. Roomi, T. Kalinovsky, M. Rath and A. Niedzwiecki

Dr. Rath Research Institute, Santa Clara, CA, USA

ABSTRACT

Influenza remains a major health threat among infectious diseases, affecting one fifth of the world's population. Current vaccines and drugs have limited efficacy and there is an urgent need for effective therapies. Influenza virus A not only infects susceptible (alveolar) cells in the lungs, it also manifests in extrapulmonary areas, which require basement membrane disruption by matrix metalloproteinases (MMPs) capable of degrading collagen type IV. Hence an effective strategy in fighting influenza must be targeted not only in blocking virus replication, but also protecting disruption of the connective tissue and inhibiting virus spread without inflicting toxicity to host cells. We have developed a unique micronutrient mixture, containing ascorbic acid, green tea extract, lysine, proline, N-acetyl cysteine, and selenium, which was shown to be effective in controlling critical steps in influenza virus infection. We evaluated its actions on cell-free influenza A virus, viral multiplication in infected cells and induction of cellular metalloproteinases following virus infection. Application of the nutrient mixture to Vero or MDCK cells post infection resulted in dose-dependent inhibition of viral nucleoprotein production in infected cells. Pretreatment of virus with the nutrient mixture enhanced the antiviral effect. Incubation of cell-free virus with the mixture resulted in dose-dependent inhibition of associated neuraminidase. Additionally, the micronutrient mixture inhibited extracellular invasive parameters such as MMP-2 and MMP-9 secretion and Matrigel invasion. In conclusion, a non-toxic micronutrient mixture tested in our investigation has potential in influenza treatment by not only decreasing viral multiplication in infected cells but also by blocking the enzymatic degradation of the extracellular matrix to limit virus spread.

INTRODUCTION

Incidence, Pathogenesis and Impacts on Health of Influenza Infection

Influenza, a febrile, acute viral disease of the respiratory tract, affects 20% of the world's population, posing a serious health problem, leading to significant morbidity and mortality, and subsequent economic costs [1]. Influenza infections occur annually in the United States as epidemics each winter affecting 5% to 20% of the population and resulting in an estimated 36,000 deaths and more than 200,000 hospitalized patients each year [1]. Recent events, such as avian flu-associated human deaths, have caused concern over the possibility of pandemics, suggesting the need for preventive/therapeutic strategies to effectively combat the emergence of the flu.

Current Treatments and Limitations: The Need for Effective Non-Toxic Therapy

Currently vaccination is the primary strategy for prevention of influenza, especially in high-risk populations. However, vaccines are often ineffective, due to the ability of influenza to evade the immune response through antigenic drift and re-assortment of genomic RNA in the virus, rendering it less effective to seasonal or pandemic outbreaks. Therefore, intense focus has shifted to developing therapeutic and/or prophylactic approaches to controlling influenza.

One approach involves the use of antiviral agents aimed at inhibiting specific steps in virus multiplication. Currently two classes of drugs are approved for the treatment or prophylaxis of influenza infections: the adamantanes (amantadine and its derivative rimantadine) and the newer neuraminidase (NA) inhibitors (oseltamivir and zanamivir). However, current therapies are not optimal and new treatments are needed. Adamantanes interfere with viral uncoating inside the cell and are effective only against influenza A. They are associated with several toxic side effects and with drug-resistant variants [2]. Neuraminidase inhibitors such as oseltamivir and zanamivir block the function of virus-encoded neuraminidase enzyme, preventing the release of virus from the host cell surface. Although neuraminidase inhibitors are effective against all strains of influenza, they must be administered early, since replication of influenza virus in the respiratory tract reaches its peak between 24–72 hours after the onset of the disease. Tamiflu (oseltamivir), a neuraminidase inhibitor, has been reported to reduce illness by one to two days and to have few adverse effects (nausea, vomiting, abdominal pain in 5%). However, Tamiflu does not prevent the flu and is reported only to reduce the length and severity of symptoms [2]. Additionally, recent reports on the use of the drug in normal flu cases in Japan—a country where Tamiflu is prescribed ten times more often than in the US—described bizarre psychiatric problems in children treated with the drug, leading to death [3]. In addition, in a recent study in Japan, 9 out of 50 treated children harbored viruses with mutations in the neuraminidase gene that encoded drug-resistant neuraminidase proteins, a serious concern since children are an important source of the spread of influenza in the community [2]. More recently, the FDA recommended new warnings about possible dangerous psychiatric side effects of influenza drugs Tamiflu and Relenza. Other approaches in the field of influenza antiviral research have involved the application of RNA viral interference through the use of short interfering RNA (siRNA) or microRNA [4,5]. Additionally, neutralizing monoclonal antibodies capable of binding to non-variant regions of the influenza hemagglutinin (surface protein) were shown recently to neutralize a broad-spectrum of influenza group 1 viruses [6]. Although still in their infancy, the therapeutic potential of these experimental approaches remains unknown.

Nutritional Approaches in Influenza

There is a well-established connection between malnutrition and low immunity. It is well known that nutritional deficiency lowers immunity and predisposes to infection [7]. In the developing world, malnutrition, accompanied by poverty and poor sanitation, is common and associated with infectious diseases that pose the greatest health risk, including death. Worldwide, failing immunity as a consequence of malnutrition is the leading cause of death of children, the elderly, and adults [8]. Micronutrient deficiencies are also prevalent in various human populations in the industrialized countries including elderly persons, people affected by various diseases, children, smokers, and those exposed to various pollutants.

In sharp contrast to nutritional deficiency, nutritional supplementation can modulate immunity and increase resistance to infection [9,10]. Most nutrients tested in influenza are antioxidants since reactive oxygen species have been implicated in the pathological damage resulting from infection [11]. However, new comprehensive approaches are needed which address other aspects associated with viral infection. In this respect we have developed a micronutrient-based approach that simultaneously targets several cellular mechanisms associated with influenza.

Importance of Defining New Targets: Connective Tissue, Virus Spread

Influenza virus not only affects lung areas, causing interstitial pneumonitis and the presence of leukocytic cell infiltrate in the submucosa of the airways and in alveolar septae [12], but also manifests in extrapulmonary areas, such as in the involvement of the central nervous system [13], pericarditis [14] and myocarditis [15]. Influenza virus in the bloodstream (viremia) has also been reported [16]. Yeo et al. [17] postulated that in order for a virus to reach the stromal compartment and blood vessels, the basement membrane must be disrupted by matrix metalloproteinases (MMPs) capable of degrading collagen type IV: MMP-2 and MMP-9. As viruses do not have any proteinases to disrupt the membrane, they suggested that infected loci, such as inflammatory cells at the infected site might release MMPs. For example, in bronchiectasis, neutrophils and mononuclear phagocytes release type IV collagenases. They proposed that MMP-2 and MMP-9 from infected epithelial cells might help the destruction of the integrity of the epithelial cell layer and basement membrane and demonstrated induction of type IV collagenases in Vero and MDCK cells from influenza A virus infection. Influenza virus induced production of MMP-2 or MMP-9 depending on the cell line infected. Viral infection increased MMP-9 expression in Vero cells but decreased it in MDCK cells [17]. The approach we have used involves inhibiting connective tissue breakdown and virus spread using naturally occurring nutrients.

Micronutrients and Nutrient Synergy

In 1992 Rath postulated that nutrients such as vitamin C and lysine play a critical role in various pathological conditions, which are associated with destruction of connective tissue, such as atherosclerosis, cancer and viral or bacterial infections [18]. Lysine and vitamin C are necessary for maintaining optimum connective tissue integrity through many mechanisms, including inhibition of proteases digesting various connective tissue components and regulation of collagen synthesis and structure. We have developed a nutrient mixture (NM) encompassing these and other nutrients, which has shown to be effective in inhibition of critical cellular mechanisms associated with cancer, cardiovascular disease and other pathological conditions. Our studies demonstrated that this synergy-based nutrient mixture (NM) containing lysine, proline, ascorbic acid, green tea extract, N-acetyl cysteine (NAC), selenium, and other micronutrients has potent antiviral [19-21], anti-carcinogenic [22] and anti-atherogenic [23] activity in vitro and in vivo.

Rationale for Application of Nutrient-Synergy in Viral Diseases Such as Influenza

All nutrients work in our bodies in harmonious synergy, not in isolation. Nutrient synergy maximizes the health benefits of micronutrients by combining small quantities of vitamins, minerals, amino acids and trace elements instead of using single nutrients in large quantity. It is based on the concept that maximum health benefits are derived from nutrients working in teams rather than in isolation.

Many of the constituents of NM have been reported in the literature to have an inhibitory effect on replication of influenza virus and other viruses [24-32]. Ascorbate has been reported to inhibit the replication of rhinovirus (linked to the common cold) [33] and more recently shown to inhibit influenza A viral antigen production in a dose-dependent manner [19]. Ascorbate levels were found to be reduced in influenza virus-infected mice [28], which displayed increased oxidative stress in the lungs [11]. Ascorbic acid was also reported to inhibit HIV replication in lymphocytic cells [26, 27], an effect that was localized to a post-transcriptional step in virus replication [34]. Ascorbate has been shown previously to selectively kill cancer cells through a pro-oxidant effect [35, 36].

In a review of clinical evidence from 21 placebo-controlled studies of vitamin C and the common cold, Hemilä reported that in each of the studies vitamin C (at a dosage of > or = 1g/d) reduced the duration of episodes and the severity of the common cold symptoms by an average of 23% [37]. In a more recent Cochrane review of placebo-controlled trials in which at least 0.2 g/d of vitamin C was used, a similar conclusion was reached [38]. The data also suggested that high doses of vitamin C were more beneficial than low doses.

Another key component of NM, green tea extract, which is enriched in polyphenols such as epigallocatechin gallate (EGCG), has been shown to be a promising agent in controlling angiogenesis, metastasis, and other aspects of cancer progression [39]. Furthermore, EGCG and epicatechin gallate were found to be potent inhibitors of influenza virus replication in MDCK cell culture [31, 29] and viral RNA synthesis in MDCK cells and neuraminidase activity [31]. In addition, EGCG prevented virus from adsorbing to MDCK cells by agglutination of influenza virus in cell culture [30].

Other components in NM include amino acids (lysine, proline, arginine) and N-acetyl cysteine (NAC) and minerals that may also play a role in the suppression of influenza infection by supporting the stability of the extracellular matrix (ECM) integrity by ensuring optimal collagen formation. Collagen stability is supported by lysine [18] and also by N-acetyl cysteine through its inhibitory effect on MMP-9 activity [40] and invasive activities of tumor cells [41]. N-acetyl cysteine (NAC) was shown to significantly decrease mortality in influenza-infected mice [32]. Furthermore, in combination with ribavirin, NAC demonstrated a synergistic effect in protecting mice against a lethal influenza viral infection [42]. Manganese and copper are also essential cofactors in collagen formation. Ghandi et al. [43] reported an antiviral effect directed towards influenza A virus by copper through inhibition of the proton translocation machinery in the M2 protein of this virus. Selenium has been shown to interfere with MMP expression and tumor invasion [44] and its deficiency has been demonstrated to increase the pathogenicity of influenza virus infection in mice [24]. Increased oxidative stress from influenza virus, which results in increased NF-kB expression and enhanced TH-2 cell response and lung inflammation, was abated by adequate selenium intake, resulting in a TH-1 response after viral infection and reduced pathology.

IN VITRO EFFECTS OF NUTRIENT SYNERGY ON INFLUENZA A VIRUS

Effects of NM on Viability of Vero and MDCK Cells

We initially evaluated the effect of various concentrations of NM on the viability of Vero and MDCK cells, using the trypan blue exclusion test, to provide a working concentration range for a therapeutic effect of NM. MDCK viability was not significantly affected after treatment with NM for 48 h, showing no apparent toxicity at 50–250 µg/ml NM, with only slight lowering of viability (<15% cell death) at 500–1000 µg/ml NM (correlation coefficient r=-0.7632, p=0.077) [19]. Treatment of Vero cells with low concentrations of NM had little effect on cell viability, producing 20% lowering of viable cell count at 100-250 µg/ml of the nutrient mixture. At higher concentrations, 500–1000 µg/ml NM, approximately 60–67% lowering in viability of Vero was observed (correlation coefficient r=-0.8889, p=0.018), although it was found that NM was selectively more inhibitory to influenza virus than to uninfected cells [19].

Effect of NM on Influenza Total NP Antigen Production in Vero Cells

To delineate the antiviral effect of the nutrient mixture, Vero cells were infected with influenza A virus, exposed to various concentrations of NM, and the titer of viral NP protein was determined as described under legend to Figure 1. Trypsin treatment increased influenza A NP antigen level from 12.5 units/ml to 340 units/ml at 44-48h after virus infection, consistent with the role of trypsin in culture as a prerequisite for viral infection [19], as shown in Figure 1. NP antigen production by influenza A virus in Vero cells treated with trypsin was inhibited profoundly by exposure to NM in a dose-dependent manner (r=-0.7260, p=0.102) with 46% inhibition over control at 50 µg/ml NM (p=0.088), 93% at 100µg/ml NM (p=0.002), and 100% at 500 and 1000 µg/ml NM (p=0.001) [19]. In the absence of trypsin, influenza A virus NP production in Vero cells was inhibited slightly less but in a dose-dependent manner (r=-0.8221, p=0.045) with 40% inhibition over control at 50 μg/ml NM (p=0.01), 54% at 100 μg/ml NM (p=0.004), 72% at 500 μg/ml (p<0.0001) and 82% at 1000 μg/ml NM (p<0.0001) [19].

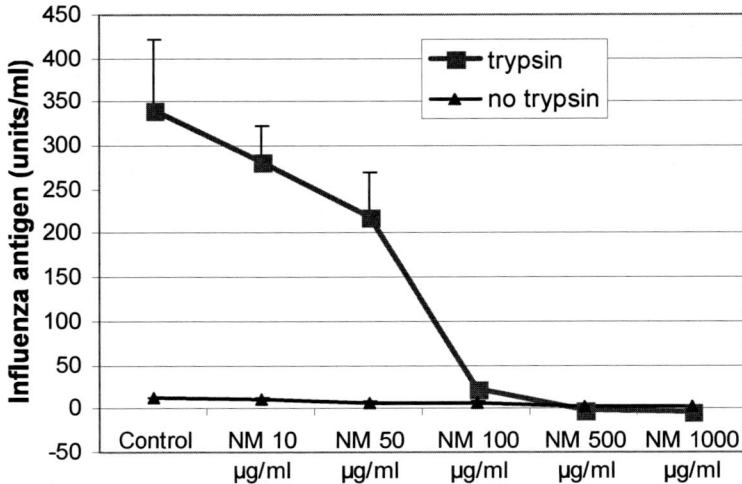

Figure 1. Effect of NM on influenza total NP antigen production in Vero cells at 44-48h. Cells (20,000/well) were inoculated with 25 μl/well influenza A virus strain A/WSN/33, MOI of 1 in the presence or absence of trypsin. Briefly, two-day old, sub-confluent monolayers of Vero cells growing at density indicated were washed with Dulbecco's PBS and exposed to human influenza A virus, (H1N1) TC-adapted (strain A/WSN/33 from ATCC) in serum-free medium at a multiplicity of infection of 1, at 33°C for one hour. The virus inoculum was left in and cells were fed serum-free medium (without or containing 1.0 μg/ml TPCK-treated trypsin) supplemented with various concentrations of nutrient mixture or components, in triplicate, and incubated further at 33°C. After 44 h, an equal volume of lysing solution (from Takara kit) was added to each well and an aliquot of the total lysate was assayed for the level of influenza A nuclear protein (NP) along with positive control (standards) using an enzyme-linked immunoassay (ELISA) kit (MK120 from Takara Mirus Bio Corp., Madison WI).

Using a Vero culture exposed to influenza virus for a shorter period (24h instead of 44h) resulted in a slightly lower NP antigen level (240 vs. 340 antigen units/ml) which was inhibited by NM in a dose-dependent manner at 24h, resulting in inhibition over control of 46% (p=0.070), 67% (p=0.027), and 87% at 50, 100, and 250 μg/ml NM [19].

Effect of NM on Influenza NP Antigen Production in MDCK Cells

The protocol for NP antigen evaluation in MDCK cells was similar to that in Vero cells. NM inhibited virus growth in a dose-dependent manner in MDCK cells, with the magnitude of inhibition dependent on the conditions of cell and virus pretreatment (Figure 2). Pretreatment of MDCK cells with NM followed by washing of cells to remove NM then exposing to influenza virus inoculum (in the absence of NM), resulted in a dose-dependent inhibition of NP antigen expression (r=-0.8784, p=0.1216) with 38% (p=0.02) reduction over control at 250 μg/ml, 55% (p=0.0037) at 500 μg/ml and 62% (p=0.0023) at 1000 μg/ml [19].

Pretreatment of virus with NM, followed by infection and post-treatment of cells with NM (after exposure to virus), resulted in dose-dependent and more profound reduction of influenza NP protein expression (r=-0.9385, p=0.0615) with 83% inhibition (p=0.004) at 500 µg/ml and 99% inhibition (p=0.003) at 1000 µg/ml [19]. No pretreatment of influenza virus or cells with NM, but adding NM to cells after virus infection resulted in more substantial inhibition than pretreatment alone but less than that observed with pre and post NM treatment (r=-0.9850, p=0.015) with 39% inhibition (p<0.0001) at 500 µg/ml and 91% inhibition (p<0.0001) at 1000 µg/ml [19].

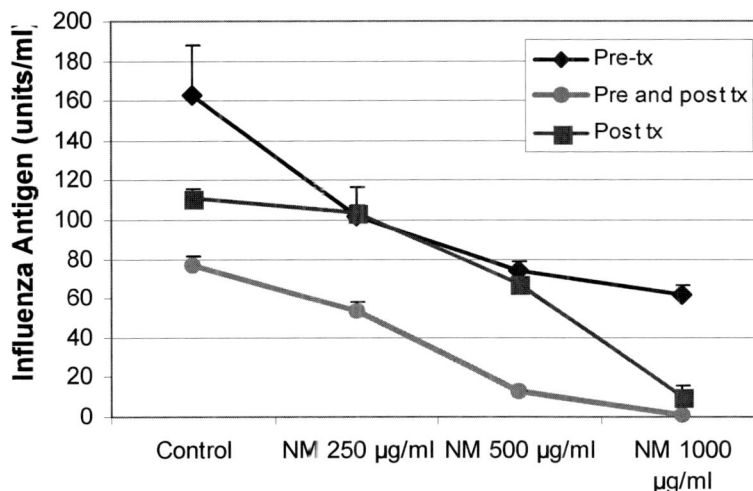

Figure 2. Effect of NM on influenza NP protein expression in MDCK cells as a function of cell or virus pretreatment. Cells (20,000/well) were inoculated with human influenza A virus strain A/WSN/33 at a MOI of 1 in the presence of trypsin under the following conditions: pretreatment of MDCK cells with NM prior to virus exposure; pretreatment of virus with NM prior to infection and treatment of cells with NM after exposure to virus; no pretreatment of cells with NM but addition of NM after exposure to virus.

Specificity of the Antiviral Effect of NM in Vero and MDCK Cells

To determine whether virus inhibition in Vero or MDCK cells was a specific effect of NM or due to the cytotoxicity of the mixture, we determined a selective index i.e. ratio of cytotoxicity value to antiviral efficacy value. Since trypan blue exclusion measures cell death but not cytostatic effects, we utilized a cytotoxicity assay based on spectrophotometric measurement of total biomass (total cell protein) by staining cellular proteins with the Sulforhodamine B dye as described by Skehan et al. [45]. In both cell lines, there was an improvement in the ratio of total cell protein to viral NP antigen with increasing concentrations of NM up to 200 µg/ml in Vero and 400 µg/ml in MDCK cells (p = 0.047 in Vero and 0.006 in MDCK at 200 µg/ml NM) [19]. These results are consistent with selectivity of the NM inhibitory effect towards influenza virus rather than due to inhibition of host cells.

Effect of Individual NM Component(s) on Virus Growth

To determine whether individual components of NM display cooperative effects on virus inhibition, we tested ascorbic acid (AA) and green tea extract (GT), individually and in combination. When tested in a higher concentration range, AA (284–710 μM) produced dose-dependent inhibition of influenza A antigen production [19]. When evaluated individually at low to moderate concentrations, 25μg/ml GT and 91 μM AA independently produced slight inhibition of NP protein production in infected MDCK, 8% and 12% respectively [19]. When these components were combined, they conferred greater inhibition (32%) of viral NP protein than either component alone [19]. This effect was also selective as evidenced from the ratio of total cell protein to viral NP antigen; the ratios for the control, GT, AA and the combination GT + AA were found to be 0.07, 0.085, 0.092 and 0.135, respectively [19].

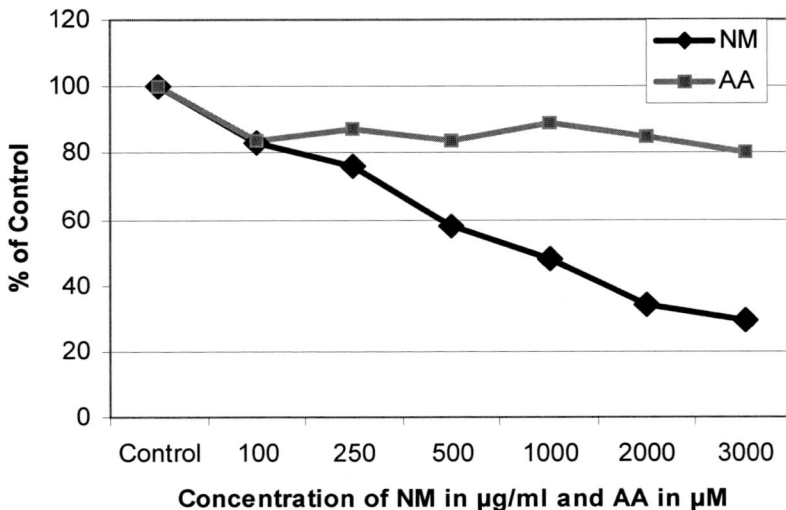

Figure 3. Effect of NM and ascorbate (AA) on human influenza A neuraminidase activity. Cell-free virus was mixed with various concentration of NM or AA and measurement of neuraminidase activity was preformed in the presence of substrate. The titer of undiluted virus stock used was $10^{5.75}TCID_{50}/0.2$ ml in 3 days on MDCK cells at 33°C with 5% CO2 by CPE. Kinetic analysis was first performed to determine optimal reaction time by incubating serial dilutions of virus in the presence of substrate solution, 1 mM 2'–(4-Methylumbelliferyl)–a–D-N-Acetylneuraminic Acid (MUN, prepared in 62.5 mM sodium acetate, pH 5.5) at 37°C for 90 mins. Reactions were stopped by addition of 150 μl of 0.1M glycine buffer (pH 10.7) containing 25% ethanol. Absorbance was read with a Schimadzu spectrophotometer at 340 nm. From the above assay, 30 mins was chosen as the reaction time for further experiments. Cell-free virus was preincubated with various concentrations of NM (50–3000 μg/ml) in substrate buffer (62.5 mM sodium acetate, pH 5.5) for 0 or 60-minute at room temperature followed by assay of residual neuraminidase activity.

Inhibitory Effect of NM and Ascorbic Acid on Influenza A Virus Neuraminidase Activity in Cell-Free System

Since pretreatment of virus affected its growth in MDCK cells, we evaluated the effect of NM and AA on neuraminidase activity of influenza A virus. Titration of NA activity was performed by the method of Potier et al. [46] using cell-free influenza A virus, subtype H1N1 as detailed under legend to Figure 3. Neuraminidase activity was determined to be linear up to 90 minutes, with coefficient of correlation r= 0.9931 (data not shown). When cell-free virus was mixed with NM in the presence of substrate and the reaction stopped at 30 mins, the viral neuraminidase activity was inhibited in a dose-dependent manner (r = -0.9221, p=0.0089), with 50% inhibition at 1000 µg/ml NM, >60% at 2000 µg/ml NM, and 70% at 3000 µg/ml, as shown in Figure 3 [19]. Ascorbic acid had minimal inhibitory effect on viral neuraminidase activity. Preincubation of cell-free virus with NM for 60 minutes versus 0 minutes demonstrated similar neuraminidase activities. In control experiments, addition of NM to the assay tube (substrate buffer) did not change the pH of the buffer, suggesting that the effect on enzyme activity by the test reagent was not due to a pH effect.

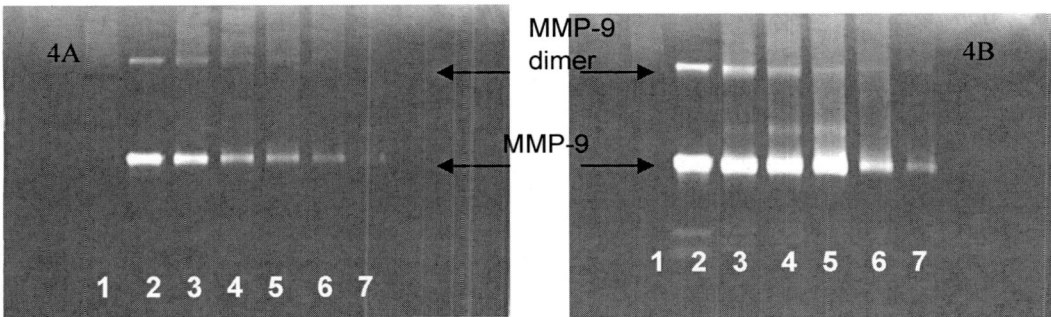

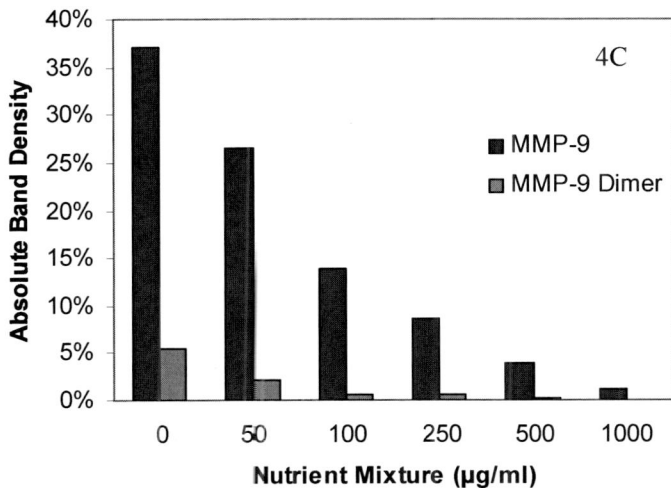

Figure 4. (Continues on next page.)

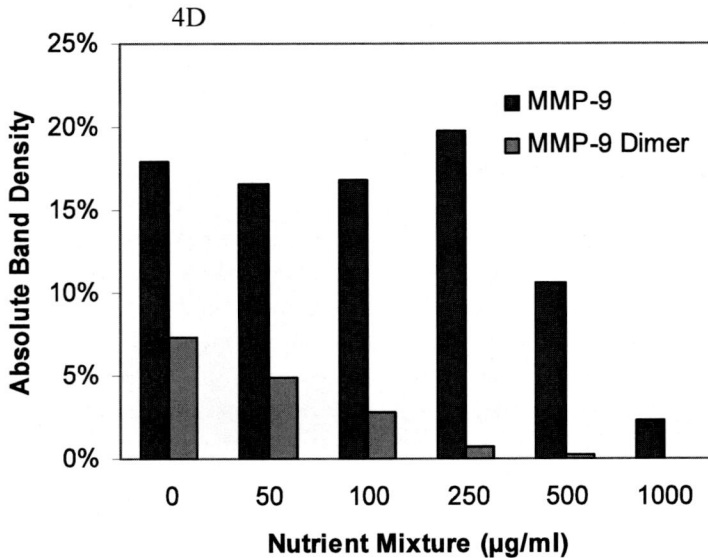

Figure 4. Effect of NM on MMP secretion by uninfected MDCK cells. Zymography demonstrated production of only MMP-9 by uninfected MDCK cells, which was enhanced by PMA treatment. NM inhibited MMP-9 secretion in a does-dependent manner. 4A – Zymogram of MDCK cells; 4B – Zymograpm of PMA (200 ng/ml)-treated MDCK cells. Legend: 1 – Markers, 2 – Control, 3–7 NM 50, 100, 250, 500, 1000 µg/ml; 4C – Denistometry MDCK cells; 4D – Densitometry of PMA-treated MDCK cells. Gelatinase zymography was performed in 10% Novex precast SDS-polyacrylamide gel (Invitrogen Corporation) in the presence of 0.1% gelatin under non-reduced conditions. Culture media (20 µl) mixed with sample buffer was loaded and SDS-PAGE was performed with tris glycine SDS buffer as described by the manufacturer (Novex). Samples were not boiled before electrophoresis. Following electrophoresis the gels were washed twice in 2.5% Triton X-100 for 30 minutes at room temperature to remove SDS. The gels were then incubated at 37°C overnight in substrate buffer containing 50 mM Tris-HCl and 10 mM CaCl2 at pH 8.0 and stained with 0.5% Coomassie Blue R250 in 50% methanol and 10% glacial acetic acid for 30 minutes and destained. Protein standards were run concurrently and approximate molecular weights were determined by plotting the relative mobilities of known proteins.

Effect of NM on MMP Secretion in Infected and Uninfected MDCK and Vero Cells

MMP secretion in conditioned media was determined by gelatinase zymography as described under Figure 4 legend. Zymography demonstrated production of only MMP-9 by uninfected MDCK cells, which was enhanced by PMA treatment. NM inhibited MMP-9 secretion in a dose-dependent manner, as shown in Figures 4A-D [20]. Zymography demonstrated production of both MMP-2 and MMP-9 by infected MDCK cells, with enhanced MMP-9 with PMA treatment (Figures 5A-D). NM inhibited MMP secretion in a dose-dependent manner above 100 µg/ml [20].

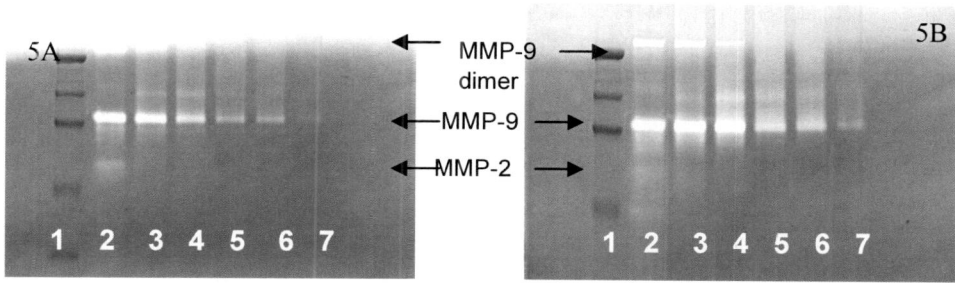

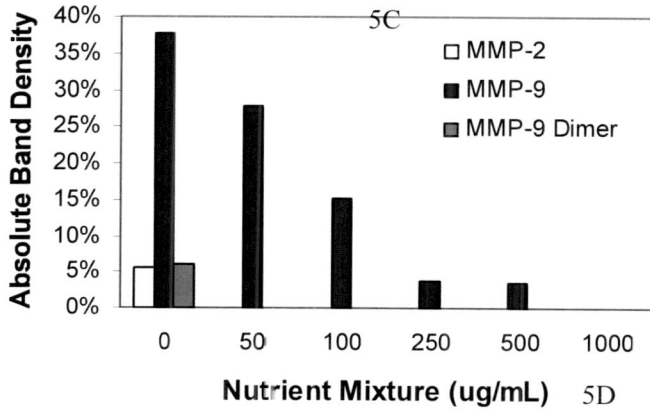

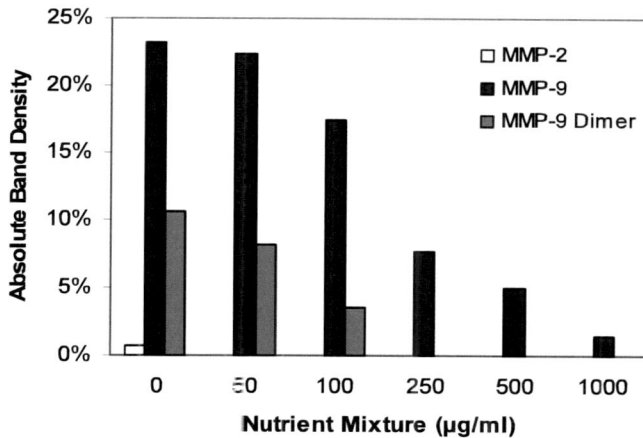

Figure 5. Effect of NM on MMP secretion by influenza virus A-infected MDCK cells. Zymography demonstrated production of both MMP-2 and MMP-9 by infected MDCK cells, with enhanced MMP-9 with PMA treatment. NM inhibited MMP secretion in a dose-dependent manner. 5A – Zymogram of infected MDCK cells; 5B – Zymogram of PMA (200 ng/ml)-treated infected MDCK cells. Legend: 1 – Markers, 2-Control, 3-7 NM 50, 100, 250, 500, 1000 µg/ml. 5C – Denistometry MDCK cells; 5D-Densitometry of PMA-treated MDCK cells.

Zymography did not detect secretion of either MMP-2 or MMP-9 by uninfected Vero cells; however, with PMA treatment, MMP-9 was visible. NM inhibited MMP-9 secretion in a dose–dependent fashion [20]. Zymography showed two bands corresponding to MMP-2 and MMP-9 secretion by influenza virus A- infected Vero cells, with significant increase in MMP-9 with PMA treatment. NM inhibited MMP secretion in a dose-dependent manner at and above 250-µg/ml concentration [20].

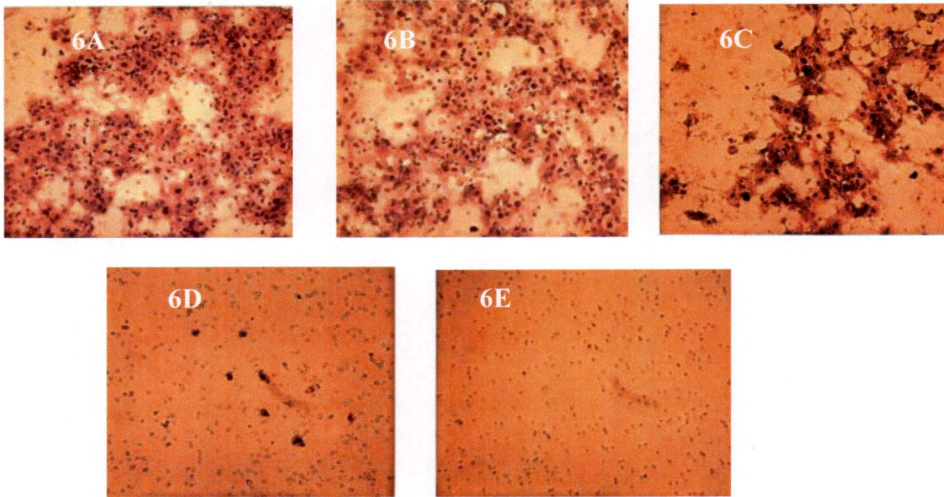

Figure 6. Effect of NM on Matrigel invasion by MDCK cells. NM inhibited MDCK cell invasion through Matrigel in a dose-dependent manner with 100% inhibition at 1000 µg/ml. 6A – Control, 6B – NM 50 µg/ml, 6C – NM 100 µg/ml, 6D – NM 500 µg/ml, 6E – NM 1000 µg/ml. Suspended in medium, MCDK and Vero cells were supplemented with NM (0–1000 µg/ml) and seeded on the insert in the well. Thus both the medium on the insert and in the well contained the same supplements. The plates with the inserts were then incubated in a culture incubator equilibrated with 95% air and 5% CO2 for 24 hours. After incubation, the media from the wells were withdrawn. The cells on the upper surface of the inserts were gently scrubbed away with cotton swabs. The cells that had penetrated the Matrigel membrane and migrated onto the lower surface of the Matrigel were stained with Hematoxylin and Eosin and visually counted under the microscope.

Effect of NM on Matrigel Invasion by MDCK and Vero Cells

Invasion studies were conducted using Matrigel (Becton Dickinson) inserts in 24-well plates as described under Figure 6 legend. NM inhibited MCDK invasion through Matrigel in a dose-dependent manner, with100% inhibition at 1000 µg/ml, as shown in Figure 6A-E [20]. NM inhibited Vero cell invasion through Matrigel in a dose-dependent manner with 100% inhibition at 500-µg/ml, as shown in Figures 7A-D [20].

Specificity of NM Inhibition of MMPs

Cell proliferation was evaluated by MTT assay 48h following incubation with test reagents as described by Mosman [47]. NM was cytotoxic to the uninfected MDCK cell line and exhibited dose-dependent toxicity (R^2=0.9553), with 19% (p=0.005) at 100 µg/ml and 80% (p<0.0001) at 1000 µg/ml with respect to the control [20]. To determine the specificity of MMP-9 inhibitory effect on MDCK cells, the selectivity index (viable cell value/MMP secretion value) was calculated. Cell value was determined using the MTT test. An increase in this ratio was observed with increased NM concentration: 2.7, 3.2, 5.7, 7.5, 17 at 0, 50, 100, 500, and 1000 µg/ml respectively [20]. NM exhibited dose-dependent toxicity (R^2=0.8947) to uninfected Vero cells with 18% (p=0.008) and 69% (p= 0.0001) cytotoxicity at 100 µg/ml and 1000-µg/ml concentration respectively [20]. To determine the specificity of MMP-9 inhibitory effect on Vero cells, the selectivity index (viable cell value/MMP secretion value) was calculated. An increase in this ratio was observed with increased NM concentration: 4.1, 4.1, 5.1, 18.5, 37 at 0, 50, 100, 250, and 500 µg/ml respectively [20].

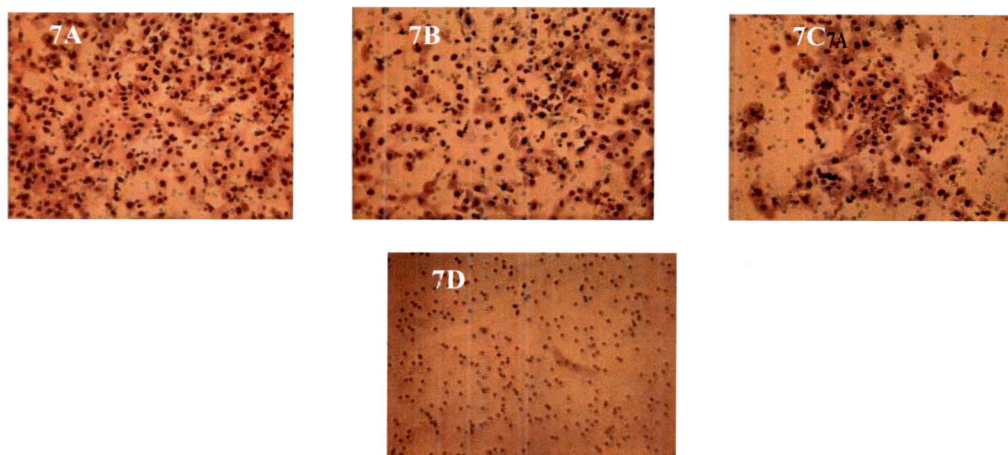

Figure 7. Effect of NM on Matrigel invasion by Vero cells. NM inhibited Vero cell invasion through Matrigel in a dose-dependent manner with 100% inhibition at 500 µg/ml. 7A – Control, 7B – NM 50 µg/ml, 7C – NM 100 µg/ml, 7D – NM 500 µg/ml.

Implications of our Findings

Therapeutic control of influenza virus infection can be directed at several targets, such as blocking viral uncoating through M2 ion channels and inhibiting virus-associated neuraminidase activity linked to infectivity. By targeting the neuraminidase enzyme, the ability of viruses to escape from host cells and infect other cells can be hindered. However, these drugs have been associated with severe toxic side effects, suggesting the need for improved therapies. Incubation of cell-free virus with NM showed dose-dependent inhibition of neuraminidase enzymatic activity. The inhibitory effect observed was not due to extraneous conditions such as pH change, since the pH of the substrate buffer in which NM was dissolved was in the 5.4 –5.5 range, the optimum pH for the enzyme reaction [46].

Another target is controlling viral growth through viral RNA, which contains all genes necessary for a virus to survive and reproduce in a host cell. The RNA is packed together with protein called NP (nuclear protein), which is needed by the virus to multiply its RNA copies [48]. In cells infected with a virus a decrease in NP protein production indicates that viral multiplication has been limited [48]. We have demonstrated that NM is a potent inhibitor of influenza A infectivity (neuraminidase secretion) and of influenza A growth (NP antigen) as tested in MDCK and Vero cell cultures [19]. This effect was not due to non-specific inhibition of viral NP resulting from NM-induced host-cell toxicity, since the selectivity index (ratio of cytotoxicity value to antiviral efficacy) increased with increasing concentration of NM indicating cell protection and selective inhibition of viral protein production. The antiviral effect was further enhanced upon pre-treatment of virus with nutrient mixture prior to infection and cell treatment with NM, suggesting the involvement of virus-associated component(s) as a possible target of action.

Although NM inhibited neuraminidase activity, it is unlikely that this is the main mechanism or the mode of inhibition of influenza virus by this mixture, since: (i) much higher concentrations of NM were required to inhibit NA activity than NP synthesis; (ii) NP inhibition was detectable within the first cycle of infection (at 24 hr), an unlikely occurrence if virion-associated neuraminidase was the sole target; and (iii) NM pre-treatment of virus alone without treatment of cells post-infection was less effective than pre plus post treatment. Other mechanisms are likely to be involved such as inhibition of a step(s) in viral replication. This is consistent with the inhibition of viral NP synthesis with individual components of NM and their known modes of action on other viruses and cancer cells.

Furthermore, since all viruses spread in the tissue and reach blood vessels by disruption of the natural collagen-rich extracellular matrix, another target would be limiting the secretion of the proteolytic enzymes, the matrix metalloproteinases, specifically MMP-2 and MMP-9, would curb the viral spread in tissue. For the virus to reach the stromal compartment and blood vessels, the basement membrane or ECM must be disrupted. MMP-2 and MMP-9 in particular have been shown to play an important role in the degradation of epithelial cell layer and ECM or basement membrane. Our results demonstrated that influenza A-infected Vero and MDCK cells secreted MMP-2 and MMP-9, which was inhibited by NM in a dose-dependent manner. Furthermore, NM significantly inhibited MDCK and Vero cell invasion through Matrigel, reaching total blockage at 1000 μg/ml and 500 μg/ml respectively.

Finally, in contrast to the toxic side effects of current influenza medications, the nutrient mixture has been shown to be a safe therapeutic agent with demonstrated utility. In a previous in vivo study addressing safety issues, we found that gavaging adult female ODS rats (weighing 250–300 gm) with the nutrient mixture (at 30, 90 or 150 mg per day for seven days), had neither adverse effects on vital organs (heart, liver and kidney), nor on the associated functional serum enzymes, indicating that this mixture is safe to use even at these high doses, which far exceed the normal equivalent dosage of the nutrient, and can be delivered in vivo [49].

CONCLUSION

In conclusion, the mixture of several micronutrients (NM) has potential in influenza treatment by its simultaneous effect on various mechanisms associated with viral infection, such as decreasing viral multiplication and infectivity and blocking the enzymatic degradation of the extracellular matrix. Further analysis of individual components of NM may provide more insight into the specific role(s) of these constituents in the inhibition of influenza virus multiplication. However, taking into account a high level of safety of these micronutrients, their intake may offer significant health benefits without a risks associated with pharmacological drugs.

ACKNOWLEDGEMENTS

We would like to thank Bhakti Gangazurkar and Nusrath Roomi for technical assistance.

REFERENCES

[1] Centers for Disease Control and Prevention. Background on influenza. http://cdc.gov/flu/professionals/background.htm, 2007

[2] Moscona, A. Neuraminidase inhibitors for influenza. *N Engl J Med* 2005; 353, 1363-1373.

[3] Moscona, A. Oseltamivir-resistant influenza? *Lancet* 2004; 364, 733-734.

[4] Ge, Q; Eisen, HN; Chen J. Use of siRNAs to prevent and treat influenza virus infection. *Virus Res* 2004; 102 (1), 37-42.

[5] Haasnoot, J; Berkhout, B. RNA interference: its use as antiviral therapy. *Handb Exp Pharmacol* 2006; 173, 117-50.

[6] Sui, J; Hwang, WC; Perez, S; Wei, G; Aird, D; Chen, LM; Santelli, E; Stec, B; Cadwell, G; Ali, M; Wan, H; Murakami, A; Yammanuru, A; Han, T; Cox, NJ; Bankston, LA; Donis, RO; Liddington, RC; Marasco, WA. Structural and functional bases for broad-spectrum neutralization of avian and human influenza A viruses. *Nat Struct Mol Biol*. 2009 Feb 22. [Epub ahead of print]

[7] Scrimshaw, NS. Historical concepts of interactions, synergism and antagonism between nutrition and infection. *J Nutr* 2003; 133(1), 316S-321S.

[8] Schofield, C; Ashworth, A. Why have mortality rates for severe malnutrition remained so high? *Bull World Health Organ* 1996; 74(2), 223-9. Review.

[9] Jariwalla, RJ. Nutrients as modulators of immune dysfunction and dyslipidemia in AIDS. *In* "AIDS and Heart Disease" (R. Watson, Ed.), 2004; pp163-175. Marcel Dekker Inc., New York, NY.

[10] Webb, AL; Villamor, E. Update: effects of antioxidant and non-antioxidant vitamin supplementation on immune function. *Nutr Rev* 2007; 65, 181-217.

[11] Buffinton, G; Christen, S; Peterhans, E; Stocker, R. Oxidative stress in lungs of mice infected with influenza A virus. *Free radical Research Communications* 1992, 16(2), 99-110.

[12] Ratcliffe, D; Migliorisi, G; Cramer, E. Translocation of influenza virus by migrating neutorphils. *Cell Mol Biol* 1992; 38, 63-70.

[13] Delorme, L; Middleton, PJ. Influenza A virus associated with acute encepahlopathy. *Am J Dis Child* 1979; 133, 822-24.

[14]   Hildebrandt, H; Maassab, HF; Willis, PW; Mich, AA. Influenza A virus pericarditis. *Am J Dis Child* 1962; 104, 179-182.

[15]   Ray, CG; Ocenogle, TB; Minnich, ML; Copeland, JG; Grogan, TM. The use of intravenous ribavirin to treat influenza virus-associated acute myocarditis. *J Infect Dis* 1989; 159: 829-836.

[16]   Mori, I; Komatsu, T; Takeuchi, K; Nakakuki, K; Sudo, M; Kimura, Y. Viremia induced by influenza virus. *Microb Pathog* 1995; 19: 237-244.

[17]   Yeo, SJ; Kim, SJ; Kim, JH; Lee, HJ; Kook, YH. Influenza A virus infection modulates the expression of type IV collagenases in epithelial cells. *Arch Virol* 1999; 144, 1361-1370.

[18]   Rath, M; Pauling, L. Plasmin-induced proteolysis and the role of apoprotein(a), lysine and synthetic analogs. *Orthomolecular Medicine* 1992; 7, 17-23.

[19]   Jariwalla, RJ; Roomi, MW; Gangapurkar, B; Kalinovsky, T; Niedzwiecki, A; Rath, M. Suppression of influenza A virus nuclear antigen production and neuraminidase activity by a nutrient mixture containing ascorbic acid, green tea extract and amino acids. *BioFactors* 2007; 31, 1-15.

[20]   Roomi, MW; Jariwalla, RJ; Kalinovsky, T; Roomi, N; Niedzwiecki, A; Rath, M. Inhibition of cellular invasive parameters in influenza A virus-infected MDCK and Vero cells by a nutrient mixture. *BioFactors* 2008; 33(1), 61-75.

[21]   Barbour, EK; Rayya EG; Shaib H; El Hakim, RG; Niedzwiecki, A; Nour, AMA; Harakeh, S; Rath, M. Evaluation of the efficacy of Epican Forte against avian flu virus. *Intern J Appl Res Vet Med* 2007, 5(1), 9-16.

[22]   Roomi, MW; Ivanov, V; Kalinovsky, T; Niedzwiecki, A; Rath, M. Inhibition of pulmonary metastasis of melanoma B16FOcells in C57BL/6 mice by a nutrient mixture consisting of ascorbic acid, lysine, proline, arginine and green tea extract. *Exp Lung Res* 2006; 32(10), 517-30.

[23]   Ivanov, V; Roomi, MW; Kalinovsky, T; Niedzwiecki, A; Rath, M. Anti-atherogenic effects of a mixture of ascorbic acid, lysine, proline, arginine, cysteine and green tea phenolics in human aortic smooth muscle cells. *J Cardiovasc Pharmacol* 2007; 49(3), 140-5.

[24]   Beck, M; Nelson, H; Shi, K; Van Dael, P; Schiffrin, E; Blum, S; Barclay, D; Levander, O. Selenium deficiency increases the pathology of an influenza virus infection. *The FASEB J*, 2001, 15, 1481-1483.

[25]   Fassina, G; Buffa, A; Benelli, R; Varnier, OE; Noonan, DM; Albini, A. Polyphenolic antioxidant (-)-epigallocatechin-3-gallate from green tea as a candidate anti-HIV agent. *AIDS* 2002, 16(6), 939-41.

[26]   Harakeh, S; Jariwalla, RJ; Pauling, L. Suppression of human immunodeficiency virus replication by ascorbate in chronically and acutely infected cells. *PNAS* 1990; 87(18), 7245-7249.

[27]   Harakeh, S; Jariwalla, RJ. Comparative study of the anti-HIV activities of ascorbate and thiol-containing reducing agents in chronically HIV-infected cells. *American Journal of Clinical Nutrition* 1991; 54(6 Suppl), 1231S-1235S.

[28]   Hennet, T; Peterhans, E; Stocker, R. Alterations in antioxidant defenses in lung and liver of mice infected with influenza A virus. *J Gen Virol* 1992; 73(1) , 39-46.

[29]   Imanishi, N; Tuji, Y; Katada, Y; Maruhashi, M; Konosu, S; Mantani, N; Terasawa, K; Ochiai, H. Additional inhibitory effect of tea extract on the growth of influenza A and B viruses in MDCK cells. *Microbiol Immunol* 2002; 46, 491-494.

[30]   Nakayama, M; Suzuki, K; Toda, M; Okubo, S; Hara, Y; Shimamura, T. Inhibition of the infectivity of influenza virus by tea polyphenols. *Antivir Res* 1993; 21, 289-299.

[31]   Song, JM; Lee, KH; Seong. BL. Antiviral effect of catechins in green tea on influenza virus. *Antivir Res* 2005; 68, 66-74.

[32]   Ungheri, D; Pisani, C; Sanson, G; Betani, A; Schloppacassi, G; Delgado, R; Sironi, M; Ghezzi, P. Protective effect of n-acetyl cysteine in a model of influenza infection in mice. *Int J Immunopathol Pharmacol*. 2000; 13, 123-128.

[33]   Schwerdt PR, Schwerdt CE. Effect of ascorbic acid on rhinovirus replication in WI-38 cells. *Proc Soc Exp Biol Med* 1975;148(4), 1237-43.

[34]   Harakeh, S; Niedzwiecki, A; Jariwalla, RJ. Mechanistic aspects of ascorbate inhibition of human immunodeficiency virus. *Chemico-Biological Interactions* 1994; 91, 207-215.

[35]   Chen, Q; Espey, MG; Krishma, MC; Mitchell, JB; Corpe, CP; Buettner, GR; Shacter E; Levine, M. Pharmacologic ascorbic acid concentrations selectively kill cancer cells: Action as a pro-drug to deliver hydrogen peroxide to tissues. *PNAS* 2005, 102(38), 13604-13609.

[36]   Maramag, C; Menon, M; Balaji, KC; Reddy, PG; Laxmanan, S. Effect of vitamin C on prostate cancer cells in vitro: effect on cell number, viability and DNA synthesis. *Prostate* 1997; 32, 188-95.

[37]   Hemilä H. Does vitamin C alleviate the symptoms of the common cold?--a review of current evidence. *Scand J Infect Dis* 1994; 26(1),1-6. Review.

[38]   Douglas, RM; Hemilä, H; D'Souza, R; Chalker, EB; Treacy, B. Vitamin C for preventing and treating the common cold. Cochrane Database Syst Rev 2004; (4), CD000980.

[39]   Hara, Y. *Green tea: Health Benefits and Applications*, Marcel Dekker, New York, Basel, 2001.

[40]   Kawakami, S; Kageyama, Y; Fujii, Y; Kihara, K; Oshima,. H. Inhibitory effects of N-acetyl cysteine on invasion and MMP 9 production of T24 human bladder cancer cells. *Anticancer Res* 2001; 21, 213-219.

[41]   Morini, M; Cai, T; Aluigi, MG; Noonan, DM; Masiello, L; De Flora, S; D'Agostini, F; Albini, A; Fassina, G. The role of the thiol N-acetyl cysteine in the prevention of tumor invasion and angiogenesis. *Int J Biol Markers* 1999; 4, 268-271.

[42]   Ghezzi, P; Ungheri, D. Synergistic combination of N-acetyl cysteine and ribavirin to protect from lethal influenza viral infection in a mouse model. *Int J Immunopathol Pharmacol* 2004; 17, 73-79.

[43]   Ghandi, CS; Shuck, K; Lear, JD; Dieckmann, GR; De Grado, WF; Lamb, RA; Pinto, LH. Cu(II) inhibition of the proton translocation machinery of the influenza A virus by gentian violet (GV) and GV-dyed cotton cloth, and bacteriological activities of these agents *J Infect Chemother*1999; 12, 73-79.

[44]   Yoon, SO; Kim, MM; Chung, AS. Inhibitory effects of selenite on invasion of HT 1080 tumor cells. *J Biol Chem* 2001; 276, 20085-92.

[45]   Skehan, P; Storeng, R; Scudiero, D; Monks, A; McMahon, J; Vistica, D; Warren, JT; Bokesch, H; Kenney, S; Boyd, MR. New colorimetric cytotoxicity assay for anti-cancer drug screening. *J Natl Cancer Inst* 1990; 82, 1107-1112.

[46] Potier, M; Mameli, L; Belisie, M; Dallaire, L; Melancon, SB. Fluorometric assay of neuraminidase with a sodium, (4-methylumbelliferyl-alpha-D-N-acetylneuraminate) substrate. *Anal Biochem* 1979; 94(2), 287-96.

[47] Mosmann, T. Rapid colorimetric assay for cellular growth and survival: application to proliferation and cytotoxicity assays. *J Immunol Methods* 1983; 65(1-2), 55-63.

[48] Wiley, DC; Skehel, JJ. The structure and function of the hemagglutinin membrane glycoprotein of influenza virus. *Annu Rev Biochem* 1987; 56, 356-94.

[49] Roomi, MW; Ivanov, V; Netke, SP; Niedzwiecki, A; Rath, M. Serum markers of the liver, heart, and kidney and lipid profile and histopathology in ODS rats treated with nutrient synergy. *J Am Coll Nutr* 2003; 22 (5), 477, Abstract #86.

PART VII:
PREVENTION POLICIES AND
THEIR APPLICATIONS

In: Global View of Fight against Influenza
Editor: Petar M. Mitrasinovic

ISBN: 978-1-60741-952-5
© 2009 Nova Science Publishers, Inc.

Chapter 16

THE IKARUS SYNDROME IN THE POULTRY INDUSTRY AND THE CONCERN ABOUT A NEW GREAT INFLUENZA PANDEMIC: WHAT TO LEARN FROM IKARUS' CRASH

Sievert Lorenzen
Zoological Institute, University of Kiel, Germany

ABSTRACT

Evidence is presented that, with respect to the development and spread of highly pathogenic avian influenza viruses (AI viruses), wild birds and small-scale poultry operations are much more biosecure than large-scale industrial poultry operations. Based on reports that more than 250 humans have succumbed to highly pathogenic strains of the avian influenza H5N1 Asia, there is concern that one strain could adapt to humans to cause a disastrous pandemic surpassing the Great Influenza of 1918. According to evidence available, the Great Influenza was largely man-made, and at least two young persons of the 250 supposed victims of H5N1 Asia actually died due to medical treatment against this virus rather than of avian influenza. The new term *Ikarus Syndrome* is explained, pointing to the problem that a glamorous series of successes may increase carelessly taken risks of crashing. The poultry industry seems to suffer from this syndrome. Measures are suggested of how to avoid a crash in the poultry industry and lower the risk of influenza pandemics that might be caused by a highly pathogenic strain of the AI virus H5N1.

INTRODUCTION

For biologists, 2009 is a Darwin year. Charles Darwin was borne in 1809, and his most fundamental work, *The Origin of Species by Means of Natural Selection,* appeared in 1859. It is based on the crucially important wisdom that unlimited growth is impossible when based upon the dissipation of resources. The reason for this is that the availability of all resources is limited in our limited world. Therefore, the further the limits of growth are exceeded, the greater will be the risk of catastrophes such as a severe influenza pandemic.

We can find this wisdom even in the Greek mythology. Prior to flying away from Crete to the Greek mainland by using wings made of feathers, wax and thread, Daedalus instructed his son Ikarus not to fly too low to prevent his wings from touching the water surface and not to fly too high to prevent the wax of the wings from getting melted by the sun's rays. Any disregard of these instructions would be disastrous. To put Daedalus' instructions into other words: If you do not want to not perish, you must work sufficiently hard without getting slaphappy. Ikarus did not take his father's words seriously. He flew higher and higher, his success exceeded all of his expectations, and made him so giddy that he did not notice that the wax of his wings had begun to melt. When enough wax had melted, Ikarus crashed. Did he fall victim to the sun's rays? No, he had fallen victim to his complacence. If he had only listened to his father's instructions, the sunrays would have been harmless to him. The syndrome of exceeding limits of growth carelessly, thus increasing the risk of a crash, is therefore referred to as the Ikarus Syndrome in the following.

The global finance industry, which had been infested with the Ikarus Syndrome, has just experienced its crash. Prior to this crash, it had lived through many years of glamorous success without noticing that the "wax of its wings" had begun to melt. So, the finance industry has not fallen victim to some kind of "sunrays" but rather to its uncured Ikarus Syndrome.

THE IKARUS SYNDROME IN THE POULTRY INDUSTRY

The poultry industry also looks back on a remarkable success story. It has grown impressively in the last 30 years. It achieved much success by increasing the numbers of farmed birds; by crowding as many farm birds as possible into limited space; by growing big, really big; through increasing degrees of industrialization; and by integrating many farms, slaughterhouses, and feed mills, etc., into mighty, vertically-integrated companies. By these means, poultry products became cheap mass products.

However, the "wax of its wings" has begun to melt. Increased industrialization has had severe effects on farm birds, such as overcrowding stress and increased susceptibility to diseases, and created severe problems of hygiene within the farmhouses. As a result, a daily poultry mortality of up to 1% of the flock is now regarded as quite normal. It was hoped that the hygiene problem would be solved by adopting the *all-in-all-out* principle which allows a farmhouse to be cleaned thoroughly only in the short period between removal of the older poultry stock and bringing in the younger one. But in between, during the fattening period, poultry and hygiene problems grow jointly. Particularly affected are long-lived farm birds— such as turkeys—that need a relatively long time (> 100 days) to reach their final weight. This obverse side of the poultry industry creates the most suitable conditions for low pathogenic (LP) strains of avian influenza viruses (AI viruses) to evolve into highly pathogenic (HP) strains. That is, poultry factories also serve as disease factories. This was evidenced strikingly in Chile in 2002, when a low pathogenic AI H7N3 virus evolved rapidly (from May to June 2002) into a highly pathogenic strain within a single broiler breeder flock (Suarez et al., 2004).

In nature, pathogens are subject to a fundamental tradeoff between virulence (making the host sick) and transmission (infecting new hosts) (Muzaffar et al., 2006). This tradeoff is invalidated in the poultry industry, where populations of pathogens may evolve into highly virulent strains without reducing their chances of transmission, which is taken over by the many movements of the integrated poultry industry (Sharkey et al., 2007).

Through these practices, the poultry industry has created a further problem which may affect the human population. According to the World Health Organization (WHO, 2009), 407 confirmed human cases of avian influenza A/(H5N1) resulting in 254 deaths were reported to the WHO up to 27 January 2009. Fortunately, no strain of H5N1 adapted to humans has yet been found that could be transmitted from human to human, but there is considerable concern that such a strain could emerge in the next few years and cause a pandemic (worldwide epidemic) in the human population with up to 150 million deaths (e.g., Liu et al., 2006; Chen et al., 2006). Should this pandemic emerge, it would clearly be man-made.

What is to be done? Prior to answering this question, the circumstances that have caused the AI problem and the pandemic concern need to be analysed in more detail.

EVOLUTION AND SPREAD OF HIGHLY PATHOGENIC STRAINS OF THE AI VIRUS H5N1 ASIA

The evolution of highly pathogenic strains of the AI virus H5N1 Asia began in Southeast Asia. It was promoted by combining practices of industrial poultry farming with the tradition of selling live poultry destined for slaughter on markets: If birds infected with AI are brought to a market, they may infect there other birds. If those newly-infected birds are not sold on the market, they are brought back to their farms, carrying a high risk of infecting other birds within their flock. Therefore, the markets served and still serve (Amonsin et al., 2008) as exchange sites for AI viruses. Additionally, following advice from the Food and Agriculture Organization (FAO), chicken waste was released directly into adjacent waters to fertilize them. That way, highly pathogenic AI viruses could be released directly into waters through which wild water birds and outdoor poultry could become infected. Even dead chickens were released as fish food into the water (Williams 2006).

The conditions described above allowed the prototype of the highly pathogenic AI virus H5N1 Asia to evolve. It was discovered first in 1996 on a goose farm in Guangdong in southern China and was designated *GS/GD* (Goose/Guangdong) (Xu et al., 1999). Li et al. (2004) found evidence that this strain must have repeatedly come into contact with other influenza viruses, thereby exchanging genes with them (gene reassortment). A strain hence derived from *GS/GD* was responsible for the avian influenza epidemic in poultry holdings in Hong Kong (close to Guangdong) in 1997 (Guan et al., 2002). Over 1.5 million poultry were culled on that occasion, but the virus survived and continued to evolve in southern China, where it cleaved into 12 variants (Li et al., 2004). One of them, whose genotype the authors named Z, became dominant between January 2002 and 2004.

In 2004 and 2005, Chen et al. (2006) observed the diversity of H5N1 strains in southern China to be greater than anywhere else in the world, although the incidences were low (0.26% for chickens, 1.83% for domestic ducks, 1.90% for domestic geese, 0.34% for wild ducks). Additionally, many other avian influenza subtypes were found to circulate both in poultry markets (H3, H6, H9, H11 and others) and among migrating wild ducks (H1, H3, H4, H5, H6, H10); clinically, all infected birds looked healthy at the moment of taking the samples. Faced with the extraordinarily high diversity of AI viruses in southern China, the authors concluded that this region could become the epicentre from where a terrifying pandemic of human influenza could spread all over the world.

Apart from circulating in southern China, AI viruses of the genotypes Z and V were also found 600 km further north on the huge Poyang Lake (surface area up to 5070 sq km depending on the water level), where they were isolated in January and March 2005 from six birds out of a sample of 4,316—apparently healthy—overwintering migratory ducks (not further identified) and from poultry of farms nearby the lake (Chen et al., 2006). The authors found evidence that the viruses had spread from the domestic to the wild birds rather than the other way around.

In May 2005, 1,700 km further west around the even larger Qinghai Lake (5,700 sq. km), a salt lake at 3,200 m altitude with no outlet, some 6,000 wild water birds—mostly bar-headed geese—died from a highly pathogenic avian influenza caused by a new H5N1 strain, whose genotype was a mixture of the Z and V strains previously found at the Poyang Lake (Yasué et al., 2006; Chen et al., 2006). It is unknown where and how the Qinghai strain originated.

Only the Qinghai strain of H5N1 Asia (clade 2.2. of the phylogenetic H5N1 Asia tree) (WHO/OIE/FAO 2008) spread westwards to reach Europe in October 2005 and Africa in February 2006 (Kilpatrick et al., 2006), whereas all other H5N1 Asia strains (clades 0, 1, 2.1., 2.3, 2.4, and 3 to 9 of the phylogenetic tree) remained confined to the far east.

Assuming that the Qinghai Lake was far away from the poultry industry, Chen et al. (2006) blamed migratory wild water birds for having carried the Qinghai strain or its two precursors from the Poyang Lake to the Qinghai Lake and further to Europe and Africa, not in a single journey, of course, but in a sort of relay race, causing outbreaks of Avian Influenza in various places along the route through Mongolia, Siberian Russia, Europe, and Africa.

This hypothesis collapsed like a house of cards once it was realized that, from 2003 on, bar-headed geese were reared on various farms close to the Qinghai Lake, some for farming purposes, others destined for release into the wild (Butler, 2006). The deaths of large numbers of wild bar-headed geese in 2005 occurred close to these farms. Furthermore, tourism and economic development have been heavily promoted in the region. A railway links the Qinghai Lake with the large town Lanzhou situated 170 km away, which is a hub for traffic via air, railway and highways; particularly, there are routes linking Lanzhou with the Poyang Lake in the East and with Siberia and Europe in the West. Along these routes, AI viruses were found, whose HA-genes matched that of the Qinghai type to 99.6 to 99.8 % (Petermann, 2008).

The new findings strongly support the hypothesis that the H5N1 Qinghai strain was spread from East to West by movements of poultry or poultry products rather than by migratory birds.

The same holds for spreads within Europe. Most spectacular was a case in January 2007, when a specific H5N1 strain struck first two goose farms in Hungary and two weeks later—1,300 km away—a turkey farm in Suffolk (Southeast England). Initially, European authorities blamed migratory birds for having carried the virus from Hungary to the English factory farm, although migration of wild birds was not observed in that midwinter time. Later, an epidemiological study by a group from the British government revealed that the owner of the farm in Suffolk regularly received semi-processed turkey meat from the H5N1-affected Hungarian area for further processing in his slaughter house adjacent to his turkey farm affected. Hence, the British group concluded that the H5N1 virus was most likely introduced to England via importation of turkey meat from Hungary (DEFRA, 2007).

Despite this and equivalent other evidences, authors of the famous German Friedrich-Loeffler-Institute insisted and still insist that "wild birds play an important role in the global infection affairs and in the spread of HPAIV H5N1" (Schoene et al., 2009).

WILD BIRDS AND OUTDOOR POULTRY SUFFER FROM INDUSTRIAL POULTRY FARMING, NOT THE CONTRARY

According to multiple evidences, highly pathogenic AI viruses may be released from poultry factories into nature where they can infect wild birds and free-ranging poultry. The other way around, there is no conclusive evidence that wild birds or outdoor poultry infected with highly pathogenic AI viruses could have introduced these viruses directly or indirectly (via contaminated feed or straw) into indoor poultry operations, although infected wild birds were evidenced to have carried such viruses over distances of up to 1,000 km until they died (Petermann, 2008; Schoene et al., 2009).

How biosecure wild birds and backyard farming are is impressively demonstrated in Laos (GAIN 2005): Although this country is situated sandwich-like between Vietnam, Cambodia and Thailand, who have suffered much from bird flu outbreaks, Laos was affected only insignificantly. The few outbreaks occurred primarily on commercial enterprises in metropolitan areas and secondarily in smallholder flocks nearby. The commercial enterprises were integrated with foreign poultry companies, importing day-old chicks mainly from Thailand. The measure Laos took against bird flu was to cull all birds within 3 km of identified outbreak sites and to ban imports of day-old chicks and other poultry products from neighbouring countries struck by bird flu No measures were taken against rural poultry flocks which account for 87 % of the total poultry production in Laos. These birds are bred, raised and consumed locally. They are not fed with imported feed and are allowed to run freely among village homes, where they have frequent chances to mix with wild birds. They remained unaffected by bird flu. Hence, "backyard farming is a solution, not the problem" (GRAIN 2006 a).

In view of the evidence referred to, it is unfair to point the finger of blame at migratory birds and poor people's backyard birds saying: "We cannot control migratory birds but we can surely work hard to close down as many backyard farms as possible" (Margaret Say, Southeast Asian director for the USA Poultry and Egg Export Council, see GRAIN 2006 a), or to state: "Charoen Pokphand (CP) will succeed in turning a crisis into an opportunity of development" (Sooksunt Jiumjaiswanglerg, Präsident der CP Vietnam Livestock, see GRAIN 2007). When bird flu broke out in Egyptian industrial poultry farms, Egypt's prime minister took the same line and said: "The world is moving towards big farms because they can be controlled under veterinarian supervision ... The time has come to get rid of the idea of breeding chickens on the roofs of houses" (GRAIN 2006 b), a plan which was realized with a military-style cleansing operation.

By television, we all became witnesses of such actions: Men in white rubber suits and gas masks grasped chickens in rural villages and put them live into plastic sacs for destruction, while wild birds flying across the sky were blamed for being carriers of AI viruses. Pictures from industrial poultry practices were usually suppressed in such reports.

As a sad result, the senseless mass slaughters of free-ranging poultry have deprived very many poor people of their main source of animal protein. That way, the problem of hunger in the world was increased.

THE PROBLEM OF BIOSECURITY AND ITS MISMATCH IN GERMANY

In Germany, the Friedrich Loeffler Institute (FLI) advises the Germany government on animal diseases. By doing so, the interests of industrial farmers were apparently protected against those of small holders. Only one example may serve as an illustration (Lorenzen 2008): From June to November 2007, a novel strain of the AI virus H5N1 Asia (subclade 2.2.3 in the phylogenetic tree; see Starick et al., 2007) struck wild birds and industrial poultry operations in the Czech Republic, central Germany and France. Outbreaks occurred over a distance of 900 km from east to west (Newman et al., 2007). Germany's largest duck farm in Wachenroth (Bavaria) was affected (outbreak on 24 August 2007), and 285 black necked grebes (*Podiceps nigricollis*) fell victim to the virus on the Kelbra water reservoir in Thuringia/Saxony-Anhalt (August 2007) (Petermann, 2007).

These incidents prompted the FLI (15 October 2007) to blame exclusively wild birds for having spread the novel virus strain, because "at least an indirect causal involvement of wild birds in the latest outbreaks of HPAIV-infections cannot be excluded. The risk that wild birds can introduce HPAIV H5N1 into domestic bird flocks is therefore considered to be *high*." This argument is utterly meaningless, because other causes for the above-mentioned outbreaks "cannot be excluded" either, for example that the new virus strain was spread by human activities. Although the FLI did not disprove this possibility, it insisted that "the risk of transmission as a result of movements of people and vehicles appears to be *negligible*" and, hence, "deserves no further consideration".

Based on this error of judgement, the German government decided (Avian Bird Flu Order of 18 October 2007): "Owners of poultry must keep their birds in closed barns or in enclosures sealed above and at the sides against the entry of wild birds (safety device)." Exceptions to this order can and must be granted by local authorities, "provided that efforts to combat avian influenza are not hindered, and an outbreak of this epidemic must not be feared". Obviously, owners of factory farms are not affected by this order, although factory farming is heavily involved in the evolution and spread of highly pathogenic H5N1 viruses. By its misleading argumentation, the FLI spared the German poultry industry unwanted control measures.

There is much talk of biosecurity in connection with epizootics, of which avian influenza is only one. Biosecurity is understood as "any practice or system that prevents the spread of infectious agents from infected to susceptible animals, or prevents the introduction of infected animals into a herd, region, or country in which the infection has not yet occurred" (Otte et al., 2007). In other words, biosecurity measures are aimed at preventing the spread of an epizootic. According to the evidence presented herein, wild birds, free-ranging poultry and independent farms reach a much higher level of biosecurity than industrial poultry farms, particularly if the latter are integrated into the network of big companies.

A PANDEMIC CAUSED BY H5N1? A RETROSPECTIVE VIEW ON THE 1918 INFLUENZA PANDEMIC

The 1918 influenza pandemic, also known as the Great Influenza, the Spanish Influenza or the mother of all pandemics (Taubenberger & Morens, 2006), caused 20 to 50 millions deaths and led John Oxford (2004, in the famous scientific journal, *Nature*) to accuse nature of being "the greatest bioterrorist of our world", who had killed "more people than the Nazis, more than the atomic bomb, and more than the First World War" by making use of "the twentieth century's weapon of mass destruction"—influenza. We all should be cautious with such foolhardy statements, particularly when they refer to the Great Influenza. We all owe our life to nature. We need to live with nature rather than against it. We need to accept that we cannot eradicate influenza viruses. Instead, we need to accept them as natural components of our environment. What we can do at most is to prevent low pathogenic influenza virus strains from evolving into highly pathogenic strains in our poultry operations and, if they should emerge, to take effective rather than ineffective measures against them.

The Great Influenza swept over the continents in three waves (Taubenberger & Morens 2006). The first and smallest one started in March 1918 "in Kansas and in military camps throughout the US" (Billings, 1997). The second and biggest wave started in September 1918, and the third and medium-sized in February 1919. In contrast to the first wave, the second and third were characterized by their "rapid progressions from uncomplicated influenza infections to fatal pneumonia" (Taubenberger & Morens, 2006). Mainly affected were Europe, the USA and India (Billings, 2005). The geographic origin of the Great Influenza is still a matter of debate (Oxford, 2004): It might have originated in army camps in the US, from where it was transported to Europe in 1918, when the US Army entered into the final stage of World War I. Alternatively, it might have originated in British army camps in France and Britain in 1916 and 1917, when so many soldiers had to bear bad and brutal conditions of life. The causative agent isolated from victims of the second Great Flu wave was identified to be a strain of the avian influenza virus H1N1 adapted to humans (Taubenberger & Morens, 2006)

Extraordinary characteristics of the Great Influenza were the following four paradoxes:

1. Unlike "normal" influenza, the Great Influenza produced rapid deaths (Billings 1997):

     "People were struck with illness on the street and died rapid deaths. One anecdote shared of 1918 was of four women playing bridge together late into the night. Overnight, three of the women died from influenza (Hoagg). Others told stories of people on their way to work suddenly developing the flu and dying within hours. (Henig). One physician writes that patients with seemingly ordinary influenza would rapidly "develop the most viscous type of pneumonia that has ever been seen" and when cyanosis appeared in the patients, "it is simply a struggle for air until they suffocate" (Grist, 1917). Another physician recalls that the influenza patients "died struggling to clear their airways of blood-tinged froth that sometimes gushed from their nose and mouth, (Starr, 1976)."

According to Bauer (1957), "The death rate appeared to parallel the pneumonia attack rather than that of influenza itself."

2. Classically, influenza causes relatively high mortality peaks in very young and very old, while comparatively low death frequencies are found at all ages in between. In contrast, the Great Influenza caused much more deaths than any other influenza, and high death frequencies were reported not only from very young and very old, but from young adults (15 – 40 years of age) as well. Many of these young adults, well trained soldiers included, were completely fit and healthy days before their rapid death (Collins, 1957; Taubenberger & Morens, 2006). Graphically, the curve of influenza deaths by age at death is U-shaped in the case of "normal" influenza, while it was W-shaped in the case of the Great Influenza (Collins, 1957) (Figure 1).

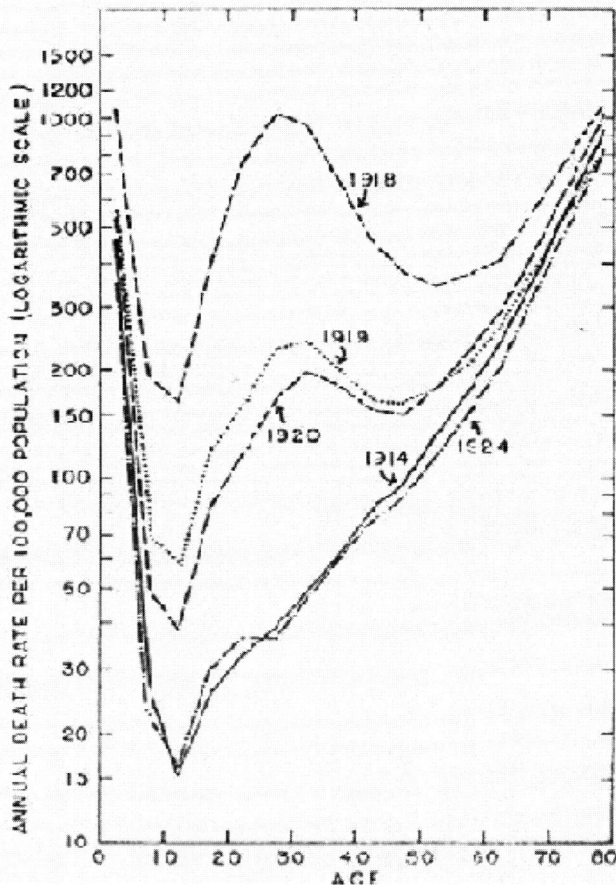

Figure 1. A singular feature of the 1918 influenza pandemic was that not only the very young and the very succumbed to it, but very many young adults as well. As a result, the curve of influenza deaths by age at death is W-shaped in the case of the 1918 influenza pandemic rather than U-shaped as in the case of "normal" influenza epidemics. Taken from Collins (1957).

3. Normally, a pandemic is a highly infectious disease. That is, the infectious agent can be transmitted rather easily from sick to healthy humans. In the case of the Great Influenza, however, five attempts failed to demonstrate the sick-to-well transmission (Cannel et al., 2008). Volunteers in these five experiments were seronegative incarcerated soldiers who "were repeatedly exposed to hospital patients exhibiting influenza-like symptoms in an attempt to make them contract the disease. ... [All] 118 men failed to develop influenza" (Gernhart, 1999). If at all, they developed only minor illness (Cannel et al., 2008).

4. In 1918 and 1919, very many US soldiers and civilians were vaccinated against the Great Flu. Unexpectedly, however, increasing vaccination rates were translated into increasing rather than decreasing illness rates (Cannel et al., 2008). This paradox was confirmed by personal experiences of McBean (1997). Her family had refused all 14 to 20 vaccinations that were strongly recommended at that time. The whole family did not contract the Great Influenza, although the parents went from house to house to look after the sick. She added: "As far as I could find out, the flu hit only the vaccinated. Those who had refused the shots escaped the flu." As a result, McBean suggested that millions of people had fallen victim to a vaccination catastrophe.

McBean's conclusion permits to explain the four paradoxes referred to much more consistently than other hypotheses suggested that deal, for instance, with intrinsically high virulence of the H1N1 strain (Taubenberger & Morens, 2006), vitamin D deficiency (Cannell et al., 2008) or the bad battle conditions during World War I (Ahmed et al., 2007). Rather than to explain the four paradoxes, these hypotheses produce additional ones. Hence, Oxford's accusation of nature to be "the greatest bioterrorist of our world" lacks substantial support, as the Great Influenza appears to be a largely man-made catastrophe. If at all, man can be accused to be "the greatest bioterrorist of our world".

This suggestion does not invalidate the concern that highly pathogenic strains of the AI virus H5N1 might cause a terrible human pandemic. However, the analysis of the Great Influenza may advise us to approach reports on fatal human cases of H5N1 avian influenza with scientific scepticism. How urgent that is will be underlined by the following two cases.

1. "On 9 May, 1997, a previously healthy 3-year-old boy, who was resident in Hong Kong, developed a sore throat, dry cough and fever. He was diagnosed with pharyngitis and prescribed antibiotics and aspirin. The child continued to be symptomatic and febrile and was hospitalized on 15 May. ... His laboratory tests were most remarkable for leukopenia (2000 white blood cells per cubic millimeter). ... The next day, he was transferred to another hospital, where he developed progressive respiratory distress associated with hypoxemia, consistent with progressive distress syndrome. He also became increasingly unresponsive. ... Despite mechanical ventilation and broad antibiotic coverage, the child died on 21 May with several complications, including respiratory failure, renal failure, and disseminated intravascular coagulopathy" (Subbarao et al., 1998). Shortly before he died, on 19 May 1997, a tracheal aspirate sample was taken, from which an avian H5N1 influenza virus was isolated.

2. In Thailand, a 6-year-old boy suffered from "a progressive viral pneumonia that led to acute respiratory distress syndrome and death 17 days after the onset of illness. He

was initially treated with multiple broad-spectrum antimicrobial agents. Virological diagnosis of H5N1 infection was made on day 7 of illness. After oseltamivir became available in Thailand, he was treated on day 15 of his illness with this agent until he died. He was also treated with methylprednisolone on day 15 until death and with granulocyte colony-stimulating factor for leukopenia from day 5 to day 10 of illness" (Uiprasertkul et al., 2005).

The two cases give rise to the hypothesis that the little patients might have succumbed to the medical treatment against the H5N1 virus rather than to the virus itself, as even laymen know that antibiotics are used to combat bacteria rather than viruses and that cocktails of strong medicines may produce unwanted harmful to fatal side effects.

WHAT WE CAN LEARN FROM IKARUS' CRASH TO MASTER THE INFLUENZA PROBLEM

Ikarus might have avoided his crash if he had followed his father's instructions and had not flown too high, thus not giving the sunrays any chance of melting the wax of his wings.

To cure the poultry industry from its Ikarus Syndrome and, hence, to master the influenza problem, biosecurity appears to be the most appropriate measure to be taken. The costs this measure will certainly be lower than costs for culling millions of birds and for fighting against a pandemic should it emerge by the adaptation of a highly pathogenic strain of the AI virus H5N1 Asia to humans.

Measures to increase the biosecurity of the poultry industry need to include the following ones:

- Both the numbers of birds per farmhouse and per square metre need to be reduced noticeably to reduce the birds' susceptibility to infectious diseases.
- Instead of cleaning farmhouses thoroughly only in the short period between *all-out* and *all-in* of poultry flocks, they need to be cleaned thoroughly also during *all-in* periods. Such additional cleanings are particularly important in the case of rather long-lived birds such as turkeys for cutting short the chains of infection that low pathogenic AI virus strains need to evolve into highly pathogenic strains
- The degree of networking within the poultry industry needs to be lowered, and efforts should be encouraged to grow poultry in independent operations, many smallholdings of poultry included. This measure serves to reduce the risk of spreading AI viruses over short and long distances, thus avoiding large AI outbreaks and endemic AI infections (Sharkey et al., 2007).
- The national and international poultry trade, which is essentially out of control, needs to be controlled rigidly to prevent AI-viruses to be spread by trade movements suggested to be legal.
- When humans are reported to have died from an H5N1 virus strain, information on the medical treatment is needed for permitting an examination of whether these humans might have succumbed to the virus or to the medical treatment against it.

Once the poultry industry will be cured of its Ikarus Syndrome, there will be no need to worry any more about a catastrophic influenza pandemic that might be caused by a highly pathogenic strain of the AI virus H5N1 Asia.

REFERENCES

Ahmed, R., Oldstone, M.B.A., Palese, F. (2007): Protective immunity and susceptibility to infectious diseases: lessons from the 1918 influenza pandemic. *Nature Immunology* 8, 1188-1193.

Amonsin, A., Choatrakol, C., Lapkuntod, J. et al. (2008): Influenza virus (H5N1) in live markets and food markets, Thailand. Emerging Infectious Diseases 14, 1739-1742.

Bauer, C.C. (2005): The Pandemic of Influenza in 1918-1919. www.history.navy.mil/library /online/influenza%20pan.htm

Billings, M. (2005): The Influenza Pandemic of 1918. http://virus.stanford.edu/uda

Butler, D. (2006): Blogger reveals China's migratory goose farms near site of flu outbreak. *Nature* 441, 263.

Cannell, J.J., Zasloff, M., Garland, C.F., Scragg, R., Giovannucci, E. (2008): On the epidemiology of influenza. *Virology Journal* 5:29, http://www.viologyj.com/content5/ 1/29

Collins, S.D. (1957): Influenza in the United States, 1887 – 1956. Extract from "Review and study of illness and medical care with special reference to long-time trends." Public Health Monographs No. 48. Http://www.histrory.navy.mil/library/online/influenza_ collins.htm

Chen, H., Smith, G.J.D., Li, K.S. et al. (2006): Establishment of multiple sublineages of H5N1 influenza virus in Asia: Implications for pandemic control. PNAS 103, 2845-2850, 2006.

DEFRA /2008): Outbreak of highly pathogenic H5N1 avian influenza in Suffolk in January 2007. A report of the epidemiological findings by the national emergency epidemio logical group. news.bbc.co.uk/1/shared/bsp/hi/pdfs/20_04_07_defra_bird.pdf

GAIN (2005): Laos poultry and products avian influenza. http://www.fas.usda.gov.gainfiles/ 200503/146119131

Gernhart, G. (1999): A forgotten enemy: PHS's fight against the 1918 influenza pandemic. *Public Health Reports* 114: 559-561. Online: www.history.navy.mil/library/online/ influenza_forgot.htm

GRAIN (2006 a): Fowl play. The poultry industry's central role in the bird flu crisis. www. grain.org/go/birdflu

GRAIN (2006 b): The top-down global response to bird flu. http://grain.org/articles /index.cfm?id=12

GRAIN (2007): Bird flu: a bonanza for 'Big Chicken'. http://www.grain.org/articles/index. cfm?id=22

Guan, Y., Peiris, S.M., Lipatov, A.S. et al. (2002): Emergence of multiple genotypes of H5N1 avian influenza viruses in Hong Kong SAR. *PNAS* 99, 8950-8955.

Kilpatrick, A.M., Chmura, A.A., Gibbons, D.W. et al. (2006): Predicting the global spread of H5N1 avian influenza. *PNAS* 103, 19368-19373.

Li, K.S., Guan, Y., Wang, J. et al. (2004): Genesis of a highly pathogenic and potentially pandemic H5N1 influenza virus in eastern Asia. *Nature* 430, 209-213.

Liu, J., Xiao, H., Lei, F. et al. (2005): Highly pathogenic H5N1 Influenza virus infection in migratory birds. *Science* 309, 1206.

Lorenzen, S. (2008): Evolution und Ausbreitung des Vogelgrippe-Virus H5N1 Asia sowie Aspekte der Biosicherheit. *Tierärztliche Umschau* 63, 333-339.

McBean, E. I. (1997): Swine Flu expose, chapter 2: The Spanish Influenza Epidemic of 1918 was caused by vaccinations. www.whale.to/vaccine/sf1.html

Muzaffar, S.B., Ydenberg, R.C., Jones, I.L. (2006): Avian influenza: An ecological and evolutionary perspective for waterbird scientists. *Waterbirds* 29, 243-257.

Newman, S., Pinto, J., DeSimone, L. et al. (2007): HPAI in Europe 2007: Concurrent outbreaks in Poultry and wild birds. www.fao.org/docs/eims/upload/ 231765/EW_ Europe_aug07_ai

Oxford, J. (2004): Nature's biological weapon. The 1918 flu pandemic killed 50 million people – and it could happen again. *Nature* 429: 345-346.

Petermann, P. (2008): Das Rätsel der "Vogelgrippe": Geflügelpest oder Wildvogelseuche? Anzeiger des Vereins Thüringer Ornithologen 6, 117-141.

Petermann, P. (2007): 285 tote Schwarzhalstaucher, ein Nachruf und ein dringender Aufruf. www.netzwerk-phoenix.net

Schoene, C., Harder, T., Globis, A., Conraths, F.J., Mettenleiter, T.C. (1009): Die Wildvogel-Frage: Welche Rolle spielen Wildvögel im Infektionsgeschehen der hochpathogenen aviären Influenza? *Tierärztliche Umschau* 64, 77-83.

Sharkey, K.J., Bowers, R.G., Morgan, K.L. et al. (2007): Epdemiological consequences of an incursion of highly pathogenic H5N1 avian influenza into British poultry flock. *Proc. R. Soc. B*: doi:10.1098/rspb.2007.1100.

Starick, E., Beer, M., Hoffmann, B. et al. (2007): Phylogenetic analyses of highly pathogenic avian influenza virus isolates from Germany in 2006 and 2007 suggest at least three separate introductions of H5N1 virus. VETMIC 3852, doi: 10.1016/j.vetmic.2007.10.012.

Suarez, D.L., Senne, D.A., Banks, J. et al. (2004): Recombination resulting in virulence shift in avian influenza outbreak, Chile. *Emerging Infection Diseases* 10, 693-699.

Subbarao, K., Klimov, A., Katz, J. et al. (1998): Characterization of an Avian Influenza A (H5N1) Virus isolated from a child with a fatal respiratory illness. *Science* 279, 393-396.

Taubenberger, K.K., Morens, D.M. (2006): 1918 Influenza: the mother of all pandemics. *Emerging Infectious Diseases* 12, 15-22.

Uiprasertkul, M., Puthavathana, P., Sangsiriwut, K. et al. (2005): Influenza A H5N1 replication sites in humans. *Emerging Infectious Diseases* 11, 1036-1041.

WHO (2009): Cumulative number of confirmed human cases of avian influenza A/(H5N1) reported to WHO. http://www.who.int/csr/disease/avian_influenza/country/cases_tab

WHO/OIE/FAO/ H5N1 (2008): Toward a unified nomenclature system for highly pathogenic avian influenza virus (H5N1).http://www.cdc.gov/eid/content/14/7/e1-T2.htm

Williams, M. (2006): Farm fish fed dead chickens a risk for H5N1 influenza in Indonesia? www.drmartinwilliams.com/conservation/catfish-farm.html

Xu, X., Subbarao, K., Cox, N.J., Guo, Y. (1999): Genetic characterization of the pathogenic influenza A/Goose/Guangdong/1/96 (H5N1) Virus: Similarity of its hemagglutinin gene to those of H5N1 viruses from the 1997 outbreaks in Hong Kong. *Virology* 261, 15-19.

Yasue, M., Feare, C.J., Bennun, W., R, Fiedler, W. (2006): The epidemiology of H5N1 Avian Influenza in wild birds: Why we need better ecological data. *BioScience* 56-11, 1-7.

In: Global View of Fight against Influenza
Editor: Petar M. Mitrasinovic

ISBN: 978-1-60741-952-5
© 2009 Nova Science Publishers, Inc.

Chapter 17

THEORETICAL ASPECT OF PREVENTION POLICIES AGAINST INFLUENZA PANDEMIC

Shingo Iwami[1*], *Yasuhiro Takeuchi*[1], *Xianning Liu*[2],
Andrei Korobeinikov[3], *Eunok Jung*[4] *and Tae-Chang Jo*[5]

[1]Graduate School of Science and Technology, Shizuoka University, Japan
[2]School of Mathematics and Statistics, Southwest University, China
[3]Department of Mathematics and Statistics, University of Limerick, Ireland
[4]Department of Mathematics, Konkuk University, Korea
[5]Department of Mathematics, Inha University, Korea

ABSTRACT

Outbreaks of highly pathogenic H5N1 avian influenza in Southeast Asia, Europe, and Africa have devastating consequences for poultry, and have resulted in numerous infections in humans. Although these infections from the animal reservoir continue to accumulate, the virus does not seem to spread extensively among humans. However, a genetic reassortment could occur in a human who, for example, is co-infected with avian influenza A virus and a human strain of influenza A virus. The resulting new virus might then be able to easily infect humans, spread from human to human and lead to a global pandemic. Thus, currently, a major public health concern is the next influenza pandemic, yet it remains unclear how to control such a crisis. In this chapter, by using simple mathematical models, we consider the effectiveness of intervention policies (elimination of infected birds and quarantine of infected humans) against influenza pandemic and warn about the risks of the disease spread caused by the interventions. Further, we propose strategies to mitigate the damage of the pandemic.

---

[*] E-mail address: yukitadahara@yahoo.co.jp

1. INTRODUCTION

The 1918–1919 influenza pandemic, called "Spanish influenza", killed 20–40 million people worldwide, and is seen as a worst-case scenario for pandemic planning [20, 67]. Like other pandemic influenza strains, the 1918–1919 H1N1 strain spread extremely rapidly. The cause of this 1918–1919 pandemic is unknown, as it is unknown whether that was linked to avian or swine influenza [59]. For example, the 1918–1919 nucleoprotein (NP) gene sequence is similar to that of viruses found in wild birds at the amino acid level but very divergent at the nucleotide level, which suggests considerable evolutionary distance between the sources of the 1918–1919 NP and of currently sequenced NP genes in wild bird strains [60]. However, recently, the emergence of the highly pathogenic avian influenza strain H5N1 has raised concerns of an imminent influenza pandemic comparable with the Spanish influenza because of its adaptive mutations, or recombinations with human influenza viruses, and immunological pressure of pharmaceutical policies [9, 19, 22, 49, 56]. Therefore, development of strategies for mitigating the severity of a new influenza pandemic is now a top global public health priority [17, 18, 38, 46, 64, 69, 70].

1.1. Avian Influenza

Avian influenza virus usually refers to influenza A virus, which is found mainly in birds. Type A influenza viruses can be highly pathogenic to birds. Avian influenza virus are subtyped by characterization of hemagglutinin (HA) and neuraminidase (NA) glycoproteins, located on the outer surface of the envelope [73]. Sixteen HA and nine NA subtypes have been identified in influenza A, which implies that 144 subtypes can exist. Several avian influenza subtypes have already spread over the world causing outbreaks among poultry [9, 14, 20, 61, 67, 73]. A risk of direct passing of avian influenza virus to humans is generally very low. Nevertheless, a number of confirmed cases of human infection with several subtypes (H5N1, H5N2, H7N7, H7N3, H9N2) of avian influenza from infected birds have been reported in several region of the world particularly in Southeast Asia since 1997 at Hong Kong [14, 15, 61, 62, 71]. According to the cases reported to the World Health Organization (WHO) on September 10, 2008, the H5N1 virus has already infected 387 humans and has killed 245 patients worldwide, with a mortality rate exceeding 50% [72]. Most human cases represent rare events of direct transmission from infected domestic birds [7, 9, 20], whereas a few instances of probable human-to-human transmission have been documented in Thailand, Indonesia, and China so far [34, 50, 55, 63]. Actually, these human-to-human cases are caused by close contacts within a family and can not be considered as an evidence of the effective transmission among humans. To be transmitted efficiently from human to human, a zoonotic virus must overcome a series of obstacles (impairment of viral entry and/or virus replication, inhibitory immune response, etc.) that might lead interspecies passage to a dead end [66]. Therefore, for a pandemic to occur, three conditions must be met: a new influenza virus subtype must emerge, this must infect humans and cause serious disease, and finally spread easily among humans [19, 30, 50, 55, 65]. The first two conditions have already been met, but, fortunately, there is no evidence to-date of the easy human-to-human transmission that is key for a pandemic. With the emergence of highly pathogenic avian influenza H5N1 strain, which is now widespread in Southeast Asia and which diffused recently in some areas of the Balkans region and Western Europe, the threat of an influenza pandemic seems to be real and inevitable [9, 10, 20, 33, 50, 55, 56, 59].

1.2. Elimination Policy

In the European Union (EU), the regulations for the control of avian influenza strains are imposed by EU council directive 92/40/EEC [8]. The U.S. Department of Agriculture (USDA) provides overall guidance for the containment of an avian influenza outbreak [64]. Common methods used to manage infected birds (and their carcasses) and associated materials include composting, burial, incineration, rendering, and so on [8, 57, 64]. Virus output is reduced by the killing and removal of infected birds (elimination). This approach was applied in the most countries where outbreak of the avian influenza occur: for instance, during outbreaks in Italy (1999–2000) [40], in the Netherlands (2003) [14, 15, 57], in most countries in Asia (2003–2004) [30, 61], and in the United States (2003–2004) [40]. The elimination of infected birds is often accompanied by the depopulation (killing and removal) of uninfected birds in the vicinity of the infected bird (preemptive culling) and other veterinary measures, such as a ban on the transport of poultry and poultry products and hygienic measures [57]. Elimination of the infected birds is supposed to reduce the potential for genetic mutations and transmission of viruses to humans.

1.3. Quarantine Policy

Vaccines and antiviral drugs are the two most important medical interventions for reducing morbidity and mortality during the pandemic, but will not be available in adequate supplies [49]. Authorities of all countries must be prepared to make the most of the available non-pharmaceutical policies to reduce morbidity, mortality, and social disruption [17, 18, 38]. For example, quarantine and isolation of persons are implemented to reduce the number of infective contacts and delay geographical spread (isolation means the (physical) separation of infected person from uninfected person; quarantine means the separation and restriction of the movement of the persons who, while not yet ill, have been or may have been exposed to an infectious agent and therefore may become infectious) [17, 18, 31]. The WHO and scientists consider that the interventions that increase social distance might include closing schools and workplaces, a ban on mass gatherings, and travel restrictions [13, 17, 18, 31, 69, 70]. During the 2003 severe acute respiratory syndrome (SARS) outbreak in Hong Kong, it is believed that the community hygienic and social distancing measures could have significantly reduced the incidence of various respiratory viral infections [36]. Thus, the quarantine of infected humans can reduce transmission of viruses among humans. The WHO has also produced guidance on the use of the distancing policies that must be applied at different stages at the start of a pandemic and after its international spread [69, 70].

It remains unknown from where a pandemic strain, having sustained human-to-human transmission ability, may emerge: current attention is directed at Vietnam, Thailand, and, more recently, Indonesia and China [10]. It is also is generally believed that a pandemic strain will emerge soon [19, 50, 55]. While preventing the emergence of the pandemic virus appears to be impossible, we can and have to prepare in advance the best plans that are aimed to prevent its internal and international spread, and to mitigate the morbidity and mortality of the virus to the minimum under the worst situation. We need to clarify the effectiveness and risks of the prevention policies to develop effective mitigation strategies. We study relations between a virulence evolution of avian influenza and an effectiveness of pandemic control measures by a simple mathematical model after the emergence of mutant avian influenza [24, 25, 26]: one is an elimination policy of infected birds with avian influenza and the other is a quarantine policy of infected humans with mutant avian influenza. In addition, we investigate an impact of execution costs of the prevention policies [27].

2. METHODS

Herein, we describe a combination model with avian influenza transmission dynamics among birds and humans (Figure 1). Recent outbreaks of emerging infectious diseases such as SARS and H5N1 avian influenza have underlined the fact that the infectious disease of wild animals might acquire the ability to spread efficiently among the humans [2]. Therefore, in order to capture an essence of invasion and transmission of avian influenza, we consider both bird and human worlds.

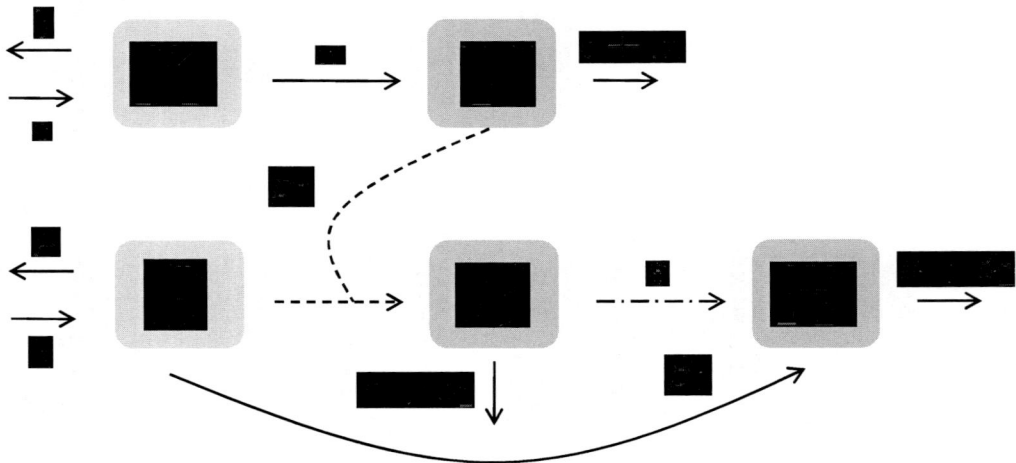

Figure 1. Model structure for avian influenza after an emergence of mutant avian influenza: all birds and humans in the effective population are divided into several compartments, respectively including susceptible birds (X), birds infected with wild avian influenza (Y), susceptible humans (S), humans infected with wild avian influenza (B), and humans infected with mutant avian influenza (H). The interactions between X and Y represent wild avian influenza transmission among birds. On the other hand, the interactions between S , B and H represent wild and mutant avian influenza transmission among humans. Note that wild avian influenza can only be transmitted into humans through Y and S interactions. We now simply assume that within the infected human hosts the virus of wild avian influenza evolves at a sufficiently small constant rate (ε) to the mutant virus. See Mathematical model for corresponding equations.

All birds in the effective population are divided into two compartments, respectively including susceptible birds (X) and birds infected with wild avian influenza (Y). We assume that susceptible birds are born or restocked at a rate of c per day and that all birds are naturally dead or removed from the effective population at a rate of b per day. Among birds, transmission occurs at a rate that is directly related to the number of infectious birds with transmission rate constants ω from infected birds with avian influenza virus (wild avian influenza strain). The infectiousness of wild strain is assumed to be exponentially distributed with mean durations of $1/(b+m)$ days.

On the other hand, all humans are divided into three compartments, respectively including susceptible humans (S), humans infected with wild avian influenza (B), and humans infected with mutant avian influenza (H). Susceptible humans are born or immigrated at a rate of λ per day and that all humans are naturally dead or migrated at a rate of μ per day. Wild avian influenza can be transmitted directly from birds or from avian virus-contaminated environments to humans [6, 7, 9, 14, 15, 20, 61, 62, 71]. We postulate, therefore, that transmission of wild strain for humans which is restricted from birds to humans occurs at a rate $\beta_1 Y$. And also many experts expect the emergence of mutant avian influenza, which can be easily transmitted among humans. The transmission rate of mutant strain among humans is β_2. The infectiousness of wild and mutant strains are assumed to be exponentially distributed, respectively, with mean durations of $1/(\mu+d_1)$ and $1/(\mu+d_2)$ days. Note that d_1 and d_2 respectively signify virulence of wild and mutant strains.

Actually, mutant avian influenza is resulted in mutation and selection process of a number of mutant strains which can increase fitness [3, 4]. Therefore if we consider the mutation process under a realistic situation, we might have to involve the detailed process. However, our results are robust for any mutation process of mutant avian influenza (see Results), we now simply assume, therefore, that within the infected human hosts the virus of wild avian influenza evolves at a sufficiently small constant rate to the mutant virus which can beat other strains in the mutation and selection process. That is, humans infected with wild avian influenza become those with mutant avian influenza at a sufficiently small constant rate ε.

2.1. Mathematical Model

We extended the standard susceptible − infective model [1] combining with avian influenza transmission dynamics among birds and humans. Our mathematical model is given by the following equations:

$$
\begin{aligned}
X' &= c - bX - \omega XY, \\
Y' &= \omega XY - (b+m)Y, \\
S' &= \lambda - \mu S - (\beta_1 Y + \beta_2 H)S, \\
B' &= \beta_1 SY - (\mu + d_1 + \varepsilon)B, \\
H' &= \beta_2 SH + \varepsilon B - (\mu + d_2)H.
\end{aligned}
\tag{1}
$$

Here we investigate relations between an evolution of virulence (d_1 and d_2: the virulence of mutant avian influenza relative to wild avian influenza) and efficacy of pandemic control measures during a pandemic. Further we evaluate impacts of recovery and execution costs of the policies which play an important role in an influenza pandemic on the efficacy of the intervention policies.

2.2. Reproduction Numbers

A measure of transmissibility and of the stringency of control policies required to stop an epidemic is the basic reproduction number, which is the number of secondary cases produced by each primary case (i.e., all individuals are susceptible) during his/her period of infectiousness [1]. We obtained two basic reproduction numbers, r_0 for infected birds with wild avian influenza and R_0 for infected humans with mutant avian influenza from model (1). Here we define

$$r_0 = \frac{\omega}{b+m}\frac{c}{b}, \quad R_0 = \frac{\beta_2}{\mu+d_2}\frac{\lambda}{\mu}.$$

However, for mutant avian influenza we are unable to describe adequately the spread of the infection by applying these usual basic reproduction numbers. The reason is that avian influenza is already endemic, particularly in Asian poultry. Note that some portion of humans have already been infected with wild avian influenza and are dead (and some portion have cross-immunity to mutant avian influenza in the extended model which includes a possibility of recovery) after avian influenza is endemic among birds. For the case that the mutation rate is sufficiently small ($\varepsilon = 0$), we have an invasive reproduction number for the mutant strain,

$$\overline{R}_0 = \frac{\beta_2}{\mu+d_2}\frac{\lambda}{\mu+\beta_1(c/(b+m)-b/\omega)},$$

which means an expected number of new infectious cases after avian influenza becomes endemic among birds (that is, after r_0 becomes larger than 1). Therefore, $\overline{R}_0$ can capture these situations and model (1) can deal with the essence of the spread of mutant avian influenza among humans.

2.3. Estimation of Epidemiological Parameters

Baseline values of model parameters and their respective ranges used for simulations are presented in Table 1. These parameters are based on previous epidemics among birds (the H5N1 2004 epidemic [21, 61, 62]) and influenza pandemics among humans (the H1N1 1918-1919 pandemic [11, 12, 41, 45, 51, 68]).

We assume that wild avian influenza transmission among birds is similar to the H5N1 epidemic which was confirmed in 2004 in Thailand [21, 61, 62].

Table 1. Description of transmission, mutation, and demography parameters of model (1) with their baseline values and ranges used for simulations. These parameters are based on previous epidemics among birds (the H5N1 2004 epidemic [21, 61, 62]) and influenza pandemics among humans (the H1N1 1918-1919 pandemic [11, 12, 41, 45, 51, 68]).

Symbol	Meaning	Value (Range)
c/b	Initial bird population size	5.00×10^2 individuals
m	Inverse of mean infectious period of infected bird	0.10 /day
ω	Transmission rate of wild avian influenza among birds	4.10×10^{-4} /day
r_0	Basic reproduction number of wild avian influenza	1.86
λ/μ	Initial human population size	1.00×10^3 individuals
d_1	Inverse of mean infectious period (virulence) of wild avian influenza	0.10 /day ($[0,0.2]$)
d_2	Inverse of mean infectious period (virulence) of mutant avian influenza	0.07 /day ($[0,0.2]$)
β_1	Transmission rate of wild avian influenza among humans	2.00×10^{-4} /day · individual
β_2	Transmission rate of mutant avian influenza among humans	2.80×10^{-4} /day · individual
ε	Mutation rate of wild avian influenza	5.50×10^{-4} /day
R_0	Basic reproduction number of mutant avian influenza	3.79
$\overline{R}_0$	Invasive reproduction number of mutant avian influenza	1.50

Estimated basic reproduction numbers of infected birds during the 2004 epidemic in Thailand range from 1.71 to 5.00 [62]. Here we use a relatively small basic reproduction number $r_0 = 1.86$. This is because we should consider a comparatively mild situation for wild avian influenza among birds since the wild strain has already become endemic. An initial bird population size is assumed to be $c/b = 5.00 \times 10^2$ individuals. Usually mean lifespan of poultry is about 2 years, but we consider that the mean duration of bird being in effective population is about $1/b = 100$ days because of migration or marketing. Therefore, birth or restocking rate of birds are $c = 5$ individuals per day. Because estimated mean infectious periods of infected birds range from 5 to 17.6 [44, 57, 62], we assume that the mean infectious period is about $1/(b+m) = 9.1$ days (i.e., $m = 0.10$ day^{-1}). Now we can estimate that transmission rate of the wild strain among birds is $\omega = 4.10 \times 10^{-4}$ day^{-1} individual^{-1}.

On the other hand, we consider parameters that are in line with the H1N1 1918-1919 pandemic situation for mutant avian influenza transmission among humans. Actually, well-known estimated 1918-1919 pandemic basic reproduction numbers vary very widely, ranging from 1.2 to 20 [11, 12, 41, 45, 51, 68]. For example, the basic reproduction number of the 1918-1919 influenza pandemic in Geneva, Switzerland has been estimated at 1.5 for the summer wave and 3.8 for the fall wave using case notification data [11], and in the major United State cities the number has also been estimated to range from 2 to 4 using mortality data [45] (a recent comprehensive review of estimates of the 1918–1919 influenza pandemic is given by G. Chowell and H. Nishiura in [12]). Here the basic reproduction number is assumed to be $R_0 = 3.79$ which is relatively large. This is because we should consider a comparatively severe situation for mutant avian influenza. An initial human population size is set in $\lambda/\mu = 1.00 \times 10^3$ individuals. We assume that mean duration of humans being in the effective population is about $1/\mu = 365$ days (mean lifespan of human is about 60 years) because of rapid human migration, transportation and so on. This implies that birth or immigration rate of humans are $\lambda = 2.7$ individuals per day. It is considered that estimated mean infectious period of infected humans with wild avian influenza is about 9 days ([30, 71]). And also, in general, the virulence of the mutant strain decreases, which implies that mean infectious period of infected humans with the mutant strain increases [1, 42, 47]. Therefore we assume that the mean infectious period of wild and mutant avian influenza are $1/(\mu + d_1) = 9.74$ days and $1/(\mu + d_2) = 13.76$ days, respectively, for baseline parameter values (the virulence of wild and mutant avian influenza virus are $d_1 = 0.1$ day^{-1} and $d_2 = 0.07$ day^{-1}). Note that, however, since we are interested in a mutation of avian influenza virulence from wild to mutant strain for the evaluation of prevention policies (see Results), the virulence parameters d_1 and d_2 are variable ranging from 0 to 0.2 in Figures 2, 3 and 4, respectively, because the expected virulence of the mutant strain is unknown. Now we can estimate that transmission parameter for the mutant strain among humans is $\beta_2 = 2.80 \times 10^{-4}$ day^{-1} individual^{-1}. Further, we assume that the transmission rate of the wild strain among humans (i.e., from infected birds to susceptible humans: the transmission rate between species, in general, seems to be smaller than one within species) is $\beta_1 = 2.00 \times 10^{-4}$ day^{-1} individual^{-1}. And also we consider that mean duration that wild avian influenza viruses do not mutate among humans is about 5 years (i.e., the rate of the wild strain mutating to the mutant strain within infected human is $\varepsilon = 5.5 \times 10^{-4}$ day^{-1}). Actually we do not have any justification for β_1 and ε, because there are not any data or paper about it, but these values are not biologically unreasonable.

2.4. Epidemiological Scenarios

We have mentioned that avian influenza is already endemic in the bird world [9, 33, 61, 67]. Therefore, we have to conclude that, unless a policy aimed at reducing r_0 is applied, $r_0 > 1$ holds in real world.

If the probability of mutation is low and the mutation rate is sufficiently small, then a long period without recurrent mutations follows after an occurrence of a single mutation. Then we can neglect the mutation process, and approximate the spread of mutant avian influenza in humans by model (1) with $\varepsilon = 0$ because there is hardly continuous mutations. In this case, $\overline{R}_0 \leq 1$ means that the mutant virus will not spread widely or cause a global pandemic. That is, even if mutant avian influenza occurs, infected humans with mutant avian influenza will disappear. On the other hand, if the probability of a mutation is comparatively high, the mutation must be considered as a continuous process, that is we postulate that $\varepsilon > 0$. In this case, even if $\overline{R}_0 \leq 1$, mutant avian influenza becomes endemic at a low level because of the mutation process from infected humans with wild avian influenza. However, the sustained human-to-human transmission and global pandemic of mutant avian influenza do not occur in the situation with $\overline{R}_0 \leq 1$, since mutant avian influenza will not spread in human world. Although there is no evidence of sustained human-to-human transmission yet, we must consider the situation with $\overline{R}_0 > 1$, which means that mutant avian influenza will spread widely among humans.

We therefore assume the following conditions for reproductive numbers without any prevention policies (our baseline parameter values are satisfied with these assumptions):

$$r_0 > 1, \overline{R}_0 > 1.$$

2.5. Prevention Policies

We will evaluate the effectiveness of prevention policies by mathematical analysis after the emergence of the mutant influenza under $r_0 > 1$ and $\overline{R}_0 > 1$.

One of the policies is an elimination of infected birds called ``elimination policy". This policy (time-independently or time-dependently) increases the effective additional death rate of infected birds (or reduces the number of infective contacts among birds) and thus decreases the value of r_0, which can be potentially reduced to $r_0 \leq 1$. We remark that the elimination policy is always effective for the case without the emergence of mutant avian influenza because it can prevent the spread of wild avian influenza among humans.

Another policy is a ``quarantine policy" which reduces the number of infective contacts among humans. In terms of model (1), this policy (time-independently or time-dependently) reduces the transmission parameter for mutant avian influenza β_2, which results in decreasing of $\overline{R}_0$. The quarantine policy is complete when $\overline{R}_0 < 1$. The complete quarantine policy very effectively prevents spreading of the mutant strain after the policy is applied. We remark that to prevent the spread of mutant avian influenza does not need to reduce the value of R_0 below 1 because of $\overline{R}_0 < R_0$. However, in the real life situation we can hardly expect that the execution of the complete quarantine policy would be possible. The incomplete quarantine policy, that is, the case when the reduced value still satisfies $\overline{R}_0 > 1$, appears to be more realistic.

3. RESULTS

We investigate how a difference of the virulence between wild and mutant avian influenza could influence on an efficacy of the (time-independent) prevention policies in terms of both human morbidity and mortality at the final phase of the disease spread (i.e., equilibrium state) and how an execution cost of the (time-dependent) prevention policies could change the disease control over the disease spreads. The virulences of wild and mutant avian influenza are represented by d_1 and d_2 (i.e., the inverse of the mean infectious period of wild and mutant avian influenza, respectively). The case $d_1 < d_2$ corresponds to ``higher virulent mutation", and $d_1 > d_2$ corresponds to ``lower virulent mutation". While evolutionary theory predicts that a virulence of H5N1 decreases in the absence of a trade-off with transmission rate [1], there is an evidence that the pathogenicity of H5N1 in mammals is increasing [9]. Actually, the expected virulence of a pandemic form of H5N1 is uncertain, which means that the mutant strain might be more or less virulent than the wild strain. Therefore we have to consider the situations of both higher and lower virulent mutations. Our evaluations can be considered strictly in virulence space (d_1-d_2 space) of the wild and mutant strains. The detailed mathematical and computational analyses are given in [24, 25, 26, 27].

3.1. Evaluation of the Prevention Policies

We calculate the total number of infected humans ($B + H$) at the equilibrium when one of the time-independent prevention policies is executed. Note that, here, we assume that the "elimination policy" always reduces r_0 to less than 1 and the "quarantine policy" is incomplete in the time-independent case. Interestingly, the optimal choice of the policy depends on the mutation rate and the virulence evolution (see Figure 2). When the relation of the virulence of wild and mutant avian influenza lies on the black region, the policy increases the total number of infected humans. On the other hand, when the relation lies on the white region, the policy can decrease the total number of infected humans. Note that the boundary line between black and white region can be obtained exactly by mathematical analysis (see Appendix in [26]). From these figures, we can obtain some tendencies about the effectiveness as follows: if the lower virulent mutation occurs, then the quarantine policy is effective: otherwise the elimination policy is effective.

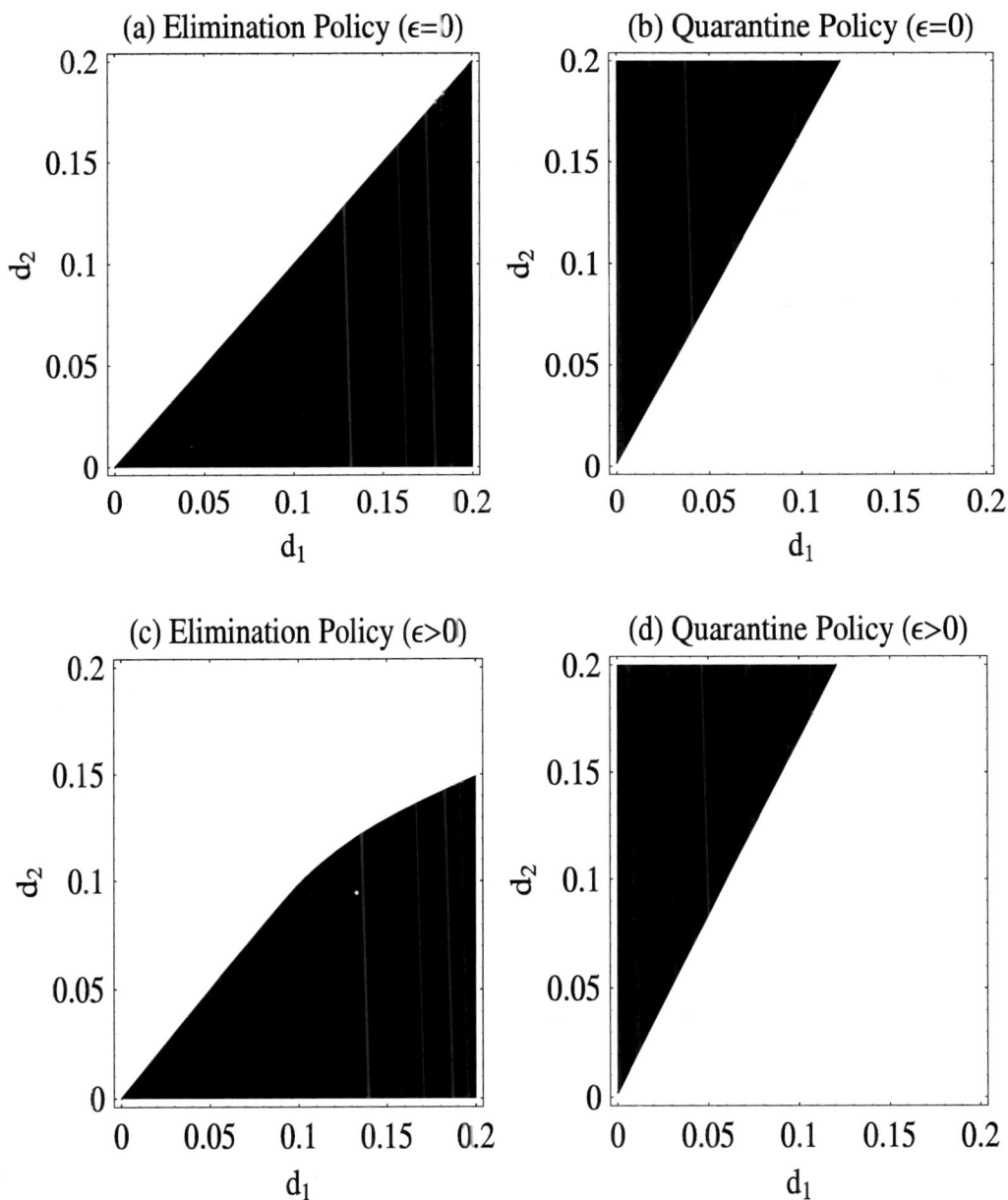

Figure 2. Evaluation of the effect of the prevention policies on total infected humans ($B+H$) at the equilibrium: the white region represents that the policy can decrease the total number of infected humans, the black region represents that the policy increases the total number of infected humans. The optimal choice of a policy depends on the mutation rate and the evolution of virulence. The horizontal axis represents the virulence of wild avian influenza and the vertical axis represents one of mutant avian influenza. The virulence of the wild and mutant strain (d_1 and d_2) are variable ranging from 0 to 0.2 and the other parameters are referred to Table 1.

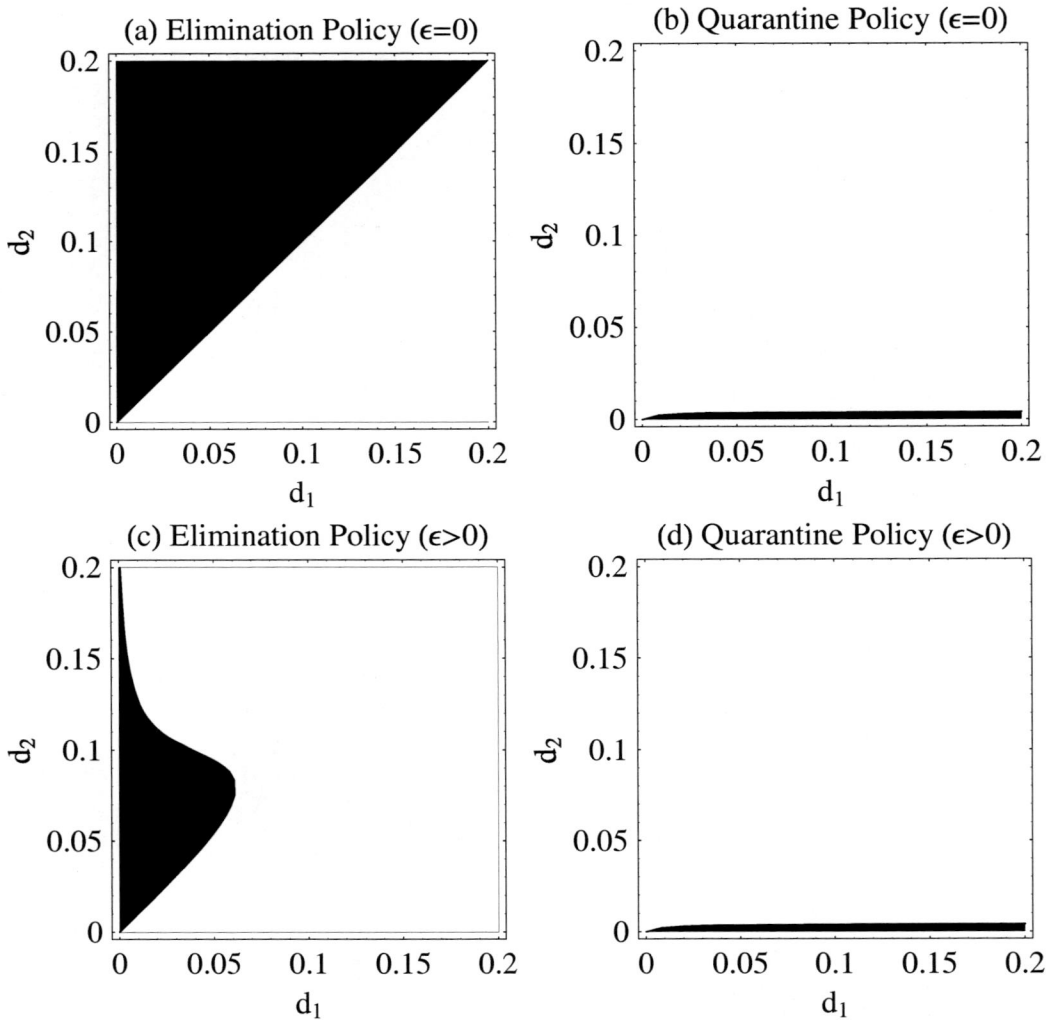

Figure 3. Evaluation of the effect of prevention policies on total dead humans ($d_1 B + d_2 H$) at the equilibrium: the white region represents that the policy can decrease the total number of the dead humans, the black region represents that the policy increases the total number of the dead humans. The optimal choice of a policy also depends on the mutation rate and the evolution of virulence. The horizontal axis represents the virulence of wild avian influenza and the vertical axis represents one of mutant avian influenza. The virulence of the wild and mutant strain (d_1 and d_2) are variable ranging from 0 to 0.2 and the other parameters are referred to Table 1.

Next, we calculate the total number of dead humans ($d_1 B + d_2 H$) at the equilibrium (see Figure 3). It can be readily seen from Figure 3, that in this case the optimal choice of the policy also depends on the mutation rate and the virulence evolution. The black and white regions in Figure 3 represent the regions where the policy is ineffective or effective regions, respectively. Interestingly, from these figures, we can obtain some counter tendencies about the effectiveness as follows: if the lower virulent mutation occurs, then the elimination policy is effective: otherwise the quarantine policy is effective.

These results stress that the evolutionary trend of the virulence of avian influenza has a crucial influence on prevention policies, because this trend determines the choice of the prevention policy. We also have to mention that the range of d_1 and d_2 (i.e., $[0,0.2]$) that was used in Figures 2 and 3 is not critical for our results: in fact, the boundary of the regions are analytically derived in Appendix in [26], and it is reasonable to expect that the qualitative features in Figures 2 and 3 will be preserved for any feasible ranges.

3.2. How to Prevent the Spread of Avian Influenza

The tendencies about the effectiveness of the prevention policies for decreasing the total number of infected humans go in the opposite direction to tendencies about the total number of dead humans. These counter results imply that controlling a next pandemic will not be so simple because we can not decide easily whether we should prioritize decreasing of the total number of infected humans or dead humans. However, fortunately, we can choose an effective policy which decreases both the total number of infected humans and dead humans. From Figures 2 and 3, we have only to consider the single mutation case ($\varepsilon = 0$) for the choice of the prevention policy because the mutation process always decreases the bad region and we must prepare for the worst situation for pandemic influenza planning.

Note that the single mutation case is a simply good modeling approach to evaluate the effect of prevention policies. Usually, in the real world, as only a low number of humans is infected by wild avian influenza and the probability that a mutation occurs is low as well, the mutation process should be analyzed in the context of a stochastic description. However, even if the stochastic approach is applied to the mutation process (εB) of model (1), we have only to consider the single mutation case to evaluate the effect of prevention policies because we can expect that the stochastic mutation process similarly decreases the bad region.

From Figure 2 (a), (b) and 3 (a), (b), we can conclude as follows: the elimination policy always has the bad face for the effectiveness because if the policy can reduce the total number of infected humans, then the policy increases the total number of dead humans, and the reverse is also true. On the other hand, the quarantine policy can reduce both the total number of infected and dead humans, in particular, when the virulence between wild and mutant avian influenza will hardly change by the antigen drift or shift, which means the relation of the virulence of wild and mutant avian influenza lies around $d_2 = d_1$. Therefore, the above qualitative results which are robust for any change of epidemiological parameters (note that the qualitative features in Figures 2 and 3 are preserved for any parameter sets) demonstrate that the best plan to limit damage by the pandemic at the minimum is the quarantine policy.

3.3. Change of Initial Phase by Prevention Policies

An emerging infection is a state that is far from equilibrium state. Our proposal for pandemic preparedness are based on analyzing the equilibria of model (1). Usually, the efficacy of intervention policies for equilibrium morbidity and mortality does not necessarily equal one for the morbidity and mortality at an initial phase of the influenza spread. In order to understand how the intervention policies influence on a transient dynamics of the disease spread (in particular, at the initial phase) we simulate model (1) using baseline epidemiological parameter values in Table 1 and realistic starting conditions.

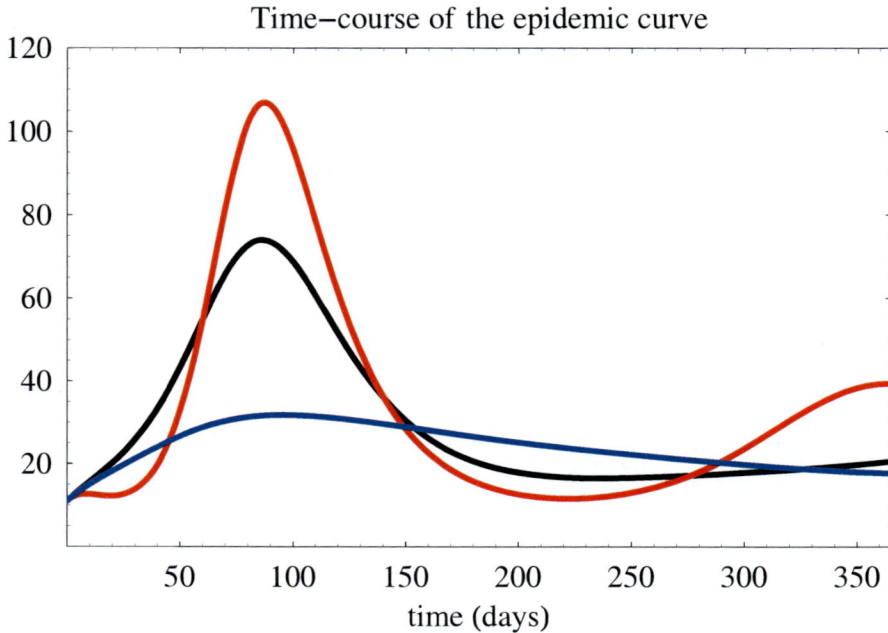

Figure 4. The effect of prevention policies for the time-course of the epidemic curve: the basic reproduction numbers and the invasive reproduction number are $r_0 = 1.86$, $R_0 = 3.79$ and $\overline{R}_0 = 1.50$, respectively. The black line shows the spread of the disease without any prevention policies. The red line shows the effect of the elimination policy ($r_0 = 0.93$) and the blue line shows the effect of the quarantine policy ($\overline{R}_0 = 1.13$) on the disease spread. We can see that the evaluation of prevention policies at the equilibria seems to be useful for prediction of the efficacy of the policies on human morbidity at the initial phase in the reasonable situation.

Since avian influenza is already endemic in bird world and some portion of humans have already been infected with wild avian influenza or are dead, we assume that the initial values are $X(0) = 300$, $Y(0) = 15$, $S(0) = 500$, $B(0) = 10$ and $H(0) = 1$. Note that the initial values are near the situation that wild avian influenza becomes endemic among humans. In Figure 4, the black line shows the spread of the disease for 365 days after the emergence of pandemic influenza without any prevention policies. The basic reproduction numbers and the invasive reproduction number are $r_0 = 1.86$, $R_0 = 3.79$ and $\overline{R}_0 = 1.50$, respectively. The red line shows the spread of the disease with the elimination policy ($r_0 = 0.93$). The policy increases the total number of infected humans at an initial phase (at around 100 days). On the other hand, the blue line shows the effect of the quarantine policy ($\overline{R}_0 = 1.13$) on the disease spread. The policy effectively decreases the total number of infected humans at the initial phase. We remark that, for baseline parameters, the mutant strain has a less virulence than the wild strain (lower virulent mutation) because of $d_1 > d_2$. These results reflect the efficacy of prevention policies at the equilibria (see Figure 2 (c) and (d)). We can conclude that the elimination policy can increase the epidemic curve in both initial and endemic phase but the quarantine policy can decrease one in the both phases when the lower virulent mutation occurs. Thus the evaluation of prevention policies at the equilibria seems to be useful for prediction of the efficacy of the policies on human morbidity at the initial phase in the reasonable situation.

3.4. Effect of Recovery

One of the important factors which can influence on dynamics, morbidity, mortality of influenza disease and even on an evolution of influenza virus is host immunity [16, 29]. Usually, humans infected with influenza A virus can recover from their infection within a week [41, 58]. In order to investigate the effect of recovery on the prevention policies we include recovery classes into model (1). Here, because wild avian influenza represents high pathogenesis for birds [30, 62], we neglect a possibility of recovery for infected birds. We simply assume that infected humans with wild and mutant avian influenza can recover and become immune with a rate δ_1 and δ_2, respectively (see Appendix in [26] for corresponding equations). However, actually, almost infected humans with wild avian influenza die within 10 days after the infection [30, 71]. Therefore we assume that the recovery rate from the infection of wild avian influenza is very small $\delta_1 \approx 0$ (once a human is infected with wild avian influenza, the human remain infected until dying from disease or dying naturally). On the other hand, humans infected with mutant avian influenza might recover from the infection [51, 58]. We assume that $\delta_2 = 0.05$ (the human can recover from the infection in 20 days on average). Since we are interested in the worst situation, we have also only to focus on the single mutation case (Figures 2 (a), (b) and 3 (a), (b)).

We evaluate how the recovery effect $\tilde{\delta}_2$ changes the efficacy of prevention policies (i.e., the boundaries between white and black regions). In Figures 5 (a) and (c), for the elimination policy, the black region reduces in both the total number of infected and dead humans cases. On the other hand, for the quarantine policy, the black region expands in Figures 5 (b) and (d). The recovery effect seems to strongly influence on the total number of dead humans rather than the total number of infected humans. Further, generally, the effect of recovery promotes the efficiency of the elimination policy, while the effect reduces the efficiency of the quarantine policy (the boundary lines move under the recovery effect (see Appendix in [26])). This is because the effect of recovery leads to some advantage to wild avian influenza virus, since the recovery rate reduces the basic reproduction number and the invasive reproduction number of the mutant strain.

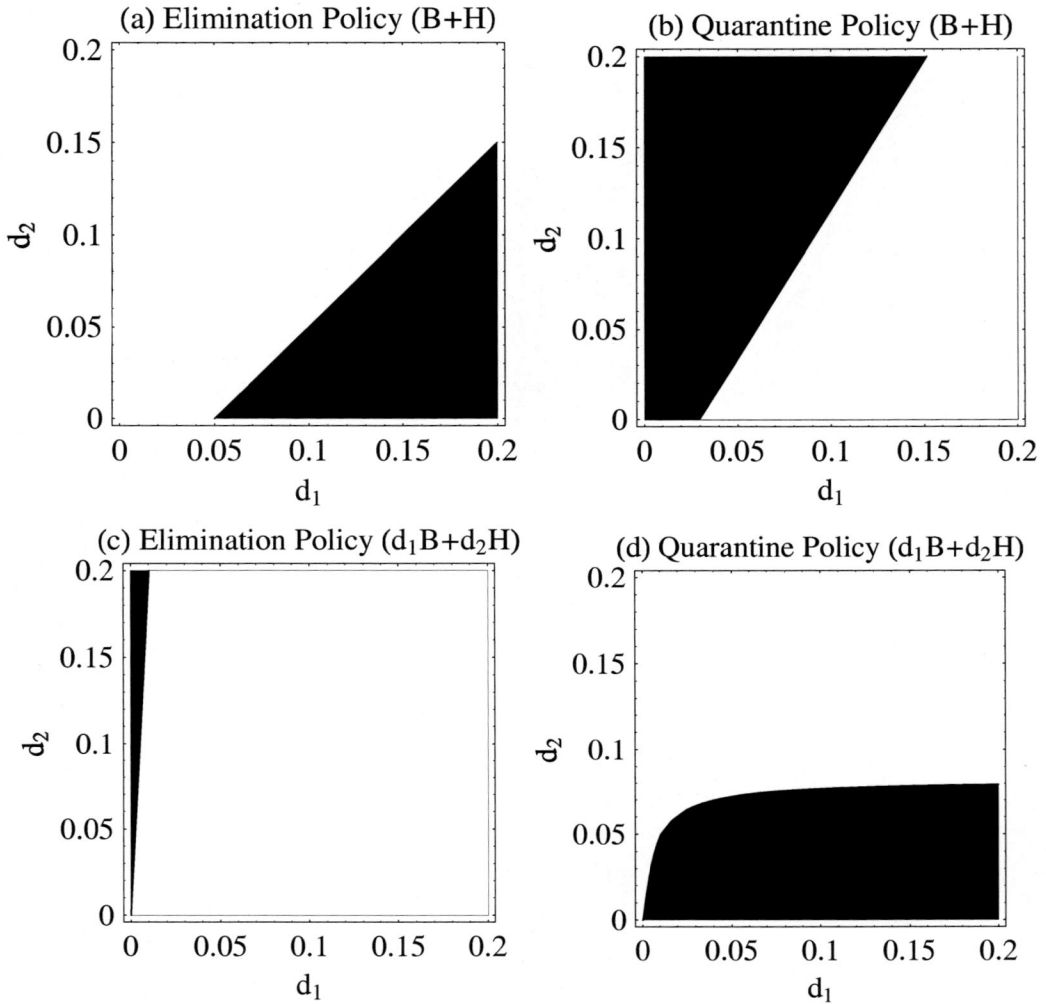

Figure 5. Effect of recovery on the prevention policies with the single mutation case ($\varepsilon = 0$): the white (black) region represents that the policy can decrease (increase) the total number of infected humans or dead humans. The horizontal axis represents the virulence of wild avian influenza and the vertical axis represents one of mutant avian influenza. The recovery rate from wild and mutant avian influenza is $\delta_1 \approx 0$ and $\delta_2 = 0.05$, respectively. The virulence of the wild and mutant strain (d_1 and d_2) are variable ranging from 0 to 0.2 and the other parameters are referred to Table 1.

3.5. Execution Cost of Prevention Policy

Most of economic studies on avian influenza have so far concentrated on the impact of the disease, more studies are needed to assess the impact of its control strategy in term of sustainability and efficacy [23, 49, 52, 53]. Epidemiological models including economic aspects are needed to estimate impacts of execution costs of prevention policies [49]. Actually, even mitigating programs which execute the same intervention policies have different unit execution costs depending on various situations. To project the potential economic impact of pandemic influenza mitigation strategies, we consider optimal control strategies associated with elimination policy and quarantine policy including execution costs based on previous combination model (1).

The US General Accounting Office estimated the human consequences of a pandemic in the US. These consequences includes 200 million Americans infected, 90 million clinically ill and 2 million dead. The study also estimates that 30% of all US workers would become ill and 2.5% would die, with 30% of workers missing a mean of 3 weeks of work, and a subsequent decrease in the US Gross domestic product of 5% [50]. Thus, influenza produces several costs due to lost productivity and associated medical treatment, as well as execution costs of preventative policies [23, 50, 53]. In the US, influenza is responsible for a total cost of over 10 billion per year and further it has been estimated that a future pandemic could cause hundreds of billions of dollars in the above costs [48]. In particular, the costs associated with vaccination, elimination of birds, hospitalization, quarantine of persons, transport restriction and so on can be great. The choice of intervention policy sometimes should be considered from an economic perspective [49]. Actually, financial ruin for poor poultry farmers has caused some to commit suicide and many others to stop cooperating with efforts to deal with avian influenza. And also, recently, new concerns have arisen regarding the illegal use of vaccines obtained from "underground" or "black" markets because of its price [49]. The illegal use of avian influenza vaccine hardly induces immune response and protects against the infection. These uncooperative behaviors increase the human morbidity and mortality, the spread of the disease and the chances for a pandemic mutation [48]. Thus, because many poor countries might not execute a costly strategy [43, 46], we should investigate impacts of direct cost (e.g., price of vaccine dose, culling of poultry, hospitalization, school closure, etc.) and indirect cost (e.g., export ban, commercial campaign, transport restriction, etc.) of intervention policies.

We extended the previous combination model (1) to evaluate the time-dependent optimal prevention policies considering its execution cost [27]. Our mathematical model is given by the following equations:

$$X' = c - bX - (1 - u_1(t))\omega XY,$$
$$Y' = (1 - u_1(t))\omega XY - (b + m)Y,$$
$$S' = \lambda - \mu S - \beta_1 YS - (1 - u_2(t))\beta_2 HS, \qquad (2)$$
$$B' = \beta_1 SY - (\mu + d_1)B,$$
$$H' = (1 - u_2(t))\beta_2 SH - (\mu + d_2)H.$$

Note that we explained the effect of time-independent prevention policies at the final phase of mutant avian influenza spread without an execution cost in previous sections. Here we investigate how we should time-dependently execute the prevention policies in order to minimize the number of total infected humans ($B(t) + H(t)$) keeping the execution cost of the policies low during the spread. We use our baseline parameter values in Table 1 for a ``lower virulence case ( $d_1 > d_2$ )". In addition, we consider $d_1 = 0.05$ day$^{-1}$ as a ``higher virulence case ($d_1 < d_2$)". Actually, durations of infectiousness of infected human with wild avian influenza are distributed on range from 6 to 30 days (i.e., d_1 ranges from 0.03 to 0.16 day^{-1} and our assumptions are satisfied with the range) [30, 71]. We investigate the optimal strategy of prevention policies based on these two cases in the same scenario ($r_0 > 1$ and $\overline{R}_0 > 1$) as previous sections. Further, because wild avian influenza is already endemic among birds and some portion of humans have already been infected with wild avian influenza or are dead, we also assume that $X(0) = 300$, $Y(0) = 15$, $S(0) = 500$, $B(0) = 10$ and $H(0) = 1$.

The control functions, $u_1(t)$ and $u_2(t)$, are bounded, Lebesgue integrable functions. The coefficient with "elimination control", $u_1(t)$, is the effort to reduce the number of infected birds. The "quarantine control", $u_2(t)$, represents the effort to reduce the number of contacts with humans infected with mutant avian influenza. For example, when the quarantine control u_2 is large, there is low infective contacts rate and high implementation costs. Note that the controls, $u_1(t)$ is bounded in [0,1] and $u_2(t)$ is bounded in [0, a], where $0 < a < 1$. The upper bound a is determined by the basic reproductive number of mutant avian influenza R_0 (see later). The time-dependent optimal prevention policies can be obtained by minimizing the following objective functional:

$$J(u_1, u_2) = \int_0^{t_f} [B(t) + H(t) + \frac{B_1}{2} u_1^2(t) + \frac{B_2}{2} u_2^2(t)] dt.$$

The costs of the elimination and quarantine policies are nonlinear and take quadratic forms. Here the coefficients B_1 and B_2, respectively, represent balancing cost factors due to size and importance of the other three parts of the objective functional. Therefore, for example, large (small) values of B_1 and B_2 imply expensive (cheap) unit execution costs of elimination and quarantine policies because $B_1 u_1^2/2$ and $B_2 u_2^2/2$ become large (small). We assume the balancing factor B_2 associated with control u_2 is bigger than B_1 associated with a control u_1 because to restrict human activity is more difficult than to eliminate infected birds. Here, although the weight of unit execution cost might be different on the situation, we fixed that $B_1 = 10$ and $B_2 = 100$ as default values of our control problem (we preserve B_2 is order 10 greater than B_1 in other cost situations). Our goal is to find an optimal control pair, $u_1^*(t)$ and $u_2^*(t)$, such that

$$J(u_1^*, u_2^*) = \min_{\Omega} J(u_1, u_2),$$

where $\Omega = \{(u_1, u_2) \in L^1(0, t_f) \mid 0 \le u_1 \le 1, 0 \le u_2 \le a\}$. We use Pontryagin's Maximum Principle [28, 54] to solve the optimal control problem and fix $t_f = 180$.

The basic reproductive numbers can be rewritten during the optimal prevention policies as follows:

$$r_0^*(t) = \frac{\omega(1 - u_1^*(t))}{b + m} \frac{c}{b}, \quad R_0^*(t) = \frac{\beta_2(1 - u_2^*(t))}{\mu + d_2} \frac{\lambda}{\mu}.$$

The optimal elimination policy, $u_1^*(t)$, decreases the value of $r_0^*(t)$. Similarly, the optimal quarantine policy, $u_2^*(t)$, reduces the value of $R_0^*(t)$. Therefore, we can expect that the policies always effectively decrease the epidemic curves unless the policies are terminated. However, in the real life situation we can hardly expect that the quarantine policy reduces $R_0^*(t)$ to the value less than 1. We assume that the reduced value still satisfies $R_0^*(t) > 1$, which implies that

$$R_0^*(t) > 1 \Leftrightarrow u_2(t) < 1 - \frac{1}{R_0} = a.$$

Note that we consider the both complete and incomplete quarantine policies in the time-dependent case because we might be able to transiently execute complete quarantine policy. Thus the upper bound a of control function u_2 is determined. Since $R_0 = 3.79$ in Table 1, we can determine the upper bound $a = 0.74$.

The dashed curves of the top figures in Figures 6 and 7 represent the epidemic curve of total infected humans without any policy in the lower and higher virulence cases, respectively. We can see that mutant avian influenza leads to a pandemic of the disease in the both cases. The solid curves of the top figures in Figures 6 and 7 represent the epidemic curve of total infected humans with optimal prevention policies. If we can execute the optimal strategy, the epidemic curve (in particular, at the pandemic phase) is dramatically reduced in the both cases. However, the total number of infected humans increases at around 140 days in the both cases. This is because the prevention policies (u_1 and u_2) are terminated at the end of the optimal strategy (see the bottom figures of Figures 6 and 7) because of these costs. Therefore, the infected humans can not be eradicated by the optimal policies and the remainder re-spreads the disease. However, if these unit execution costs are cheaper, the total number remains at lower level over 180 days (see Figure 8). The bottom figures of Figures 6 and 7 show the time-dependent optimal strategy of prevention policies u_1 and u_2 in the lower and higher virulence cases, respectively. In the lower virulence case (the bottom figures in Figure 6), the quarantine policy is more important than the elimination policy, because u_2 remains at high level for a long time than u_1, even if the unit cost of the quarantine policy is

10 times as expensive as one of the elimination policy. On the other hand, in the higher virulence case (the bottom figures in 6 and 7), the effort of the elimination policy u_1 is greater than the effort in the lower virulence case. Therefore, the elimination policy becomes more effective in the higher virulence case. In addition, in the higher virulence case, the quarantine policy is also more important to prevent the disease spread.

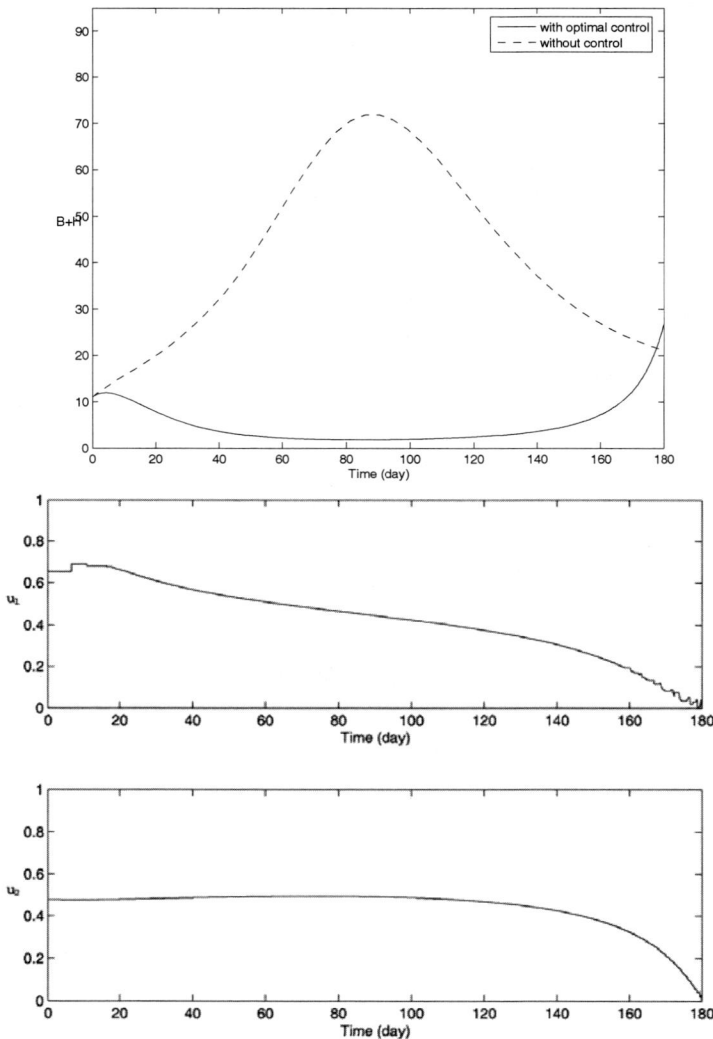

Figure 6. Time-course of disease spread with optimal prevention policies for 180 days after the emergence of mutant avian influenza virus in the lower virulence case: the top figure shows that the epidemic curves of total infected humans without (dashed curve) and with (solid curve) optimal prevention policies. The bottom two figures show the time-dependent optimal strategy of u_1 and u_2. The optimal policies dramatically reduce the epidemic curve (in particular, at the pandemic phase). We can see that the quarantine policy is more important than one of elimination policy even if the unit execution cost of u_1 is cheaper than one of u_2. Here we assume that $B_1 = 10$ and $B_2 = 100$.

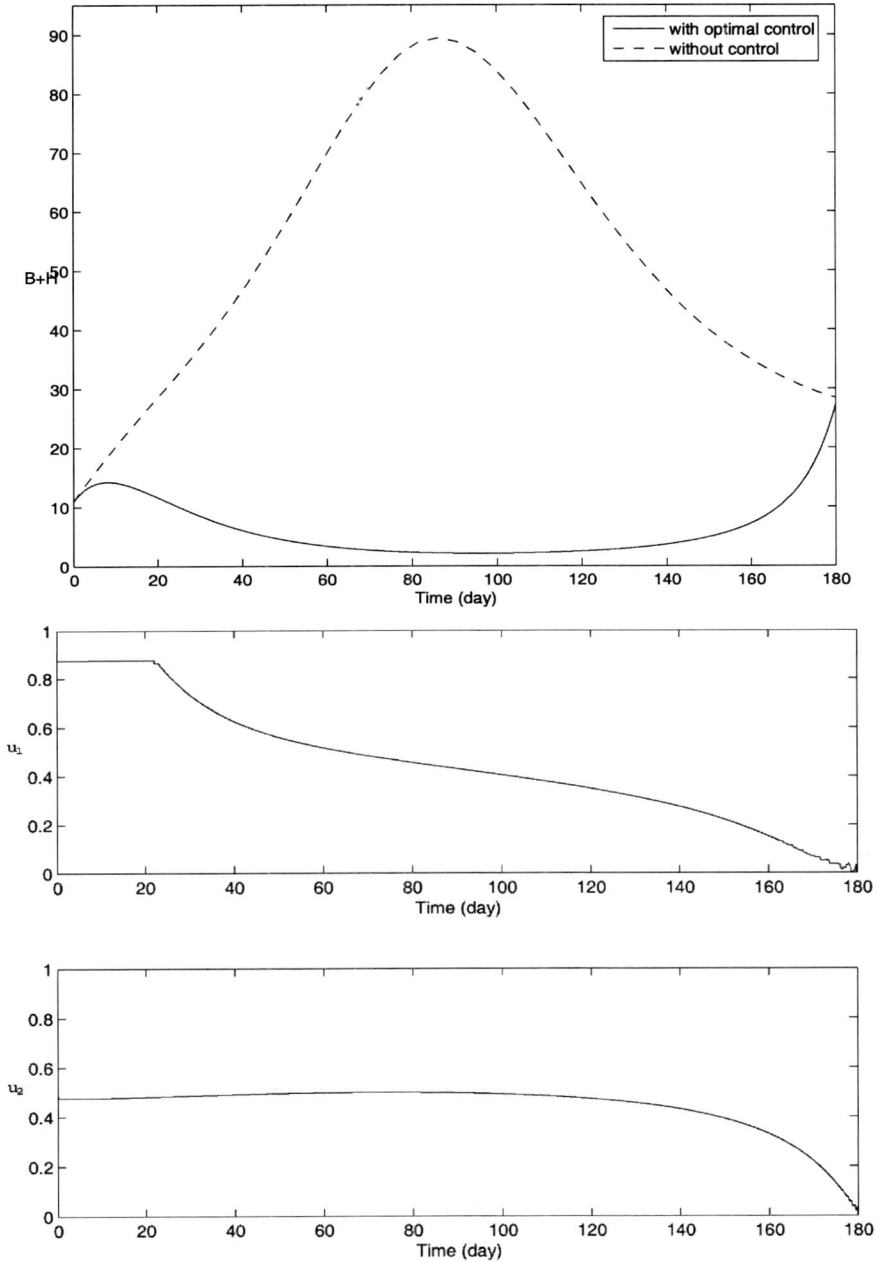

Figure 7. Time-course of disease spread with optimal prevention policies for 180 days after the emergence of mutant avian influenza virus in the higher virulence case: the top figure shows that the epidemic curves of total infected humans without (dashed curve) and with (solid curve) optimal prevention policies. The bottom two figures show the time-dependent optimal strategy of u_1 and u_2. The optimal policies also dramatically reduce the epidemic curve (in particular, at the pandemic phase). The effort of the elimination policy (u_1) is greater than the effort in the lower virulence case (Figure 6). Here we assume that $B_1 = 10$ and $B_2 = 100$.

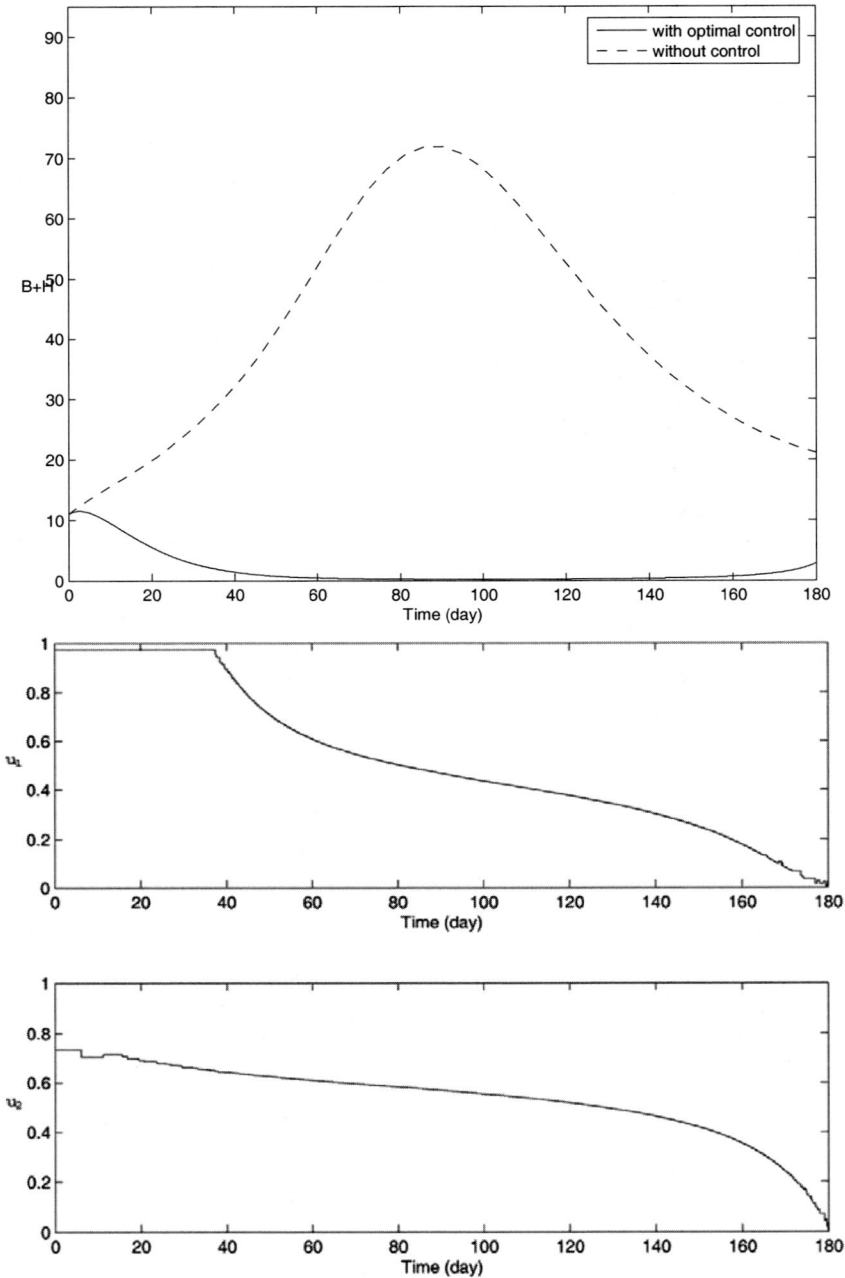

Figure 8. Time-course of disease spread with optimal prevention policies for 180 days in the lower virulence and the cheap cost case: the top figure shows that the epidemic curves of total infected humans without (dashed curve) and with (solid curve) optimal prevention policies. The bottom two figures show that the time-dependent optimal strategy of u_1 and u_2. Because the unit costs are cheaper, we can execute the prevention policies easily compared with our default case. The optimal policies dramatically reduce the overall epidemic curve and almost subdue the disease spread. Here we assume that the case with $B_1 = 1$ and $B_2 = 10$ is considered as the cheap cost case.

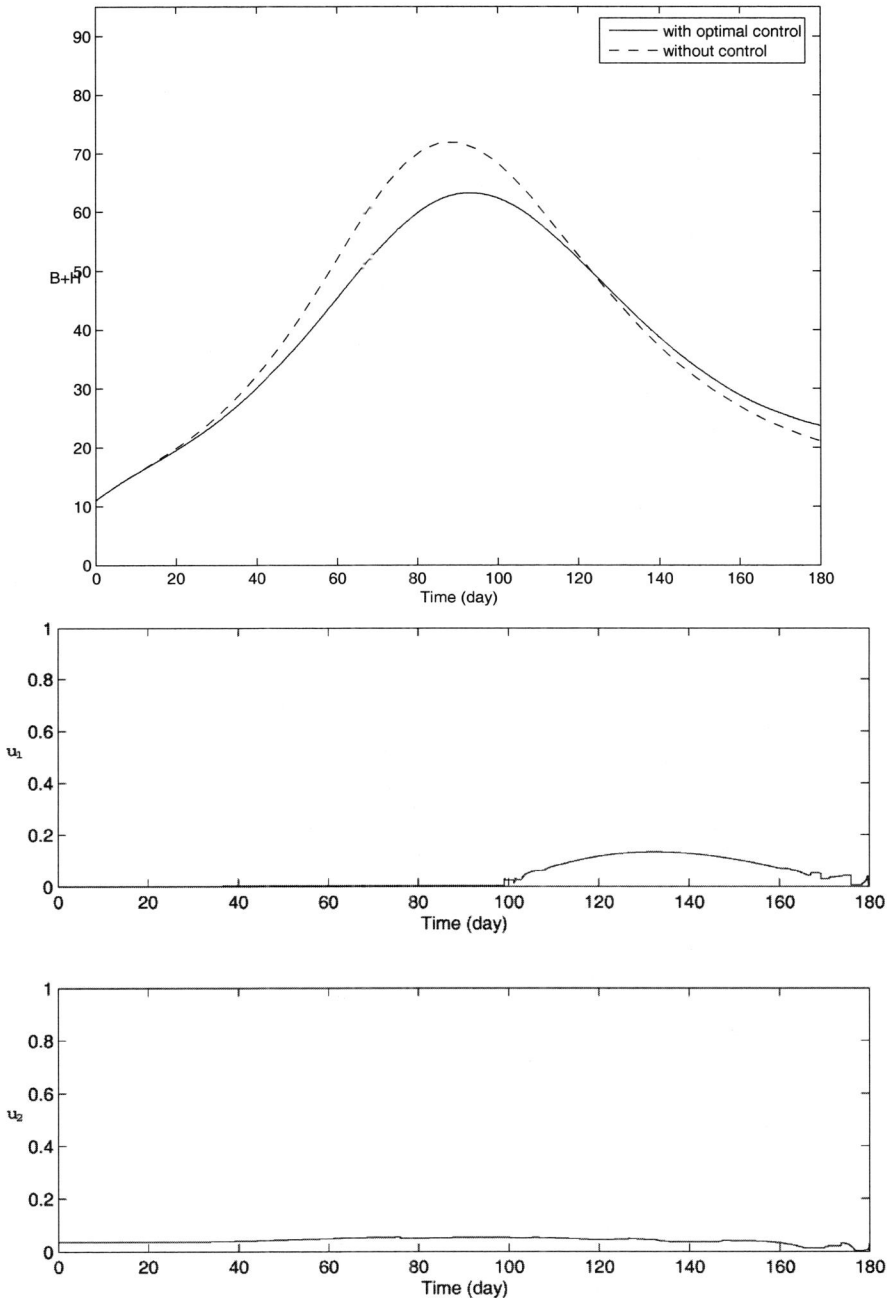

Figure 9. Time-course of disease spread with optimal prevention policies for 180 days in the lower virulence and the expensive cost case: the top figure shows that the epidemic curves of total infected humans without (dashed curve) and with (solid curve) optimal prevention policies. The bottom two figures show that the time-dependent optimal strategy of u_1 and u_2. Because the unit costs are more expensive, we can hardly execute the prevention policies compared with our default case. The optimal policies no longer reduce the epidemic curve and can not prevent the disease spread, even if we can execute the optimal control strategy. Here we assume that the case with $B_1 = 100$ and $B_2 = 1000$ is considered as the expensive cost case.

Next, we investigate an impact of the unit execution cost of prevention policies on the optimal strategy. Assume that $B_1 = 1$ and $B_2 = 10$ are a cheap cost case and $B_1 = 100$ and $B_2 = 1000$ are an expensive cost case in Figures 8 and 9, respectively. We consider that the virulence of mutant avian influenza is lower than one of wild strain (the lower virulence case: $d_1 = 0.1$ and $d_2 = 0.07$). We do not consider the higher virulence case here but the conclusion for this case is qualitatively the same. When the unit execution costs are cheap comparing with our default case, the prevention policies can be easily executed (the bottom figures in Figure 8: both u_1 and u_2 become larger than ones in Figure 6) and therefore the overall epidemic curves of total infected humans with the optimal policies (the solid curve of the top figure in Figure 8) is dramatically reduced compared with that without any policy (the dashed curve of the top figure in Figure 8). Thus the disease spread is effectively prevented by the optimal policies. And also we can see that the quarantine policy is more important than the elimination policy (note that the upper bound a for u_2 is 0.74). On the other hand, if the unit costs become expensive, we can hardly execute the prevention policies compared with our default case (the bottom figures in Figure 9: both u_1 and u_2 become smaller) and the optimal strategy becomes very complex (i.e., the optimal strategy of the elimination policy becomes non-monotonic). In particular, the effort of the quarantine policy significantly decreases because of its expensive cost. The optimal policies no longer reduce the epidemic curve and can not prevent the disease spread, even if we can execute the complex optimal control strategy. Thus, when the unit execution cost of the interventions is a serious problem, it becomes difficult to prevent the disease spread.

4. CONCLUSION

General theory of evolution postulates that the trend of evolution is to increase the fitness of an evolving species. That is, in the case of the evolution of virulence, the trend is to increase the basic reproduction number of the evolving virus [1, 42, 47]. From the perspective of maximization of $\overline{R}_0$, the mutation should lead to a lower virulence if there is no functional relationship between the virulence and the transmission rate. However, if there is some functional relationship between the virulence and the transmission rate, then the higher virulence of the mutant strain optimizes the basic reproduction number [1, 47]. Moreover, for the models that include further complications, such as superinfection and vertical transmission, the mutant virus with a higher virulence is selected [32, 35]. It is noteworthy that there is some experimental evidence supporting the possibility of the mutation to a strain with a higher virulence [9, 39]. Further, it is reported that the virulence of the virus circulating in South Asia gradually increases [9]. Thus, the expected virulence of mutant avian influenza is uncertain.

We found that the evolutionary trend of the virulence significantly influences the efficacy of the time-independent prevention policies because the effective policy depends on the trend (Figures 2 and 3). Based on equilibrium analysis, we confirmed that each of the prevention policies could be ineffective for human morbidity (see Figure 2) and for human mortality (see Figure 3). Further, interestingly, the same intervention might, under the same conditions, increase human morbidity and decrease human mortality, or vice versa (Figures 2 and 3). These results are caused by a competition between the wild strain (infected birds with the wild strain Y) and the mutant strain (infected humans with the mutant strain H) for susceptible humans. Our practical findings are that quarantine policy can decrease both human morbidity and mortality but elimination policy increases either human morbidity or mortality at the equilibria in the worst situation. Also, by considering the effect of recovery from mutant avian influenza infection (Figure 5), we showed that our conclusions about the efficacy of prevention policies on human morbidity and mortality are reasonable if the recovery rates of infected humans δ_1 and δ_2 are sufficiently small compared with the virulences d_1 and d_2. In particular, the recovery rate from infection of the mutant strain (δ_2) seems to be significantly important because the recovery rate from infection of the wild strain is almost negligible ($\delta_1 \approx 0$) [30, 71].

In addition to clarifying the effectiveness and risk of the prevention policies, we investigated the impact of their execution costs. When the unit execution costs are relatively low, the optimal time-dependent prevention policies can dramatically reduce the epidemic curves (the top figures of Figures 6, 7, 8). On the other hand, when the unit costs become expensive, the disease spread cannot be prevented even if the complex prevention policies can be executed (Figure 9). Thus, the execution cost seems significantly to affect the optimal control strategy and the prevention of disease spread. We found that decreasing the unit execution cost promotes the effort of the prevention policies (the bottom figures of Figure 8) and efficiently suppresses the disease spread.

Further, in the context of considering time-dependent prevention policies with the execution costs, we showed that the quarantine policy seems to be very important rather than the elimination policy during the disease spread, even if the unit execution cost of the quarantine policy is more expensive than that of the elimination policy in both virulence cases (the bottom figures in Figures 6, 7, 8). This result is partially different from our conclusions obtained at the final phase of the disease spread in Figure 2 (because we concluded that the quarantine policy might increase the total number of infected humans at the equilibrium in the higher virulence cases). Although for the elimination policy we can see the same tendency of previous results (in particular, at the beginning) about the optimal prevention policies (i.e., the effort of the elimination policy is relatively large in the higher virulence case), in general the quarantine policy is more important than the elimination policy in order to maximize the effect of prevention policies even in the higher virulence case. Further, as the unit execution cost of the quarantine policy decreases, we can expect that the effort of the quarantine policy increases and the optimal prevention policies efficiently reduce the total number of infected humans during the disease spread (numerical simulations are not shown). In order to succeed in prevention, the unit execution cost of the quarantine policy should be reduced.

The WHO recommends that all countries undertake urgent action to prepare for a pandemic influenza. Some of the world's most skilled mathematical modelers have turned their attention to pandemic influenza [17, 18, 37, 51, 58]. These models allow us to study the impact of particular interventions, including vaccines, antivirals, and social distancing and to understand the expectations for the magnitude and spread of the disease [5]. We pointed out potential risks of two major interventions (i.e., elimination of birds and quarantine of humans) related to the virulence evolution of avian influenza by model (1). To determine the effective interventions, monitoring the virulence of pandemic strain is an important factor. In addition to development of effective interventions, we have to know the impacts of execution cost of prevention policies. If the execution cost of the interventions is expensive in developing countries or poor areas, the interventions might not attain effective levels to contain the disease spread. Epidemiological models, including economic aspects, would help decision makers in their choice of the best strategy to implement according to the specific socioeconomic context of the country/area [49]. We investigated the impact of the unit execution cost of the two major interventions by model (2). To achieve the execution of effective interventions, cooperating with local communities, public health authorities, media, and the government to reduce the unit execution cost are required. Because the region most likely to be the source of a new pandemic might be a developing country, international support for executing the interventions in developing countries is most important in stopping the pandemic and the worldwide spread of the disease.

REFERENCES

[1]   R. M. Anderson and R. M. May (1991) Infectious disease of humans: dynamics and control, *Oxford University Press*.

[2]   R. Antia, R. R. Regoes, J. C. Koella, and C. T. Bergstrom (2003) The role of evolution in the emergence of infectious diseases, *Nature*, 426, 658-661.

[3]   S. Bonhoeffer and M. A. Nowak (1994) Mutation and the evolution of virulence, *Proc. R. Soc. Lond B*, 258, 133-140.

[4]   J. J. Bull, L. A. Meyers, and M. Lachmann (2005) Quasispecies made simple, *PLoS Comp. Biol.*, 1(6), e61.

[5]   J. D. Campbell (2007) Pandemic flu vaccine: are we doing enough?, *Nature*, 82, 633-635.

[6]   Centers for Disease Control and Prevention (2005) Transmission of influenza A viruses between animals and people, http://www.cdc.gov/flu/avian/gen-info/pdf/spread.pdf, October 17.

[7]   Centers for Disease Control and Prevention (2006) Key facts about avian influenza (bird flu) and avian influenza A (H5N1) virus, http://www.cdc. gov/flu/avian/gen-info/pdf/avianfacts.pdf, June 30.

[8]   Council of the European Communities (1992) Community measures for the control of avian influenza, *Off. J. Eur. Commiss.*, 167, 1-15.

[9]   H. Chen, G. Deng, Z. Li, G. Tian, Y. Li, P. Jiao, L. Zhang, Z. Liu, R. G. Webster, and K. Yu (2004) The evolution of H5N1 influenza viruses in ducks in southern China, *Proc. Nant. Acad. Sci. U.S.A.*, 101, 10452-10457.

[10]   H. Chen, G. L. Smith, K. S. Li, J. Wang, X. H. Fan, J. M. Rayner, D. Vijaykrishna, J. X. Zhang, L. J. Zhang, C. T. Guo, C. L. Cheung, K. M. Xu, L. Duan, K. Huang, K. Qin, Y. H. Leung, W. L. Wu, H. R. Lu, Y. Chen, N. S. Xia, T. S. Naipospos, K. Y. Yuen, S. S. Hassan, S. Bahri, T. D. Nguyen, R. G. Webster, J. S. Peiris, and Y. Guan (2006) Establishment of multiple sublineages of H5N1 influenza virus in Asia: implications for pandemic control, *Proc. Nant. Acad. Sci. U.S.A.*, 103, 2845-2850.

[11] G. Chowell, C. E. Ammon, N. W. Hengartner, and J. M. Hyman (2006) Transmission dynamics of the great influenza pandemic of 1918 in Geneva, Switzerland: Assessing the effects of hypothetical interventions, *J. Theor. Biol.*, 241, 193-204.

[12] G. Chowell and H. Nishiura (2008) Quantifying the transmission potential of pandemic influenza, *Phy. Life Rev.*, 5, 50-77.

[13] V. Colizza, A. Barrat, M. Barthelemy, A.-J. Valleron, and A. Vespignani (2007) Modeling the worldwide spread of pandemic influenza: baseline case and containment interventions, *PLoS Med.*, 4(1), e13.

[14] A. R. Elbers, T. H. Fabri, T. S. de Vries, J. J. de Wit, A. Pijpers, and G. Koch (2004) The highly pathogenic avian influenza A (H7N7) virus epidemic in The Netherlands in 2003 - lessons learned from the first five outbreaks, *Avian Dis.*, 48, 691-705.

[15] A. R. Elbers, G. Koch, and A. Bouma (2005) Performance of clinical signs in poultry for the detection of outbreaks during the avian influenza A (H7N7) epidemic in The Netherlands in 2003, *Avian Pathol.*, 34, 181-187.

[16] N. M. Ferguson, A. P. Galvani, and R. M. Bush (2003) Ecological and immunological determinants of influenza evolution, *Nature*, 422, 428-433.

[17] N. M. Ferguson, D. A. T. Cummings, S. Cauchemez, C. Fraser, S. Riley, A. Meeyai, S. Iamsirithaworn, and D. S. Burke (2005) Strategies for containing an emerging influenza pandemic in Southeast Asia, *Nature*, 437, 209-214.

[18] N. M. Ferguson, D. A. T. Cummings, C. Fraser, J. C. Cajka, P. C. Cooley, and D. S. Burke (2006) Strategies for mitigating an influenza pandemic, *Nature*, 442, 448-452.

[19] A. Gambotto, S. M Barratt-Boyes, M. D de Jong, G. Neumann, and Y. Kawaoka (2008) Human infection with highly pathogenic H5N1 influenza virus, *Lancet*, 371, 1464-1475.

[20] W. W. Gibbs and C. Soares (2005) Preparing for a pandemic, *Sci. Amer.*, November

[21] M. Gilbert, X. Xiao, J. Domenech, J. Lubroth, V. Martin, and J. Slingenbergh (2006) Anatidae migration in the Western Palearctic and spread of highly pathogenic avian influenza H5N1 virus, *Emer. Infec. Dise.*, 12, 1650-1656.

[22] F. G. Hayden (2001) Perspectives on antiviral use during pandemic influenza, *Phil. Trans. R. Soc. Lond. B*, 356, 1877-1884.

[23] W. Hogg, D. Gray, P. Huston, and W. Zhang (2007) The costs of preventing the spread of respiratory infection in family physician offices: a threshold analysis, *BMC Health Serv. Res.*, 7, 181.

[24] S. Iwami, Y. Takeuchi, and X. Liu (2007) Avian-human influenza epidemic model, *Math. Bios.*, 207, 1-25.

[25] S. Iwami, Y. Takeuchi, A. Korobeinikov, and X. Liu (2008) Prevention of avian influenza epidemic: what policy should we choose?, *J. Theor. Biol.*, 252, 732-741.

[26] S. Iwami, Y. Takeuchi, and X. Liu, Avian flu pandemic: can we prevent it?, *J. Theor. Biol.*, In Press.

[27] E. Jung, S. Iwami, Y. Takeuchi, and T-C. Jo, Optimal control strategy for prevention of avian influenza pandemic, In Review.

[28] M. I. Kamien and N. L. Schwarz (1991) Dynamic optimization: the calculus of variations and optimal control, *North Holland*, Amsterdam.

[29] K. Koelle, S. Cobey, B. Grenfell, and M. Pascual (2006) Epochal evolution shapes the phylodynamics of interpandemic influenza A (H3N2) in humans, *Science*, 314, 1898-1903.

[30] T. T. Lam, C. C. Hon, O. G. Pybus, S. L. Kosakovsky Pond, R. T. Wong, C. W. Yip, F. Zeng, and F. C. Leung (2007) Evolutionary and transmission dynamics of reassortant H5N1 influenza virus in Indonesia, *PLoS Pathog.*, 4(8), e1000130.

[31] P. Y. Lam (2008) Avian Influenza and Pandemic Influenza Preparedness in Hong Kong, *Ann. Acad. Med. Singapore*, 37, 489-496.

[32] S. A. Levin and D. Pimentel (1981) Selection of intermediate rates increase in parasite-host system, *Amer. Nat.*, 117, 308-315.

[33] K. S. Li, Y. Guan, J. Wang1, G. J. D. Smith, K. M. Xu, L. Duan, A. P. Rahardjo, P. Puthavathana, C. Buranathai, T. D. Nguyen, A. T. S. Estoepangestie, A. Chaisingh, P. Auewarakul, H. T. Long, N. T. H. Hanh, R. J. Webby, L. L. M. Poon, H. Chen, K. F. Shortridge, K. Y. Yuen, R. G. Webster, and J. S. M. Peiris (2004) Genesis of a highly pathogenic and potentially pandemic H5N1 influenza virus in eastern Asia, *Nature*, 430, 209-213.

[34] N. T. Liem, World Health Organization International Avian Influenza Investigation Team, Vietnam and W. Lim (2005) Lack of H5N1 avian influenza transmission to hospital employees, Hanoi, 2004 *Emer. Infec. Dise.*, 1, 210-215.

[35] M. Lipsitch and M. A. Nowak (1995) The evolution of virulence in sexually transmitted HIV/AIDS, *J. Theor. Biol.*, 174, 427-440.

[36] M. Lipsitch, T. Cohen, B. Cooper, J. M. Robins, S. Ma, L. James, G. Gopalakrishna, S. Chew, C. C. Tan, M. H. Samore, D. Fisman, and M. Murray (2003) Transmission dynamics and control of severe acute respiratory syndrome, *Science*, 300, 1966-1970.

[37] M. Lipsitch, T. Cohen, M Murray, and B. R. Levin (2007) Antiviral resistance and the control of pandemic influenza, *PLoS Med.* 4(1), e15.

[38] I. M. Longini Jr., A. Nizam, S. Xu, K. Ungchusak, W. Hanshaoworakul, D. A. T. Cummings, and M. E. Halloran (2005) Containing Pandemic Influenza at the Source, *Scince*, 309, 1083-1087.

[39] T. R. Maines, X. H. Lu, S. M. Erb, L. Edwards, J. Guarner, P. W. Greer, D. C. Nguyen, K. J. Szretter, L. M. Chen, P. Thawatsupha, M. Chittaganpitch, S. Waicharoen, D. T. Nguyen, T. Nguyen, H. H. Nguyen, J. H. Kim, L. T. Hoang, C. Kang, L. S. Phuong, W. Lim, S. Zaki, R. O. Donis, N. J. Cox, J. M. Katz, and T. M. Tumpey (2005) Avian Influenza (H5N1) viruses isolated from humans in Asia in 2004 exhibit increased virulence in mammals, *J. Virol.*, 79, 11788-11800.

[40] S. Marangon, M. Cecchinato, and I. Capua (2008) Use of vaccination in avian influenza control and eradication, *Zoo. Pub. Health*, 55, 65-72.

[41] J. D. Mathews, C. T. McCaw, J. McVernon, E. S. McBryde, and J. M. McCaw (2007) A biological model for influenza transmission: pandemic planning implications of asymptomatic infection and immunity, *PLoS ONE*, 2(11), e1220.

[42] R. M. May and R. M. Anderson (1983) Epidemiology and genetics in the coevolution of parasites and hosts, *Proc. R. Soc. Lond B*, 219, 281-313.

[43] A. McLeod, J. Rushton, A. Riviere-Cinnamond, B. Brandenburg, J. Hinrichs and L. Loth (2007) Economic issues in vaccination against highly pathogenic avian influenza in developing countries, *Dev. Biol. (Basel)*, 130, 63-72.

[44] A. L. Menach, E. Vergu, R. F. Grais, D. L. Smith, and A. Flahault (2006) Key strategies for reducing spread of avian influenza among commercial poultry holdings: lessons for transmission to humans, *Proc. R. Soc. Lond B*, 273, 2467-2475.

[45] C. E. Mills, J. M. Robins, and M. Lipsitch (2004) Transmissibility of 1918 pandemic influenza, *Nature*, 432, 904-906.

[46] D. Normile (2006) Avian influenza. WHO proposes plan to stop pandemic in its tracks, *Science*, 311, 315-316.

[47] M. A. Nowak (2006), Evolutionary dynamics, *Harvard University Press*.

[48] The New York Times (2006) In the Nile delta, bird flu preys on ignorance and poverty, April 13.

[49] M. Peyre, G. Fusheng, S. Desvaux, and F. Roger (2008) Avian influenza vaccines: a practical review in relation to their application in the field with a focus on the Asian experience, *Epidemiol. Infect.*, 14, 1-21.

[50] G. A. Poland, R. M. Jacobson, and P. V. Targonski (2007) Avian and pandemic influenza: an overview, *Vaccine*, 25, 3057-3061.

[51] R. R. Regoes and S. Bonhoeffer (2006) Emergence of drug-resistant influenza virus: population dynamical considerations, *Nature*, 312, 389-391.

[52] J. Rushton, R. Viscarra, E. Guerne Bleich and A. McLeod (2005) Impact of avian influenza outbreaks in the poultry sectors of five South East Asian countries (Cambodia Indonesia Lao PDR Thailand Viet Nam) outbreak costs responses and potential long term control, *World's Poultry Science Journal*, 61, 491-514.

[53] B. Sander, A. Nizam, L. P. Garrison, M. J. Postma, M. E. Halloran, and I. M. Longini (2008) Economic evaluation of influenza pandemic mitigation strategies in the United States using a stochastic microsimulation transmission model, *Value. Health*, Jul. 30.

[54] S. Sethi and G. L. Thompson (2000) Optimal control theory: applications to management science and economics. *Kluwer Academic*, Boston.

[55] N. Skeik and F. I. Jabr (2008) Influenza viruses and the evolution of avian influenza virus H5N1, *Int. J. Infec. Dise.*, 12, 233-238.

[56] G. J. D. Smith, X. H. Fan, J. Wang, K. S. Li, K. Qin, J. X. Zhang, D. Vijaykrishna, C. L. Cheung, K. Huang, J. M. Rayner, J. S. M. Peiris, H. Chen, R. G. Webster, and Y. Guan (2006) Emergence and predominance of an H5N1 influenza variant in China, *Proc. Nant. Acad. Sci. U.S.A.*, 103, 16936-16941.

[57] A. Stegeman, A. Bouma, A. R. W. Elbers, M. C. M. de Jong, G. Nodelijk, F. de Klerk, G. Koch, and M. J. van Boven (2004) Avian influenza A virus (H7N7) epidemic in The Netherlands in 2003: course of the epidemic and effectiveness of control measures, *J. Infect. Dis.*, 190, 2088-2095.

[58] N. I. Stilianakis, A. S. Perelson, and F. G. Hayden (1998) Emergence of drug resistance during an influenza epidemic: insights from a mathematical model, *J. Infec. Dis.*, 177, 863-873.

[59] J. K. Taubenberger, A. H. Reid, and T. G. Fanning (2005) Capturing a killer flu virus, *Sci. Amer.*, January.

[60] J. K. Taubenberger, and D. M. Morens (2006) 1918 Influenza: the mother of all pandemics, *Emer. Infec. Dis.*, 12, 15-22.

[61] T. Tiensin, P. Chaitaweesub, T. Songserm, A. Chaisingh, W. Hoonsuwan, C. Buranathai, T. Parakamawongsa, S. Premashthira, A. Amonsin, M. Gilbert, M. Nielen, and A. Stegeman (2005) Highly pathogenic avian influenza H5N1, Thailand, 2004, *Emerg. Infect. Dis.*, 11, 1664-1672.

[62] T. Tiensin, M. Nielen, H. Vernooij, T. Songserm, W. Kalpravidh, S. Chotiprasatintara, A. Chaisingh, S. Wongkasemjit, K. Chanachai, W. Thanapongtham, T. Srisuvan, and

A. Stegeman (2007) Transmission of the highly pathogenic avian influenza virus H5N1 within flocks during the 2004 epidemic in Thailand, *J. Infec. Dis.*, 196, 1679-1684.

[63] K. Ungchusak, P. Auewarakul, S. F. Dowell, R. Kitphati, W. Auwanit, P. Puthavathana, M. Uiprasertkul, K. Boonnak, C. Pittayawonganon, N. J. Cox, S. R. Zaki, P. Thawat-supha, M. Chittaganpitch, R. Khontong, J. M. Simmerman, and S. Chunsutthiwat (2005) Probable person-to-person transmission of avian influenza A (H5N1), *N. Engl. J. Med.*, 352, 333-340.

[64] United States Environmental Protection Agency (2007) Disposal of domestic birds infected by avian influenza-an overview of considerations and options, http://www.epa.gov/epaoswer/homeland/flu.pdf, July 8.

[65] D. Vijaykrishna, J. Bahl, S. Riley, L. Duan, J. X. Zhang, H. Chen, J. S. Peiris, G. J. Smith, and Y. Guan (2008) Evolutionary dynamics and emergence of panzootic H5N1 influenza viruses, *PLoS Pathog.*, 4(9), e1000161.

[66] R. Webby, E. Hoffmann, and R. G. Webster (2004) Molecular constraints to interspecies transmission of viral pathogens, *Nat. Med.*, 10, S77-S81.

[67] R. G. Webster, M. Peiris, H. Chen, and Y. Guan (2006) H5N1 Outbreaks and enzootic influenza, *Emer. Infec. Dise.*, 12, 3-8.

[68] L. F. White and M. Pagano (2008) Transmissibility of the influenza virus in the 1918 pandemic, *PLoS ONE*, 3(1), e1498.

[69] The World Health Organization (2005) Responding to the avian influenza pandemic threat, http://www.who.int/csr/resources/publications/influenza/WHOCDSCSRGIP058-EN.pdf, August.

[70] The World Health Organization (2005) Global influenza preparedness plan, http://www.who.int/csr/resources/publications/influenza/WHOCDSCSRGIP20055.pdf.

[71] The Writing Committee of the World Health Organization (WHO) Consultation on Human Influenza A/H5 (2006) Avian influenza A (H5N1) infection in humans, *N. Engl. J. Med.*, 353, 1374-1385.

[72] The World Health Organization (2008) Cumulative Number of Confirmed Human Cases of Avian Influenza A/(H5N1) Reported to WHO, http://www.who.int/csr/disease/avianinfluenza/country/casestable20080910/en/index.html, September.

[73] K. S. Yee, T. E. Carpenter, and C. J. Cardona (2008) Epidemiology of H5N1 avian influenza, *Comp. Immun. Microbiol. Infect. Dis.*, In Press.

In: Global View of Fight against Influenza
Editor: Petar M. Mitrasinovic

ISBN: 978-1-60741-952-5
© 2009 Nova Science Publishers, Inc.

Chapter 18

THE IMPACT OF AN EMERGING AVIAN INFLUENZA VIRUS (H5N1) IN A SEABIRD COLONY

Suzanne M. O'Regan[1], Thomas C. Kelly[2], Andrei Korobeinikov[3], Michael J. A. O'Callaghan[1] and Alexei V. Pokrovskii[1]

[1]Department of Applied Mathematics, Aras na Laoi,
University College Cork, Ireland
[2]Department of Zoology, Ecology and Plant Science,
Distillery Fields, North Mall, University College Cork, Ireland
[3]MACSI, Department of Mathematics and Statistics,
University of Limerick, Limerick, Ireland

ABSTRACT

Emerging and re-emerging pathogens pose a significant threat to the health status of man, of domestic animals and of wildlife. Therefore, it is important to know how such pathogens spread in immunologically naive host populations. In this Chapter, we study mathematical models for the long-term dynamics of an emerging pathogen H5N1 in a mixed population of marine birds. Seabirds are highly colonial and form densely-packed colonies containing thousands of individuals. A SEIR (Susceptible-Exposed-Infected-Recovered) model is developed that incorporates the population biology of seabirds and the H5N1 virus. By employing the theory of integral manifolds, it was possible to reduce the SEIR model to a simpler system of two differential equations based exclusively on the infected and recovered populations; this is termed the IR model. The SEIR and IR models are shown to agree closely. Moreover, by employing Lyapunov's direct method, it has been proved that the equilibria of the SEIR and IR models are globally asymptotically stable in the positive quadrant. The effect of seasonality is also investigated by considering a seasonally perturbed variant of the IR model. This system exhibits complex dynamics as the amplitude of the seasonal perturbation term is increased. A rigorous proof of the existence of chaos in the seasonally perturbed IR system is established, using methods from topological degree theory and split-hyperbolicity. To our knowledge, this is the first time that this method has been used to prove the existence of chaos in an epidemiological model.

Key words: avian influenza, mathematical model, emerging pathogen, global properties, chaos, seabird colonies

AMS Subject Classification: 92D30, 34D20.

1. INTRODUCTION

Emerging infectious diseases (EIDs) continue to pose a major threat to man, agriculture and wildlife populations [32, 37]. Mathematical modelling is a powerful technique that can be employed to describe the dynamics of infectious disease. In addition, it may be deployed to devise mitigating measures to combat the negative impacts of spreading invading pathogens. Epidemiological modelling, for example, was instrumental in containing the spread of the Foot and Mouth virus in Britain in 2001, and led to its eventual elimination [10, 18, 36]. H5NI is one of a number of zoonotic emerging infectious diseases that threaten the world's public health systems. Avian influenza, or "bird flu", is a zoonotic micropathogen that belongs to the A group of influenza viruses. Several major pandemics involving this type of virus have occurred in recent human history, the most serious being the so-called Spanish flu (H1N1) which became epidemic in 1918 and, over a period of less than one year, is believed to have killed approximately 40 million people [61].

An outbreak of the novel and highly pathogenic avian influenza strain H5N1 was first detected in Hong Kong in 1997 where 18 people became infected, with six fatalities [30]. However, by 2003, this virus was known to be widely established among domestic poultry in Southeast Asia [8]. Moreover, international concern has been raised about the risk of a new global influenza pandemic following outbreaks of the disease in humans in several countries in Asia, Africa and Europe. Wild bird mortality has also been detected. More than 1,500 migratory waterbirds—mainly bar headed geese, *Anser indicus*—were found to have died from being infected with the H5N1 strain of avian influenza at Qinghai Lake in western China in April and May 2005 [8]. Such mass die-offs, caused by a recently emerged virulent and zoonotic strain of the influenza virus, are alarming and emphasise the need for a strategy to curtail, or halt, the spread of the disease [33].

The goal of this Chapter is to model the introduction and spread of the H5N1 virus in a seabird colony. Colonial animals, generally, and marine birds in particular, are at risk from both micro- and macro-pathogens [7, 32, 49, 65]. Outbreaks of disease among colonial-nesting bird populations are known to have a marked effect upon their survival [51, 59]. Seabirds, such as the Northern Gannet (*Morus bassanus*) and Guillemot (*Uria aalge*), have unusual life histories in that they have exceptionally low reproductive output, deferred breeding and long life expectancy. In addition, they form large colonies that may contain thousands, and sometimes, millions of birds [12] on inaccessible mainland cliffs and offshore islands. Nests are often in close proximity to each other and it is interesting that, despite the apparently ideal conditions for the direct transmission of micropathogens, epidemics involving the mass mortalities of seabirds are rarely reported.

2. SEIR MODEL

2.1. Modelling Assumptions

The Kermack and McKendrick model [38], widely used in analysing the spread of infectious disease, involves dividing a population into the following disjoint classes: those susceptible to the infection, those infected and those recovered from the disease. The resulting Susceptible-Infected-Recovered (SIR) model, which leads to a set of ordinary differential equations, has been used successfully in modelling the spread of infections such as Foot and Mouth disease [18], Severe Acute Respiratory Syndrome (SARS) [46] and West Nile virus [66].

In constructing our model to investigate the effect of the H5N1 influenza virus on an isolated seabird colony, we divide the total population $N = N(t)$, at time t years, into four disjoint subclasses - those above - susceptible $S(t)$, infectious $I(t)$, and recovered $R(t)$ - with the addition of a latently infected class, $E(t)$, comprising those birds already infected with the virus but not yet infectious. We assume that the size of a colony is constrained by the available nesting space and we assume that this available space is constant. Thus, we assume that the total population, N, remains constant, i.e., at any time t the equality

$$S(t) + E(t) + I(t) + R(t) = N \qquad (1)$$

holds.

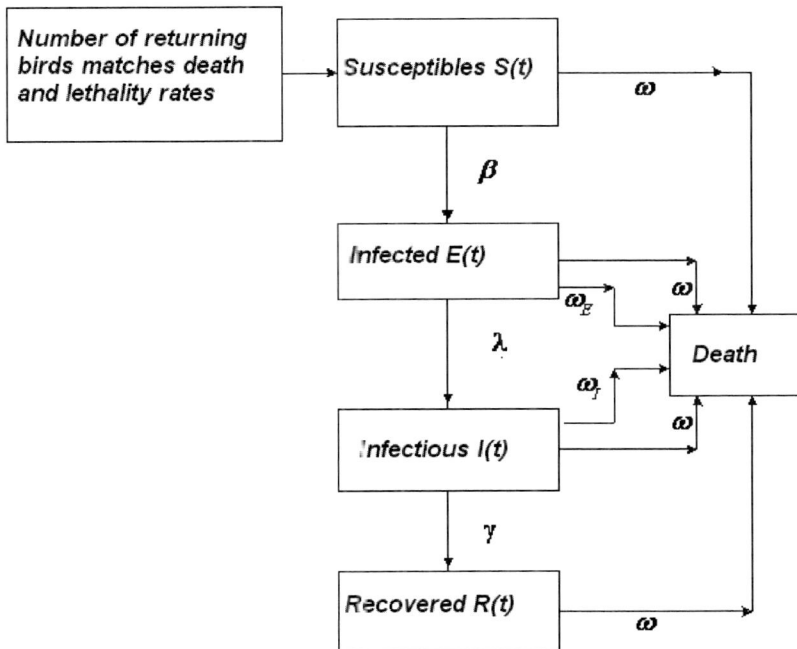

Figure 1. The transfer diagram for the SEIR model describing the introduction of H5N1 into an adult seabird population.

The flow chart in Figure 1 represents a summary of our model. The more obvious parameters in the diagram are ω, the natural death rate, and ω_E and ω_I, the death rates due to the lethality of the disease in the E and I classes respectively. These parameters are assumed to be constant in time and in space. We further assume that the members of the latently infected E class become infectious at a constant rate λ. The time from the instant of infection to the beginning of the state of infectiousness is the latent period and thus has value $1/\lambda$ years. The birds recover at a constant rate γ.

Susceptible individuals become infected through disease transmission. To model this for a directly transmitted pathogen, such as avian influenza H5N1, note first that there has to be contact between susceptible and infected individuals. Furthermore, we assume frequency-dependent (or mass-action) transmission in which the number of contacts between susceptibles (S) and infectives (I) is independent of relevant population size. The transmission term then takes the simple form βSI where we further assume that the (constant) β is positive. This transmission parameter combines many epidemiological, environmental and social factors and cannot be measured directly.

A key assumption in this model is that the recruitment rate of the susceptibles is equal to the number of the vacant nesting spots; that is, the recruitment of the new susceptibles balances the number of seabird deaths in the colony. For example, when a guillemot chick is born, it remains in the colony for about 22 days before leaving the colony. These chicks then return to the colony as adults after 4-5 years to breed [11]. We assume that all of these birds return as susceptibles. However, since the colony is densely inhabited and space is scarce, these birds must wait for an appropriate nesting site. We make the assumption that when a bird in the colony dies, a bird in the "queue" will immediately take the space vacated by the dead bird. Hence, $S(t)$ is maintained by a return rate which matches the total number of adults dying, both naturally, and as a result of the disease.

We focus only on the adult seabird population. The colony is mainly comprised of breeding adults because chicks leave the colony and non-breeders (that is, the birds aged 2-4 years) tend to occupy exposed rocks at the edge of the colony [11]. Clancy et al. [9] formulated two SEIR models which described the dynamics of the adult and chick populations respectively. Numerical experiments have indicated that the chicks have negligible impact on the overall dynamics of the disease in the colony. In addition, concentrating on the adult population alone enables us to analyse the long-term dynamics of the disease.

Therefore, for $t \geq 0$, the system can be described by the following set of ordinary differential equations, which are readily derived from an examination of Figure 1:

$$\dot{S} = \omega(S + E + I + R) + \omega_E E + \omega_I I - \beta SI - \omega S,$$

$$\dot{E} = \beta SI - (\lambda + \omega + \omega_E)E, \qquad (2)$$

$$\dot{I} = \lambda E - (\gamma + \omega + \omega_I)I,$$

$$\dot{R} = \gamma I - \omega R.$$

Here a dot denotes the time derivative (i.e., $\dot{S} \equiv \dfrac{dS}{dt}$, etc.). This system must satisfy the additional restriction

$$S(t) + E(t) + I(t) + R(t) = S(0) + E(0) + I(0) + R(0) = N. \tag{3}$$

2.2. The Basic Reproduction Number

One of the most important concepts in epidemiological modelling is the so-called *basic reproduction number*, R_0, of a pathogen. The basic reproduction number of a pathogen is defined to be the average number of secondary cases arising from a primary case in an entirely susceptible population. Clearly, when $R_0 < 1$, each infected individual produces, on average, less than one infected individual, and hence one can expect that the infection will eventually be no longer sustained within the population. If $R_0 > 1$, however, we can expect that the virus will establish itself and remain in the population. There is no definitive method for calculating the basic reproduction number. Heffernan, Smith and Wahl [27] give a comprehensive overview of the various methods used to calculate R_0. We assume that the host population is *homogeneously mixed*, i.e., epidemiological properties (e.g., genetic make-up) are intrinsically similar in the host population. The following formula, suggested by Anderson and May [3], is used in this paper to calculate R_0

$$R_0 = N/S_*, \tag{4}$$

where S_* is the susceptible population at the unique positive equilibrium state $Q_* = (S_*, E_*, I_*, R_*)$. It is easy to see that for system (2) this definition leads to

$$R_0 = \frac{\beta \lambda N}{ab}, \tag{5}$$

where $a = \lambda + \omega + \omega_E$ and $b = \gamma + \omega + \omega_I$.

2.3. Parameter Values

Numerical values for each of the parameters in system (2) were required to perform numerical simulations of the system.

Colonies of seabirds tend to be quite large; for example, there are more than 13,000 pairs of the Northern Gannet on Stac Lee, a small 180m high sea rock at St Kilda, Western Isles off the coast of Scotland   [64]. With this information, we conservatively chose the bird population N to be 10,000.

Seabirds are known to have long lifespan and high survival rates. Sandvik et al. [57] show that the annual survival rates for the Common Guillemot in an island colony in Norway is over 90%. Wanless *et al.* [63] give a similar rate for the annet. Thus, let $\omega = 0.1$.

Gani et al. [20] take the latent period to be 2 days and the infectious period to be 4 days in their model of an influenza pandemic. Tiensin *et al.* [62] cite a latent period of 1-2 days and an infectious period of 2-6 days. Here, we assume that the latent period to be 2 days, i.e., $\lambda = 365/2$, and the infectious period to be 4 days giving $\gamma = 365/4$.

It is difficult to quantify the rate of lethality induced by the H5N1 strain. Clancy *et al.* [9] varied the lethality parameters ω_E and ω_I in their model of the dynamics of the H5N1 virus in an isolated seabird colony to study their influence. They found that these lethality parameters governed the length of time between the outbreaks of the disease—the higher the lethality, the closer the occurrences. Clancy et al. [9] initially assumed that $\omega_E = 0.5$ and $\omega_I = 0.75$; these are reasonable estimates of the lethality rates. We will assume the same values here.

Finally, we require the transmission parameter β. From equation (4) we have

$$\beta = \frac{(\lambda + \omega + \omega_E)(\gamma + \omega + \omega_I)R_0}{\lambda N}. \tag{6}$$

Therefore, we can find a value for β by inputting a value for R_0. A precise value of R_0 for the H5N1 strain of avian influenza is not known. Tiensin et al. [62] estimated R_0 to be between 2.2 and 2.7 during the 2004 H5N1 avian flu epidemic among chicken flocks in Thailand. Clancy et al. [9] varied R_0 from 2 up to 10 and examined the resulting dynamics.

3. THEORETICAL ANALYSIS OF THE SEIR MODEL

3.1. General Comments

By (3), the quantity $N = N(S, E, I, R) = S + E + I + R$ is the first integral (constant of motion) of system (2). Thus, for a given value of N, system (2) is equivalent to the reduced system

$$\dot{S} = \omega N + \omega_E E + \omega_I I - \beta SI - \omega S,$$

$$\dot{E} = \beta SI - (\lambda + \omega + \omega_E)E, \tag{7}$$

$$\dot{I} = \lambda E - (\gamma + \omega + \omega_I)I,$$

satisfying

$$\mathcal{S}_0 + \mathcal{E}_0 + \mathcal{I}_0 \le N. \tag{8}$$

It is hardly surprising that the basic reproduction number R_0 of this system coincides with that of system (2) and is given by (5). For any non-negative $\mathcal{S}_0, \mathcal{E}_0, \mathcal{I}_0$, satisfying (8), system (7) has the unique non-negative solution $(S(t), E(t), I(t))$, satisfying the initial condition

$$S(0) = \mathcal{S}_0, \quad E(0) = \mathcal{E}_0, \quad I(0) = \mathcal{I}_0,$$

and it satisfies

$$S(t) + E(t) + I(t) \le N, \quad t \ge 0.$$

This solution is strictly positive, if $\mathcal{E}_0 > 0$ or $\mathcal{I}_0 > 0$.

Lemma 3.1 *If the basic reproduction number $R_0 > 1$, then system (7) has the unique strictly positive equilibrium state*

$$(S_*, E_*, I_*) = \left(\frac{ab}{\beta\lambda}, \frac{b\omega(\beta\lambda N - ab)}{\beta\lambda(ab - b\omega_E - \lambda\omega_I)}, \frac{\omega(\beta\lambda N - ab)}{\beta(ab - b\omega_E - \lambda\omega_I)} \right). \tag{9}$$

The system also always has a nonnegative equilibrium $(S_{**}, E_{**}, I_{**}) = (N, 0, 0)$. If $R_0 \le 1$, then this latter equilibrium is the only non-negative equilibrium of the system.

The proof of this is straightforward: just note that $R_0 > 1$ is equivalent to $ab < \lambda\beta N$.

Now we may formulate some further interesting propositions. System (7) is called *persistent* if any solution with strictly positive initial $E(0)$ condition is, for all $t \ge \tau > 0$, at some positive distance from the boundary [29].

Proposition 3.1
(a) The interval

$$J = \{ (S, 0, 0) : 0 \le S < N \}$$

is a trajectory of the system. The trajectory J is a local attractor for $0 \le S < S_* = N/R_0$, and it is a local repeller for $S_* < S < N$.

(b) System (7) is persistent if $R_0 > 1$ holds (i.e, if this system has strictly positive equilibrium), and it is not persistent if $R_0 \le 1$.

(c) *The positive equilibrium* (S_*, E_*, I_*), *if this exists, is exponentially asymptotically stable.*

Let us comment briefly on 3.1(a). From a mathematical point of view, it means that the trajectory J is a canard in the terminology described in [6, 15]; this canard exhibits, in particular, a delayed loss of stability [48]. From a practical point of view, we observe an apparent disappearance effect. For some time, both the number of latently infected E and infective I decrease exponentially; afterwards, we observe explosive epidemics. We emphasize that this effect is significant only when λ is reasonably small.

3.2. Proof of Proposition 3.1

The linearization matrix M for system (7) is

$$M(S, E, I) = \begin{pmatrix} -\beta I - \omega & \omega_E & \omega_I - \beta S \\ \beta I & -a & \beta S \\ 0 & \lambda & -b \end{pmatrix}. \tag{10}$$

In particular, for the interval J,

$$M(S, 0, 0) = \begin{pmatrix} -\omega & \omega_E & \omega_I - \beta S \\ 0 & -a & \beta S \\ 0 & \lambda & -b \end{pmatrix}. \tag{11}$$

This implies Proposition 3.1(a).

Clearly, the boundary of the simplex

$$\sigma(N) = \{(S, E, I) : S, E, I \geq 0, S + E + I \leq N\},$$

except for the line $(S, 0, 0)$, $0 \leq S \leq N$, is a repeller when it is approached from the interior of $\sigma(N)$. Then, by definition, the velocity of the phase flow near the attractive part of the interval J is separated from zero. It remains to consider behaviour close to the second equilibrium $(S_{**}, E_{**}, I_{**}) = (N, 0, 0)$. By definition,

$$M(N, 0, 0) = \begin{pmatrix} -\omega & \omega_E & \omega_I - \beta N \\ 0 & -a & \beta N \\ 0 & \lambda & -b \end{pmatrix}. \tag{12}$$

Consider the characteristic polynomial of this matrix,

$$P(z) = \det \begin{pmatrix} -\omega - z & \omega_E & \omega_i - \beta N \\ 0 & -a - z & \beta N \\ 0 & \lambda & -b - z \end{pmatrix} = -(\omega + z)(z^2 + (a+b)z + (ab - \beta \lambda N)).$$

This polynomial has all roots in the left hand side of the complex plane if $ab > \beta \lambda N$ (that is, when $R_0 < 1$), and it has at least one root with negative real part if $ab < \beta \lambda N$ (that is when $R_0 > 1$). In the first case, the equilibrium (S_{**}, E_{**}, I_{**}) is an attractor, and thus system (7) is not persistent. In the second case, the equilibrium (S_{**}, E_{**}, I_{**}) is a repeller, and the proof of persistence (proposition 3.1(b)) is finalized in the usual way.

Let us prove proposition 3.1(c). In this case,

$$M(x_*, y_*) = \begin{pmatrix} -\beta I_* - \omega & \omega_E & \omega_I - \beta S_* \\ \beta I_* & -a & \beta S_* \\ 0 & \lambda & -b \end{pmatrix}, \tag{13}$$

and, using the identity $\beta \lambda S_* - ab = 0$, we can write the corresponding characteristic polynomial

$$P_*(z) = \det \begin{pmatrix} -\beta I_* - z - \omega & \omega_E & \omega_I - \beta S_* \\ \beta I_* & -a - z & \beta S_* \\ 0 & \lambda & -b - z \end{pmatrix},$$

as

$$P_*(z) = z^3 + Az^2 + Bz + C,$$

where

$$A = \beta I_* + \omega + a + b,$$

$$B = b(\beta I_* + \omega) + (\lambda + \omega \beta I_* + a\omega),$$

$$C = \beta I_*(-b\omega_E - \lambda \omega_I + ab) = \beta I_*(\gamma(\lambda + \omega) + \omega(\lambda + \omega + \omega_I)).$$

Firstly, we note that

$$A > 0, \qquad B > 0, \qquad C > 0.$$

It remains to verify the inequality

$$AB - C > 0.$$

This difference may be clearly represented as

$$AB - C = \beta^2 I_*^2 [(\gamma + \lambda + 2\omega + \omega_I) + \omega(\gamma + \lambda + 2\omega + \omega_E + \omega_I)(\gamma + \lambda + 3\omega + \omega_E + \omega_I)]$$

$$+ \beta I_* [\gamma^2 + \lambda^2 + 5\lambda\omega + 7\omega^2 + \lambda\omega_E + 3\omega\omega_E + (2\lambda + 5\omega + \omega_E)\omega_I$$

$$+ \omega_I^2 + \gamma(\lambda + 5\omega + \omega_E + 2\omega_I)] > 0,$$

which completes the proof.

3.3. Global Stability of the SEIR Model for the Case $\omega_E = 0$

For the particular case $\omega_E = 0$, the direct Lyapunov method enables us to analytically establish the global asymptotic properties of the model. The assumption $\omega_E = 0$ implies that there is no disease-induced death from the exposed compartments E, and that all the disease-induced deaths are from the infectious compartment I. Such an assumption appears to be fairly well justified for a SEIR model.

Theorem 3.1 *Let* $\omega_E = 0$, *and assume that there exists a strictly positive equilibrium* Q_*. *Then the positive equilibrium state* Q_* *is globally asymptotically stable in* $\mathbb{R}_+^4$.

Proof. To establish the properties of the model (2), it suffices to consider system (7). We consider a Lyapunov function

$$V(S, E, I) = S - S_* \ln S + B(E - E_* \ln E) + C(I - I_* \ln I),$$

where $B = 1 - \omega_I / \beta S_*, C = B(\lambda + \omega)/\lambda$. The point Q_* is the only stationary point of this function and is its global minimum. This function satisfies

$$\dot{V} = \omega N + \omega_I I - \beta SI - \omega S - \omega N \frac{S_*}{S} - \omega_I I \frac{S_*}{S} + \beta S_* I + \omega S_*$$

$$+ B\left(\beta SI - (\lambda + \omega)E - \beta SI \frac{E_*}{E} + (\lambda + \omega)E_* \right)$$

$$+ C\left(\lambda E - (\gamma + \omega + \omega_I)I - \lambda E \frac{I_*}{I} + (\gamma + \omega + \omega_I)I_* \right).$$

Using the simultaneous relationships $\omega N + \omega_I I_* = \beta S_* I_* + \omega S_*$, $\beta S_* I_* = (\lambda + \omega)E_*$ and $C\lambda E_* - C(\gamma + \omega + \omega_I)I_* = B(\lambda + \omega)E_*$, we obtain

$$\dot{V} = (\omega S_* + \omega_I I)\left(2 - \frac{S}{S_*} - \frac{S_*}{S}\right)$$

$$+ B\beta I_* S_*\left(3 - \frac{SE_* I}{S_* EI_*} - \frac{EI_*}{E_* I} - \frac{S_*}{S}\right).$$

Here,

$$\frac{SE_* I}{S_* EI_*} + \frac{EI_*}{E_* I} + \frac{S_*}{S} \geq 3, \qquad \frac{S}{S_*} + \frac{S_*}{S} \geq 2$$

for all $S, E, I \geq 0$, because the arithmetic mean is greater than, or equal to the geometric mean. Therefore, $\frac{dV}{dt} \leq 0$ holds for all $S, E, I \geq 0$, provided that S_*, E_*, I_* are non-negative, where the equality $\frac{dV}{dt} = 0$ holds only on the straight line $S = S_*, I/I_* = E/E_*$. It is easy to see that, for this system, Q_* is the only equilibrium state on this line. Therefore, by the Lyapunov-La Salle asymptotic stability theorem [5, 42], the positive equilibrium state Q_* is globally asymptotically stable in the positive region R_+^3.

This completes the proof.

4. REDUCING THE SEIR MODEL TO THE IR MODEL

Recall that the latent period of an infection is the time interval from the instant of infection to the beginning of the state of infectiousness. The latent period of avian flu is short, approximately two days [20, 62], relative to the other time scales in the SEIR model (2). The latently infected population $E(t)$ become infectious at a constant rate $\lambda = 365/2$. This parameter is large relative to the other parameters in the SEIR system, and thus $1/\lambda$ is small. Hence, the latently infected population decreases at a much faster rate relative to the proportions of the susceptible, infected and recovered populations.

Clearly, system (2) is a system containing ODEs which exhibit dynamic behaviour evolving on different time scales. This makes it difficult to analyse the system both theoretically and numerically. Therefore, it is desirable to reduce system (2) to a smaller system without loss of accuracy [22]. Due to the short duration of the latent period, it is reasonable to combine the latently infected and infectious classes. The theory of integral manifolds may then be employed to analyse the resulting system. Goldfarb et al. [22] and Sobolev [58] provide comprehensive introductions to this theory.

Setting $U = E + I$, we have

$$\dot{S} = \omega(S + U + R) - \omega S + (\beta S + \omega_E - \omega_I)E + (\omega_I - \beta S)U,$$

$$\dot{E} = \beta SU - (\beta S + \lambda + \omega + \omega_E)E, \tag{14}$$

$$\dot{U} = (\beta S - \gamma - \omega_I - \omega)U - (\beta S - \gamma - \omega_I + \omega_E)E,$$

$$\dot{R} = \gamma U - \gamma E - \omega R.$$

We note that λ is the dominant parameter in the equation for the derivative of E and thus, E is decreasing rapidly. Let $1/\lambda = \varepsilon \ll 1$. Then the system may be written as:

$$\varepsilon \dot{E} = \varepsilon \beta SU - [1 + \varepsilon(\beta S + \omega + \omega_E)]E,$$

$$\dot{S} = \omega(S + U + R) - \omega S + (\beta S + \omega_E - \omega_I)E + (\omega_I - \beta S)U, \tag{15}$$

$$\dot{U} = (\beta S - \gamma - \omega_I - \omega)U - (\beta S - \gamma - \omega_I + \omega_E)E,$$

$$\dot{R} = \gamma U - \gamma E - \omega R.$$

System (15) is a singularly perturbed system of ordinary differential equations. The system of equations

$$\dot{S} = \omega(S + U + R) - \omega S + (\beta S + \omega_E - \omega_I)E + (\omega_I - \beta S)U,$$

$$\dot{U} = (\beta S - \gamma - \omega_I - \omega)U - (\beta S - \gamma - \omega_I + \omega_E)E, \tag{16}$$

$$\dot{R} = \gamma U - \gamma E - \omega R$$

represents the slow subsystem, and the equation

$$\varepsilon \dot{E} = \varepsilon \beta SU - [1 + \varepsilon(\beta S + \omega + \omega_E)]E$$

represents the fast subsystem. The theory of integral manifolds allows us to replace system (15) by another system on an integral manifold with dimension equal to that of the slow subsystem. That is, in this case, we can replace system (15) by a system of three ordinary differential equations.

The slow manifold $E = E(S,U,R,\varepsilon)$ of (15) can be found as an asymptotic expansion,

$$E = E(S,U,R,\varepsilon) = E_0(S,U,R) + \varepsilon E_1(S,U,R) + O(\varepsilon^2).$$

Noting that

$$\varepsilon \frac{dE}{dt} = \varepsilon \left[\frac{\partial E}{\partial S} \dot{S} + \frac{\partial E}{\partial U} \dot{U} + \frac{\partial E}{\partial R} \dot{R} \right],$$

and substituting the asymptotic expansion of E into the fast subsystem of (15), we obtain

$$\varepsilon \beta SU - [1 + \varepsilon(\beta S + \omega + \omega_E)](E_0 + \varepsilon E_1 + \ldots) =$$

$$\varepsilon [\frac{\partial E_0}{\partial S} \{ \omega(S + U + R) - \omega S + (\beta S + \omega_E - \omega_I)E_0 + (\omega_I - \beta S)U \} \tag{17}$$

$$+ \frac{\partial E_0}{\partial U} \{ (\beta S - \gamma - \omega_I - \omega)U - (\beta S - \gamma - \omega_I + \omega_E)E_0 \}$$

$$+ \frac{\partial E_0}{\partial R} \{ \gamma U - \gamma E_0 - \omega R \}] + O(\varepsilon^2).$$

From (17), by equating respective orders of ε, we obtain

$$\varepsilon^0 : E_0 = 0,$$
$$\varepsilon^1 : \beta SU - (\beta S + \omega + \omega_E)E_0 - E_1 = 0 \Rightarrow E_1 = \beta SU.$$

Thus, the slow integral manifold $E = E(S,U,R,\varepsilon)$ of (15) is given by

$$E = E(S,U,R,\varepsilon) = \varepsilon \beta SU + O(\varepsilon^2), \tag{18}$$

and consequently, $I = U - \varepsilon \beta SU + O(\varepsilon^2)$. Therefore, on substituting equation (18) into system (16), we have

$$\dot{S} = \omega(S + U + R) - \omega S + (\omega_I - \beta S)U + \varepsilon \beta SU(\beta S + \omega_E - \omega_I) + O(\varepsilon^2),$$

$$\dot{U} = (\beta S - \gamma - \omega_I - \omega)U - (\beta S - \gamma - \omega_I + \omega_E)\varepsilon \beta SU + O(\varepsilon^2), \tag{19}$$

$$\dot{R} = \gamma U - \omega R - \gamma \varepsilon \beta SU + O(\varepsilon^2).$$

In the limiting case, i.e., for $\varepsilon \to 0$, system (19) becomes

$$\dot{S} = \omega(S + U + R) - \omega S + (\omega_I - \beta S)U,$$

$$\dot{U} = (\beta S - \gamma - \omega_I - \omega)U,$$

$$\dot{R} = \gamma U - \omega R.$$

Since $I = U - \varepsilon\beta SU + O(\varepsilon^2)$, then in the limiting case, $I \approx U$. Thus, we may replace U with the more intuitively-clear variable I, representing the infected (and infectious) population, to obtain a Susceptible-Infected-Recovered (SIR) system,

$$\dot{S} = \omega(S + I + R) - \omega S + (\omega_I - \beta S)I,$$

$$\dot{I} = (\beta S - \gamma - \omega_I - \omega)I, \tag{20}$$

$$\dot{R} = \gamma I - \omega R.$$

Finally, since we have assumed the total population N to be constant (equation (1)), it suffices to consider a two-dimensional system, omitting one of these three equations. Usually, it is the equation for $R(t)$ which is omitted; however, the actual choice makes no difference, and here, we prefer to omit the equation for $S(t)$. Thus, we obtain the following set of differential equations, which we term the IR model:

$$\dot{I} = (\beta(N - I - R) - \gamma - \omega_I - \omega)I, \tag{21}$$

$$\dot{R} = \gamma I - \omega R.$$

We examine the convergence of the SEIR system to the IR system using the mathematical software package *Mathematica*, by increasing λ incrementally. Figure 2 indicates that the SEIR model and IR models are in close agreement. The latent period of the disease becomes shorter with increasing values of λ, and in Figure 2, the convergence of the SEIR system to the IR system becomes more pronounced as the latent period tends to zero. Figure 2 also shows that there is a significant outbreak of the disease in the first year after the pathogen is introduced into the colony. This observation agrees with the results of numerical simulations of the SEIR model conducted by Clancy et al. [9].

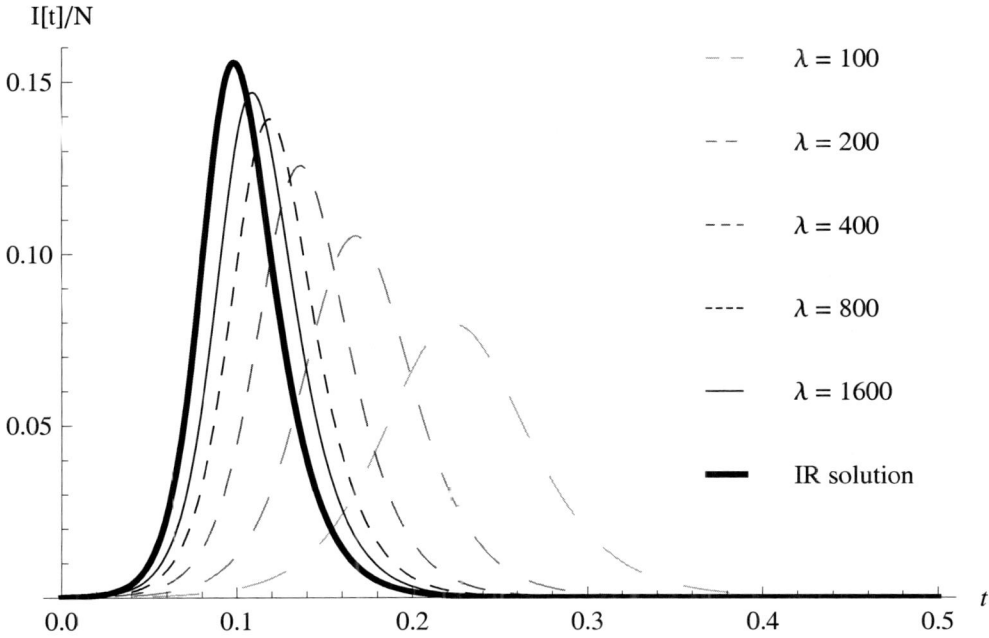

Figure 2. The fraction of the infected hosts in time: comparing solutions of the SEIR model to the IR solution for various λ values, for $t = [0,0.5]$. The convergence of the SEIR solution to the IR solution becomes more pronounced as λ grows. Parameters: $N_0 = 10000$, $R_0 = 2$, $\beta = 0.01848$, $\gamma = 365/4$, $\omega = 1/10$, $\omega_E = 1/2$, $\omega_I = 3/4$,

4.1. Analysis of the IR Model

An elegant Lyapunov function may be constructed for the IR model. Consider the rate of change of the infected population in system (21):

$$\dot{I} = \beta(N - I - R)I - (\gamma + \omega + \omega_I)I.$$

Set $p_0 = \beta N - (\gamma + \omega + \omega_I)$. Then p_0 is a positive constant and system (21) may be written as

$$\dot{I} = (p_0 - \beta I - \beta R)I, \tag{22}$$

$$\dot{R} = \gamma I - \omega R.$$

The coordinates of the positive equilibrium state of system (22) are given by

$$I_* = \frac{\omega p_0}{\beta(\gamma + \omega)}, \qquad R_* = \frac{\gamma p_0}{\beta(\gamma + \omega)}.$$

On substituting these coordinates into system (22) we obtain

$$\dot{I} = I(\beta(I_* - I) + \beta(R_* - R)),$$ (23)

$$\dot{R} = \gamma(I - I_*) - \omega(R - R_*).$$

It can be shown that the function

$$V(I, R) = I - I_* \ln I + (\beta/2\gamma)(R - R_*)^2$$ (24)

is a Lyapunov function for system (23) (see [50] for details). The derivative of function (24),

$$\dot{V}(I, R) = -(\beta/\gamma)\omega(R - R_*)^2 - \beta(I - I_*)^2,$$

is strictly negative for I, $R > 0$ and for $(I, R) \neq (I_*, R_*)$. Moreover,

$$V(I, R) \to \infty \text{ as } I \to 0, I \to \infty \text{ and } V(I, R) \to \infty \text{ as } R \to 0, R \to \infty.$$

Therefore, the equilibrium (I_*, R_*) of system (21), is globally asymptotically stable in the positive quadrant.

Numerical simulations confirm this result. It is important to investigate what will happen when a pathogen is introduced into a population in which there is no existing herd immunity. We assume that at $t = 0$, there is a single infectious bird and thus, $I(0) = 1$, and $R(0) = 0$. Then $S(0) = N - 1$ since all other birds are susceptible to the virus. Using the parameters mentioned in Section 2.3 and $R_0 = 2$ and 10, the IR system of equations was solved using *Mathematica*. Figure 3 shows solutions of the IR model, for $R_0 = 2$ (Figure 3(a)) and $R_0 = 10$ (Figure 3(b)).

As predicted by the theoretical analysis, the infectious population tends to an asymptotically stable positive equilibrium in the long-term. Thus, the disease persists in the population. Note that the numerical simulations shown in Figure 2 and 3 are scaled by a factor of $1/N$ (that is, these Figures show the infectious fractions of the population).

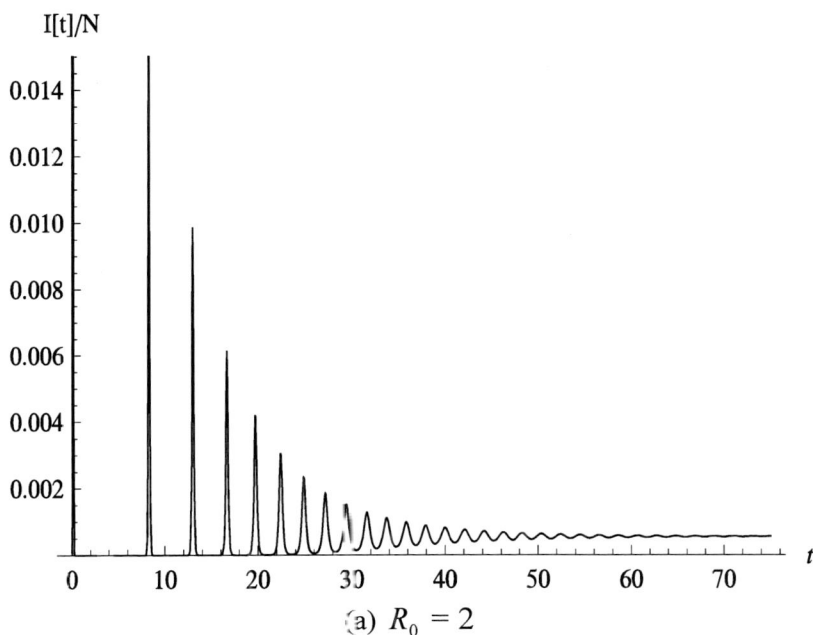

(a) $R_0 = 2$

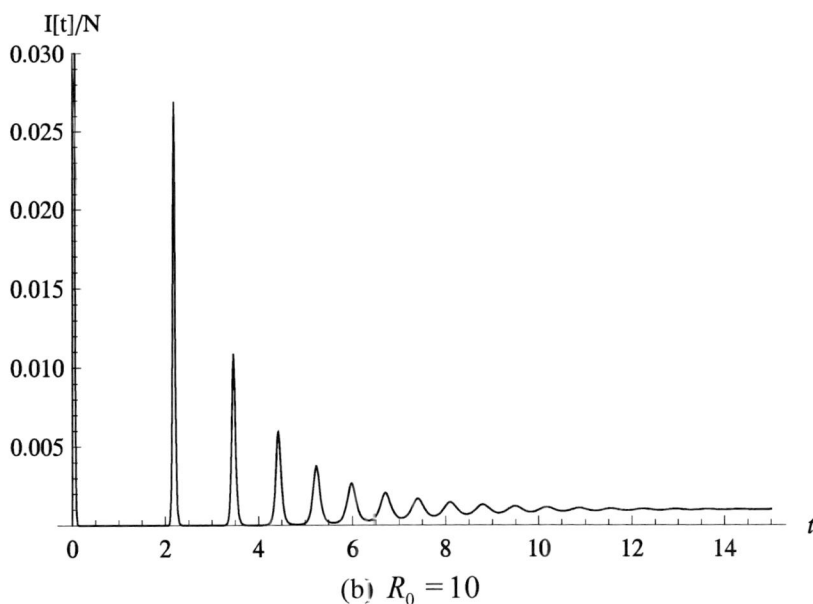

(b) $R_0 = 10$

Figure 3. The infectious fraction of the population in time for IR model. Here we use the following parameters: for (a) $N_0 = 10000$, $R_0 = 2$, $\beta = 0.01848$, $\gamma = 365/4$, $\omega = 1/10$, $\omega_E = 1/2$, $\omega_I = 3/4$, $t = [0,75]$; for (b) $R_0 = 10$, $\beta = 0.0924$, $\gamma = 365/4$, $\omega = 1/10$, $\omega_E = 1/2$, $\omega_I = 3/4$, $t = [0,15]$.

5. SEASONALLY PERTURBED MODEL

5.1. Seasonality

Wild birds, like the rest of the animal kingdom, are dependent upon, and influenced by, seasonal changes. Seasonal variations may affect a variety of processes in a seabird colony, e.g., changes in flocking and social mixing, the recruitment of susceptibles through annual pulses of births and deaths [2], and the timing of the breeding cycle [26]. Seasonality may significantly drive the dynamics of an epidemic by affecting components of the basic reproduction number R_0 [2] and the rate of transmission [23]. For these reasons, it is important to investigate the effect of seasonality on the spread of avian influenza in a seabird population.

A major source of seasonality arises from seasonal changes in social grouping of seabirds. Seabirds tend to congregate in large numbers at the beginning of the breeding season, over a short period of time [26]. A sudden onset of increased contact may increase the transmission rate of a disease [2]. Such a phenomenon has been observed in house finches, *Carpodacus mexicanus*, whereby social aggregation during the winter has coincided with changes in transmission dynamics of mycoplasmal conjunctivitis in North America [31]. In addition, the timing of the breeding cycle depends on seasonal factors such as temperature, wind and food availability. For example, some seabird species delay nesting during cold weather [26]. Nesting may also be delayed if there is not enough food available. Once the breeding season has finished, seabirds tend to disperse away from the colony. The behaviour of seabirds during the winter season is not well observed; the colony is primarily occupied during the breeding season but there may be social aggregation during the winter as well.

Seasonal changes in susceptibility to infection may be another important factor. Seasonal changes in immunity may reduce host recovery rates [2]. Environmental stresses such as physiologically challenging weather conditions are known to increase susceptibility to diseases while simultaneously decreasing the rate of reproduction in hosts [43]. Climatic extremes may affect the breeding success of seabirds [26]. Seasonal fluctuations in seabird food may also affect the dynamics of disease incidence. There is likely to be increased competition for food during the breeding season [19, 26, 44]. Such seasonal variations may considerably affect the transmission rate and the basic reproduction number of an infection. It is also important to emphasise that multiple seasonal drivers may interact in complex ways [2].

In this Section, we investigate the effect of seasonal variations on the dynamics of H5N1 avian influenza virus in a seabird colony. A seasonally forced variant of the IR model is derived and analysed in detail. Such a model may allow us to better capture a more realistic pattern of recurrent epidemics [37], in contrast to the unforced model, system (21), which, as we demonstrated earlier in this Chapter, predicts oscillations that are damped towards equilibrium.

The usual method of introducing seasonality in a SIR model is to subject it to periodical external forcing. Seasonally perturbed SIR models may induce a wide range of population dynamics, including annual oscillations, high-order cycles and chaos [4, 16, 17, 35]. Perturbing the transmission parameter β is a common method of introducing seasonality to a model [2, 4, 35, 37, 60]. In this Chapter, we assume that the seasonally perturbed quantity is the total population $N(t)$ of the colony. That is, instead of assuming the conservation law (1), we assume that

$$S(t) + E(t) + I(t) + R(t) = N(t), \qquad (25)$$

where $N(t)$ is a given (non-constant) 1-periodic function, that is, $N(t+1) = N(t)$ holds. System (2), for $t \geq 0$, takes now the form

$$\dot{S} = \omega N(t) + \omega_E E + \omega_I I - \beta SI - \omega S,$$

$$\dot{E} = \beta SI - (\lambda + \omega + \omega_E)E, \qquad (26)$$

$$\dot{I} = \lambda E - (\gamma + \omega + \omega_I)I,$$

$$\dot{R} = \gamma I - \omega R,$$

with an additional constraint, $S(0) + E(0) + I(0) + R(0) = N(0)$. This is equivalent to the three dimensional system,

$$\dot{E} = \beta(N(t) - (E + R + I))I - (\lambda + \omega + \omega_E)E, \qquad (27)$$

$$\dot{I} = \lambda E - (\gamma + \omega + \omega_I)I,$$

$$\dot{R} = \gamma I - \omega R,$$

with the constraint,

$$E(0) + I(0) + R(0) \leq N(0). \qquad (28)$$

Correspondingly, the reduced IR model (22) may be written as

$$\dot{I} = (p(t) - \beta I - \beta R)I, \qquad (29)$$

$$\dot{R} = \gamma I - \omega R.$$

Here, the parameter $p_0 = \beta N - (\gamma + \omega + \omega_I)$ in system (22) is subjected to external forcing. This parameter combines seasonal variations of the transmission parameter β, the recovery rate γ, the death rates ω, ω_I and, in particular, the population N. We assume that $p(t)$ is a given 1-periodic function and is defined by the equation

$$p(t) = p_0(1 + \varepsilon(t)), \tag{30}$$

where the constant p_0 is the mean value of the periodic function $p(t)$, and

$$|\varepsilon(t)| < p_0. \tag{31}$$

The perturbation $\varepsilon(t)$ may be any type of function; however, the seasonal forcing term is usually assumed to be a sinusoidal or step function [4, 14, 60]. System (29) will be referred to as the *Seasonally Perturbed IR Model*.

Setting $\dot{I} = 0$, we obtain

$$p(t) = \beta(1 + \varepsilon(t))I_* + \beta(1 + \varepsilon(t))R_*,$$

where (I_*, R_*) is the positive equilibrium state of system (21) and for $\dot{R} = 0$, we have $\gamma I_* - \omega R_* = 0$. Consequently, we may rewrite the seasonally perturbed IR model in the following way:

$$\dot{I} = I\{\beta[(1 + \varepsilon(t))I_* - I] + \beta[(1 + \varepsilon(t))R_* - R]\}, \tag{32}$$

$$\dot{R} = \gamma(I - I_*) - \omega(R - R_*).$$

Employing the Lyapunov function (24), we find $\dot{V}(I, R)$ with respect to system (32),

$$\dot{V}(I, R) = -(\beta / \gamma)\omega(R - R_*)^2 - \beta[(I - I_* - b(t))^2 - b(t)^2], \tag{33}$$

where $b(t) = \varepsilon(t)(I_* + R_*)/2$. Expression (33) defines a family of ellipses with the size of each ellipse controlled by the parameter $\varepsilon(t)$, through $b(t)$. Together with function (24), expression (33) describes a bound for the region in which trajectories enter and remain for all time.

5.2. Numerical Simulations of the Seasonally Perturbed IR Model

To examine the dynamics of the seasonally perturbed IR model, numerical simulations of system (29) were required. In these simulations, we set the forcing as follows:

$$p(t) = p_0(1 - p_1 \sin 2\pi t).$$

Thus, $p(t)$ is periodic with a period of 1 year. Varying the amplitude of the perturbed transmission term may have a strong effect on the dynamics of the system [2, 4, 14]. Here, however, the effect of varying the amplitude p_1 of the forcing function $p(t)$ is examined, whilst keeping all other parameters fixed. Table 1 gives the parameter values that were used for the experiments shown in Figures 4, 5(a) and 6(a).

Table 1. Fixed parameter values for simulations of system (29)

N	R_0	β	γ	ω	ω_1	p_0
10000	10	0.0924	91.25	0.1	0.75	831.928

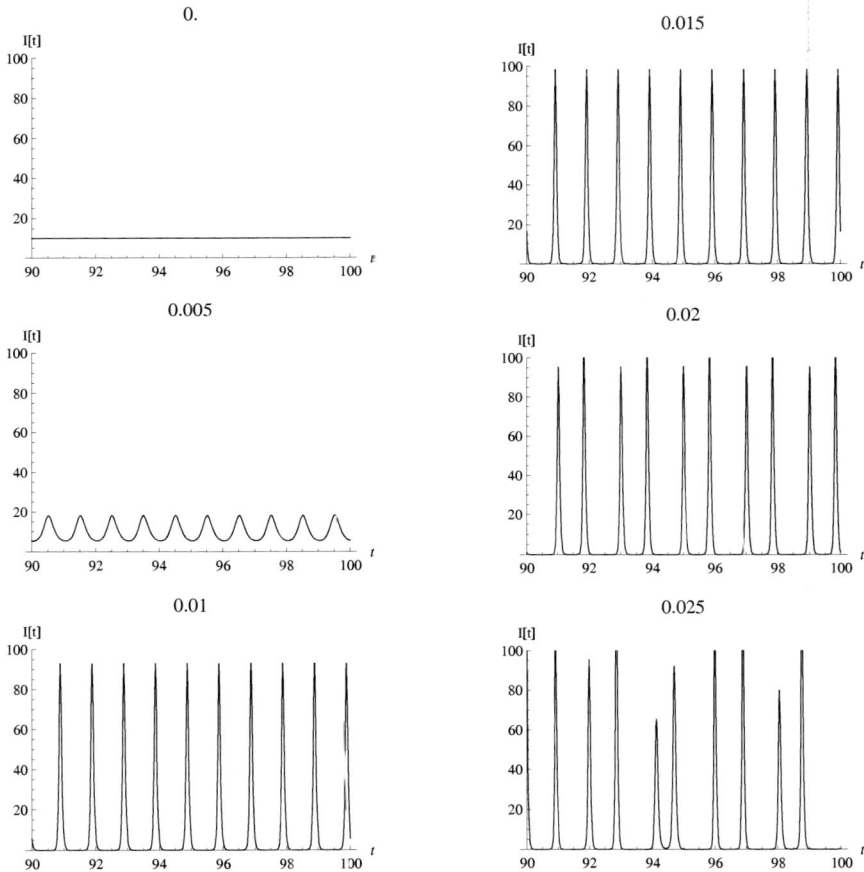

Figure 4. Progression from stable to more complicated behaviour as the amplitude p_1 of $p(t)$ increases. The value of p_1 is indicated above each graph. Note the appearance of period-doubling for $p_1 = 0.02$ and, apparently, irregular dynamics for $p_1 = 0.025$.

Figure 4 shows the long-term dynamics of the seasonally perturbed IR model for a range of values of p_1 (the value of p_1 is indicated on the top of each graph). The Figure indicates that the seasonally perturbed IR system can exhibit complex dynamics as the amplitude p_1 is increased. The infected population oscillates with a period of 1 year for $p_1 = 0.005, 0.01, 0.015$ and it oscillates with a period of 2 years for $p_1 = 0.02$. However, for $p_1 = 0.025$, the infected population oscillates in a seemingly random manner. Clearly, very modest levels of variation of the parameter p_0 (in this case, these are of magnitude of about 0.003%) can translate into large amplitude fluctuations in the observed outbreaks. These results are in striking contrast with the observation in Section 4.1 that all solutions of system (21) converge to a globally asymptotically stable positive equilibrium in the long-term.

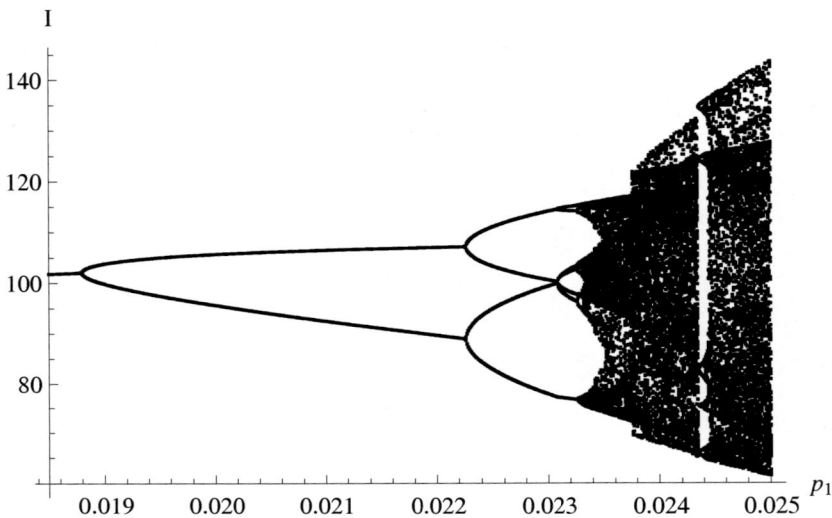

(a) Bifurcation diagram for the seasonally perturbed IR model.

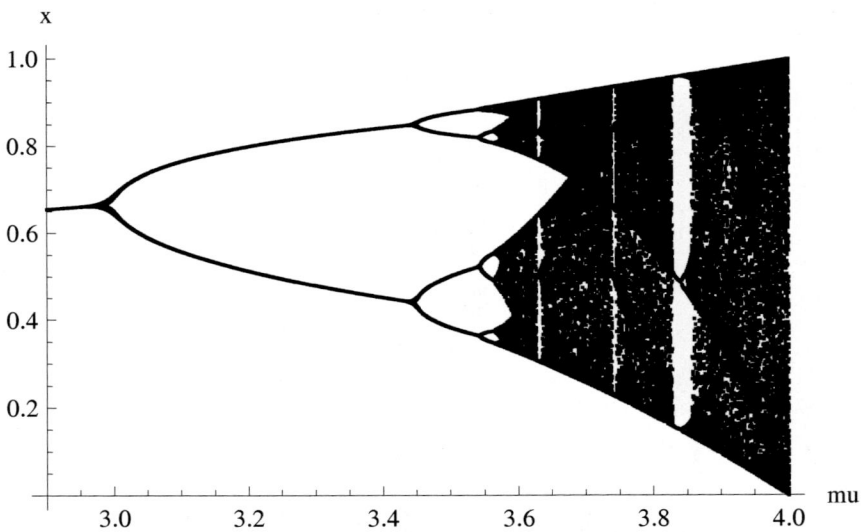

(b) Bifurcation diagram for the logistic mapping, $x_{n+1} = \mu x_n (1 - x_n)$

Figure 5. Figure 5(a) shows a cascade of period-doubling bifurcations and eventually, transition to chaos. This bifurcation diagram is remarkably similar to that of the logistic mapping (Figure 5(b)).

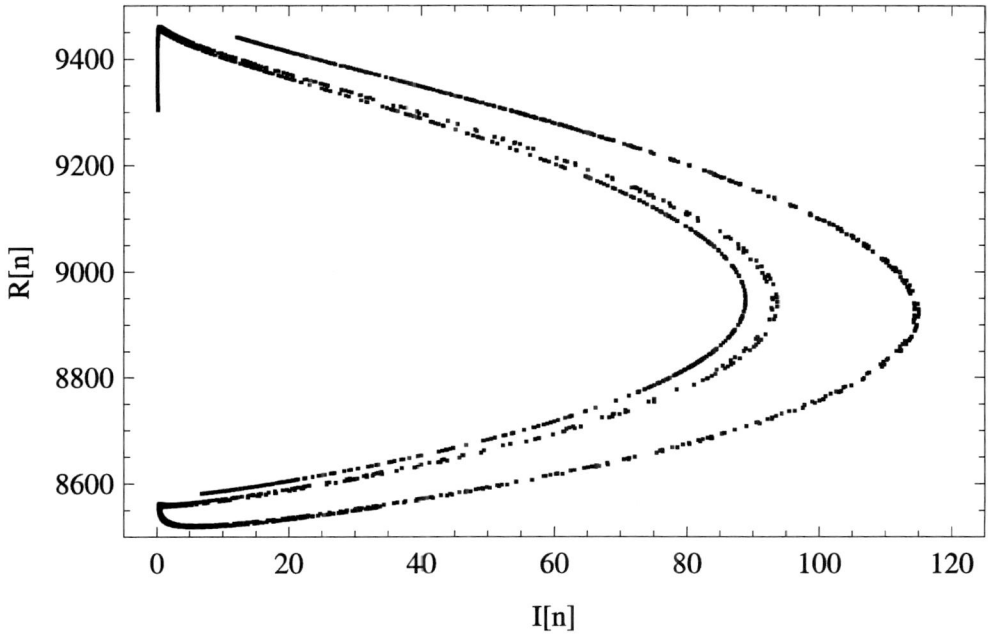

(a) Henon-type attractor observed in system (29) for $\varepsilon(t) = 0.025 \sin 2\pi t$.

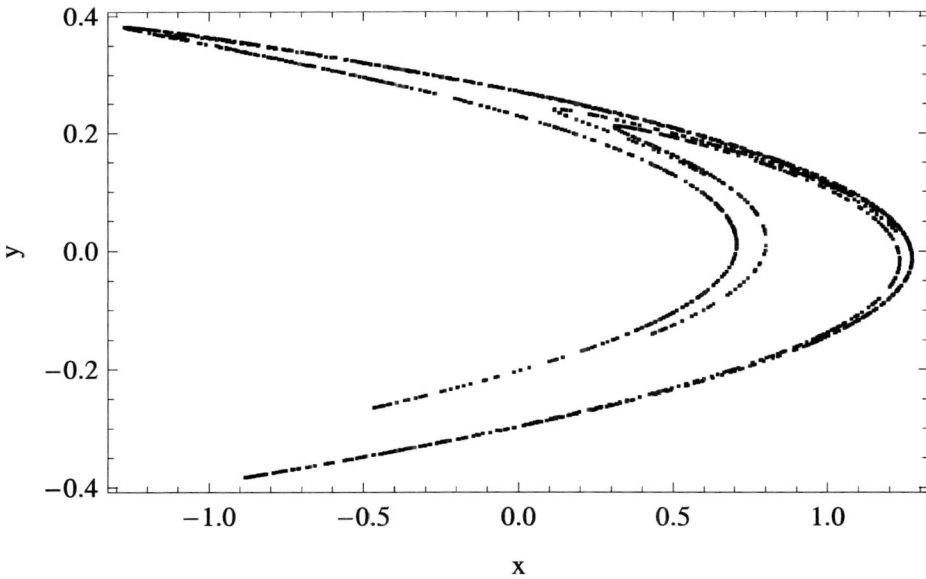

(b) Chaotic attractor of the Hénon mapping, $f(x, y) = (1 - ax^2 + y, bx)$, for $a = 1.4, b = 0.3$.

Figure 6. Numerical evidence of chaos in the seasonally perturbed IR model. The set generated by the output of the seasonally perturbed system (29) in (a) closely resembles the chaotic attractor of the Hénon mapping, shown in (b) for comparison.

(a) Bifurcation diagram for the seasonally perturbed IR model, $R_0 = 1.25$.

(b) Close-up of Figure 7.

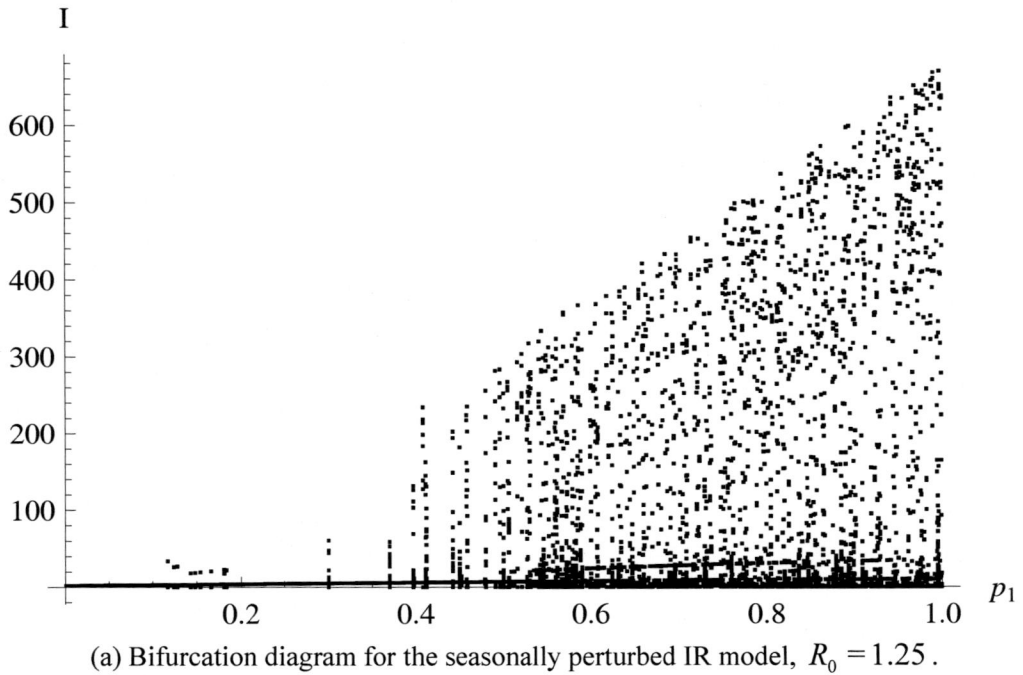

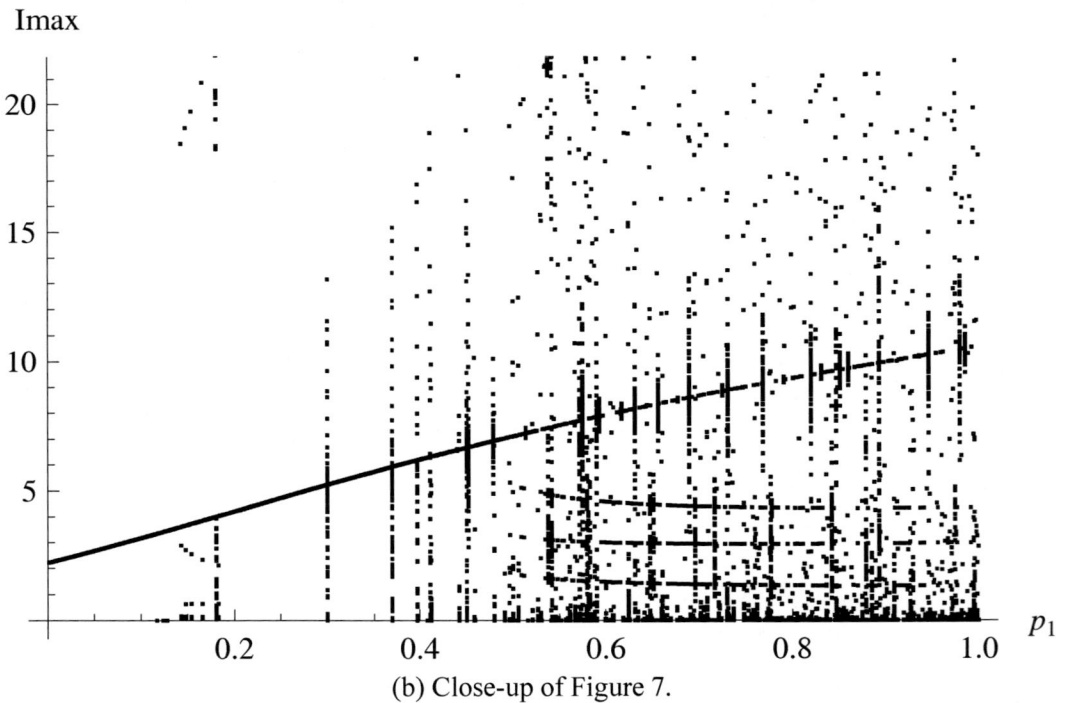

Figure 7. Further experimental evidence of chaos in the seasonally perturbed IR model: the period-doubling route to chaos is not observed for $R_0 = 1.25$. Here, all parameters are the same as in Table 1, except for p_0 and β; these depend on R_0.

The bifurcation diagram of the system (Figure 5(a)) clearly shows a transition to unstable dynamics as the bifurcation parameter p_1 is increased from 0.0185 to 0.025. In Figure 5(a), for each value of p_1, 900 years of transients were discarded before the maximum value of the infected population was recorded each year for 100 years. In this Figure, for p_1 approximately greater than 0.0188, biennial dynamics are observed, which subsequently give way to a cascade of the period-doubling bifurcations, eventually leading to chaos when the amplitude of seasonality exceeds, approximately, 0.0235. The period-doubling route to chaos has also been observed in other seasonally-forced SIR models [4, 14] and famously, in the logistic map [1] (the bifurcation diagram for the logistic map is given in Figure 5(b) for comparison).

Figure 6(a) shows a set in the IR plane which was obtained for the seasonally perturbed IR system (29) for $p_1 = 0.025$. It is easy to see that this closely resembles the famous strange attractor of the Hénon mapping [28], shown in Figure 6(b) for comparison. The set in Figure 6(a) was produced by running the simulation for 1500 years and recording the values of the infected and recovered populations at the end of each year after discarding the first 500 transient years. More precisely, the output of the *translation operator* [40] for time $t = 1$ along a trajectory of system (29), starting from $I(0) = 1, R(0) = 0$, was plotted after discarding the transients. We denote by F the time $t = 1$ translation operator along trajectories of the seasonally perturbed IR system. The output of this operator is the solution of system (29) shifted by time 1. The translation operator F is well-defined. In particular, solutions do not explode to infinity. This is easy to see from the derivative of the Lyapunov function (24). Indeed, from inequality (33), it is easy to see that for sufficiently large values of $I - I_*$ and $R - R_*$, the derivative of function (24) is always negative, and hence, there is a compact positive invariant set in the phase space of the system that contains the equilibrium of the unperturbed system as its inner point.

Finally, it should be noted that not all values of R_0 result in a cascade of period-doubling bifurcations. Figure 7 shows unstable dynamics for $R_0 = 1.25$, but in this case, the exact nature of the bifurcations to chaotic behaviour is unclear, even on closer inspection (Figure 7(b)). In Figure 7 all parameters are the same as for Fig. 4 except for the transmission rate β and p_0 because these values depend on R_0. This phenomenon is observed because the natural period of oscillations of system (21) for $R_0 = 1.25$ is much larger than the period of the seasonal perturbation.

6. RIGOROUS COMPUTER-AIDED ANALYSIS OF THE LONG-TIME BEHAVIOUR OF THE SEASONALLY PERTURBED IR MODEL

The graph in Figure 6(a) indicates the presence of potentially chaotic behaviour in the seasonally perturbed IR model for $p_1 \geq 0.025$. This observation provides the foundation for a rigorous proof of chaos in the model, for $p_1 = 0.025$ and the parameter values in Table 1.

To prove this fact, we employ methods from topological degree theory and split-hyperbolicity [54]. It is noteworthy that the method of proving the existence of chaos in a dynamical system employed in this Chapter has not been, to our knowledge, previously applied to an epidemiological model. Melnikov's method [24], for proving the existence of chaotic trajectories, has been applied to SIR models [13, 21]. However, the systems analysed in those papers have used a nonlinear incidence function similar to that discussed by Liu et al. [47], which has the effect of making the SIR system a perturbation of a Hamiltonian system. However, Melnikov-type methods will not work for system (29) because it is not a disturbance of a Hamiltonian system.

6.1. Problems with Computer Implementations

The system (29) is simple from an analytical point of view, and it also seems simple for the computer implementation. However, this impression is somewhat deceptive. The difficulty is the system is rather stiff for the parameter values defined in Table 1. In particular, this system has a rather large logarithmic norm.

Recall that the logarithmic norm L of a square matrix Q is defined, with respect to the Euclidean metric, by

$$L(Q) = \lim_{h \to 0, h > 0} \frac{\|I + hQ\| - 1}{h},$$

where I is the identity matrix and $\|\cdot\|$ is the operator norm of the matrix. The quantity $e^{L(Q)}$ characterizes the Lipschitz constant of the translation operator for the time of order 1 along trajectories of the linear differential equation $\dot{x} = Qx$; the quantity $e^{L(Q)}h^n$, loosely speaking, describes the local precision of the Runge-Kutta method of order n (see further relevant detail in [25], p. 60, Theorem 10.6.) For a nonlinear dynamical system, $\dot{x} = f(t,x)$, an analogous role is played by the quantity

$$L(f, x(\cdot)) = \int_0^1 e^{L(f'(t, x(t)))} dt,$$

where $x(t)$ is a (numerical) trajectory of the differential equation, and f' denotes the Jacobian.

In our case the value $L(f, x(\cdot))$ for a typical interesting trajectory is of the order of 15 (after optimal adjustment of the norm in $\mathbf{R}^2$). The net result of this observation is that we may be sure of the result of computer-aided analysis for times of order 1, but not for times of the order of 10 or even of 5 (and this estimate is in line with our experiments). Therefore, the rigorous conclusions from computer experimentation with system (29) should rely upon analysis of the translation operator for the time of order 1.

6.2. Topological Hyperbolicity: Informal Discussion

Topological hyperbolicity is a useful tool in computer-aided analysis of long periodic trajectories and chaotic behaviour. Informally, a parallelogram P is said to be *topologically hyperbolic* if P and its image under a continuous mapping F, $F(P)$, form a distorted cross-shape with one another (Figure 8(a)). From the two dimensional version of topological degree theory [41], it follows that, there exists a fixed point of the mapping F in the intersection of P and $F(P)$ (Figure 8(b)). Next, suppose we have a chain of parallelograms where the image of the previous parallelogram in the chain crosses the next parallelogram in the chain. Figure 8(c) shows three parallelograms, P_1, P_2 and P_3, and their images under the mapping F. In this Figure, the image of P_1, $F(P_1)$, crosses P_2, $F(P_2)$ crosses P_3 and $F(P_3)$ crosses P_1. Then the Product Theorem [41] guarantees that there exists a periodic trajectory with minimal period, in this case, with period 3, whose elements belong to the corresponding intersections (see Figure 8(d)). Of course, this assertion is true for a chain of parallelograms of arbitrary length $p > 1$.

Now suppose that in addition to this chain of parallelograms, the image of the third parallelogram is in a cross-type position with respect to itself, as shown in Figure 8(e). Then, by the Product Theorem [41], there exist periodic orbits with any given period that are greater than or equal to 3, (Figures 8(f) and 8(g)). Again, this assertion is true for a chain of parallelograms of arbitrary length $p > 1$.

6.3. Topological Hyperbolicity: The Formal Definition

Fix two positive integers d_u, d_s such that $d_u + d_s = d$. The indices "u" and "s" signify "unstable" and "stable" respectively. Let V and W be bounded, open and convex product-sets

$$V = V^{(u)} \times V^{(s)} \subset \mathbf{R}^{d_u} \times \mathbf{R}^{d_u}, \quad W = W^{(u)} \times W^{(s)} \subset \mathbf{R}^{d_u} \times \mathbf{R}^{d_s},$$

satisfying the inclusions $0 \in V, W$, and let $f : \overline{V} \to \mathbf{R}^{d_u} \times \mathbf{R}^{d_s}$ be a continuous mapping. It is convenient to treat f as the pair $(f^{(u)}, f^{(s)})$ where $f^{(u)} : V \to \mathbf{R}^{d_u}$ and $f^{(s)} : V \mapsto \mathbf{R}^{d_s}$. Denote the topological degree of a mapping f with respect to a set Ω by $\deg(f, \Omega)$ and the closure of a set S by $\overline{S}$.

Definition 6.1 *The mapping* f *is* (V, W)-*hyperbolic, if the equalities*

$$f^{(u)}\left(\partial V^{(u)} \times \overline{V}^{(s)}\right) \cap \overline{W}^{(u)} = \varnothing, \quad f(\overline{V}) \cap \left(\overline{W}^{(u)} \times (\mathbf{R}^{d_s} \setminus W^{(s)})\right) = \varnothing \tag{34}$$

hold, and $\deg(f^{(u)}, V^{(u)}) \neq 0$.

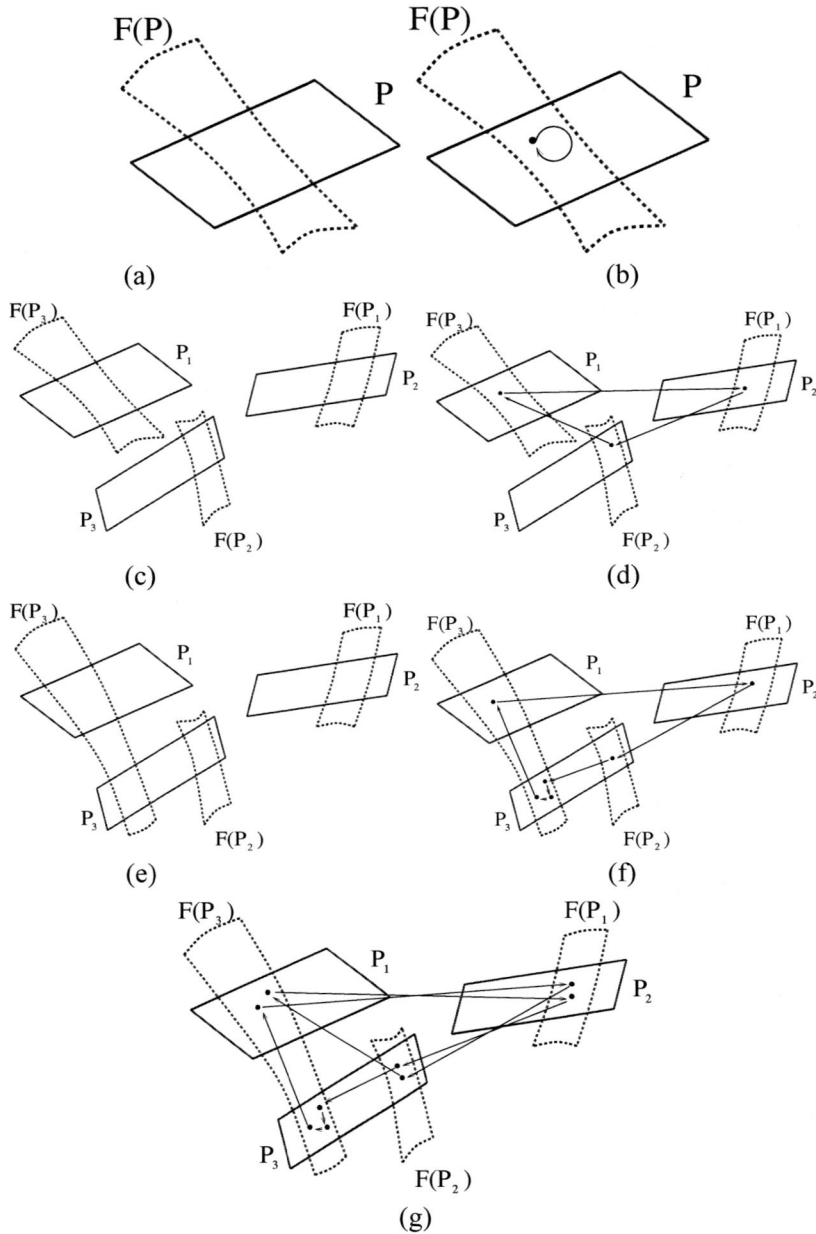

Figure 8. (a) Topologically hyperbolic parallelogram P and its image $F(P)$. (b) A topologically hyperbolic parallelogram always contains a fixed point of the mapping. (c) Topologically hyperbolic chain of three parallelograms, P_1, P_2 and P_3. (d) A topologically hyperbolic chain of three parallelograms will always contain a 3-periodic orbit. (e) Topologically hyperbolic chain of three parallelograms, in which the parallelogram P_3 is also topologically hyperbolic. (f) In a topologically hyperbolic chain of three parallelograms, in which the parallelogram P_3 is also topologically hyperbolic, there exist periodic orbits with any given period that are greater than or equal to 3. This is an example of a 6-periodic orbit. (g) This is an example of a 9-periodic orbit.

The first condition of (34) means geometrically that the image of the "unstable" boundary, $\partial V^{(u)} \times \overline{V}^{(s)}$ of V, does not intersect the infinite cylinder $C = \overline{W}^{(u)} \times \mathsf{R}^{d_s}$. The second condition of (34) means that the image of the entire set $f(V)$ can intersect the cylinder C only through its central fragment $\overline{W}^{(u)} \times W^{(s)}$. Thus, (34) means that the mapping "expands" in a rather weak sense along the first, unstable "u"-coordinate in the Cartesian product $\mathsf{R}^{d_u} \times \mathsf{R}^{d_s}$, and "contracts" along the second, stable "s"-coordinate.

Establishing the (V, W)-hyperbolicity of sets provides information on the existence of long periodic trajectories of a particular mapping. The following Theorem and Corollary rely upon the (V, W)-hyperbolicity property of a certain group of sets:

Theorem 6.1 *Let* $f : \mathsf{R}^d \to \mathsf{R}^d$ *be a continuous mapping. Let there exist homeomorphisms* h_i *and product sets* V_i *such that* $h_j^{-1} f h_i$ *is* (V_i, V_j)-*hyperbolic for all* $j = i+1 \bmod p$, *and let the family* U *of connected components of the union set* $\bigcup h_i(V_i)$ *have more than one element. Then the mapping* f *has a periodic orbit with minimal period* p. *If, in addition* $h_1^{-1} f h_1$ *is* (V_1, V_1)-*hyperbolic, then there exist periodic orbits with all minimal periods greater than* p.

Corollary 6.2 *Let* $\mathsf{F} : \mathsf{R}^2 \to \mathsf{R}^2$ *be a translation operator for time 1 along trajectories of system (29). Let there exist homeomorphisms* h_i *and product sets* V_i *such that* $h_j^{-1} \mathsf{F} h_i$ *is* (V_i, V_j)-*hyperbolic for all* $j = i+1 \bmod p$. *Then system (29) has a periodic orbit with minimal period* p. *If, in addition* $h_1^{-1} \mathsf{F} h_1$ *is* (V_1, V_1)-*hyperbolic, then there exist periodic orbits with all minimal periods greater than* p. *Moreover, this is true also for the three dimensional system (27) for sufficiently large* λ.

Proof. The part of statement before "moreover" is straightforward. The rest follows in a usual way from asymptotic analysis.

Theorem 6.1 is a formal analogue of the informal discussion in Section 6.2. The sets $h_i(V_i)$ describe parallelograms P_i.

6.4. Main Assertion

Figures 9 and 10 show a topologically hyperbolic sequence of 15 parallelograms, $\mathsf{P}_1, \ldots, \mathsf{P}_{15}$ and their images (the distorted quadrilaterals) under the translation operator F along trajectories of system (29) for time of order 1. The image of each parallelogram, $\mathsf{F}(\mathsf{P}_i)$, crosses the next parallelogram, P_{i+1}, in the sequence for $i = 1, \ldots, 14$. Furthermore, the image of the fifteenth parallelogram crosses P_1 (see the bottom right-hand corner in Figure 10) and the image of the first parallelogram $\mathsf{F}(\mathsf{P}_1)$ also crosses P_1 (see the top left-hand corner in Figure 9). Note that the unstable boundaries of the parallelograms and the images of these boundaries are indicated by the bold lines in these Figures. The stable boundaries and the images of these are indicated by the dashed lines.

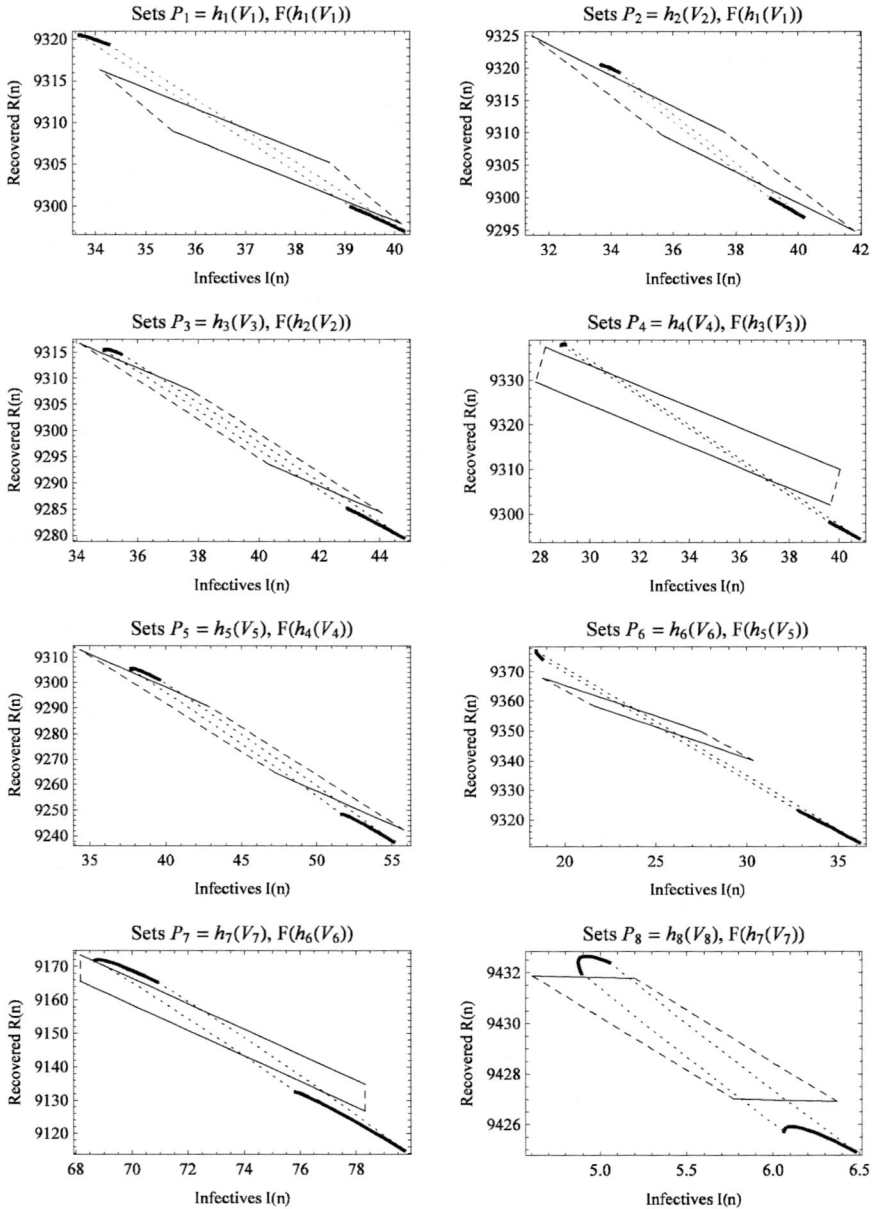

Figure 9. The first graphic (top left-hand corner) shows the mapping $F(h_1(V_1))$ and parallelogram P_1; The other 7 show the mappings $F(h_i(V_i))$ and parallelograms P_{i+1} for $i = 1, \ldots, 7$. The unstable boudaries of the parallelograms and their images under the mapping F are indicated by the bold lines and the stable boundaries are indicated by the dashed lines.

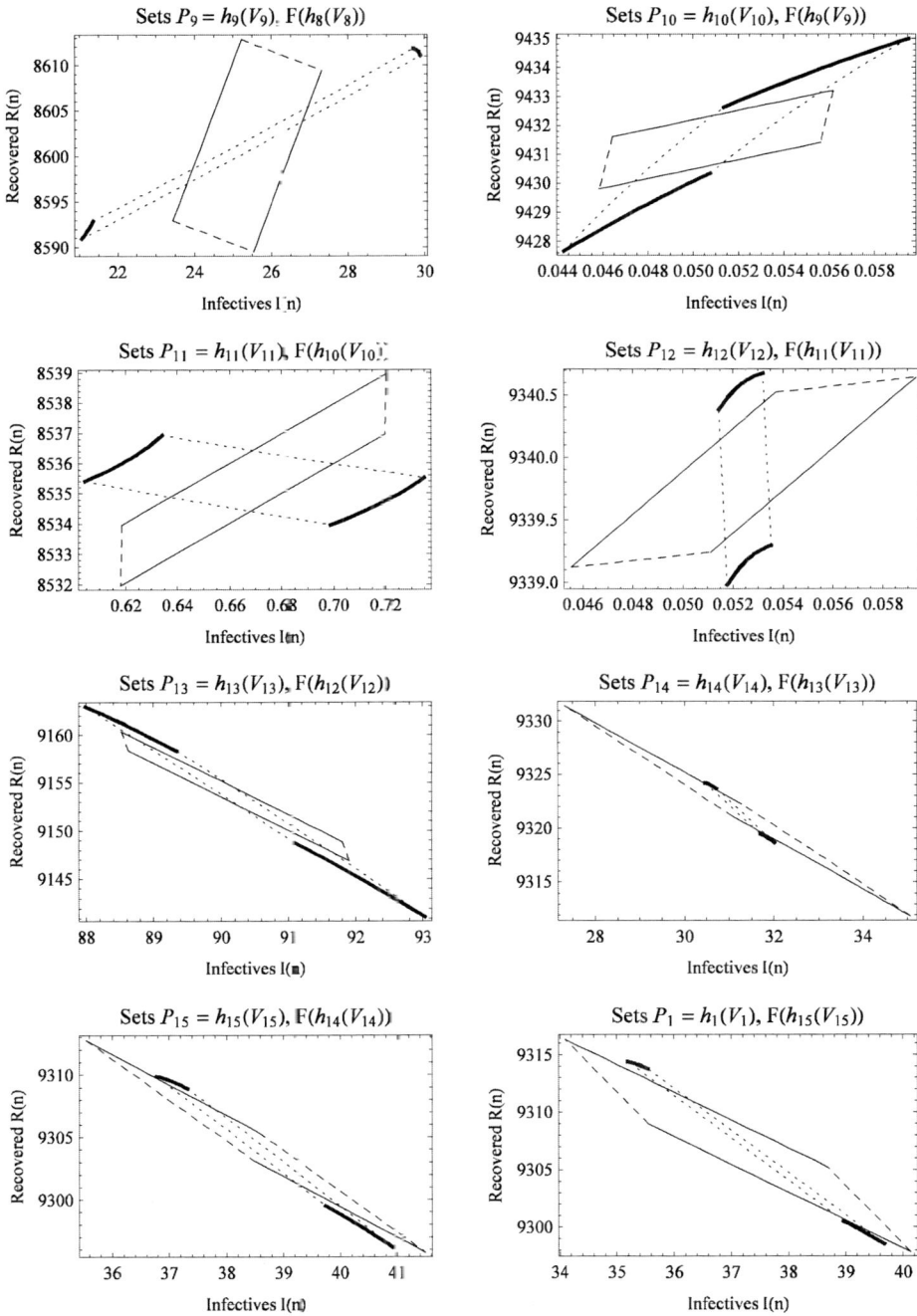

Figure 10. The mappings $F(h_i(V_t))$ and parallelograms P_{i+1} for $i = 8,\ldots,14$; the final graphic (bottom right-hand corner) shows the mapping $F(h_{15}(V_{15}))$ and parallelogram P_1. The unstable boundaries of the parallelograms and their images under the mapping F are indicated by the bold lines and the stable sides are indicated by the dashed lines.

Based on the informal discussion in Section 6.2, we may suspect that the following assertion is true:

Theorem 6.3 *The system (29) has periodic orbits with all minimal periods greater than 15. This is also true for the three dimensional system (27) for sufficiently large λ.*

Proof. To prove this assertion rigorously, we should switch to the formal definition of topological hyperbolicity.

Firstly, we give the analytic definition for the parallelograms P_i around our points $x_i = (I_i, R_i)$:

$$P_i = \{x_i + \kappa_1 a_i^{(u)} x_i^{(u)} + \kappa_2 a_i^{(s)} x_i^{(s)}\},$$

where $|\kappa_1|$, $|\kappa_2| < 1$. The coordinates of the points x_i and the sizes $(a_i^{(u)}, a_i^{(s)})$ of the corresponding parallelograms are presented in Table 2. The vectors $x_i^{(u)}$ and $x_i^{(s)}$ are defined in Table 3.

Table 2. Numerical values I_i, R_i, $a_i^{(u)}$ and $a_i^{(s)}$

i	I_i	R_i	$a_i^{(u)}$	$a_i^{(s)}$
1	37.113	9307.1	3.75	6
2	36.6294	9309.91	8	8
3	39.0891	9300.52	12	5
4	33.9295	9319.77	4	15
5	45.0663	9277.67	25	12
6	24.5481	9354.05	5	10
7	73.2449	9150.18	4	20
8	5.48759	9429.4	2.5	0.3
9	25.3733	8601.2	2	10
10	0.0510245	9431.51	0.9	0.8
11	0.66918	8535.46	1	2.5
12	0.0524238	9339.88	0.06	0.7
13	90.2127	9153.63	1	6
14	31.1815	9321.67	5.5	5
15	38.515	9304.28	5	4

We define homeomorphisms $h_i : \mathbb{R}^2 \to \mathbb{R}^2$, $i = 1, \ldots, 15$, that map the two vectors, i and j, in the standard $\mathbb{R}^2$ basis to the vectors $x_i + x_i^{(u)}$ and $x_i + x_i^{(s)}$ respectively, as follows:

$$h_i : \mathbb{R}^2 \to \mathbb{R}^2, \quad (a_i^{(u)}, a_i^{(s)}) \mapsto x_i + a_i^{(u)} x_i^{(u)} + a_i^{(s)} x_i^{(s)}.$$

Table 3. Vectors defining orientations of parallelograms P_i

i	$x_i^{(u)}$	$x_i^{(s)}$
1	(-0.193582, 0.981084)	(0.381538, -0.924353)
2	(-0.263371, 0.964558)	(0.384224, -0.92324)
3	(-0.25983, 0.965654)	(0.375556, -0.9268)
4	(-0.0495462, -0.998772)	(-0.394077, 0.919077)
5	(-0.257906, 0.96617)	(0.355469, -0.934688)
6	(0.287037, -0.957919)	(-0.435555, 0.900162)
7	(-0.000440847, 1.)	(0.254311, -0.967123)
8	(0.234038, -0.972215)	(-0.987824, 0.155575)
9	(0.521902, -0.853006)	(0.0888201, 0.996048)
10	(-0.000324325, -1.)	(-0.00610066, -0.999981)
11	(-0.000228771, -1.)	(-0.0203626, -0.999793)
12	(0.0466627, 0.998911)	(0.00586125, 0.999983)
13	(-0.051018, 0.998698)	(0.273534, -0.961862)
14	(-0.342414, 0.939549)	(0.396575, -0.918002)
15	(0.291732, -0.9565)	(-0.378975, 0.925407)

Note that these homeomorphisms map the product sets (rectangles) $V_i = \{(a_i^{(u)}, a_i^{(s)}) \in \mathbf{R}^2\}$ into lines in $\mathbf{R}^2$ which define the sides of parallelograms P_i. Figures 11 and 12 show the product sets V_i and the image of each parallelogram, $P_i = h_i(V_i)$, under the mapping, $h_{i+1}^{-1} \circ F$, for $i = 1, \ldots, 14$. In addition, the graphic in the top left-hand corner of Figure 11 shows the mapping $h_1^{-1}(F(h_1(V_1)))$ and the product set V_1, i.e., $h_1^{-1}Fh_1$ is (V_1, V_1)-hyperbolic. Furthermore, the mapping $h_1^{-1}Fh_{15}$ is (V_{15}, V_1)-hyperbolic, see the bottom right-hand corner graphic in Figure 12.

Figures 11 and 12, together with routine error analysis, prove the following statement:

Lemma 6.1 *The mapping $h_j^{-1}Fh_i$ is (V_i, V_j)-hyperbolic for all $j = i + 1 \mod 15$; furthermore, the mapping $h_1^{-1}Fh_1$ is (V_1, V_1)-hyperbolic.*

Thus, Corollary 6.2 holds, and we arrive at Theorem 6.3.

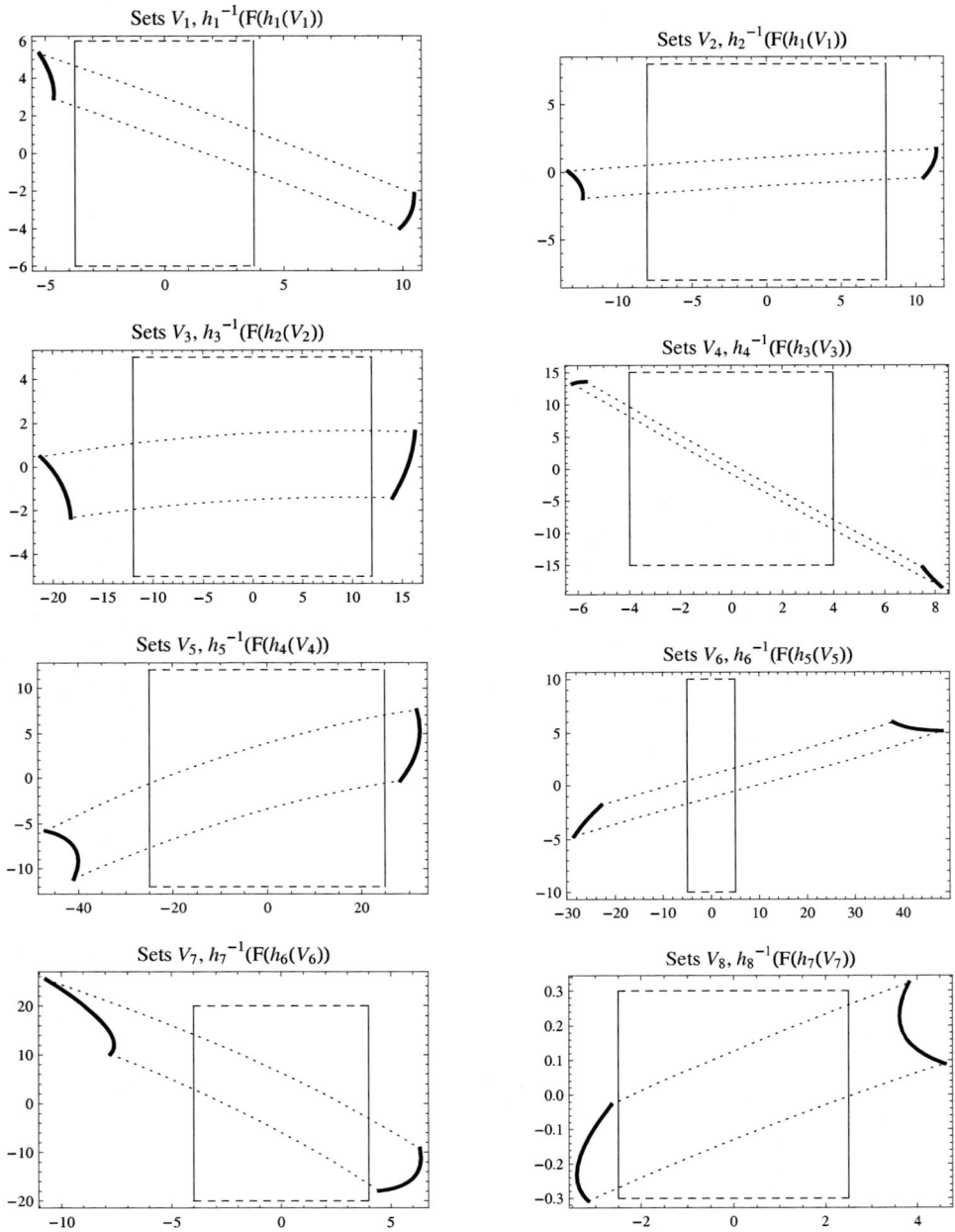

Figure 11. The first graphic (top left-hand corner) shows the mapping $h_1^{-1}(\mathsf{F}(h_1(V_1)))$ and product set V_1; the other 7 show the mappings $h_{i+1}^{-1}(\mathsf{F}(h_i(V_i)))$ and product sets V_{i+1} for $i=1,\ldots,7$. The unstable sides of the product sets and unstable boundaries of the mappings are indicated by the bold boundaries and the stable sides are indicated by the dashed boundaries.

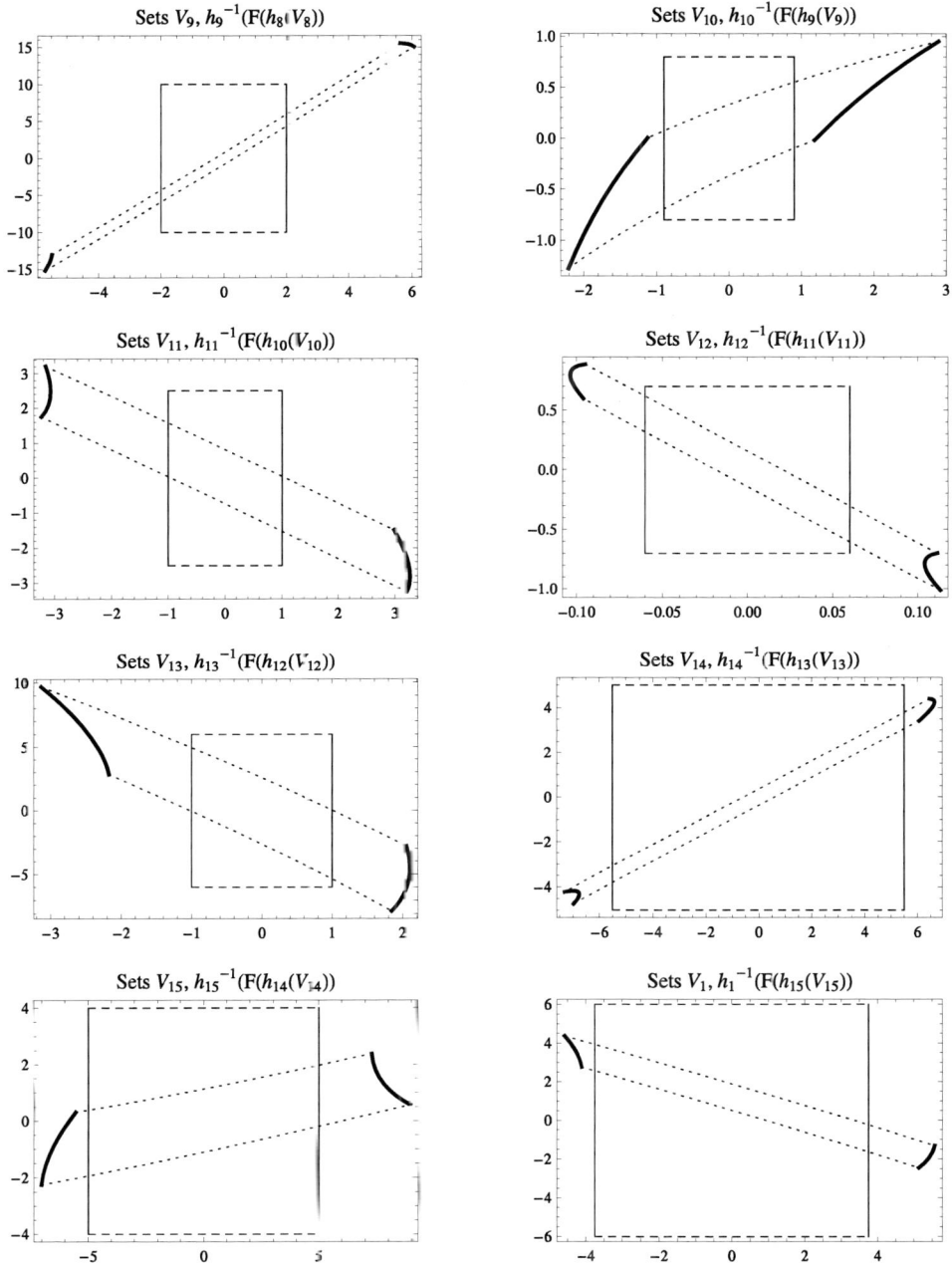

Figure 12. The mappings $h_{i+1}^{-1}(F(h_i(V_i))$ and product sets V_{i+1} for $i = 8,\ldots,14$; the last graphic (bottom right-hand corner) shows the mapping $h_1^{-1}(F(h_{15}(V_{15}))$ and product set V_1. The unstable boundaries of the product sets and the unstable boundaries of the mappings are indicated by the bold lines and the stable boundaries are indicated by the dashed lines.

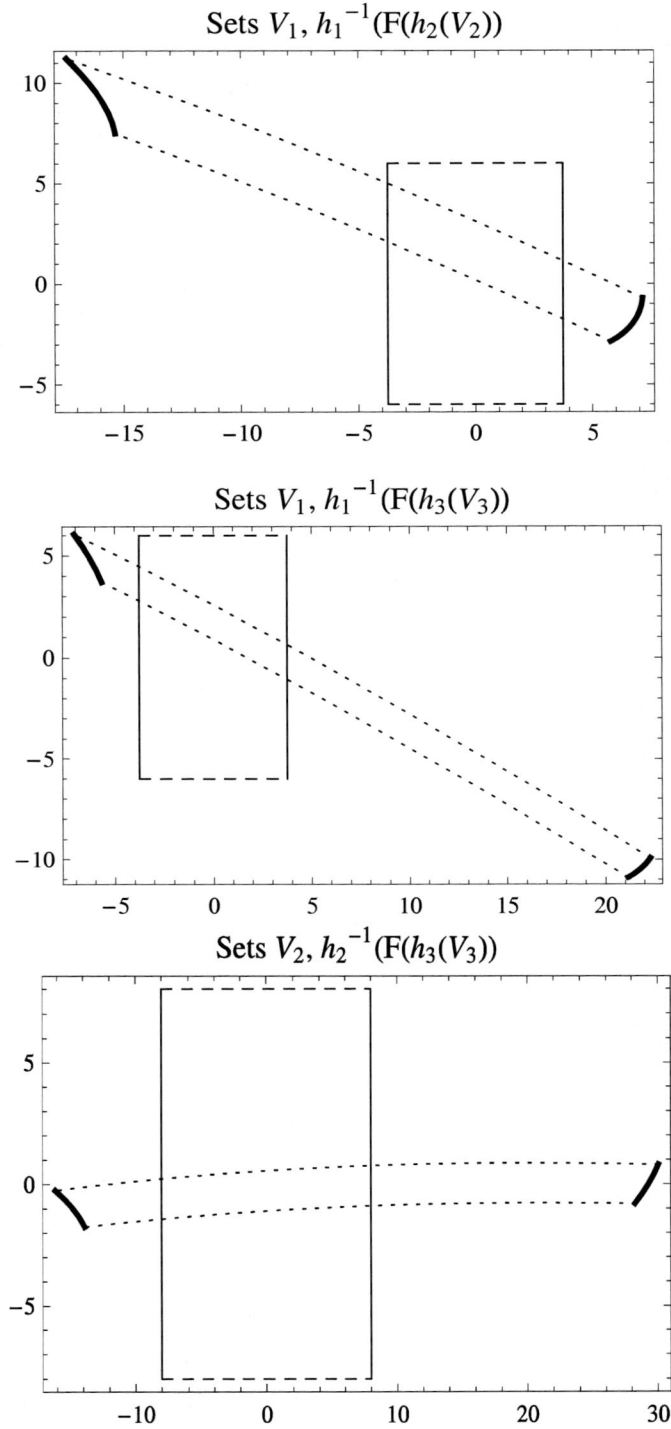

Figure 13. Additional crossings V_1 and $h_1^{-1}(\mathcal{F}(h_2(V_2)))$; V_1 and $h_1^{-1}(\mathcal{F}(h_3(V_3)))$; V_2 and $h_2^{-1}(\mathcal{F}(h_3(V_3)))$.

6.5. How the Topologically Hyperbolic Parallelograms Were Located

The procedure for generating a sequence of topologically hyperbolic parallelograms depends largely on trial and error. Due to the stiffness of system (29), finding a suitable sequence of topologically hyperbolic sets is a non-trivial task.

The first step in identifying potentially suitable sets is to find a quasi-periodic orbit of length p of the mapping F, the translation operator of time $t = 1$ along trajectories of system (29). Given a continuous mapping, parallelograms oriented around these points will be useful in obtaining a topologically hyperbolic chain of sets. The orbit should have elements x_i, $i = 1, \ldots, p$, in a small vicinity of a fixed point of F and have elements that are far away from this fixed point. The fixed point was found using the broken orbits method [54, 55]. However, due to the stiffness of (29), this method was not precise enough for identifying a suitable quasi-periodic point close to the fixed point of F. Instead, an alternative procedure was used. A small rectangle around the fixed point was identified. The iterated mapping F^p was defined. A loop was used to search for a suitable quasi-periodic points x_p such that $|x_p - F^p(x_p)| \ll 1$. By using smaller rectangles, this point was refined by choosing the point with the smallest norm.

Once a suitable quasi-periodic point had been found, a linearisation of the iterated mapping F^p about the point x_i, $i = 1, \ldots, p$ was obtained. The solution of the linearised system at x_i is a 2×2 matrix. The eigenvectors of this matrix were used as first approximations of the orientations of the parallelograms. The vectors $x_i^{(u)}$, $x_i^{(s)}$, $i = 1, \ldots, 15$ in Table 3 are the eigenvectors of the linearisation matrix except for the following:

- The vectors $x_8^{(u)}, x_9^{(u)}$ were obtained by rotating the eigenvector by 10 degrees anti-clockwise.
- The vector $x_{14}^{(s)}$ was obtained by rotating the eigenvector by 20 degrees anti-clockwise.

However, the sizes $(a_i^{(u)}, a_i^{(s)})$ of the parallelograms must be varied to obtain suitable results. The mapping F is topologically hyperbolic if the procedure has been successful.

6.6. Further Consequences of Existence of Parallelograms

Important attributes of chaotic behavior of a mapping $f : R^d \to R^d$ include sensitive dependence on initial conditions, an abundance of periodic trajectories and an irregular mixing effect, i.e., the existence of a finite number of disjoint sets which can be visited by trajectories of f in any prescribed order.

Let $U = \{U_1, \ldots, U_m\}$, $m > 1$, be a family of disjoint subsets of $\mathbf{R}^d$ and let us denote the set of one-sided sequences $\omega = \omega_0, \omega_1, \ldots$ by Ω_m^R. Sequences in Ω_m^R will be used to prescribe the order in which sets U_i are to be visited. For $x \in \bigcup_{i=1}^m U_i$ we define $I(x)$ to be the number i satisfying $x \in U_i$.

A mapping f is called (U, k)-chaotic, if there exists a compact f-invariant set $S \subset \bigcup_i U_i$ with the following properties:

(p1) for any $\omega \in \Omega_m^R$ there exists $x \in S$ such that $f^{ik}(x) \in U_{\omega_i}$ for $i \geq 1$;

(p2) for any p-periodic sequence $\omega \in \Omega_m^R$ there exists a p-periodic point $x \in S$ with
$$f^{ik}(x) \in U_{\omega_i};$$

(p3) for each $\eta > 0$ there exists an uncountable subset $S(\eta)$ of S, such that the simultaneous relationships

$$\limsup_{i \to \infty} | I(f^{ik}(x)) - I(f^{ik}(y)) | \geq 1, \quad \liminf_{i \to \infty} | f^{ik}(x) - f^{ik}(y) | < \eta$$

hold for all $x, y \in S(\eta)$, $x \neq y$.

The above defining properties of chaotic behavior are similar to those in the Smale transverse homoclinic trajectory theorem [56] with an important difference being that we do not require the existence of an invariant Cantor set. Instead, the definition includes property (p2), which is usually a corollary of uniqueness, and (p3), which is a form of sensitivity and irregular mixing as in the Li-Yorke definition of chaos [45], with the subset $S(\eta)$ corresponding to the Li-Yorke scrambled subset S_0. We recall that a set S_0 is called scrambled [45], if for any $x, y \in S_0$

(1) $\limsup_{n \to \infty} | f^n(x) - f^n(y) | > 0$,

(2) $\liminf_{n \to \infty} | f^n(x) - f^n(y) | = 0$

(the original paper [45] contained a third property, which is known to be redundant).

Lemma 6.2 *The family U of connected components of the set $\bigcup_{i=1}^{15} P_i$ has 9 elements.*

Proof. This is clear from the definition of the parallelograms P_i and Figure 14.

Theorem 6.4 *The mapping F is $(U, 26)$-chaotic, where U is the family of connected components of the set $\bigcup_{i=1}^{15} P_i$. For sufficiently large λ, this is also true for the three dimensional system (27).*

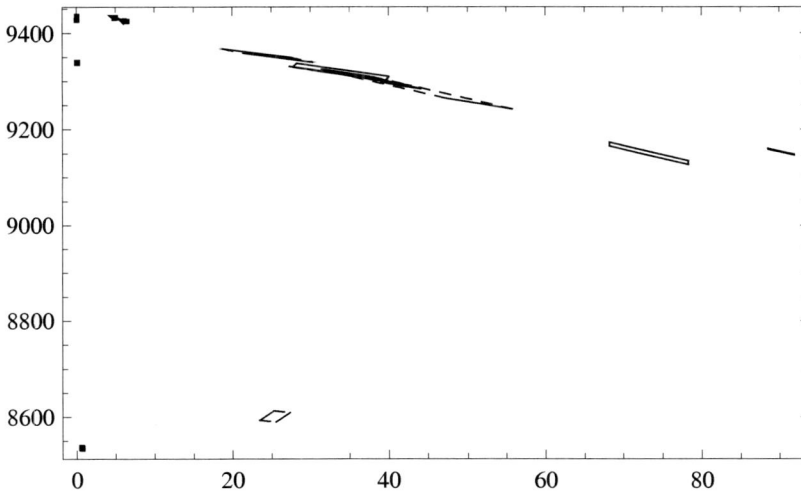

(a) The 9 connected components of the set $\bigcup_{i=1}^{15} P_i$.

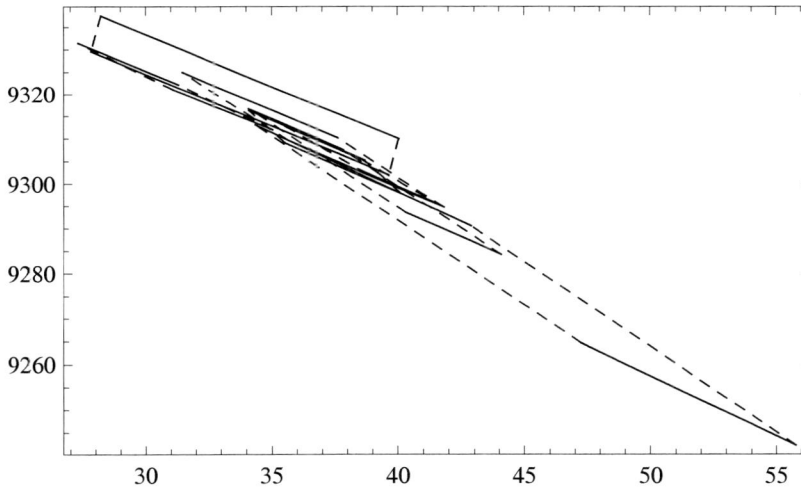

(b) Close-up view of sets $P_1, P_2, P_3, P_4, P_5, P_{14}$ and P_{15}.

Figure 14. The connected components of the set $\bigcup_{i=1}^{15} P_i$ are shown in (a). Figure 14(b) shows one connected component of the set $\bigcup_{i=1}^{15} P_i$. These graphics provide a geometric proof of Lemma 6.2.

The proof relies on Figure 13 and the results from [54]. The proof is similar to the proof of Theorem 1 from [54]. Finally, a lower bound on the topological entropy of the mapping F, which we will denote by $E^{op}(F)$, may be calculated. The topological entropy is a way of quantifying chaos in a dynamical system. In particular, it is a positive quantity for chaotic systems and it is zero for non-chaotic systems [52]. The topological entropy of a mapping is discussed in [52]. The maximal eigenvalue, λ_{max}, of a k-transitive matrix A, which represents the hyperbolicity properties of F (see Theorem 1 in [54] for the definition of A), was calculated. The topological entropy is greater than or equal to the natural logarithm of

λ_{max}. Thus, a lower bound on the topological entropy of the chaotic attractor of trajectories of F is given by:

$$\mathsf{E}^{top}(\mathsf{F}) \geq \ln(\lambda_{max}) = 0.693168.$$

7. Conclusion

The introduction of H5N1 avian influenza to a seabird colony with no existing herd-immunity is an issue of concern to marine conservationists and population ecologists because of the potentially destabilizing impact of additive mortality among adults. In addition, zoonotic emerging infectious diseases, such as H5N1 avian influenza, are a significant growing threat to global health, with the majority of EID events caused by pathogens acquired from vertebrate animals [34]. Furthermore, migratory birds have been implicated as a potential pathway by which the H5N1 virus could be carried between countries [39, 53]. Therefore, an insight into the dynamics of H5N1 in a densely populated seabird colony is inherently interesting and the probable dynamics of the epidemic are relevant to public and veterinary health.

In this Chapter, we formulated a SEIR model which incorporates the main features of the spread of the H5N1 avian influenza virus in a seabird colony. Using the theory of integral manifolds, we rigorously reduced this SEIR model to a SIR model, and then to the IR model, a system dependent on the infected and recovered populations only. By constructing Lyapunov functions, we analysed the long-term behaviour of the SEIR model (for a particular case when the disease-induced mortality of the exposed hosts is absent), and the IR model. It was proved that for these models all trajectories tend to a globally asymptotically stable positive equilibrium, meaning that the disease, once introduced, persists in the population in the long-term. These findings establish a process in which micropathogens persist in seabird populations.

From the results of numerical experiments, we saw that the IR model retains the essential features of the SEIR model. Figure 2 shows that a major epidemic occurs in the first year: for $R_0 = 2$, the number of infectives rises sharply to a maximum of 1,500 and then decreases to almost zero in a period of 0.2 years. Subsequent outbreaks are smaller, and damped oscillations of the infective and recovered populations are observed. The size and frequency of these outbreaks depend upon the value of R_0. If $R_0 = 2$, outbreaks are smaller and less frequent but it may take a long time, i.e., up to 75 years, for the system to reach equilibrium. However, if $R_0 = 10$, outbreaks are more severe and occur more frequently, and thus, the infected and recovered populations damp to equilibrium in a much shorter time frame, about 15 years. Once an individual enters the R class, it acquires permanent immunity from the disease. Since more individuals become infected when R_0 is large, consequently, more individuals recover and cannot return to the susceptible class. Thus, the pool of susceptibles becomes exhausted in a much shorter time frame, and it is hardly surprising, therefore, that for larger R_0 the system approaches equilibrium faster.

In the case of H5N1 in a seabird colony, the SEIR system is a multi-scaled system: influenza dynamics in seabirds exhibit fast dynamics at the individual and colony levels when compared to seabird demography. The average lifespan of a seabird (about 10–20 years) is thousands of times greater than the duration of the latent period of H5N1 (about 1–2 days). For such a case, singular perturbation theory enables us to greatly simplify the four-dimensional SEIR system by reducing it to a two dimensional system. The analysis of the resulting two-dimensional IR model is much simpler compared to the corresponding analysis for the original SEIR system. Reducing the SEIR model to the IR system also enables us to develop and analyse interesting and relevant variants of the basic model. In particular, the IR model may be subject to seasonal perturbations. Seasonality is a complex force in nature, and much theoretical and computational work is required to obtain a basic understanding of how seasonality affects various processes in a seabird colony, such as recruitment of susceptibles, changes in social behaviour and the timing of the breeding season. Seasonality may cause changes in food availability which may, in turn, delay the breeding season of seabirds and increase their susceptibility to disease. Seasonal variations such as these may have a considerable effect on the transmission dynamics of a pathogen. It is, therefore, important for marine conservationists to understand how seasonality interacts with these processes.

Numerical simulations of the IR model show that seasonality has a significant effect on the dynamics of the disease. The numerical simulations show that seasonal forcing of comparatively small magnitude can generate very complex dynamics. For sufficiently large amplitudes of perturbation, epidemics of unpredictable magnitude and duration may occur (Figures 4, 5(a), 7(a)). In particular, the period-doubling route to chaos was observed in this system. However, it should be noted that, for smaller values of R_0, a cascade of period-doubling bifurcations may not occur.

In this Chapter, we employed Lyapunov's direct method to find a convex region of stability for the seasonally perturbed IR model. Thereafter, using methods from topological degree theory and split-hyperbolicity, the existence of chaotic trajectories for the seasonally perturbed IR model was rigorously proved. This is a significant result because, to our knowledge, this is the first time that this method has been used to prove the existence of chaos in an epidemiological system. To prove the existence of such complex behaviour in a simple, yet realistic, model is a very exciting development. Therefore, problems in epidemiology may lead to new and interesting mathematical work. In turn, mathematics can help biologists understand the mechanisms leading to outbreaks of disease.

In conclusion, we also have to stress that the models and methods used in this chapter, and to some extent the result obtained, can be readily applied to a comparable scenario in which a novel pathogen is introduced to a crowded population.

ACKNOWLEDGEMENTS

Suzanne O'Regan was supported by the Irish Research Council for Science, Engineering and Technology (IRCSET), under the Embark Initiative Postgraduate Funding Scheme. Andrei Korobeinikov is supported by the Mathematics Applications Consortium for Science and Industry funded by the Science Foundation Ireland Mathematics Initiative Grant 06/MI/005. Alexei Pokrovskii is supported by Grant 06-01-72552 of the Russian Foundation of Basic Researches. The authors wish to gratefully acknowledge the valuable contributions of Prof. Elena Schepakina and Prof. Vladimir Sobolev, University of Samara, Russia.

REFERENCES

[1] Alligood, KT; Sauer, TD; Yorke, JA. *Chaos An Introduction to Dynamical Systems*. New York: Springer-Verlag; 1997

[2] Altizer, S; Dobson, A; Hosseini, P; Hudson, P; Pascual, M; Rohani, P. Seasonality and the dynamics of infectious diseases. *Ecology Letters*, 2006 9, 467-484

[3] Anderson, RM; May, RM. *Infectious Diseases of Humans: Dynamics and Control*. Oxford: Oxford University Press; 1992

[4] Aron, JL; Schwartz, IB. Seasonality and period-doubling bifurcations in an epidemic model. *Journal of Theoretical Biology*, 1984 110, 665-679

[5] Barbashin, EA. *Introduction to the theory of stability*. Groningen: Wolters-Noordhoff; 1970

[6] Benot, E; Callot, JL; Diener, F; Diener, M. Chasse au canard. *Collectanea Mathematica*, 1981–1982 31-32, 37-119.

[7] Brown, CR; Brown, MB. *Coloniality in the Cliff Swallow—The Effect of Group Size on Social Behaviour*. Chicago and London: The University of Chicago Press; 1996

[8] Chen, H; Smith, GJD; Zhang, SY; Qin, K; Wang, J; Li, KS; Webster, RG; Peiris, JSM; Guan, Y. H5N1 virus outbreak in migratory waterfowl. *Nature*, 2005 436, 191-192

[9] Clancy, CF; O'Callaghan, MJA; Kelly, TC. A multi-scale problem arising in a model of avian flu virus in a seabird colony. *Journal of Physics: Conference Series*, 2006 55, 45-54. doi: 10.1088/1742-6596/55/1/004

[10] Clery, D. David King interview: U.K. science adviser offers some parting shots. *Science*, 2007 318, 1862-1863

[11] Crespin, L; Harris, MP; Lebreton, JD; Frederiksen, M; Wanless, S. Recruitment to a seabird population depends on environmental factors and on population size. *Journal of Animal Ecology*, 2006 75, 228-238

[12] Croxall, JP., Ed. *Seabirds: Feeding Ecology and Role in Marine Ecosystems*. Cambridge: Cambridge University Press; 1987

[13] Diallo, O; Koné, Y. Melnikov analysis of chaos in a general epidemiological model. *Nonlinear Analysis: Real World Applications*, 2007 8, 20-26

[14] Dietz K. The incidence of infectious diseases under the influence of seasonal fluctuations. In: Berger J; Buhler W; Repges R; Tautu P, editors. *Lecture Notes in Biomathematics*. vol. 11. Berlin: Springer; 1976. p.1-15

[15] Dumortier, F; Roussarie, R. Canard cycles and center manifolds. *Memoirs of the American Mathematical Society* 1996 121(577)

[16] Dushoff, J; Plotkin, JB; Levin, SA; Earn, DJB. Dynamical resonance can account for seasonality of influenza epidemics. *Proceedings of the National Academy of Sciences of the United States of America*, 2004 101, 16915-16916

[17] Earn, DJD; Rohani, P; Bolker, BM; Grenfell, BT. A simple model for complex dynamical transitions in epidemics. *Science* 2000 287, 667-670

[18] Ferguson, NM; Donnelly, CA; Anderson, RM. The Foot and Mouth epidemic in Great Britain: Pattern of spread and impact of interventions. *Science*, 2001 292, 1155-1160

[19] Furness, RW; Birkhead, TR. Seabird colony distributions suggest competition for food supplies during the breeding season. *Nature*, 1984 311, 655-656

[20] Gani, R; Hughes, H; Fleming, D; Griffin, T; Medlock, J; Leach, S. Potential impact of antiviral drug use during influenza pandemic. *Emerging Infectious Diseases*, 2005 11, 1355-1362

[21] Glendinning, P; Perry, LP. Melnikov analysis of chaos in a simple epidemiological model. *Journal of Mathematical Biology*, 1997 35, 359-373

[22] Goldfarb, I; Goldshtein, V; Maas, U. Comparative analysis of two asymptotic approaches based on integral manifolds. *IMA Journal of Applied Mathematics*, 2004 69, 353-374

[23] Grassly, NC; Fraser, C. Seasonal infectious disease epidemiology. *Proceedings of the Royal Society B: Biological Sciences*, 2006 273, 2541-2550

[24] Guckenheimer, J; Holmes, P. *Nonlinear oscillations, dynamical systems, and bifurcations of vector fields*. New York: Springer; 1983

[25] Hairer, E; Nørsett, SP; Wanner, G. *Solving Ordinary Differential Equations I Nonstiff Problems*. Berlin and New York: Springer-Verlag; 1987

[26] Hamer, KC; Schreiber, EA; Burger, J. Breeding biology, life histories, and life history—environment interactions in seabirds. In: Schreiber EA; Burger J, editors. *Biology of Marine Birds*. Florida: CRC Press; 2001. p. 217-263

[27] Heffernan, JM; Smith, RJ; Wahl, LM. Perspectives on the basic reproductive ratio. *Journal of the Royal Society Interface*, 2005 2, 281-293

[28] Hénon, M. A two-dimensional mapping with a strange attractor. *Communications in Mathematical Physics*, 1976 50, 69-77

[29] Hofbauer, J; Sigmund, K. *The Theory of Evolution and Dynamical Systems: Mathematical Aspects of Selection*. Cambridge: Cambridge University Press; 1988

[30] Horimoto, T; Kawaoka, Y. Influenza: Lessons from past pandemics, warnings from current incidents. *Nature Reviews Microbiology*, 2005 3, 591-600

[31] Hosseini, PR; Dhondt, AA; Dobson, A. Seasonality and wildlife disease: how seasonal birth, aggregation and variation in immunity affect the dynamics of *Mycoplasma gallisepticum* in house finches. *Proceedings of the Royal Society B: Biological Sciences*, 2004 271, 2569-2577

[32] Hudson, PJ; Rizzoli, A; Grenfell, BT; Heesterbeek, H; Dobson, AP. *The Ecology of Wildlife Diseases*. Oxford: Oxford University Press; 2002

[33] Iwami, S; Takeuchi, Y; Korobeinikov, A; Liu, X. Prevention of avian influenza epidemic: What policy should we choose? *Journal of Theoretical Biology*, 2008 252, 732-741

[34] Jones, KE; Patel, NG; Levy, MA; Storeygard, A; Balk, D; Gittleman, JL; Daszak, P. Global trends in emerging infectious diseases. *Nature*, 2008 451, 990-994

[35] Keeling, MJ; Rohani, P; Grenfell, BT. Seasonally forced disease dynamics explored as switching between attractors. *Physica D: Nonlinear Phenomena*, 2001 148, 317-335

[36] Keeling, MJ. Models of foot-and-mouth disease. *Proceedings of the Royal Society B: Biological Sciences*, 2005 272, 1195-1202

[37] Keeling, MJ; Rohani, P. *Modeling Infectious Diseases in Humans and Animals*. Princeton, New Jersey: Princeton University Press; 2008

[38] Kermack, WO; McKendrick, AG. A contribution to the mathematical theory of epidemics. *Proceedings of the Royal Society of London Series A*, 1927 115, 700-721

[39] Kilpatrick, AM; Chmura, AA; Gibbons, DW; Fleischer, RC; Marra, PP; Daszak, P. Predicting the global spread of avian influenza. *Proceedings of the National Academy of Sciences of the United States of America*, 2006 103, 19368-19373

[40] Krasnosel'skii, MA. *The operator of translation along the trajectories of differential equations*. vol. 19 of Translation of Mathematical Monographs. Providence RI: American Mathematical Society; 1968

[41] Krasnosel'skii, MA; Zabreiko, PP. *Geometrical methods of nonlinear analysis*. Berlin: Springer-Verlag 1984

[42] La Salle, J; Lefschetz, S. *Stability by Liapunov's direct method with applications*. New York: Academic Press; 1961

[43] Lafferty, KD; Holt, RD. How should environmental stress affect the population dynamics of disease? *Ecology Letters*, 2003 6, 654-664

[44] Lewis, S; Sherratt, TN; Hamer, KC; Wanless, S. Evidence of intra-specific competition for food in a pelagic seabird. *Nature*, 2001 412, 816-819

[45] Li, TY; Yorke, JA. Period three implies chaos. *American Mathematical Monthly*, 1975 82, 985-992

[46] Lipsitch, M; Cohen, T; Cooper, B; Robins, JM; Ma, S; James, L; Gopalakrishna, G; Chew, SK; Tan, CC; Samore, MH; Fisman, D; Murray, M. Transmission dynamics and control of Severe Acute Respiratory Syndrome. *Science*, 2003 300, 1966-1970

[47] Liu, WM; Hethcote, HW; Levin, SA. Dynamical behavior of epidemiological models with nonlinear incidence rates. *Journal of Mathematical Biology*, 1987 25, 359-380

[48] Neishtadt, AI. Asymptotic investigation of the loss of stability by an equilibrium as a pair of eigenvalues slowly cross the imaginary axis. *Uspekhi Matematicheskikh Nauk*, 1985 40, 190-191

[49] Nuttall, PA; Kelly, TC; Carey, D; Moss, SR; Harrap, KA. Mixed infections with tick-borne viruses in a seabird colony in Eire. *Archives of Virology*, 1984 79, 35-44

[50] O'Regan, SM; Kelly, TC; Korobeinikov, A; O'Callaghan, MJA; Pokrovskii, AV. Qualitative and numerical investigations of the impact of a novel pathogen on a seabird colony. *Journal of Physics: Conference Series*, 2008 138. doi: 10.1088/1742-6596/138/1/012018

[51] Österblom, H; Van Der Jeugd, HP; Olsson, O. Adult survival and avian cholera in common guillemots *Uria aalge* in the Baltic Sea. *Ibis*, 2004 146, 531-534

[52] Ott, E. *Chaos in dynamical systems*. Cambridge and New York: Cambridge University Press; 2002

[53] Peterson, AT; Benz, BW; Papes, M. Highly pathogenic H5N1 avian influenza: Entry pathways into north america via bird migration. *PLoS ONE*, 2007 2. e261. doi:10.1371/journal.pone.0000261

[54] Pokrovskii, AV; Szybka, SJ; McInerney, JG. Topological degree in locating homoclinic structures for discrete dynamical systems. *Preprints of INS*, UCC 01-001, 2001

[55] Pokrovskii, AV; Rasskazov, OA. On the use of the topological degree theory in broken orbits analysis. *Proceedings of the American Mathematical Society*, 2004 132, 567-577

[56] Ruelle, D. *Elements of differentiable dynamics and bifurcation theory*. Boston: Academic Press; 1989

[57] Sandvik, H; Erikstad, KE; Barrett, RT; Yoccoz, NG. The effect of climate on adult survival in five species of North Atlantic seabirds. *Journal of Animal Ecology*, 2005 74, 817-831

[58] Sobolev V. Geometry of singular perturbations: critical cases. In: Mortell MP; O'Malley RE; Pokrovskii A; Sobolev V, editors. *Singular perturbations and hysteresis*. Philadelphia, USA: Society for Industrial and Applied Mathematics; 2005. p. 153-207

[59] Sovada, MA; Pietz, PJ; Converse, KA; King, DT; Hofmeister, EK; Scherr, P; Ip, HS. Impact of West Nile virus and other mortality factors on American white pelicans at breeding colonies in the northern plains of North America. *Biological Conservation*, 2008 141, 1021-1031

[60] Stone, L; Olinky, R; Huppert, A. Seasonal dynamics of recurrent epidemics. *Proceedings of the Royal Society B: Biological Sciences*, 2007 446, 533-536

[61] Taubenberger, JK; Reid, AH; Fanning, TG. The 1918 influenza virus: A killer comes into view. *Virology*, 2000 274, 241-245

[62] Tiensin, T; Nielen, M; Vernooij, H; Songserm, T; Kalpravidh, W; Chotiprasatintara, S; Chaisingh, A; Wongkasemjit, S; Chanachai, K; Thanapongtham, W; Srisuvan, T; Stegeman, A. Transmission of the highly pathogenic avian influenza virus H5N1 within flocks during the 2004 epidemic in Thailand. *Journal of Infectious Diseases*, 2007 196, 1679-1684

[63] Wanless, S; Frederiksen, M; Harris, MP; Freeman, SN. Survival of Gannets *Morus bassanus* in Britain and Ireland, 1959-2002. *Bird Study*, 2006 53, 79-85

[64] Wanless, S; Murray, S; Harris, MP. The status of northern gannet in Britain and Ireland in 2003/04. *British Birds*, 2005 98, 280-294

[65] Wittenburger, JF; Hunt, GL. jr. The adaptive significance of coloniality in birds. In: Farner DS; King JR; Parkes KC, editors. *Avian Biology*. vol. 8. New York: Academic Press; 1985. p. 1-78

[66] Wonham, MJ; de Camino-Beck, T; Lewis, MA. An epidemiological model for West Nile virus: invasion analysis and control applications. *Proceedings of the Royal Society B: Biological Sciences*, 2004 271, 501-507

Chapter 19

CONTROL OF INFLUENZA AT HEALTHCARE FACILITIES IN RESOURCE-LIMITED SETTINGS

Thana Khawcharoenporn,[1] Anucha Apisarnthanarak[1] and Linda M. Mundy[2]*

[1]Division of Infectious Diseases and Infection Control, Faculty of Medicine,
Thammasart University Hospital, Pratumthani, Thailand,
[2]Saint Louis University School of Public Health, St. Louis, MO, USA

ABSTRACT

Influenza is a common acute respiratory tract infection, generally caused by influenza A or B viruses. Similar to most other viral infections, influenza A and B infections are self-limited in healthy persons. However, influenza has well-recognized complications and mortality, especially in at-risk populations, and outbreaks and pandemics of influenza occur worldwide. The recent emergence of avian influenza (H5N1) virus infections has posed significant threats to human and animal health. The potential of the often lethal avian influenza (H5N1) viral infection as the point source of the next devastating influenza pandemic has prompted global influenza surveillance and preparedness strategies that include infection-control practice and policy.

Healthcare facilities are at risk for complex transmission dynamics of influenza given the close proximity of patients and varied encounter types among patients, visitors, and healthcare personnel (HCP). Patients with risk factors for influenza-related complications benefit from healthcare within a facility that employs early influenza detection via appropriate specimen procurement, transport, and testing as well as early interventions for treatment and prevention. Antiviral therapy for influenza control should be prescribed based on indications, local influenza epidemic and resistance data, host-immunization status, and tolerability of adverse reactions. Influenza vaccination plays an

---

* Correspondence to: Anucha Apisarnthanarak, MD., Division of Infectious Diseases, Faculty of Medicine, Thammasart University Hospital, Pratumthani, Thailand, 12120. Tel: 6681-987-2030, Fax: 662-443-8533; E-mail: anapisarn@yahoo.com.

important role and is shown to be effective in minimizing illness, if not preventing infection. Although few data support the cost-effectiveness of annual influenza vaccination in resource-limited settings, immunization is beneficial to high-risk patients and HCP at long-term care facilities and in intensive care units.

Five components of influenza preparedness plans are recommended at healthcare facilities in resource-limited facilities. These components include appropriate infection-control measures using existing infrastructure, targeted educational programs, administrative support, access to a nationally-coordinated laboratory system for early and rapid influenza detection, and adequate stocks of antiviral therapy and vaccinations.

INTRODUCTION

Influenza is an acute, febrile illness caused by influenza viruses that belong to the family *Orthomyxoviridae*. The viruses are classified into three different types—influenza A, influenza B, and influenza C—based on differences of the major surface antigens. Several distinct genetic and molecular characteristics of these three influenza viruses influence the epidemiology, clinical manifestations, and global economic impact of infected populations [1]. Influenza is usually a self-limited respiratory illness, yet variation in attack rates and attributable mortality have been documented in pandemics and interpandemics over the past 400 years [2,3].

During the twentieth century, there were three notable influenza pandemics that each attributed to the emergence of a novel influenza A virus. The first and greatest influenza A pandemic occurred in 1918. The emergence of Spanish influenza virus (swinelike H1N1 subtype influenza A virus) spread worldwide and resulted in an estimated 50 million deaths [4]. The second influenza A pandemic occurred in 1957 when a new H2N2 influenza virus emerged in several Asian countries and was associated with an estimated one million deaths. The last influenza A pandemic of the twentieth century occurred in 1968, caused by a new human H3N2 virus. This pandemic occurred in Asian Pacific countries and was associated with an estimated one million deaths [5]. The emergence of the new influenza virus strains in these three influenza A pandemics involved gene reassortment of two proximal viruses and virus mutation in response to adapting pressures to facilitate replication [4,5]

Over the past decade, the emergence of avian influenza A (H5N1) virus has threatened human lives, public health, and infection-control practices worldwide. The capacity of viral adaptation from animals to humans, along with plausible human-to-human transmission, enhances global concerns for avian influenza H5N1 as the potential source of the next influenza pandemic. Prevention and control of spread of influenza has become an important global issue with the goals of reduction in the impact of infection and effective preparedness for the next influenza pandemic. This chapter reviews the epidemiology of influenza in healthcare facilities, risk factors for influenza acquisition and transmission, clinical manifestation of influenza, rapid diagnosis and five key components of strategic infection-control preparedness for influenza, especially in resource-limited settings.

EPIDEMIOLOGY

Influenza epidemics usually occur in the winter in the northern and southern hemispheres and may be seen year round in the tropics, with peak activity during the rainy season. The epidemics result in significant morbidity and mortality, usually reported as pneumonia, influenza-related hospitalizations, and deaths. Globally, it is estimated that 3 to 5 million cases of severe illnesses and approximately 250,000 to 500,000 deaths are caused by influenza each year [6]. The majority of cases are in vulnerable populations such as the elderly or the very young. In the United States (US), influenza has caused more than 100,000 hospitalizations and nearly 51,000 deaths annually [7,8]. Because of the lack of efficient surveillance programs in resource-limited settings, the impact of influenza on morbidity and mortality is difficult to assess in these settings [9]. In Thailand, 64–91 cases per 100,000 persons were reported annually during the years 1993–2002, and the annual rate of influenza-related hospitalizations was estimated to be 21 per 100,00 persons [10]. The lower rate of morbidity and mortality in Thailand compared with that of the US likely reflects the underreporting of milder cases, lack of routine testing for influenza, and limitations associated with national surveillance [9]. Nonetheless, this population-based estimate permits a benchmark comparison with US surveillance data and serves as an estimate of influenza burden in an avian influenza (H5N1) endemic region.

Influenza A viruses circulate worldwide. The influenza A subtype H3N2 is predominant and associated with outbreaks in most countries, while a lower magnitude of circulating influenza A (H1) and B viruses may attribute to less frequent outbreaks from these strains [1]. In the US, influenza surveillance during 2004-2005 detected 75.4% of isolates were influenza A and 24.6% were influenza B [11]. Among the influenza A isolates, 99.7% were subtype H3N2 and 0.3% were subtype H1. During the same period, surveillance in Thailand revealed that influenza A and B account for 74.0% and 26.0% of all isolates respectively. H3N2 was the predominant subtype (66.2%), followed by H1 (31.7%) and H5N1 avian influenza (2.1%) [12]. An excess in influenza-related hospitalizations and deaths has been observed during epidemics of influenza A H3N2, whereas influenza B and to a less extent influenza A H1N1 viruses have occasionally been associated with excess mortality [1].

An influenza epidemic is usually confined to one geographic location such as a city, town, county, or community. The outbreaks usually begin abruptly, reach a peak in 2–3 weeks, and last about 5–6 weeks. The first indicator of an influenza epidemic is usually case detection of respiratory tract infections in children and/or nursing home residents, followed by cases of influenza-like illnesses among adults and eventually hospital admissions for pneumonia, chronic obstructive pulmonary disease exacerbation, and congestive heart failure [1]. A single strain of influenza virus usually prevails during an epidemic. However, two different strains with a single subtype, or two different influenza A subtypes, occasionally circulate simultaneously [13]. Rarely, concomitant outbreaks of influenza A and B or simultaneous outbreaks of influenza A and other respiratory viruses have been reported [14].

In healthcare settings, influenza outbreaks have predominantly been reported among patients in either acute-care or long-term care facilities. Outbreaks in acute-care settings have involved patients in pediatric, neonatology, transplantation, oncology, and intensive care units (ICUs), while older persons are commonly infected in long-term care facilities [15,16]. The transmission of influenza virus in these settings is dynamic and complex given the relatively close proximity of sick persons cared for by small groups of HCP in confined geographic units. Patients admitted with community-acquired influenza are usually the main source of the nosocomial spread of the virus, especially if case detection is delayed or does not prospectively occur – hence delaying the initiation of effective infection-control measures. Additionally, persons in contact with the infected patients, such as HCP and visitors, are important source of influenza infection and viral transmission [15,17,18]. One study reported that up to 35.3% of unvaccinated HCP may develop influenza during community epidemics with a majority (76.6%) continuing to work while ill [18]. In a study from Thailand the attack rates for influenza A subtype H3N2 were 18-24% among HCP during three healthcare-associated outbreaks [15].

Table 1. Risk factors associated with excess hospitalization, morbidity, and mortality from community–associated and healthcare-associated influenza viruses

Community- and healthcare-associated acquisition	Healthcare-associated acquisition
Cardiopulmonary diseases	Prolonged hospitalization
Neuromuscular disorders	Low birth weight infant
Renal diseases	Low gestational age infant
Chronic metabolic diseases	Prolonged mechanical ventilator support
Hemoglobinopathies	Crowded wards
Malignancy	Understaffing
Immunocompromised status	
HIV infection	
Women in the 2nd or 3rd trimester of pregnancy	

Risk factors for influenza acquisition. The highest incidence of influenza infection is among children who subsequently serve as reservoirs for transmission of infection to adults [16]. However, mortality is generally highest among older adults [1]. Risk factors related to hospitalization, morbidity, and mortality for both community-associated and healthcare-associated influenza infections are summarized in Table 1. Chronic medical morbidities and immunocompromised status are important risk factors for both community- and healthcare-associated influenza [1,16,17,19], while prolonged hospitalization, ventilator support, crowded wards, and understaffing predispose to healthcare-associated influenza infection [16,17]

Routes of transmission. Influenza A and B can be transmitted from person-to-person via a number of routes [6,20]. The primary transmission route is via large contagious respiratory droplets (>5 μm) as a consequence of coughing or sneezing by infected hosts with subsequent exposure to the nasal mucosa, conjunctiva, or mouth of susceptible persons usually defined as persons within a three-foot radius of the infected host. Second, airborne transmission may occur by the inhalation of small droplets (<5 μm) that persist in the air for prolonged periods of time. Lastly, transmission can occur via direct interpersonal contact between the infected person and an unvaccinated person, e.g., hand-shaking, or indirect contact via contact with viable influenza virus on contaminated, common-touch surfaces.

H5N1 avian influenza. Influenza A avian influenza (H5N1) virus has transitioned from infectivity of poultry to humans in Asia, Africa, and the Middle East. Despite widespread environmental and animal exposures, avian influenza H5N1 infection among humans remains very rare [21]. Global efforts to minimize human exposures include international surveillance, rapid-test diagnostics, and aggressive culling of infected animals. Human case detection of avian influenza (H5N1) is a key activity for the World Health Organization, with attributable mortality estimated at 50–90% worldwide. Most confirmed cases have been associated with either sick poultry or contaminated environmental exposures in community settings [5]. Human-to-human transmission remains theoretically plausible, although only one possible case has been reported to date [22]. There have been no reports of healthcare-associated transmission or outbreak of H5N1 influenza. However, low yet existent anti-H5 antibody titers have been detected in HCP exposed to patients infected with avian influenza H5N1 [23,24]. Risk factors for acquisition of H5N1 virus include history of close contact with live or dead domestic fowl and wild birds, traveler from endemic areas, unprotected contact with persons suspected fro H5N1 virus infection, history of travel to a country or territory with reported H5N1 virus activity, and occupational exposure in a domestic fowl worker, worker in a domestic fowl processing plant, domestic fowl culler, worker in a live animal market, chef working with live or recently killed domestic fowl, dealer or trader in pet birds, HCP, and laboratory technician processing samples possibly containing influenza A (H5N1) virus [25]. It is important that patients with potential exposures or clinical suspicion of avian influenza infection be triaged and cared for with appropriate infection-control practices.

CLINICAL MANIFESTATION

Clinical manifestations of influenza infection are protean and range from asymptomatic illnesses to multi-system organ failure to death. Early case detection of avian influenza H5N1 clinical presentations is crucial to successful treatment and the potential for abrogating viral spread in healthcare settings.

Uncomplicated cases. Typical presentations of influenza begin with an abrupt onset of high fever, chills, headache, myalgias, arthralgias, malaise, and anorexia after a one- to two-day incubation period. Upper respiratory symptoms such as a dry cough, sore throat, nasal obstruction, and nasal discharge may also be present at the onset of illness, yet only 50% of infected adults have both systemic and respiratory symptoms [20]. Furthermore, otitis media, febrile seizures, and gastrointestinal symptoms can be found in infants and young children while older adults may present with high fever and confusion without any respiratory complaints [1,16]. Fever typically lasts three days but may persist for up to eight days or recur as a second peak on the third and fourth days in a small number of cases. Systemic symptoms usually resolve by the time the fever subsides. However, a dry cough and clear nasal discharge may persist for one to two weeks [16]. Flushed face, moist and hot skin, watery and reddened eyes, clear nasal discharge, hyperemic nasopharyngeal membranes, and small, tender cervical lymph nodes are common physical findings. Children tend to have higher peak temperatures and more cervical lymphadenopathy than adults [26]. Abnormal chest findings such as rhonchi and localized rales are uncommon. Illnesses caused by influenza B are usually milder or similar to that described for influenza A infection while influenza C infection often causes an afebrile, common-cold syndrome and rarely produces systemic symptoms [1].

Complicated cases. Pulmonary complications are the most common amongst complicated influenza infections. The illness begins with typical symptoms of influenza, followed by a rapid progression to cough, dyspnea, hypoxemia, and typical clinical presentations of either primary influenza viral pneumonia or secondary bacterial pneumonia. The etiologies of bacterial pneumonias are usually *Streptococcus pneumoniae, Hemophilus influenzae,* or *Staphylococcus aureus.* Bilateral rhonchi or rales on physical examination and bronchioalveolar infiltrates on chest radiograph can be evident in cases with primary influenza viral pneumonia while localized areas of rales, consolidation and alveolar infiltration are typical for secondary bacterial pneumonia. Other complications include croup, exacerbation of chronic obstructive pulmonary disease, myositis, myocarditis, pericarditis, cardiomyopathy, Guillian-Barré syndrome, transverse myelitis, encephalitis, and Reye's syndrome [1,16,20]. In severe cases, acute respiratory distress syndrome and multi-system organ failure occur and are associated with higher risk for death. Patients with more severe infection and immunocompromised conditions such as malignancies, bone marrow transplantation, solid organ transplantation, and HIV infection have more prolonged clinical illnesses, higher mortality, and longer episodes of viral shedding than immunocompetent hosts [27-29].

H5N1 avian influenza. Mild cases of infection have been more likely to be reported in young children whereas case detection in adults has primarily been hospital-based [30]. Early clinical presentations are similar to those associated with influenza A and B except for more frequent watery diarrhea. Atypical manifestations include diarrhea, nausea, vomiting, seizures, and rapid clinical progression to coma [31,32]. Chest radiograph findings for primary avian influenza pneumonia are more varied than those of influenza A and B and include interstitial infiltration, patchy lobar infiltration, lobar collapse, air bronchograms, and diffuse bilateral ground-glass opacities [5].

DIAGNOSIS

Early recognition of an epidemic of influenza in the community is essential to control and prevent spread of the virus into healthcare settings. Definitive diagnosis of influenza is warranted to guide infection-control practices and policies in healthcare settings [20]. For patients coming from a community where an influenza outbreak has been identified, the triad clinical presentations of fever, respiratory symptoms, and constitutional symptoms had a diagnostic sensitivity of 60% for influenza [33]. Nonetheless, clinical presentations should prompt diagnostic testing via one of several available laboratory tests including rapid antigen detection assays, nucleic acid amplification methods, immunofluorescence, serology titers, or viral cultures. Various types of respiratory specimens can be obtained - nasopharyngeal swab, throat swab, nasal wash, nasal aspirate, sputum, bronchial wash, or sera. Notably, multiple, adequate, technically-correct, pretreatment specimens should be procured to minimize false-negative diagnoses [34].

Rapid antigen detection. A variety of techniques have been used to speed the diagnosis of influenza. Rapid antigen detection tests using immunological methodologies are widely used in point-of-care settings such as emergency departments, ICUs, physicians' offices, and as a component of surveillance [20]. These tests are relatively simple to perform and have turn-around results within 0.5 to six hours [1,16]. The tests are very specific (85–100%) but of 40–80% sensitivity [35-38]. Higher sensitivity has been noted in children compared with adults, in earlier phases of influenza illness, and in nasal swab and aspirates relative to lower respiratory tract specimens [1,38].

Nucleic acid amplification. Nucleic acid hybridization and polymerase chain reaction (PCR) amplification are gaining widespread use due to sensitivity and specificity approaching 100% as well as capacity for multi-pathogen detection. However, the PCR techniques are more labor intensive, technically-demanding, require specialized laboratory equipment, and results need to be interpreted carefully as specimen contamination may occur and positive results may represent non-viable, non-infectious viruses [16,39-41].

Viral culture. The viral culture is the gold standard test for definitive influenza diagnosis [20]. Over 90% of positive cultures can be detected within three days and the remainder within five to seven days [1,20]. The culture is helpful in defining the etiology of local outbreaks and provides information about serotype and genotype for the annual preparation of vaccines as well as antiviral drug resistance [1,16, 20]. However, culture-based methods are time-consuming and culture is not an appropriate point-of-care diagnostic test in acute-care settings.

Serology. Confirmatory diagnostic testing of influenza infection can be conducted by testing sera for IgM and IgG antibodies using complement fixation or hemagglutination inhibition. The usefulness of the serology in point-of-care settings is limited, since paired acute and convalescent sera obtained over a 7–21 day interval is required.

H5N1 avian influenza. PCR has been the best rapid method for the initial diagnosis of H5N1 influenza [42]. Specimens obtained as tracheal aspirates have higher viral loads and diagnostic yields than those from the upper respiratory tract, with results available in four to six hours [21]. Multiple pretreatment nasal and tracheal specimens are recommended for higher diagnostic yields [42]. Commercially-available rapid influenza antigen detection assays for H5N1 influenza have poor clinical sensitivity and are significantly less sensitive than viral culture [21,43]. The detection of serum anti-H5 antibodies is used for retrospective diagnostic confirmation and epidemiological investigations with the same limited utility for rapid diagnosis in acute-care settings as serologic tests for influenza A and B [21].

INFLUENZA PREPAREDNESS AND CONTROL

Control of influenza in resource-limited healthcare settings can be accomplished by five components of influenza preparedness: 1) appropriate infection-control measures using existing infrastructure, 2) targeted educational programs, 3) healthcare administrative support, 4) access to a nationally-coordinated laboratory system for early and rapid influenza detection, and 5) adequate stocks of antiviral therapy and vaccinations. These strategies can readily be adjusted according to resource allocation in each healthcare setting.

1. Appropriate infection-control measures using existing infrastructure. Appropriate infection-control strategies are keys to prevention and control of influenza in healthcare settings and the main goal is to minimize the risk of influenza transmission within the facilities. Although recommendations for influenza control are available from the US Centers for Disease Control and Prevention (CDC) and the World Health Organization (WHO), adopting or modifying these recommendations has practical challenges that need to be considered [44,45]. In middle-income and developing countries, infection-control resources may vary considerably depending on hospital policies, disease prevalence, local priorities, personnel availability, and financial constraints [46,47]. Relevant infection-control measures for influenza include

   A. ***Basic infection-control measures.*** Droplet precaution is generally required for influenza prevention while air-borne precaution may be necessary for H5N1 avian influenza given the unclear nature of transmission dynamics [48]. The basic measures include hand hygiene and personal protection equipment (PPE) such as masks, gowns and gloves. Hand washing with water and soap or alcohol-based antiseptics should be performed before and after patient contact [49]. PPE should be strictly used in cases with confirmed or suspected influenza [45]. Compliance to these basic measures and correct use of PPE are necessary for reducing influenza transmission and needs to be monitored [17].

   B. ***Precautions for households and close contacts.*** Individuals with household or close contacts with suspected or confirmed influenza either in a community or a healthcare facility should be informed of the index case's diagnosis and received appropriate vaccine and/or antiviral prophylaxis. If and when infections develop, these individuals should be treated with antiviral therapy and advised to wear a face mask, reduce social interactions, and avoid contact with at-risk patients. Restrictions in visitation of family members and friends should be prudently assessed to minimize risk of transmission.

   C. ***Environmental control.*** Viral shedding of influenza can occur for seven days after the onset of symptoms in adults and for weeks in infants and immunocompromised individuals [6,49]. Hence, environmental control of influenza is difficult in healthcare facilities, especially since influenza viruses can persist after drying, become re-aerosolized during floor sweeping, and survive for 24–48 hours on nonporous surfaces [50]. A viable virus can be spread to the skin and lead to cross-infection of patients via the hands of HCP [51]. Per the Healthcare Infection Control Practice Advisory Committee of the CDC, Environmental Protection Agency (EPA)-approved disinfectant or detergent-disinfectant is recommended for decontamination of environmental surfaces contaminated with influenza viruses [52]. However, there are no clinical trials specifically assessing the efficacy of environmental cleaning for reduction of influenza transmission and illnesses in healthcare settings.

   D. ***Involvement of specialists.*** The interdisciplinary expertise of specialists from infectious diseases, pulmonary medicine, critical care medicine, and emergency care promote best practices for screening of suspected cases of influenza and early recognition of typical and atypical cases [48]. Since healthcare providers with the least experience are often the first to evaluate and encounter influenza cases, delayed recognition of early case detection and missed opportunities to minimize disease transmission can potentially occur. Additionally, early involvement of specialists promotes procurement of adequate specimens for diagnostics, correct interpretation of laboratory results, early treatment, appropriate prophylaxis, and control of viral spread.

   2. Targeted educational programs, ongoing preparedness training, and effective systems of communication. Although HCP play an important role in minimizing influenza transmission in healthcare settings, opportunities exist to promote health education and health behavior related to hand hygiene, use of PPE, and receipt of annual influenza vaccines [46,48,53]. Education and training programs for influenza control should be implemented for all HCP prior to the first day of work and may be tailored into the occupational health and safety programs and continuous medical education programs of the healthcare setting. Each healthcare facility should effectively communicate with HCP about influenza outbreaks, influenza strains, antiviral resistance, effective control measures, problems encountered at other institutions, and public health initiatives. These examples of streamlined communication promote early case detection and implementation of appropriate pharmaceutical and non-pharmaceutical interventions [54].

3. Healthcare administrative support. Implementation of effective infection control and occupational-health strategies is needed within healthcare settings for influenza control. Healthcare administrative support should include routine occupational health and safety program for HCP, appropriate infection-control expertise, provision of adequate supplies for hand hygiene and PPE for HCP, and epidemiological resources for the prevention and control of influenza. Capacitance building for healthcare systems in resource-limited settings is a challenge yet the number of physicians, nurses, laboratory technicians, and hospital beds estimated for an influenza pandemic need to be considered. In addition, the availability of sufficient essential medical supplies, such as gloves, masks, gowns, syringes, antipyretics, and antimicrobial agents needs to be anticipated for pandemic preparedness.

4. Access to a nationally-coordinated laboratory system for early and rapid influenza detection. Early detection of influenza-exposed individuals can be enhanced by surveillance and monitoring programs. Although cost-benefit analyses of such programs have not been conducted in resource-limited settings, a nationally-conducted laboratory system for influenza is feasible in these settings, increases the number of adequate confirmatory tests, decreases the median time for specimen procurement, and decreases the specimen transfer times [55]. Additionally, information about emerging influenza virus strains and antiviral resistance patterns can be shared and expedite collaborations for annual vaccine and antiviral treatment recommendations [46]. Individuals, especially unvaccinated HCP exposed to infected cases, should be monitored for influenza and influenza-like illnesses and provided with appropriate vaccine and/or antiviral prophylaxis. As a component of occupational health and safety, all exposed HCP who become ill should be furloughed. Patients with suspected or confirmed influenza should be isolated from high-risk patients and received antiviral therapy. While preparedness varies among countries and gaps in secure systems exist even in developed countries, coordinated laboratory systems are feasible [57]. The WHO urges countries to develop and implement national pandemic preparedness plans to mitigate the health and social effects of a pandemic [56].

5. Adequate stocks of antiviral therapy and influenza vaccination

- **Antiviral therapy**

Four antiviral agents are available for prevention and treatment of influenza—two adamantanes (amantadine and rimantadine) and two neuraminidases inhibitors (NI; zanamivir and oseltamivir). Zanamivir is administered by inhalation and the other three drugs are only available in oral form. The adamantanes are only effective for influenza A infections while the NI are active against both influenza A and B viruses. Adverse reactions associated with the NI are usually mild and include nausea and emesis for oseltamivir and bronchospasm for zanamivir. The adamantanes reportedly have a 13–17% discontinuation rate due to central nervous system side effects such as anxiety, insomnia, impaired thinking, confusion, lightheadedness, and hallucination especially in the elderly [58,59]. Notably, these side effects are not as frequently observed in rimantadine as in amantadine [58]. Given the potential for influenza A drug resistance, the use of adamantanes is limited [60]. In the US, adamantane resistance increased significantly from ≤2% during 1995–2002 to 92% during 2005–2006 for influenza A (H3N2) after which the CDC recommendations were not to use the drugs for treatment and prevention of influenza until evidence of susceptibility is reestablished [20,61,62]. In a global-based assessment of influenza A isolates from 1994–2005, 61% of adamantane-resistant isolates were from Asia. The potential contributors to adamantane resistance may be the overuse of over-the-counter antiviral drugs, alleged administration of the drugs to poultry, and adamantine use during the severe acute respiratory syndrome (SARS) epidemic [63,64]. However, the emergence of resistance may vary depending on the viral strains. In one study there was no antiviral resistance in influenza A (H1N1) viral isolates compared with a 65% rate of resistance in influenza A (H3N2) strains [65]. Compared to the adamantanes, NI resistance is much lower. Influenza A (H1N1) oseltamivir resistance differed by geographic region—20% in Europe, 13% in Canada, 9% in the US, and 5% in Japan [66]. The resistance to oseltamivir is attributable to point mutations commonly occurring in the N1 neuramiidase [67]. This phenomenon occurs in the absence of selective drug pressure, was effectively transmitted from person to person, and observed in oseltamivir-resistant influenza A (H5N1) isolates [67,68]. In contrast, zanamivir retains its full activity against oseltamivir-resistant influenza A (H5N1) isolates [67].

Table 2. Targeted groups and recommended antiviral agents for influenza prophylaxis

Influenza A and B		Avian influenza (H5N1)
Targeted groups	Doses	Targeted groups (and doses)
• Individuals at high risk who receive influenza vaccine within two weeks of influenza case detection in community • Individuals expected to mount an inadequate response to the vaccine, such as immunocompromised patients, advanced HIV-infected patients • Individuals at high risk who receive vaccine with strain poorly-matched to circulating influenza strains • Individuals at high risk in whom the vaccine is contraindicated • Non-immunized close contacts of high-risk individuals • Care providers to those at high risks, e.g., unvaccinated or received vaccine strains poorly-matched to circulating influenza strains • Unvaccinated individuals in influenza outbreaks in close settings or institutions	Oseltamivir[a] • 30 mg/day (wt. ≤15 kgs) • 45 mg/day (wt. >15–23 kgs) • 60 mg/day (wt. >23–40 kgs) • 75 mg/day (wt. >40 kgs) Zanamivir[b] • 10 mg/day (inhalation) Amantadine and rimantadine[c] • 5 mg/kg/day (not >150 mg/day; age 1–9 years) • 100 mg twice daily (age 10–64 years) • 100 mg/day (age ≥65 years)	Recommended: • Household contacts or family of a patient with H5N1 influenza infection (oseltamivir 75 mg/day) Considered: • Individuals involving in handling sick animals or decontaminating affected environments without appropriate protection • Individuals in contact with sick animals infected with H5N1 influenza or implicated in human cases • Healthcare workers with close exposure (e.g., intubation) to a patient with diagnosed H5N1 influenza or a suspected case • Laboratory workers with unprotected exposure to a virus-containing sample

NOTE:

[a] For individuals aged ≥ 1 year old

[b] For individuals aged ≥ 5 years old

[c] Centers of Disease Control and Prevention has recommended against the use for influenza prophylaxis in the US.

Antiviral agents for influenza prophylaxis. Influenza chemoprophylaxis with antiviral drugs is needed in individuals who have not been immunized. The drugs can be administered simultaneously with the trivalent inactivated vaccine (TIV) to provide protection until post-vaccination host-immunity develops. In healthcare settings, antiviral prophylaxis can be used in different schemes, including post-exposure prophylaxis for close contacts, outbreak-initiated prophylaxis, and prophylaxis for high-risk patients. Targeted groups and recommended doses of antiviral drugs for influenza A and B are shown in Table 2 [21,61,69]. The duration of prophylaxis is 7–10 days after exposure to infected individuals and 2 weeks for unvaccinated, high-risk individuals and for persons in outbreaks who could not receive the vaccines or did not develop adequate post-vaccine immune response [69,70]. For avian influenza A (H5N1), household contacts of the infected patients should receive prophylaxis for 7–10 days [21]. Prophylactic therapy with oseltamivir or zanamivir was shown to reduce the odds of developing influenza A and B by 70-90% depending on the population and adopted strategies [71]. However, the effectiveness of oseltamivir in H5N1 avian influenza prevention has not been studied in humans. The recommendation is based on studies of prophylaxis for seasonal influenza [71].

Table 3. Recommended doses and duration of antiviral therapy for influenza

Antiviral agents		Influenza A	Influenza B	H5N1 influenza
Oseltamivir[a]	Doses	30 mg twice daily (wt. ≤15 kgs) 45 mg twice daily (wt. >15–23 kgs) 60 mg twice daily (wt. >23–40 kgs) 75 mg twice daily (wt. >40 kgs)		75 mg twice daily 150 mg twice daily[b]
	Duration	5 days		5-10 days[c]
Zanamivir[d]	Doses	10 mg inhale twice daily		No data
	Duration	5 days		No data
Amantadine and rimantadine[e]	Doses	• 5 mg/kg/day (not >150 mg/day; age 1–9 yrs) • 100 mg twice daily (age 10–64 yrs) • 100 mg/day (age ≥65 yrs)	No activity	No data
	Duration	5 days		

NOTE:
[a] For individuals aged ≥ 1 year old, no pediatric dose recommended for H5N1 influenza
[b] Dose considered in severe cases
[c] Prolonged duration considered in severe cases
[d] For individuals aged ≥ 7 years old
[e] Centers of Disease Control and Prevention has recommended against the use for influenza treatment in the US.

Antiviral agents for influenza therapy. The recommended doses and duration of antiviral therapy for influenza A and B are shown in Table 3 [21,61,69]. Treatment with oseltamivir within 36–48 hours of the onset of symptoms provides benefits in terms of reduction in length of illnesses by 0.5–1.5 days, prevention of secondary complications related to influenza and minimization of risk for viral transmission in healthcare settings [60]. Zanamivir was associated with a 2-day reduction in time-to-resolution of symptoms in high-risk patients aged $\geq$ 60 years old and in children aged 5–12 years [71,72]. Given the high levels of resistance to the adamantanes in recent years, these antiviral agents should be used for influenza A treatment only if the susceptibility is clearly established among circulating viruses. For the avian influenza (H5N1) infections, early treatment with oseltamivir is recommended due to the benefits of improved survival [21]. A higher dose and more prolonged duration of therapy may be required given the high levels of viral replication [21]. However, the optimal doses and duration of oseltamivir therapy remain unknown. In geographic areas where H5N1 viruses are likely to be susceptible to adamantanes, combination therapy of oseltamivir and amantadine is reasonable, especially for severe cases given the higher survival rates and inhibition of viral replication in internal organs compared with monotherpy in animal models [21,73]. Zanamivir may be an alternate treatment option. However, it has not been studies in humans and suboptimal drug delivery via inhalation route is a concern for patients with severe infection and pulmonary comorbidities [21].

In resource-limited settings, the availability of antiviral agents is limited and the stockpiles of these drugs are small and insufficient for prevention and treatment during an influenza epidemic or pandemic [46]. The use of NI, especially oseltamivir, may not be feasible for low-income countries given the costs and availability of drugs. Limited data regarding the emergence of drug resistance in influenza strains in these settings poses a significant risk of using inactive antiviral agents. A study from Thailand reported that physicians who believed that rapid tests reliably predicted H5N1 infections were less-likely to prescribe antiviral agents while physicians who believed that antiviral agents reduced mortality were more-likely to prescribe antiviral agents [47]. These findings suggest that appropriate early antiviral prescribing practices and belief in antiviral efficacy are necessary components of influenza preparedness planning in resource-limited settings.

- **Influenza vaccination**
  Annual vaccination against influenza is the major and most-effective measure available for control of influenza [1,16]. Advanced techniques have been used in vaccine development to increase efficacy and decrease adverse reactions to influenza A and B. Vaccine investigations for H5N1 avian influenza have focused on an optimal vaccine antigens, vaccine vectors, doses, adjuvants, and targeted antibody level production [21]. Two common types of influenza A and B vaccine currently used include the TIV and the live-attenuated vaccine (LAV). The TIV contains an influenza A (H1N1) virus, A (H3N2) virus, and influenza B virus in the form of the whole virus or split-virus preparation and is administered intramuscularly. The LAV uses a master-attenuated, cold-adopted donor virus and is administered intranasally. TIV has been shown to be effective in the prevention of influenza A and B [74-76]. The protective efficacy of the vaccine is determined by the relationship between the strains in the vaccine and the circulating epidemic viruses (closeness of "fit"). When there is a good antigenic match, the efficacy of TIV has been 50–80% in adults depending on different measurement methods to confirm the influenza diagnosis in the study population [1,74,75], while the efficacy was 70–90% in children [16,77,78]. In addition, the vaccine reduces the rates of physician visits, sick leave, antibiotic use, number of influenza-like illnesses, hospitalization for coronary heart disease and cerebrovascular diseases, risk of all-cause mortality in the elderly and is cost-effective [17,79-83]. TIV has also been shown to be protective in other high-risk groups including HCP and persons with HIV infection [80-82,84]. In children, although the efficacy of TIV in preventing asthma exacerbation is unclear

[85], vaccine administration was associated with reduction in acute otitis media and otitis media with effusion in 6-60-month old day-care children [86]. The LAV has recently been licensed for use in the US. This vaccine offers some potential advantages over TIV, including induction of a mucosal immune response mimicking the response induced by natural influenza virus infection and improved patient vaccination acceptance due to a painless procedure [1]. In one randomized double-blinded controlled trial in adult aged 18–46 years, LAV was less effective in preventing influenza A and B compared with TIV (57% vs. 77%) and the difference in efficacy between the 2 vaccines was mainly due to reduced protection of LAV against influenza B [74] However, in non-comparative studies in children, the efficacy of LAV was 95% against influenza A (H3N1) and 91% against influenza B and one meta-analysis demonstrated that the efficacy of LAV against both types of influenza viruses was approximately 80% [16,87]. Although LAV is more expensive than TIV, it may provide greater heterotypic immunity and be more protective against both well-matched and poorly-matched influenza A viruses in children compared with TIV [88].

Table 4. High-risk groups among children and adults targeted for influenza vaccination

Children	Adults
Children 6–59 months of age	Adult ≥ 50 years old
Children 5–18 years of age[a]	Adults 50–64 years of age[b]
Children who are receiving long-term aspirin therapy	Healthcare personnel at chronic healthcare facilities, providers of home care to persons at high risks[c]
Residents of nursing homes and other chronic care facilities	
Individuals who have chronic pulmonary (including asthma, bronchopulmonary dysplasia, cystic fibrosis), cardiovascular (excluding hypertension), renal, hepatic, hematologic, or metabolic disorders (including diabetes mellitus), asplenia, hemoglobinopathies, or immunocompromised status (including immunosuppression caused by medications or HIV infection)	
Individuals who have any conditions than can compromise respiratory function, or the handling of secretions, or that can increase the risk of aspiration (e.g. cognitive dysfunction, spinal cord injuries, seizure disorders, or other neuromuscular disorders)	
Individuals who will be pregnant during the influenza season	
Household contact of persons in high risk groups	
Individuals who wish to reduce the risk of becoming ill with influenza or of transmitting influenza to others	

NOTE:
[a] Recommendations for this age group to be accomplished by 2009-2010 influenza season
[b] Recommendations for this age group to increase vaccination rate among persons with high-risk conditions
[c] Risks for influenza acquisition and influenza-related complications

The 2007 Advisory Committee on Immunization Practices (ACIP) recommendations for both adults and children target reduction in incidence and transmission of influenza in high-risk patients (Table 4) [61]. Notably, a significant benefit of influenza vaccination for prevention of influenza-like illnesses has been extrapolated from an investigation of HCP at long-term care facilities [89]. Influenza vaccine is generally well-tolerated in adults, with local side effects such as soreness at the injection site documented in 60-80% of vaccinees while systemic reactions such as malaise, flu-like illnesses, and fever were uncommon [1]. The post-vaccination Guillian Barré syndrome (GBS) and GBS-related mortality have been very rare [1]. In addition, TIV is safe to administer to adults and children with asthma and does not increase the risk of exacerbation [90]. However, hypersensitivity to eggs is a contraindication for receipt of both TIV and LAV. Children less than two years of age and persons on long-term salicylate therapy, with known or suspected immunodeficiency, asthma, advanced HIV infection (CD4 <200 cells/μl.), pregnancy, history of GBS and other conditions considered to be risk factors for severe influenza infection or complications of influenza should not receive LAV [61,91,92]. Because influenza activity can peak anytime between winter and early spring and antibodies against the viruses typically develop two weeks post vaccination, the optimal time for vaccination is one to two months prior to winter in the northern and southern hemispheres. However, in tropical regions, where influenza occurs throughout the year, the vaccine can be given year round.

In resource-limited settings, there are some difficulties in influenza vaccine implementation as a measure of influenza control. First, as estimated by WHO [93], the worldwide vaccine production capacity for influenza vaccine is 350 million doses per year, which is clearly not sufficient for global vaccination coverage. To date, most vaccines are supplied to developed countries and are of limited availability in developing countries [46]. Second, in Thailand, the vaccine is available to persons who can afford it and, hence, often restricted to private healthcare settings. In addition, the vaccine is mainly distributed to university hospitals, the Thai Ministry of Public Health, and private sectors such as hotels and the airline industries [9]. It is estimated that less than 1% of the general Thai population are currently vaccinated for influenza and no systematic assessment of influenza vaccine coverage has been conducted in Thailand [9]. Third, although a study from Thailand suggests potential benefit of annual influenza vaccination of ICU HCP for protection of at-risk patients, less than 50% of HCP received the vaccine due to reported concern for adverse reactions and beliefs of not being susceptible to influenza [15, 94]. Fourth, lack of knowledge and attitude of influenza vaccine in the community is an important barrier for an effective influenza control program in healthcare settings. A study from Thailand suggested that parents of pre-school children had misperceptions that childhood influenza vaccination was not effective and caused allergic reactions and asthma [95]. Lastly, healthcare facilities in resource-limited settings experience challenges in implementing immunization programs due to limited resources in an era when vaccines and antiviral agents require full-scale implementation of pharmaceutical industries and international mechanisms to share vaccines and drugs at a low cost.

CONCLUSION

Influenza has become an important infectious disease given its worldwide clinical and economic impact on population health. Outbreaks, epidemics, and pandemics caused by influenza viruses have threatened human lives and healthcare system for centuries and require appropriate interventions and plans that are feasible according to each healthcare facility's available resources. Strategies involving early case detection entail clinical recognition, rapid laboratory testing, effective prophylactic vaccines, access to antiviral therapy, and appropriate infection-control measures. Regional, national, and international collaborations are essential to optimize global influenza preparedness.

REFERENCES

[1]   Treanor JJ. Influenza virus. In: Mandell GL, Bennett JE, Dolin R, editors. Mandell, Bennett, & Dolin: Principles and Practice of Infectious Diseases 6th ed. 2005. Available at www.mdconsult.com. Accessed October 15, 2008.

[2]   Hirsch A. *Handbook of Geographical and Historical Pathology*. 2nd ed. London: New Sydenham Society; 1883.

[3]   Thomson D, Thomson R. *Influenza*, New York, Ann Pickett-Thomas Research Labs; 1933.

[4]   Tumpey TM, Basler CF, Aguilar PV, et al. Characterization of the reconstructed 1918 Spanish influenza pandemic virus. *Science*, 2005 Oct 7, 310, 77-80.

[5]   Khawcharoenporn T, Mundy LM, Apisarnthanarak A. Epidemiology and risk factors for avian influenza. In: Tambyah P, Leung P, editors. *Bird Flu: A Rising Pandemic in Asia and Beyond?* Singapore: World Scientific Publishing; 2006; p. 53-68.

[6]   Rothman RE, Hsieh YH, Yang S. Communicable respiratory threats in the ED: tuberculosis, influenza, SARS, and other aerosolized infections. *Emerg Med Clin North Am*, 2006 Nov, 24: 989-1017.

[7]   Thompson WW, Shay DK, Weintraub E, et al. Mortality associated with influenza and respiratory syncytial virus in the United States. *JAMA*, 2003 Jan 8, 289: 179-186.

[8]   World Health Organization. Influenza. March 2003. Available at: http://www.who.int. eres.library.manoa.hawaii.edu/mediacentre/factsheets/2003/fs211/en/. Accessed January 1, 2009.

[9]   Simmerman JM, Thawatsupha P, Kingnate D, Fukuda K, Chaising A, Dowell SF. Influenza in Thailand: a case study for middle income countries. *Vaccine*, 2004 Nov 25, 23: 182-187.

[10]   Thailand Public Health Statistics. 3rd ed. Bangkok, Alpha Research; 2001.

[11]   Centers for Disease Control and Prevention. Update: Influenza activity--United States and worldwide, 2004-05 season. MMWR Morb Mortal Wkly *Rep*, 2005 Jul 1, 54: 631-634.

[12]   Waicharoen S, Thawatsupha P, Chittaganpitch M, Maneewong P, Thanadachakul T, Sawanpanyalert P. Influenza viruses circulating in Thailand in 2004 and 2005. *Jpn J Infect Dis*, 2008 Jul, 61: 321-323.

[13]   Kendal AP, Schieble J, Cooney MK, Chin J, Foy HM, Noble GR.. Co-circulation of two influenza A (H3N2) antigenic variants detected by virus surveillance in individual communities. *Am J Epidemiol*, 1978 Oct, 108: 308-311.

[14]   Falsey AR, Cunningham CK, Barker WH, et al. A comparison of respiratory syncytial virus and influenza infection in the hospitalized elderly. In: *Annual meeting of the Infectious Disease Society of America, 1993*. New Orleans, La; 1993.

[15]   Apisarnthanarak A, Puthavathana P, Kitphati R, Auewarakul P, Mundy LM. Outbreaks of influenza A among nonvaccinated healthcare workers: implications for resource-limited settings. *Infect Control Hosp Epidemiol*, 2008 Aug, 29: 777-780.

[16]   Maltezou HC, Drancourt M. Nosocomial influenza in children. *J Hosp Infect*, 2003 Oct, 55: 83-91.

[17]   Salgado CD, Farr BM, Hall KK, Hayden FG. Influenza in the acute hospital setting. *Lancet Infect Dis*, 2002 Mar, 2: 145-155.

[18]   Cunney RJ, Bialachowski A, Thornley D, Smaill FM, Pennie RA. An outbreak of influenza A in a neonatal intensive care unit. *Infect Control Hosp Epidemiol*, 2000 Jul, 21: 449-454.

[19]   Apisarnthanarak A, Puthavathana P, Mundy LM. Risk factors and outcomes of influenza A (H3N2) pneumonia in an area where avian influenza (H5N1) is endemic. *Infect Control Hosp Epidemiol*, 2007 Apr, 28: 479-482.

[20]   Beigel JH. Influenza. *Crit Care Med*, 2008 Sep, 36: 2660-2666.

[21]   Writing Committee of the Second World Health Organization Consultation on Clinical Aspects of Human Infection with Avian Influenza A (H5N1) Virus, Abdel-Ghafar AN, Chotpitayasunondh T, Gao Z, et al. Update on avian influenza A (H5N1) virus infection in humans. *N Engl J Med*, 2008 Jan 17, 358: 261-273.

[22]   Ungchusak K, Auewarakul P, Dowell SF, et al. Probable person-to-person transmission of avian influenza A (H5N1). *N Engl J Med*, 2005 Jan 27, 352: 333-340.

[23]   Chan PK. Outbreak of avian influenza A(H5N1) virus infection in Hong Kong in 1997. *Clin Infect Dis*, 2002 May 1, 34: S58-S64.

[24]   Apisarnthanarak A, Erb S, Stephenson I, et al. Seroprevalence of anti-H5 antibody among Thai health care workers after exposure to avian influenza (H5N1) in a tertiary care center. *Clin Infect Dis*, 2005 Jan 15, 40: e16-e18.

[25]   Beigel JH, Farrar J, Han AM, et al; Writing Committee of the World Health Organization (WHO) Consultation on Human Influenza A/H5. Avian influenza A (H5N1) infection in humans. *N Engl J Med*, 2005 Sep 29, 353: 1374-1385.

[26]   Jordan WS, Denny FW, Badger GF. A study of illness in a group of Cleveland families: XVII. The occurrence of Asian influenza. *Am J Hyg*, 1958 Sep, 68: 160.

[27]   Ison MG, Gnann JW Jr, Nagy-Agren S, et al. Safety and efficacy of nebulized zanamivir in hospitalized patients with serious influenza. *Antivir Ther*, 2003 Jun, 8: 183-190.

[28]   Klimov AI, Rocha E, Hayden FG, et al. Prolonged shedding of amantadine-resistant influenzae A viruses by immunodeficient patients: Detection by polymerase chain reaction-restriction analysis. *J Infect Dis*, 1995 Nov, 172:1352-1355.

[29]   Evans KD, Kline MW. Prolonged influenza A infection responsive to rimantadine therapy in a human immunodeficiency virus-infected child. *Pediatr Infect Dis J*, 1995 April, 14: 332-334.

[30]   Yuen KY, Chan PK, Peiris M, et al. Clinical features and rapid viral diagnosis of human disease associated with avian influenza A H5N1 virus. *Lancet*, 1998 Feb 14, 351: 467-471.

[31]   Apisarnthanarak A, Kitphati R, Thongphubeth K, et al. Atypical avian influenza (H5N1). *Emerg Infect Dis*, 2004 Jul, 10: 1321-1324.

[32]   de Jong MD, Bach VC, Phan TQ, et al. Fatal avian influenza A (H5N1) in a child presenting with diarrhea followed by coma. *N Engl J Med*, 2005 Feb 17, 352: 686-691.

[33] Treanor JJ, Hayden FG, Vrooman PS, et al. Efficacy and safety of the oral neuraminidase inhibitor oseltamivir in treating acute influenza: a randomized controlled trial. US Oral Neuraminidase Study Group. *JAMA*, 2000 Feb 23, 283: 1016-1024.

[34] Apisarnthanarak A, Kitphati R, Mundy LM. Difficulty in the rapid diagnosis of avian influenza A infection: Thailand experience. *Clin Infect Dis*, 2007 May 1, 44: 1252-1253.

[35] Smit M, Beynon KA, Murdoch DR, Jennings LC. Comparison of the NOW Influenza A & B, NOW Flu A, NOW Flu B, and Directigen Flu A+B assays, and immuno-fluorescence with viral culture for the detection of influenza A and B viruses. *Diagn Microbiol Infect Dis*, 2007 Jan, 57: 57-70.

[36] Weinberg A. Evaluation of three influenza A and B rapid antigen detection kits—update. *Clin Diagn Lab Immunol*, 2005 Aug, 12: 1010.

[37] Hurt AC, Alexander R, Hibbert J, Deed N, Barr IG. Performance of six influenza rapid tests in detecting human influenza in clinical specimens. *J Clin Virol*, 2007 Jun, 39: 132-135.

[38] Steininger C, Kundi M, Aberle SW, Aberle JH, Popow-Kraupp T. Effectiveness of reverse transcription-PCR, virus isolation, and enzyme-linked immunosorbent assay for diagnosis of influenza A virus infection in different age groups. *J Clin Microbiol*, 2002 Jun, 40: 2051-2056.

[39] Cox NJ, Subbarao K. Influenza. *Lancet*, 1999 Oct 9, 354: 1277-1282.

[40] Zieger T, Cox NJ. Influenza viruses. In: Murray PR, Baron EJ, Pfaller MA, Tenover FC, Yolken RH, editors. *Manual of clinical microbiology*, 7th ed. Washington, DC: American Society of Microbiology; 1999; p. 928-935.

[41] Claas EC, van Milaan AJ, Sprenger MJ, et al. Prospective application of reverse transcriptase polymerase chain reaction for diagnosing influenza infections in respiratory samples from a children's hospital. *J Clin Microbiol*, 1993 Aug, 31: 2218-2221.

[42] World Health Organization. Collecting, preserving and shipping specimens for the diagnosis of avian influenza A (H5N1) virus infection: guide for field operations. Available at http://www.who.int/csr/resources/publications/syrveillance/whocdscs redc2004. pdf. Accessed November 11, 2008.

[43] Chan KH, Lam SY, Puthavathana P, et al. Comparative analytical sensitivities of six rapid influenza A antigen detection test kits for detection of influenza A subtypes H1N1, H3N2 and H5N1. *J Clin Virol*, 2007 Feb, 38: 169-171.

[44] Fiore AE, Shay DK, Broder K, et al. Prevention and control of influenza: recommendations of the Advisory Committee on Immunization Practices (ACIP), 2008. *MMWR Recomm Rep*, 2008 Aug 8, 57: 1-60.

[45] World Health Organization. Influenza. Available at http://www.who.int/csr/disease/influenza/eml. Accessed Jan 2, 2009.

[46] Oshitani H, Kamigaki T, Suzuki A. Major issues and challenges of influenza pandemic preparedness in developing countries. *Emerg Infect Dis*, 2008 Jun, 14: 875-880.

[47] Apisarnthanarak A, Mundy LM. Antiviral therapy for avian influenza virus (H5N1) infection at 2 Thai medical centers: survey findings and implications for pandemic preparedness. *Infect Control Hosp Epidemiol*, 2008 Dec, 29: 1185-1188.

[48]   Apisarnthanarak A, Warren DK, Fraser VJ. Issues relevant to the adoption and modification of hospital infection-control recommendations for avian influenza (H5N1 infection) in developing countries. *Clin Infect Dis*, 2007 Nov 15, 45: 1338-1342.

[49]   Grayson ML, Melvani S, Druce J, et al. Efficacy of soap and water and alcohol-based hand-rub preparations against live H1N1 influenza virus on the hands of human volunteers. *Clin Infect Dis*, 2009 Feb 1, 48: 285-291.

[50]   Hota B. Contamination, disinfection, and cross-colonization: are hospital surfaces reservoirs for nosocomial infection? *Clin Infect Dis*, 2004 Oct 15, 39: 1182-1189.

[51]   Bridges CB, Kuehnert MJ, Hall CB. Transmission of influenza: implications for control in health care settings. *Clin Infect Dis*, 2003 Oct 15, 37: 1094-1101.

[52]   Sehulster L, Chinn RY. Guidelines for environmental infection control in health-care facilities. Recommendations of CDC and the Healthcare Infection Control Practices Advisory Committee (HICPAC). *MMWR Recomm Rep*, 2003 Jun 6, 52: 1-42.

[53]   Apisarnthanarak A, Phattanakeitchai P, Warren DK, Fraser VJ. Impact of knowledge and positive attitudes about avian influenza (H5N1 virus infection) on infection control and influenza vaccination practices of Thai healthcare workers. *Infect Control Hosp Epidemiol,* 2008 May, 29: 472-474.

[54]   World Health Organization. Recommendations for non-pharmaceutical public health interventions. Available at http://www.who.int/csr/resources/publications/influenza/ GIP_2005_5Eweb.pdf. Accessed Jan 17, 2009.

[55]   Kitphati R, Apisarnthanarak A, Chittaganpitch M, et al. A nationally coordinated laboratory system for human avian influenza A (H5N1) in Thailand: program design, analysis, and evaluation. *Clin Infect Dis*, 2008 May 1, 46: 1394-1400.

[56]   World Health Assembly. Strengthening pandemic-influenza preparedness and response:WHA58.5. May 2005. Available at http://www.who.int/gb/ebwha/pdf_files/ WHA58/WHA58_5-en.pdf. Accessed Jan 13, 2009.

[57]   Bartlett JG, Borio L. Healthcare epidemiology: the current status of planning for pandemic influenza and implications for health care planning in the United States. *Clin Infect Dis*, 2008 Mar 15, 46: 919-925.Ohmit SE, Victor JC, Rotthoff JR, et al. Prevention of antigenically drifted influenza by inactivated and live attenuated vaccines. *N Engl J Med*, 2006 Dec 14, 355: 2513-2522.

[58]   Dolin R, Reichman RC, Madore HP, Maynard R, Linton PN, Webber-Jones J. A controlled trial of amantadine and rimantadine in the prophylaxis of influenza A infection. *N Engl J Med*, 1982 Sep 2, 307: 580-584.

[59]   Pettersson RF, Hellström PE, Penttinen K, et al. Evaluation of amantadine in the prophylaxis of influenza A (H1N1) virus infection: a controlled field trial among young adults and high-risk patients. *J Infect Dis*, 1980 Sep, 142: 377-383.

[60]   Moscona A. Neuraminidase inhibitors for influenza. *N Engl J Med*, 2005 Sep 29, 353: 1363-1373.

[61]   Fiore AE, Shay DK, Haber P, et al. Prevention and control of influenza. Recommendations of the Advisory Committee on Immunization Practices (ACIP), 2007. *MMWR Recomm Rep*, 2007 Jul 13, 56: 1-54.

[62]   Bright RA, Shay DK, Shu B, Cox NJ, Klimov AI. Adamantane resistance among influenza A viruses isolated early during the 2005-2006 influenza season in the United States. *JAMA*, 2006 Feb 22, 295: 891-894.

[63] Bright RA, Medina MJ, Xu X, et al. Incidence of adamantane resistance among influenza A (H3N2) viruses isolated worldwide from 1994 to 2005: a cause for concern. *Lancet*, 2005 Oct 1, 366: 1175-1181.

[64] Weinstock DM, Zuccotti G. Adamantane resistance in influenza A. *JAMA*, 2006 Feb 22, 295: 934-936.

[65] Deyde VM, Xu X, Bright RA, et al. Surveillance of resistance to adamantanes among influenza A (H3N2) and A(H1N1) viruses isolated worldwide. *J Infect Dis*, 2007 Jul 15, 196: 249-257.

[66] World Health Organization. Influenza A (H1N1) virus resistance to oseltamivir – Last quarter 2007 to 06 March 2008. Available at http://www.who.int/entity/csr/disease/ influenza/Resistance%20Web%2020080305.pdf. Accessed Nov 15, 2008.

[67] Hayden F. Developing new antiviral agents for influenza treatment: what does the future hold? *Clin Infect Dis*, 2009 Jan 1, 48: S3-S13.

[68] Monitoring of neuraminidase inhibitor resistance among clinical influenza virus isolates in Japan during the 2003-2006 influenza seasons. Wkly Epidemiol Rec. 2007 Apr 27, 82: 149-150.

[69] Centers for Disease Control and Prevention. Antiviral agents for seasonal influenza: dosage. Available at http://www.cdc.gov/flu/professionals/antivirals/dosage.htm#table. Accessed Dec 16, 2008.

[70] Welliver R, Monto AS, Carewicz O, et al. Effectiveness of oseltamivir in preventing influenza in household contacts: a randomized controlled trial. *JAMA*, 2001 Feb 14, 285: 748-754.

[71] Cooper NJ, Sutton AJ, Abrams KR, Wailoo A, Turner D, Nicholson KG. Effectiveness of neuraminidase inhibitors in treatment and prevention of influenza A and B: systematic review and meta-analyses of randomised controlled trials. *BMJ*, 2003 Jun 7, 326: 1235-1240.

[72] Hedrick JA, Barzilai A, Behre U, et al. Zanamivir for treatment of symptomatic influenza A and B infection in children five to twelve years of age: a randomized controlled trial. *Pediatr Infect Dis J*, 2000 May, 19: 410-417.

[73] Ilyushina NA, Hoffmann E, Salomon R, Webster RG, Govorkova EA. Amantadine-oseltamivir combination therapy for H5N1 influenza virus infection in mice. *Antivir Ther*, 2007, 12: 363-370.

[74] Ohmit SE, Victor JC, Rotthoff JR, et al. Prevention of antigenically drifted influenza by inactivated and live attenuated vaccines. *N Engl J Med*, 2006 Dec 14, 355: 2513-2522.

[75] Meiklejohn G, Eickhoff TC, Graves P, I J. Antigenic drift and efficacy of influenza virus vaccines, 1976-1977. *J Infect Dis*, 1978 Nov, 138: 618-624.

[76] Wilde JA, McMillan JA, Serwint J, Butta J, O'Riordan MA, Steinhoff MC. Effectiveness of influenza vaccine in health care professionals: a randomized trial. *JAMA*, 1999 Mar 10, 281: 908-913.

[77] Bridges CB, Fukuda K, Uyeki TM, Cox NJ, Singleton JA. Prevention and control of influenza. Recommendations of the Advisory Committee on Immunization Practices (ACIP). *MMWR Recomm Rep*, 2002 Apr 12, 51: 1-31.

[78] Neuzil KM, Dupont WD, Wright PF, Edwards KM. Efficacy of inactivated and cold-adapted vaccines against influenza A infection, 1985 to 1990: The pediatric experience. *Pediatr Infect Dis J*, 2001 Aug, 20: 733-740.

[79] Nichol KL, Nordin J, Mullooly J, Lask R, Fillbrandt K, Iwane M. Influenza vaccination and reduction in hospitalizations for cardiac disease and stroke among the elderly. *N Engl J Med*, 2003 Apr 3, 348: 1322-1332.

[80] Hurwitz ES, Haber M, Chang A, et al. Effectiveness of influenza vaccination of day care children in reducing influenza-related morbidity among household contacts. *JAMA*, 2000 Oct 4, 284: 1677-1682.

[81] Bridges CB, Thompson WW, Meltzer MI, et al. Effectiveness and cost-benefit of influenza vaccination of healthy working adults: A randomized controlled trial. *JAMA*, 2000 Oct 4, 284: 1655-1663.

[82] Muennig PA, Khan K. Cost-effectiveness of vaccination versus treatment of influenza in healthy adolescents and adults. *Clin Infect Dis*, 2001 Dec 1, 33: 1879-1885.

[83] Molinari NA, Ortega-Sanchez IR, et al. The annual impact of seasonal influenza in the US: measuring disease burden and costs. *Vaccine*, 2007 Jun 28, 25: 5086-5096.

[84] Tasker SA, Treanor JJ, Paxton WB, Wallace MR. Efficacy of influenza vaccination in HIV-infected persons: A randomized, double-blind, placebo-controlled trial. *Ann Intern Med*, 1999 Sep, 131:430-433.

[85] Cates CJ, Jefferson TO, Bara AI, Rowe BH. Vaccines for preventing influenza in people with asthma. *Cochrane Database Syst Rev*, 2004: CD000364.

[86] Ozgur SK, Beyazova U, Kemaloglu YK, et al. Effectiveness of inactivated influenza vaccine for prevention of otitis media in children. *Pediatr Infect Dis J*, 2006 May, 25: 401-404.

[87] Negri E, Colombo C, Giordano L, Groth N, Apolone G, La Vecchia C. Influenza vaccine in healthy children: a meta-analysis. *Vaccine*, 2005 Apr 22, 23: 2851-2861.

[88] Belshe RB, Edwards KM, Vesikari T, et al. Live attenuated versus inactivated influenza vaccine in infants and young children. *N Engl J Med*, 2007 Feb 15, 356: 685-696.

[89] Thomas RE, Jefferson TO, Demicheli V, Rivetti D. Influenza vaccination for health-care workers who work with elderly people in institutions: a systematic review. *Lancet Infect Dis*, 2006 May, 6: 273-279.

[90] The American Lung Association Asthma Clinical Research Centers. The safety of inactivated influenza vaccine in adults and children with asthma. *N Engl J Med*, 2001 Nov 22, 345: 1529-1536.

[91] Centers for Disease Control and Prevention. Notice to readers: Expansion of use of live attenuated influenza vaccine (FluMist®) to children aged 2-4 years and other FluMist changes for the 2007-2008 influenza season. *MMWR Morbid Mort Wkly Rep*, 2007 Nov 23, 56: 1217-1219.

[92] U.S Food and Drug Administration. FDA approves nasal influenza vaccine for use in younger children. Available at http://www.fda.giv/bbs/topics/NEWS/2007/NEW01705. html. Accessed October 23, 2008.

[93] World Health Organization. Global pandemic influenza action plan to increase vaccine supply. Available at http://www.who.int/csr/resources/publications/influenza/WHO_CDS_EPR_GIP_2006__1/en/index.html. Accessed December 12, 2008.

[94] Evans ME, Hall KL, Berry SE. Influenza control in acute care hospitals. *Am J Infect Control*, 1997 Aug, 25: 357-362.

[95] Apisarnthanarak A, Apisarnthanarak P, Mundy LM. Knowledge and attitudes of influenza vaccination among parents of preschool children in a region with avian influenza (H5N1). *Am J Infect Control*, 2008 Oct, 36: 604-605.

In: Global View of Fight against Influenza
Editor: Petar M. Mitrasinovic

ISBN: 978-1-60741-952-5
© 2009 Nova Science Publishers, Inc.

Chapter 20

BETWEEN PANIC AND APATHY: THE FIGHT AGAINST INFLUENZA IN SOUTH AFRICA

Thomas Gstraunthaler[*]

Department of Accounting, University of Cape Town, South Africa

ABSTRACT

This chapter aims to give the reader an understanding about the fight against influenza in South Africa. The author has conducted interviews with leading South African scientists and practitioners, and viewed government policies. South Africa is mostly concerned with other communicable diseases like HIV/AIDs or TB. Still, the Strategic Plan includes the preparedness against an influenza outbreak as a strategic priority, although professionals are skeptical.

INTRODUCTION

The fight against influenza is seen as a side event next to the more prominent healthcare problems of South Africa. First and foremost, the attention is directed to keep HIV/AIDs at bay. For the longest time, South Africa has had a troublesome relationship with HIV/AIDs, especially as many of those who have returned to South Africa after the end of Apartheid from exile were infected with the virus. The main focus of the fight against communicable diseases still rests on the prevention of HIV/AIDs and on the control of TB and malaria. The Department of Health reports annually declining malaria figures and communicates this as one of their biggest success stories. Now, with the deterioration of the healthcare system in Zimbabwe, South Africa is more concerned about the control of cholera.

---

[*] E-mail: thomas.gstraunthaler@uct.ac.za

THE INSTITUTIONAL ENVIRONMENT

The Department of Health is a key player in the South African healthcare system. So far, the Department has built a bad reputation for the weaknesses of their ministers rather than the efficiency or efficacy of their work. Despite all of the negative press, South African professionals are very positive that the situation in the Department of Health is going to change for the better. Next to the National Department of Health, there are many subunits in place to enforce the public policy. Each province runs a provincial Infection Prevention & Control Committee/Unit. These committees meet at least quarterly with another committee, the District Infection Prevention & Control Committee. Each healthcare facility is supposed to set up a multidisciplinary Infection Prevention & Control Committee where appropriate, including the officer in charge of infection prevention and control in the facility, a microbiologist, heads of all relevant medical disciplines, a pharmacist, a housekeeping supervisor, a food service manager, a laundry service manager, a maintenance manager, and the hospital manager. Additional to the committee, the facility sets up an Infection Prevention & Control Team consisting of at least a clinician and a registered nurse who have been trained in infection prevention and control [1,2].

The surveillance of influenza in South Africa is based on the influenza laboratory of National Institute of Virology, together with the Department of Microbiology, University of Cape Town and Department of Virology, University of Natal. General practitioners, clinics and staff health centres act as sentinel sampling sites to allow the collection of routine upper respiratory tract specimens from patients with acute respiratory disease for virus isolation. After their collection these samples are antigenically typed by reagents of the WHO and are confirmed by the National Institute of Medical Research in the UK, which is one of the WHO reference centres. Additionally, the National Institute of Virology determines the polypeptide sequence to quickly notify changes in sequences. Other clinical material that reaches NIV for diagnostic purposes complement the system [3].

So far, the fight against both the endemic and the pandemic influenza has been strengthened by the Province of the Western Cape. Hosting the University of Cape Town and Stellenbosch University, two of the leading scientific institutions of the country, the provincial government called in a working group to prepare for the fight against influenza. Members of this group reported that it was led in a very professional way and the outcome was very satisfying. Therefore, the Department of Health took the matter into their own hands and tried to extend this plan to all nine South African provinces. Such a procedure is not unusual, taking the centralistic state model into account. Due to very slow procedures on the state level, this promising work has still not been completed.

It has already been a priority during the years 2004 to 2009 to improve management of communicable diseases and non-communicable illnesses. The National Department of Health Measureable Objectives for 2008 to 2011 now includes the target to "maintain country preparedness for an influenza pandemic". Multisectoral influenza implementation plans should be implemented in all nine provinces. The target for 2008–2009 is the conduct of a simulation for influenza, together with the implementation of a preparedness tool. Throughout the years 2009 and 2010, an evaluation of the pandemic preparedness in all nine provinces is taking place. For 2010 and 2011, refresher training of trainers to response to influenza pandemic is scheduled. The year 2010 might bring stronger awareness of communicable disease, as there is training in place to ensure preparedness for the 2010 Soccer World Cup. The mock drill is scheduled for 2009 [1].

To give an overview of the preparedness of South Africa, the potential threats should be brought to the attention of the reader. How could an influenza pandemic break out and threaten the country?

PANDEMIC INFLUENZA

South Africa has a large number of very busy ports and a large border line with its neighboring countries. Both may act as traffic routes through which both infected humans and infected livestock could enter the country. Assuring that effective controls are in place, together with ongoing training of the personnel present, have become paramount. Therefore, together with veterinarians, procedures have been set up to inform how a case of influenza is defined and how to handle it. Quick testing procedures are now in place, including the countries' chemistry facilities. Although essential for the functioning of the whole system, it took over a year to establish reliable quick testing procedures.

Another threat comes from migration birds that flock into South Africa in big numbers. To address these risks, the animal demography unit at the University of Cape Town (former Avian Demography Unit) monitors the health of migration birds, including water fowl. The idea of such an institution goes back to 1983, when a workshop was held in Johannesburg to establish a Bird Populations Data Bank for South Africa. This workshop was organized together with the "Birds and Man" symposium which was held by the Southern African Ornithological Society (now BirdLife South Africa).

A potential threat comes from domestic poultry in South Africa. Basically, ostrich farms are prone to breakouts. These occurrences happened regularly, for which the agricultural monitoring system is well managed and is seen by experts as comparable to the Western level. On account of the socioeconomic situation in South Africa, it is common that families in the poorer areas keep their own backyard poultry. These chickens are mostly bought from local factories, which are under surveillance.

If a farmer should catch the disease from infected poultry, it is likely that he or she would be properly classified and treated. The situation is less predictable in the poorer areas. If an inhabitant of a poorer community were to become infected, the threat would most likely remain undetected and the infection could spread easily. The third possible method for the spread of an influenza pandemic is via passengers travelling into South Africa. These incidences happen regularly; the South African healthcare system is well prepared for this. The virus associated with bird flu, H5N1, is meanwhile seen as endemic in West Africa. The widely-spread avian markets are hard to control, and isolated outbreaks would not reach media attention. In those countries, the media would report on these happenings if hospitals had to close down. Good indicators for the infection rates are expatriates who are diagnosed in places like South Africa.

EPIDEMIC INFLUENZA

Epidemic influenza reveals the difficulties and inequalities of the South African healthcare system. Whereas wealthier South Africans have their own general practitioners and insurance to cover the costs, the majority of those who live in the poor areas have no access to such assistance. Offering influenza immunization would offer a way to significantly cut down on infection, but this still is met with a lot of skepticism from the side of the people [3].

With the ending of the northern hemisphere influenza season, representatives of the reference centres and influenza experts review the past influenza season to evaluate the gathered data on antigenicity. This material is the basis for the estimation of the strain's A subtypes and the B influenza type virus most likely to affect the population. Out of these strains the vaccination for the next season is designed. This information, published in the *Weekly Epidemiological Record* on the last Friday of February, gives four to five months' time for manufacturers to prepare for demand in winter. During the last week in September a similar outlook for the southern hemisphere formulation is published The focus on the southern hemisphere is of vital importance to its population, as influenza epidemics last for – 12 weeks and virus isolation in South Africa takes place between May and September. The vaccination available for the southern population is therefore used with a larger time delay and might not be effective due to the possible evolution of the virus. Now, with the specific southern hemisphere formulation, this problem appears to be solved [3].

The competition against the richer industrialized countries in the north is seen by some researchers as the biggest threat. Its intensive trade relations with countries like China that have a previous history of outbreaks remain a constant threat for South Africa with its multinational population. Due to its geographical situation, South Africa is exposed to a different influenza cycle than most industrialized countries on the northern hemisphere. Again, here administration is the weakest link and might impose a big hurdle to the offering of influenza vaccinations. Timing is particularly crucial. It is an imperative to start offering immunization in April or May to render effective protection. Due to slow procedures, immunizations do not start prior to end of June. Most of the time delay is lost on administrative procedures in relation to placing orders.

What causes concern among specialists is the limited availability of vaccinations in general. In times of high demand it is assumed that South Africa would not necessarily be served on time, as the demands of the richer industrial states would get settled first. Therefore, specialists take a stand for a South African production line to ensure that enough vaccination would be available. Relying on expanding production capacity of the pharmaceutical industry is seen as a very risky method. Establishing a production line on an international level would be expensive but might pay off in times of an outbreak.

To boost the demand for vaccination, there have been initiatives to offer these vaccinations free of charge. Unfortunately, due to a lack of support from administration, the initiative was doomed to fail. Roughly 10,000 injections could not be used. Despite the vast proof of the effectiveness of the vaccination and its cost-benefit, the public is still quite skeptical about its use, particularly because of fears of negative side effects. Stories about unforeseeable side effects are common, ranging from the fear that the vaccine would cause influenza to the fear of Guillain-Barré-syndrom. Additionally, in years with low influenza activity, the illness-related absenteeism from work seems not to warrant influenza vaccination for the next years to come.

Whereas the points mentioned above are probably applicable to any other country, the skepticism against influenza vaccination leaves HIV-infected persons particularly vulnerable, especially to *Streptococcus pneumoniae* and *Haemophilus*. Even if the person seeks treatment, it often goes undetected as its symptoms are similar to opportunistic infections of HIV such as *Pneumocystis carinii*. In addition to the reasons for an underutilization of influenza vaccines that have been stated above, HIV-positive persons fear that the vaccination might stimulate T-cells and speed up HIV replication [3].

Although in other African countries outbreaks could be covered up by officials, the press system in South Africa is well established and independent, and report on any outbreak. This puts pressure on the officials in charge. Still, a great deal of healthcare work is done by NGOs and NPOs on a community level. There are no policies in place on how to assure that these people are properly trained and receive the necessary support in their job. The Department of Health has understood the importance of these workers and has reserved 1,458 billion Rand to increase the salary of 100,000 nurses.

CONCLUSION

The fight against influenza receives little attention from government officials due to more prominent threats from communicable diseases like HIV/AIDs or TB. A substantial risk is imposed on the formal and informal settlements in the Townships, where many people live closely together and the healthcare workers are not always as trained as desired. An outbreak would quickly spiral out of control and this would impose a severe challenge to the healthcare system. Still, there is a very active press which covers each and every outbreak and puts pressure on officials to respond quickly.

REFERENCES

[1]   Department of Health (2008) *Strategic Plan* 2008/09-2010/11, Pretoria
[2]   Department of Health (2007) *The National Infection Prevention and Control Policy and Strategy*, Pretoria
[3]   Schoub, B. D., & Martin, D. J. (2006). Influenza Pandemic Preparedness—a concept plan to prepare for the contingency of a major global pandemic of Influenza, www.who.int/entity/csr/disease/influenza/southafricaplan.pdf

ABOUT THE EDITOR

Petar M. Mitrasinovic, Canadian, born on November 15, 1968, obtained his B.Sc.-Dipl.Ing. (1993) in control engineering and M.Sc.-Magister (1995) in nanotechnology from the University of Belgrade, Serbia, and his Ph.D. (2002) in chemistry from Florida State University, U.S.A. He was European Union Research Scientist (2002) at the University of Mons-Hainaut, Belgium; Izaak Walton Killam Fellow (2003–04) at Dalhousie University, Canada; and Research Scientist for IBM (2005) at Henri Poincaré University, France. He is currently Senior Scientist and Professor of Biophysics at the Center for Multidisciplinary Studies, University of Belgrade; Director/Founder of the Belgrade Institute of Science and Technology; and Invited Professor of Chemistry and Biophysical Chemistry at several universities in Europe, Canada, China, and Japan. He has published more than 40 original scientific articles (of which ten as a single author in leading international journals) in chemistry, structural biology, drug design, biotechnology, materials science, and nanotechnology, six review articles, five book chapters, and two books. He has been an invited speaker at numerous international meetings worldwide and has served as reviewer for *The Journal of the American Chemical Society, The Journal of Physical Chemistry A, The Journal of Physical Chemistry B, Current Organic Chemistry, The Journal of Mass Spectrometry, Current Drug Targets, The Medical Science Monitor, Current Radiopharmaceuticals, The International Journal of Radiation Biology, The IEEE Publications,* and *The IFAC Proceedings*. He is a Guest Editor of *Current Organic Chemistry* and serves on the international editorial advisory boards of the following journals: *Current Radiopharmaceuticals, Research&Reviews in BioSciences,* and *Research&Reviews in ElectroChemistry*. He is a member of the American Chemical Society, the Foresight Institute for Molecular Nanotechnology, U.S., and the Canadian Chemical Society. He has been a peer-elected Full Member of the European Society of Computational Methods in Sciences and Engineering (MESCMSE) since 2005. He has been a recipient of the Izaak Walton Killam Memorial Award (2003–04) in recognition of outstanding academic achievement from Dalhousie University, Canada, and has been a recipient of the International Scientist of the Year 2008 award from the International Biographical Center (IBC), Cambridge, England. His bibliographical listings include the following encyclopedias: *Leading Scientists of the World* (2008) and *2000 Outstanding Scientists* (2009) published by the IBC, Cambridge, England; *Who's Who of Emerging Leaders* (2007), *Who's Who in Science and Engineering* (2008), *Who's Who in America* (2009), and *Who's Who in the World* (2009) published by the Marquis Who's Who, New Providence, U.S.A. (Web page: http://myweb.dal.ca/pmitrasi/).

CONTRIBUTORS

CHAPTER 1

Robert G. Webster, Ph.D., M.Sc., FRS
Rose Marie Thomas Chair
Division of Virology
Department of Infectious Diseases
St. Jude Children's Research Hospital
Memphis, TN, U.S.A.;
Director of the World Health Organization Collaborating Center on
the Ecology of Influenza Viruses in Lower Animals and Birds;
Fellow of the Royal Society of London;
Fellow of the Royal Society of New Zealand;
Member of the National Academy of Sciences of the United States;
2002 Bristol-Myers Squibb Award for Distinguished Achievement in
Infectious Diseases Research
E-mail: robert.webster@stjude.org

CHAPTER 2

Adrian J. Gibbs, Ph.D., FAA
Professor
School of Botany and Zoology &
The John Curtin School of Medical Research
Australian National University
Canberra, AUSTRALIA;
Fellow of the Australian Academy of Science
E-mail: adrian_j_gibbs@hotmail.com

CHAPTER 3

Graeme Laver (1929–2008), Ph.D., M.Sc., FRS
Professor
School of Biochemistry and Molecular Biology &
The John Curtin School of Medical Research
Australian National University
Canberra, AUSTRALIA;
Fellow of the Royal Society of London;
1996 Australia Prize for Excellence in Pharmaceutical Design
E-mail: pennylaver@bigpond.com (Penny G. Laver, Graeme's daughter)

CHAPTER 4

Xiu-Feng (Henry) Wan, D.V.M., Ph.D.
Principal Investigator
Molecular Virology and Vaccine Branch
Influenza Division
Centers for Disease Control and Prevention
Atlanta, GA;
Adjunct Faculty
School of Biology
Georgia Institute of Technology, Atlanta, GA;
School of Computer Science and Systems Analysis
Miami University, Oxford, OH;
Department of Microbiology
Southern Illinois University, Carbondale, IL, U.S.A.
E-mail: wanhenry@yahoo.com

CHAPTER 5

Jiang Gu, M.D., Ph.D.
Professor & Chair, Department of Pathology
Director, Infectious Disease Center
Beijing (Peking) University Health Science Center, Beijing;
Dean, Shantou University Medical College, Hong Kong;
President, Chinese Pathologist Association, CHINA;
Clinical Professor, Health Science Centre
State University of New York, New York, U.S.A
E-mail: jianggu@bjmu.edu.cn

CHAPTER 6

Yi-Ming Arthur Chen, M.D., M.Sc., Sc.D.
Professor, Institute of Microbiology and Immunology
Director, AIDS Prevention and Research Center
Director, Center of International Affairs
National Yang-Ming University;
Adjunct Investigator
Vaccine Research & Development
National Health Research Institute, Taipei, TAIWAN
E-mail: arthur@ym.edu.tw

CHAPTER 7

Noel A. Roberts, Ph.D.
Professor
School of Biosciences
University of Cardiff, Cardiff, U.K.;
1999 Pharmaceutical Research & Manufacturers of America Discoverers Award;
1997 Society of Medicines Research Award for Drug Discovery;
1995 Roche International R&D Prize
E-mail: robertsna@btinternet.com

Elena A. Govorkova, M.D., Ph.D.
Senior Scientist
Division of Virology
Department of Infectious Diseases
St. Jude Children's Research Hospital
Memphis, TN, U.S.A.
E-mail: elena.govorkova@stjude.org

CHAPTERS 8, 10 AND 11

Petar M. Mitrasinovic, Ph.D., M.Sc., Dipl.Ing., MESCMSE
Professor & Senior Scientist
Center for Multidisciplinary Studies
University of Belgrade;
Director/Founder, Belgrade Institute of Science and Technology
Belgrade, SERBIA;
Full Member of the European Society of
Computational Methods in Sciences and Engineering (MESCMSE);
Izaak Walton Killam Memorial Award (2003-04), Dalhousie University, CANADA;
International Scientist of the Year 2008 Award, IBC, Cambridge, U.K.
E-mail: petar.mitrasinovic@gmail.com

CHAPTER 9

Rupert J. Russel, Ph.D.
Lecturer
Interdisciplinary Centre for Human and Avian Influenza Research
School of Biology
University of St Andrews, St. Andrews, Fife, U.K.
E-mail: rjmr@st-andrews.ac.uk

CHAPTER 12

Slobodan Paessler, D.V.M., Ph.D.
Associate Professor, Department of Pathology;
Director, Galveston National Laboratory Preclinical Studies Core;
Scientific Director, ABSL-3 facilities, Institute for Human Infections and Immunity;
Member, WHO Collaborating Center for Tropical Diseases;
Member, Sealy Center for Vaccine Development;
University of Texas Medical Branch (UTMB)
Galveston, TX, U.S.A.
E-mail: slpaessl@utmb.edu

CHAPTER 13

Sean (Xuguang) Li, M.D., Ph.D.
Research Scientist
Center for Biologics Research
Biologics and Genetic Therapies Directorate
Health Canada, Ottawa;
Adjunct Professor
Department of Biochemistry, Microbiology, and Immunology
Faculty of Medicine, University of Ottawa, Ottawa, ON, CANADA
E-mail: sean_li@hc-sc.gc.ca

Runtao He, Ph.D.
Principal Investigator
Department of Virology
National Microbiology Lab
Public Health Agency of Canada;
Adjunct Professor
Department of Medical Microbiology
School of Medicine
University of Manitoba, Winnipeg, MB, CANADA
E-mail: Runtao_He@phac-aspc.gc.ca

CHAPTER 14

Amy E. Krafft, Ph.D.
Program Officer
Influenza Drug and Diagnostic Development
Influenza, SARS and Related Viral Respiratory Diseases Section
RDB/DMID/NIAID/National Institutes of Health/DHHS
Bethesda, MD, U.S.A.
E-mail: kraffta@niaid.nih.gov

CHAPTER 15

Aleksandra Niedzwiecki, Ph.D., FACN
Executive Vice President and
Vice President of Research, Matthias Rath, Inc.;
Board Member of the Dr. Rath Health Foundation;
Dr. Rath Research Institute
Santa Clara, CA, U.S.A.;
Fellow of the American College of Nutrition
E-mail: a.niedz@drrath.com

CHAPTER 16

Sievert Lorenzen, Dr. rer. nat.
Professor
Zoological Institute
University of Kiel, Kiel, GERMANY
E-mail: slorenzen@zoologie.uni-kiel.de

CHAPTER 17

Yasuhiro Takeuchi, Ph.D.
Professor
Department of Systems Engineering
Graduate School of Science and Technology
Shizuoka University, Shizuoka, JAPAN
E-mail: takeuchi@sys.eng.shizuoka.ac.jp

CHAPTER 18

Andrei Korobeinikov, Ph.D.
Senior Research Fellow
MACSI, Department of Mathematics and Statistics
University of Limerick, Limerick, IRELAND
E-mail: andrei.korobeinikov@ul.ie

Alexei V. Pokrovskii, Ph.D.
Professor, Department of Applied Mathematics
National University of Ireland;
Associate Director, Institute for Nonlinear Science
University College Cork, IRELAND;
Adjunct Professor, Deakin University, Geelong;
Director of European Operations,
Center for Applied Dynamical Systems, Mathematical Analysis and Probability
University of Queensland, AUSTRALIA;
Head, Group of Mathematical Methods in Control
Institute for Information Transmission Problems
Russian Academy of Sciences, RUSSIA
E-mail: a.pokrovskii@ucc.ie

CHAPTER 19

Anucha Apisarnthanarak, M.D.
Adjunct Professor
Division of Infectious Diseases and Infection Control
Faculty of Medicine
Thammasart University Hospital
Pratumthani, THAILAND
E-mail: anapisarn@yahoo.com

CHAPTER 20

Thomas Gstraunthaler, Ph.D., M.Sc.
Associate Professor
Department of Accounting
University of Cape Town, Cape Town, SOUTH AFRICA;
Vice-President of the "Association des
Formations Européennes a la Comptabilité et a l'Audit"
E-mail: thomas.gstraunthaler@uct.ac.za

INDEX

C

D

F

G

M

T

U

V

W

X